SPRINGER SERIES ON REHABILITATION

Myron G. Eisenberg, PhD, Series Editor
Veterans Affairs Medical Center, Hampton, VA

Thomas E. Backer, PhD, Consulting Editor
Human Interaction Research Institute, Los Angeles, CA

Herbert H. Zaretsky, PhD, is currently Administrator, Department of Rehabilitation Medicine at the Rusk Institute, New York University Medical Center, and Clinical Professor of Rehabilitation Medicine at the New York University School of Medicine. He received his PhD from Adelphi University. Dr. Zaretsky has published extensively in the field of rehabilitation in such areas as psychological aspects of disability, geriatric rehabilitation, learning and conditioning with the neurologically impaired and spinal-cord injured, rehabilitation psychology and long-term care of the chronically ill, chronic pain management, and behavioral medicine applications to rehabilitation. Dr. Zaretsky is a Fellow of the American Psychological Association (APA), Past President of APA's Division of Rehabilitation Psychology, and a recipient of the APA's Distinguished Contribution to Rehabilitation Psychology Award. Dr. Zaretsky was formerly Chair of the Board of Trustees of the Commission on Accreditation of Rehabilitation Facilities (CARF) and recently its Past-Chair. He is a member of the Board of Directors of the American Cancer Society's (ACS) Eastern Division (New York/New Jersey), recently served as the Board's Treasurer, is currently a National Division Delegate of the ACS National Assembly, and is the recipient of the St. George Medal, a national award from the ACS in recognition for outstanding contributions to the control of cancer.

Edwin F. Richter III, MD, is Clinical Associate Professor of Rehabilitation Medicine at New York University School of Medicine and Associate Clinical Director of the Rusk Institute of Rehabilitation Medicine. He received his MD from New York University School of Medicine and continued residency training there. He is a Fellow of the Academy of Physical Medicine and Rehabilitation. He has published and presented extensively in the field of physical medicine and rehabilitation on topics including orthopedic impairments, stroke, brain injury, pain, and wound care. He serves as director of the Stroke Rehabilitation Program, the Mild Traumatic Brain Injury Program, and the Adult Spasticity Clinic at the Rusk Institute of Rehabilitation Medicine, and is Chairman of the Advisory Board of the Brain Injury Society.

Myron G. Eisenberg, PhD, is Director of Psychological Services and Director of Research Services at the Department of Veterans Affairs Medical Center in Hampton, VA, and is Associate Professor of both Physical Medicine and Rehabilitation and of Psychiatry and Behavioral Sciences at Eastern Virginia Medical School, Norfolk. Additionally, Dr. Eisenberg is the Associate Chief of Staff for Education and Research at the Hampton VA Medical Center, and the Education Manager for the Veterans Administration's Mid-Atlantic Health Care Network which includes eight Medical Centers in Virginia, West Virginia and North Carolina. He obtained his PhD from Northwestern University and received postdoctoral training at the University of Toronto's Clarke Institute. Dr. Eisenberg has published extensively in the area of rehabilitation, holds editorial board positions on several journals, is the immediate past Editor of *Rehabilitation Psychology*, and is a member of several national task forces charged with investigating various quality-of-life issues of importance in persons with chronic disabling conditions. Dr. Eisenberg has received recognition at the local, regional, and national level for contributions he has made to the rehabilitation of persons with physical impairments. A Fellow and Past President of the American Psychological Association's Division of Rehabilitation Psychology, he is actively involved in heightening the public's awareness of the importance of rehabilitation through the promotion of research.

Medical Aspects *of* Disability

3rd Edition

A Handbook for
the Rehabilitation
Professional

HERBERT H. ZARETSKY, PhD
EDWIN F. RICHTER III, MD
MYRON G. EISENBERG, PhD
EDITORS

 SPRINGER PUBLISHING COMPANY

Springer Publishing Company, Inc.
11 West 42nd Street
New York, NY 10036-8002

Acquisitions Editor: Lauren Dockett
Production Editor: Pamela Lankas
Cover and page design by Reyman Studio

05 06 07 08 09/5 4 3 2 1

Library of Congress Cataloging-in-Publication Data

Medical aspects of disability : a handbook for the rehabilitation professional / Herbert H. Zaretsky, Edwin F. Richter, Myron G. Eisenberg, editors.-- 3rd ed.
    p. ; cm. -- (Springer series on rehabilitation)
  Includes bibliographical references and index.
  ISBN 0-8261-7973-8 (hardcover)
 1. Medical rehabilitation. 2. Chronic diseases. 3. Disability evaluation.
  [DNLM: 1. Disabled Persons--rehabilitation. 2. Disability Evaluation. 3. Rehabilitation--methods. WB 320 M48872 2005] I. Zaretsky, Herbert H. II. Richter, Edwin F. III. Eisenberg, Myron G. IV. Springer series on rehabilitation (Unnumbered)
  RM930.M42 2005
  617'.03--dc22

                                    2005005046

Printed in the United States of America by Sheridan Books

To my wife, Diane, for her love, inspiration, support, and friendship; to my daughter, Lauren; my son, Andrew; my son-in-law, Lee; and to my grandchildren, Alec, Will, and Jake.
— Herb Zaretsky

To my wife, Mary-Ann, and our son, Edwin, for all of their love and support.
— Edwin Richter

To my wife, Ellen, and our daughter, Toby
— Mike Eisenberg

Contents

PART III
Special Topics

Contributors

Steven R. Abramson, MD
Professor of Medicine and
    Pathology
New York University School of
    Medicine
Hospital for Joint Diseases
New York, NY

Francis V. Adams, MD
Clinical Assistant Professor of
    Medicine
New York University School of
    Medicine
New York, NY

Jung H. Ahn, MD
Clinical Professor of
    Rehabilitation Medicine
New York University School of
    Medicine
Rusk Institute of Rehabilitation
    Medicine
New York, NY

Harriet Udin Aronow, PhD,
Director of Research
Casa Colina Centers for
    Rehabilitation
Pomona, CA

Stefanie R. Auer, PhD
Morbus Alzheimer Association
Austria

Alan Berkman, MD
Medical Specialist
HIV Center for Clinical and
    Behavioral Studies
New York State Psychiatric
    Institute and Columbia
    University
New York, NY

Frederick A. Bevalaqua, MD
Clinical Assistant Professor of
    Medicine
New York University School of
    Medicine
New York, NY

Mary F. Bezkor, MD
Clinical Associate Professor of
  Rehabilitation Medicine
New York University School of
  Medicine
Rusk Institute of Rehabilitation
  Medicine
New York, NY

Andrew R. Block, PhD
Director
The Well-Being Group
Plano, TX

Gary R. Bond, PhD
Professor of Psychology
Indiana University—Purdue
  University at Indianapolis
Indianapolis, IN

Brian J. Boon, PhD
President/CEO
Commission on Accreditation of
  Rehabilitation Facilities
Tucson, AZ

Ludmilla Bronfin, MD
Assistant Professor of Neurology
New York University School of
  Medicine
New York, NY

Susanne M. Bruyere, PhD
Director, Program on
  Employment and Disability
School of Industrial and Labor
  Relations
Cornell University
Ithaca, NY

Kikuko Campbell
Indiana University—Purdue
University at Indianapolis
Indianapolis, IN

Esther Chachkes, DSW
Clinical Associate Professor of
  Social Work
New York University School of
  Social Work
Faculty, End of Life Certificate
  Program
Smith College School of Social
  Work
Director of Social Work and
  Therapeutic Recreation
New York University Medical
  Center
New York, NY

Roy Gordon Cole, OD, FAAO
Director of Vision Program
  Development
The Jewish Guild for the Blind
New York, NY

**Constance Saltz Corley,
  MSW, PhD**
Professor and Associate Director
  of Research
Csula Roybal Institute for
  Applied Gerontology
University of California
Los Angeles, CA

Natalie DeLuca
Indiana University—Purdue
  University at Indianapolis
Indianapolis, IN

Robert DePorto, DO
Clinical Assistant Professor of
  Rehabilitation Medicine
New York University School of
  Medicine
Rusk Institute of Rehabilitation
  Medicine
New York, NY

Leonard Diller, PhD
Professor of Rehabilitation
    Medicine
New York University School of
    Medicine
Director of Psychology
Rusk Institute of Rehabilitation
    Medicine
New York, NY

Thomas M. Dixon, PhD
Assistant Professor of Physical
    Medicine and Rehabilitation
Case Western Reserve University
Staff Psychologist
Cleveland VA Medical Center
Cleveland, OH

Jeanne Dzurenko, RN, MPH
Director of Nursing
Rusk Institute of Rehabilitation
    Medicine
New York University Medical
    Center
New York, NY

Nancy Eng, PhD
Associate Professor
Department of Speech,
    Communication Sciences,
    and Theater
St. John's University
Jamaica, NY

Ora Ezrachi, PhD
Clinical Assistant Professor of
    Rehabilitation Medicine
Department of Rehabilitation
    Medicine
New York University Medical
    Center
Manager, Program Outcomes
Rusk Institute of Rehabilitation
    Medicine
New York, NY

Robert T. Fraser, PhD, CRC
Professor
Departments of Neurology
University of Washington
Seattle, WA

Ingrid Freidenbergs, PhD
Clinical Instructor
Department of Psychiatry
New York University School of
    Medicine
Psychologist
Rusk Institute of Rehabilitation
    Medicine
New York, NY

Les Gallo-Silver, CSW-R, ACSW
New York University Medical
    Center
New York, NY

Joan T. Gold, MD
Clinical Associate Professor of
    Rehabilitation Medicine
New York University School of
    Medicine
Clinical Director of Children's
    Rehabilitation Services
Rusk Institute of Rehabilitation
    Medicine
New York, NY

Muriel Gray, PhD
Associate Professor
School of Social Work
University of Maryland
Baltimore, MD

Ilana Grunwald, PhD
Clinical Instructor of
    Rehabilitation Medicine
New York University School of
    Medicine
Rusk Institute of Rehabilitation
    Medicine
New York, NY

John C. Guare, PhD
Senior Lecturer, Department of
    Psychology
Indiana University—Purdue
    University of Indianapolis
Indianapolis, IN

Kristofer J. Hagglund, PhD
Associate Dean of Health Policy
    and Academic Affairs
Co-Director, Center for Health
    Policy
School of Health Professions
University of Missouri—
    Columbia
Columbia, MO

Andrew J. Haig, MD
Associate Professor
Physical Medicine and
    Rehabilitation and
    Orthopedic Surgery
The University of Michigan
Ann Arbor, MI

**Allen W. Heinemann, PhD,
    ABPP**
Professor, Physical Medicine and
    Rehabilitation
Feinberg School of Medicine,
    Northwestern University
Director, Center for
    Rehabilitation Outcomes
Research
Rehabilitation Institute of
    Chicago
Chicago, IL

Leonard Holmes, PhD
Veterans Affairs Medical Center
Hampton, VA

Glenn R. Jacobowitz, MD
Assistant Professor of Surgery
Division of Vascular Surgery
New York University Medical
    Center
New York, NY

Ali Javed, MD
Clinical Research Fellow
Silberstein Aging and Dementia
    Research Center
New York University School of
    Medicine
New York, NY

Esin Kaplan, MD
Clinical Associate Professor of
    Rehabilitation Medicine
New York University School of
    Medicine
Rusk Institute of Rehabilitation
    Medicine
New York, NY

Robert Allen Keith, PhD
Casa Colina Hospital for
    Rehabilitative Medicine
Pomona, CA

Sunny Kenowsky, DVM
Clinical Instructor
Department of Psychiatry
Associate Director, Fisher
    Alzheimer's Disease Program
New York University School of
    Medicine
New York, NY

Donald G. Kewman, PhD
Clinical Professor
Department of Physical Medicine
    and Rehabilitation
University of Michigan
Ann Arbor, MI

Ann M. Kremer, PhD
Medical Social Worker
Neuroscience Program
St. Mary's Mercy Medical Center
Grand Rapids, MI

Edwin F. Kremer, PhD
Senior Health Psychologist
Neuroscience Program
St. Mary's Mercy Medical Center
Grand Rapids, MI

Marcia Lawton, PhD
Associate Professor (Retired)
Department of Rehabilitation
    Counseling
School of Allied Health
Virginia Commonwealth
    University
Richmond, VA

Barry S. Layton, PhD
Assistant Professor of Physical
    Medicine and Rehabilitation
Case Western Reserve University
Cleveland, OH

Mathew H.M. Lee, MD
Chairman and Professor of
    Rehabilitation Medicine
New York University School of
    Medicine
Medical Director
Rusk Institute of Rehabilitation
    Medicine
New York, NY

Sicy H. Lee, MD
Assistant Clinical Professor of
    Medicine
New York University School of
    Medicine
Hospital for Joint Diseases
New York, NY

Patricia Kerman Lerner, MA
Director
Swallowing Disorders Center
New York University Medical
    Center
New York, NY

Jerome Lowenstein, MD
Professor of Medicine
Co-Director, Division of
    Nephrology
New York University School of
    Medicine
New York, NY

David G. Marrero, PhD
Professor of Medicine
Indiana University School of
    Medicine
Indianapolis, IN

**Diane Maydick-Youngberg,
    MS, RN, CWOCN**
New York University Medical
    Center
New York, NY

Alex Moroz, MD
Assistant Professor of
    Rehabilitation Medicine
Associate Director of Training
Department of Rehabilitation
    Medicine
New York University School of
    Medicine
New York, NY

Richard J. Morris, PhD
Meyerson Distinguished
    Professor of Disability and
    Rehabilitation
Director, School Psychology
    Program
University of Arizona, College of
    Education, Department of
    Special Education,
    Rehabilitation, and School
    Psychology
Tucson, AZ

Yvonne P. Morris, PhD
Licensed Psychologist, Private
    Practice
Tucson, AZ

Kotresha Neelakantappa, MD
Clinical Assistant Professor of
    Medicine
New York University School of
    Medicine
New York, NY

Bruce G. Raphael, MD
Professor of Clinical Medicine
New York University School of
    Medicine
New York, NY

Purva H. Rawal, MA
Pre-Doctoral Student
Division of Clinical Psychology
Northwestern University
    Feinberg Medical School

Barry Reisberg, MD
Professor, Department of
    Psychiatry
Clinical Director, Silberstein
    Aging and Dementia Research
    Center
Director, Fisher Alzheimer's
    Disease Program
New York University School of
    Medicine
New York, NY

Robert H. Remien, PhD
Clinical Psychologist and
    Research Scientist
HIV Center for Clinical and
    Behavioral Studies
New York State Psychiatric
    Institute
Columbia University
New York, NY

Mariano J. Rey, MD
Senior Associate Dean for
    Student Affairs
Associate Professor of Medicine
    and Physiology and
    Neuroscience
Director, Centers for Health
    Disparities Research
New York University School of
    Medicine
Director, Joan and Joel Smilow
    Cardiac Rehabilitation and
    Prevention Center
Rusk Institute of Rehabilitation
    Medicine
New York, NY

Steven C. Riggert, PhD
Frazier Rehabilitation Institute
Louisville, KY

Bruce P. Rosenthal, OD, FAAO
Adjunct Professor
Department of Ophthalmology
Mount Sinai Hospital
and
Distinguished Professor
State University of New York
Chief, Low Vision Program
The Lighthouse International
New York, NY

James Satriano, PhD
Director, HIV/AIDS Programs
New York State Office of Mental
    Health
New York, NY

Rose Mary Shaw
Psychology Intern
Cleveland VA Medical Center
Cleveland, OH

Sara A. Van Looy
Cornell University
Ithaca, NY

Michael Weiner, MSW
Karen Horney Clinic
New York, NY

Priscilla Bade White, MS
Doctoral Student in School
    Psychology
University of Arizona, College of
    Education, Department of
    Special Education,
    Rehabilitation, and School
    Psychology
Tucson, AZ

Nancy E. Wirth, MD
Physiatrist
Ann Arbor, MI

Introduction to the Third Edition

This third edition of *Medical Aspects of Disability: A Handbook for the Rehabilitation Professional* represents a significant update from the previous editions. There is the addition of a new co-editor, Edwin F. Richter, a prominent board-certified physiatrist, academician, and researcher, who brings an important and necessary perspective to the content of the third edition. Some of the chapters from the second edition have been completely rewritten, in some cases by new authors. Among the chapters from new authors are: "Neuromuscular Disorders" by Ludmilla Bronfin; "Ostomy Surgeries" by Les Gallo-Silver, Diane Maydick-Youngberg, and Michael Weiner; and "Burn Injuries" by Edwin F. Richter. Other chapters have been revised substantially and also include new co-authors. These updates reflect the dynamic nature of rehabilitation and medical science. New references represent advances in many aspects of evaluation and treatment of disabling conditions, and new developments in health care systems. The updated chapters on "Telerehabilitation—Solutions to Distant and International Care" by Andrew J. Haig and "The Computer Revolution and Assistive Technology" by Leonard Holmes reflect the continued convergence between clinical practice and modern technology. Consistent with the feedback from several teachers using the text in their classes, new chapters have again been included in the section on special topics: "Accreditation—A Quality Framework in the Consumer-Centric Era" by Brian J. Boon addresses the importance of the accreditation process as a fundamental component of the quality assurance and improvement process. This new special chapter will serve as a useful review of this field for the current or future clinician. "Outcomes Measurement and Quality Improvement in an Acute Inpatient Rehabilitation Setting" by Ora Ezrachi addresses important developments in the process of evaluating the performance of rehabilitation services. As medical care moves toward more use of evidence-based practices, quantitative assessments of outcome data will be increasingly important for clinical performance improvement and academic purposes.

The editors are confident that this revised edition of *Medical Aspects of Disability* will continue to present a very timely and comprehensive overview of important areas in rehabilitation service delivery. We are also confident that this new edition will enable this textbook to continue as a most useful resource in the classroom and for the practicing clinician.

Herbert H. Zaretsky, PhD

ACKNOWLEDGMENTS

The editors also wish to acknowledge Gwen Treharne, Jane Ehlers, and Petrina Rodgers for their tireless efforts and invaluable assistance in the preparation of this manuscript.

Part I

An Introduction to Key Topics and Issues

1

Comprehensive Rehabilitation: Themes, Models, and Issues

ROBERT ALLEN KEITH, PhD, AND
HARRIET UDIN ARONOW, PhD

LONG-TERM DEMOGRAPHIC and epidemiological trends in industrial societies, including the United States, have changed the face of health care. Communicable diseases, such as smallpox and measles, no longer exact a toll on life. Modern medicine, better hygiene and living conditions, and improved nutrition have had a profound effect on health. Falling birth rates have changed age profiles so that older populations make up an increasing proportion of the population. Not only are more people staying alive, they are living longer.

These two trends, more individuals staying alive and more living longer, have greatly increased chronic disease rates. A major share of health care is now devoted to treating coronary heart disease, strokes, cancer, and arthritis, to name the more prominent chronic diseases. Individuals with catastrophic injuries, such as brain injury or spinal cord injury, now survive more frequently. It has been estimated that the prevalence of disability in all adults varies from 5.2% to 18.2%, depending on the underlying condition (DeJong et al., 2002). Chronic diseases and injuries result in large numbers of people who require specialized services to regain lost functions: the role of comprehensive rehabilitation.

The focus here is on medical rehabilitation and the remediation of physical and cognitive deficits. The model guiding such services, particularly for hospital-based rehabilitation, has been the comprehensive team: physiatrists (physical medicine specialists), other physician specialists, nurses, physical therapists, occupational therapists, psychologists, speech and language specialists, social workers, recreation therapists, and orthotists (individuals who design and make assistive devices such as leg braces). With the advent of managed care, the case manager has also been added to the team, an individual charged with identifying and coordinating the most cost-effective treatment. The populations served include individuals with strokes, brain injuries, spinal cord injuries, orthopedic disorders, neuromuscular diseases, and other such conditions. The rationale for such a broad array of services is that patients present a wide span of problems that require specialized knowledge and treatment skills.

Although medical rehabilitation is a relatively small part of health care, it experienced considerable growth during the 1980s and early 1990s, as did many sectors of health care. In 1985 there were 68 rehabilitation hospitals and 386 rehabilitation units; by 2003 the numbers had grown to 214 hospitals and 1109 units (personal communication, American Medical Rehabilitation Providers Association, 2003). The tally of outpatient programs is more difficult to determine because of the lack of organized statistics and also because of the diversity of services, many of which are not comprehensive and have specialized aims. There was considerable expansion, however, during the growth era mentioned. In the last few years the growth spurt in postacute services has come to a halt; the frenetic pace of mergers and acquisitions has also slackened, principally because funds for such enterprises has dried up. Services are increasingly in the hands of large corporations, however. HealthSouth Corporation, for example, owns and operates over half of the free-standing rehabilitation hospitals (Wheatley, DeJong, & Sutton, 1998).

The provision of rehabilitation in skilled nursing facilities (SNFs), often called subacute rehabilitation, was one of the fastest growing services in the mid-1990s. Costs are considerably lower than for comprehensive hospital rehabilitation, although evidence of outcomes is mixed. The growth of SNF-based rehabilitation came to a halt with the Balanced Budget Act of 1997 with a clampdown on Medicare payments. Between the years 1998 and 2001, for example, several of the largest chains filed for bankruptcy protection or went out of business (DeJong et al., 2002).

Rehabilitation shares in the increasingly chaotic status of U.S. health care. Both managed care and Medicare reimbursement for rehabilitation services have fallen. The comprehensive nature of care is being honored in the breach. Some disciplines, such as psychology, are being excluded as not essential. State budget crises have drastically reduced payments for Medicaid and Departments of Rehabilitation. Despite this bleak economic picture, the need is still expanding, as stated above, and the professional and personal rewards for working in the field still remain.

THE ORIGINS OF REHABILITATION

THE ROAD TO legitimacy has not been an easy one for rehabilitation medicine, for either physicians in this specialty or other health professionals in the field. An acquaintance with its origins helps to understand its current status and its response to changes in health care. The history of medical rehabilitation is scattered through various journals and presentations to professional societies. The best source of early beginnings is in Gritzer and Arluke's 1985 volume The Making of Rehabilitation. Most of this account is taken from that work. The focus is on physiatry, physical therapy, and occupational therapy. Although other professions have made important contributions to medical rehabilitation, these three have had the most prominent role in shaping the origins of the field.

PHYSIATRY

THE TERM "PHYSIATRY" is a confusing one for those unacquainted with the physical medicine and rehabilitation specialty designation because it is close to psychiatry, a more widely known term. It was chosen from a combination of the Greek physis, meaning nature, and iatreia, healing.

The basis for specialization began before World War I, when a group of physicians began using electrical stimulation and eventually added the modalities of hydrotherapy, heat, massage, and exercise. During the war these physicians, who now called themselves physiotherapy physicians, joined other professionals in treating the consequences of injuries. After the conflict they returned to acute medicine.

World War II and the immediate postwar period brought significant changes to most health care professions, including physical medicine. Even though there were heavy demands for services, physical therapy physicians (yet another name) did not initially establish a claim for special competence. It remained for Howard Rusk, an internist outside physical medicine, to lay the groundwork for the modern field of physical medicine. He built a program on the use of convalescent time at an air force hospital that began to feature physician training in rehabilitation methods.

With status as a medical specialty in 1946 came a more explicit recognition of the commitment to rehabilitation. The emphasis was an important one because it marked a departure from the use of rest as the prescribed treatment during convalescence in favor of reconditioning. That emphasis has remained and, if anything, has become stronger in recent years with the general recognition of the importance of fitness.

Physical medicine and rehabilitation remain one of the smallest specialties in medicine, although the expansion of rehabilitation facilities has strengthened its position. The small number of physiatrists engaged in research is a matter of concern. The aggressive push by physical and occupational therapy for greater autonomy, particularly in independent practice, is a challenge to physician control, although the physiatrist is still acknowledged as the leader of the comprehensive treatment team.

PHYSICAL THERAPY

THE ORIGINS OF physical therapy were also heavily tied to wartime needs. During World War I those individuals who had been orthopedic assistants were designated as reconstruction physiotherapy aides, and they began to work with physical therapy physicians.

In 1921 former military aides and a few physicians formed what was soon called the American Physiotherapy Association. There then followed a period of several years in which physiotherapy aides had to battle to establish their legitimacy and independence. Relations with medicine waxed and waned, with physicians insisting that aides call themselves physiotherapy technicians to differentiate themselves from physiotherapy physicians. By 1936 the American Medical Association was accrediting physiotherapy schools. Doctors also controlled the American Registry of Physical Therapy, which restricted the opening of private offices by technicians. According to Gritzer and Arluke (1985), even though there was lack of autonomy, the field of physiotherapy benefited from this association with medicine by establishing education and training standards that excluded those with poor preparation.

World War II did much to establish the status of modern physical therapy. When physicians acquired the title of physical medicine specialists instead of physical therapy physicians, those individuals who had been called aides or technicians were able to discard these terms for the designation of physical therapist.

The later history of physical therapy shows this field to be in a very strong position on the rehabilitation scene. In the early 1980s it broke the domination of the American Medical Association in the accreditation of physical therapists and set up its own accrediting organization. The close relationship with physiatry no longer remains because most referrals to physical therapists now come from other medical specialties (Institute of Medicine, 1989). A significant number have chosen independent practice rather than an institutional setting. The perception of the importance of physical reconditioning and the expansion of rehabilitation services have made physical therapy job growth greater than that of any other allied health occupation.

OCCUPATIONAL THERAPY

GRITZER AND ARLUKE (1985) observe that the origins of occupational therapy can be traced to the belief that activity and work can be therapeutic, a connection first used for treating those with mental illness. Just prior to World War I, the first professional society for occupational therapy was formed. Early on, its members established the working principle that therapeutic activity should be physician-prescribed.

In the 1920s occupational therapy began to expand its base from mental institutions to include tuberculosis sanatoriums. The treatment of industrial accident injuries was also added to its domain. In the early years of World War II, occupational therapy still had to fight the view of its mission as diversional rather than therapeutic. Physical therapy physicians became interested in the potential of occupational therapy to bridge the gap between physical and vocational rehabilitation.

The postwar years have been marked by the push for greater autonomy and also by the continuing struggle to convey to other professionals and to the public just what it is that an occupational therapist does. The decision to opt for certification rather than licensure contributed to some ambiguity of status. It was only in 1987, for example, that occupational therapy was able to bill separately under Medicare. The inclusion of occupational therapy with physical therapy (later to include speech and language pathology) in the Medicare regulation mandating 3 hours a day of therapy has helped to consolidate occupational therapy's position in rehabilitation. Occupational therapists' unique expertise in sensory and cognitive retraining ensures that they will remain important members of the treatment team.

All of the disciplines in rehabilitation have a vigorous scientific and practice base by maintaining their own professional associations with scientific journals and web sites. An interdisciplinary association, the American Congress of Rehabilitation Medicine, publishes one of the leading journals in the field, the Archives of Physical Medicine and Rehabilitation. Another prominent journal, the American Journal of Physical Medicine and Rehabilitation, is published by the Association of Academic Physiatrists. Medical rehabilitation is also represented by a trade organization, the American Medical Rehabilitation Providers Association.

COMPREHENSIVE REHABILITATION OPERATIONS

MEDICAL REHABILITATION PROGRAMs come in many forms, and they serve a variety of clients. In spite of this diversity, there has been a common philosophy of treatment that holds that the complex problems of individuals with severe disability require the services of a team of specialists. No one profession has the knowledge and skills to address all the biological, psychological, functional, and environmental ramifications of chronic, severe disabling illnesses and injuries.

Understanding rehabilitation operations requires a description of the kinds of rehabilitation facilities and programs, the caseloads that they serve, and some idea of how rehabilitation professionals divide up their labor and distribute themselves within the continuum of rehabilitation services. The rapidly changing health care system has resulted in the modification of some of the traditional forms of rehabilitation.

THE CONTINUUM OF REHABILITATION CARE

REHABILITATION SERVICES EXIST in a continuum of post-acute care. Typically applied after the onset of an acute episode of illness or injury, post-acute care services include inpatient and outpatient rehabilitation, chronic care, skilled nursing (distinct part) care, and home and community-based health services. Rehabilitation services can be prescribed sequentially as levels of restorative care or singly as appropriate pathways from office-based or hospital-based physician care and even by self-referral.

For many years there was no defining mechanism for determining the number of rehabilitation programs in the United States. Consequently, there were no reasonable estimates of the number and kinds of rehabilitation programs in operation or of the populations they served. This uncertain identity obviously did not help the field's quest for greater visibility. It also meant that rehabilitation was not often included in health care planning or policymaking.

With the advent of a prospective payment system for acute inpatient medical and surgical hospital admissions beginning in 1983, the situation changed dramatically. The prospective payment system was based on diagnosis related groups (DRGs) within which patients had relatively similar costs for their acute hospital care. Inpatient medical rehabilitation units and hospitals were recognized to have patient populations that fell outside the typical distribution of costs of care. They were designated as exempt from the use of DRGs, and a system for qualifying as an "exempt" unit or hospital was established. The qualifications included, among other provisions, a case mix with at least 75% of patients to fall within 10 diagnoses and a coordinated multidisciplinary treatment team (Health Care Financing Administration, 1982).

Alongside the rehabilitation hospitals and units there grew an impressive array of post-acute care services to accommodate the continuing care needs of persons being discharged promptly (within the DRG limits) from acute care hospitals. There was enormous growth in distinct part (short term) units in skilled nursing facilities, home health care services, rehabilitation units and hospitals, and long-term chronic care hospitals (Liu, Gage, Harvell, Stevenson, & Brennan, 1999).

The Centers for Medicare and Medicaid Services (CMS—formally HCFA) responded to this growth with alarm—and over time have adopted systems for regulating and rationalizing the use of resources within the continuum of post-acute services, including prospective payment by Resource Utilization Groups (RUGs) in skilled facilities and impairment-based Case Mix Groups (CMGs) in acute licensed rehabilitation. In the meantime, rehabilitation services have been responding to changes in the payment incentives with the prudent dual goals to maximize rehabilitation outcomes for persons with disability while remaining fiscally solvent. The current continuum of levels of rehabilitation care is discussed in detail below.

Inpatient Acute Licensed Rehabilitation Programs

Inpatient programs receive most of their referrals from acute care hospitals. Because inpatients are still medically fragile and are severely impaired, close medical supervision and 24-hour nursing care are needed. All domains of health and function are assessed and monitored by the interdisciplinary team. Treatment programs are usually multidisciplinary and intensive, that is, with a full schedule of therapy, because hospitalization is expensive.

Inpatient rehabilitation is provided in distinct units of acute hospitals, in freestanding acute licensed rehabilitation hospitals, and in affiliated hospitals in health systems. With the trend for consolidation, there are fewer freestanding rehabilitation hospitals today than 10 years ago, while increasing numbers of units and rehabilitation hospitals are owned by chains.

Inpatient Skilled Licensed Rehabilitation Programs

Skilled nursing facilities with distinct part Medicare beds afford patients the opportunity to have an extended period of recuperation with some therapy as needed on a daily basis. SNF licensed beds providing rehabilitation services are located as units (licensed as skilled nursing or transitional care units) within acute licensed medical and surgical hospitals, within freestanding acute licensed rehabilitation hospitals, within free-standing long-term care facilities, and as freestanding skilled rehabilitation hospitals.

With SNF licensing the frequency of medical supervision and level of nurse staffing is reduced, and therefore this level of care can accommodate patients with less acute medical needs. Skilled rehabilitation is targeted mostly to older post-acute patients who may not need, or be able to tolerate, intensive programs of therapy. However, there have also emerged diagnostic specialty rehabilitation programs that are suited to this level of care. For example, there are several programs throughout the nation that specialize in emergence from coma and ventilator dependent care housed in skilled licensed facilities. Highly regulated and dependent on public funding, these programs are changing rapidly as payment policies are reformulated at CMS and the private insurance industry follows suit.

There is some controversy about the effectiveness of SNF-based rehabilitation in comparison to hospital-based programs. In examining these two settings, Kramer and colleagues (1997) found an advantage of acute rehabilitation for patients with strokes but not for those with hip fractures.

Comprehensive Day Treatment Programs

Although more commonly used for psychiatric and substance abuse treatment, comprehensive day treatment programs are also available for persons with physical and cognitive disabilities. Like their mental health counterparts, the comprehensive day rehabilitation programs have the goal of preventing long-term institutionalization while providing a quality daily program of activities. Some day rehabilitation programs provide restorative services and are geared toward therapeutic goals, a defined length of stay, and discharge to a more independent community life. The therapeutic program is intensive and targeted for persons not requiring overnight care, but not able to care for themselves at home (e.g., persons with acquired brain injury). The other main type of comprehensive day treatment program is geared more to long-term care in a maintenance model. This level of care may be distinguished from Adult Day Care for older persons with dementia by its greater medical supervision and ability to take clients who require daily nursing care and therapies.

Outpatient Rehabilitation Programs

Outpatient rehabilitation care can be provided in a wide variety of settings and programmatic models—ranging from single services provided in physician offices to licensed multidisciplinary comprehensive programs. In 2000 there were a total of 516 licensed Comprehensive

Outpatient Rehabilitation Facilities (CORFs) receiving reimbursement for patient care from the CMS. While relatively popular in the 1980s, currently there is great regional variation in the use of CORFs. Florida has the largest number of CORFS, 181, while California has just 14 (CMS, 2002). Comprehensive multidisciplinary outpatient services are also associated with acute inpatient rehabilitation facilities, providing follow-up therapies for discharged inpatients, and as post-acute community-based day programs for diagnoses that benefit from intensive multidisciplinary therapies in a more home-like setting (e.g., traumatic and acquired brain injury).

Pediatric rehabilitation is most commonly provided in outpatient settings. Increasingly, payment policies favor providing therapy to children in more ecologically appropriate settings, such as in the home with family members or in the classroom with teachers and other students present. A reverse trend, moving physician specialty clinics out of community settings and into outpatient rehabilitation settings, may also be ecologically appropriate for persons with disabling chronic diseases, such as arthritis and neurological conditions.

There are a host of care settings in which single discipline therapies are provided, including industrial and occupational health clinics, physicians' offices, and freestanding outpatient therapy clinics. Again, a recent funding decision by CMS (July 1, 2003) to limit total annual reimbursement for physical therapy to $1,950 and occupational therapy to the same amount may precipitate rapid and profound changes in the settings in which these outpatient therapies are delivered.

In addition to settings in which rehabilitation care is provided and funded by insurance, there are a growing number of settings in which therapeutic services are offered and paid for out of pocket by the consumer or in some contractual manner with an existing health care provider. These settings include sports and fitness centers that offer therapeutic classes or individualized programs, community centers, clubs, and resorts. As more "baby-boomers" age into middle and older years, we can expect to see the demand for informal and self-directed rehabilitation programs to increase.

Residential Rehabilitation Programs

Residential rehabilitation and habilitation programs provide extended therapeutic services for persons with chronic or life-long disabilities. Transitional Living programs, typically provided at the termination of acute rehabilitation treatment or after an unsuccessful re-integration into home and community life after serious injury or illness, have as their common goal successful community re-entry and participation in home and community activities. Similar services may be offered in long-term supervised and semi-independent living programs to provide residential supports and periodic restorative care for persons living and aging with disabilities.

Home and Community Programs

A final level of care in the rehabilitation continuum is provided in the home and community setting. This level of rehabilitation care has seen a recent increase in demand with the general aging of the population. Physical therapists, occupational therapists, and speech pathologists have joined the home care team for patients after orthopedic surgeries for major joint replacements, strokes, and for a host of older patients who suffer from debilitation after an episode of acute hospitalization. On the other side of the age continuum, increasing interest is being expressed for providing pediatric rehabilitation services in the school and community within the social network of family and school community. Just as this setting makes more sense for children, persons receiving rehabilitation for traumatic brain injuries may be best served in the familiar home and community settings where they will have to perform their newly restored behaviors.

POPULATIONS SERVED

JUST AS LACK of information about the definition of rehabilitation facilities hampered the development of medical rehabilitation, so too has a scarcity of caseload information been a hindrance to the understanding and rational distribution of rehabilitation resources to specific groups of persons living with disabilities.

The rehabilitation industry has begun to keep and publish statistics on the use of rehabilitation services. One of the oldest and largest efforts to maintain a minimum set of common data on patients discharged from comprehensive rehabilitation services has been managed by the State University of New York at Buffalo. The Uniform Data System for Medical Rehabilitation (UDSmr) 10th annual report described almost 300,000 rehabilitation patients discharged from 676 participating facilities in 1999 (Deutsch, Fielder, Granger, & Russell, 2002). The report shows that orthopedic conditions, primarily lower extremity fracture and joint replacement, comprised the largest group of admissions (30%) with stroke the next largest (23%). Lengths of stay have plummeted over the past 10 years, from an average of 28 days in 1990 to 16 days in 1999.

The situation in the rehabilitation industry has changed dramatically since 1999, with the implementation of the prospective payment system (PPS) for rehabilitation in 2001. More recent data, drawn from a newer data system, based on the CMS mandated Inpatient Rehabilitation Facility–Patient Assessment Instrument (IRF-PAI), reflect these current trends.

In 1999, the American Medical Rehabilitation Providers Association (AMRPA) developed an electronic data system, eRehabdata, for participating AMRPA facilities to use to model the effects of prospective payment system. Volunteer facilities submitted UDSmr data, billing abstracts, and Medicare Cost Reports to eRehabdata to produce cost benchmarking data and allow the facilities to model the costs and outcomes of patients under varying assumptions of payment and service delivery (http://www.erehabdata.com). The system received data from over 117,000 patients discharged in 2002. It has been expanded to accommodate new IRF-PAI billing, standard, and ORYX outcome data reports and other patient outcome analyses.

PROGRAM OPERATIONS

ALTHOUGH REHABILITATION PROGRAMS (inpatient and outpatient) do not all conduct their operations in the same way, they have many processes in common because of the nature of the tasks involved and the position of rehabilitation in the continuum of health care services.

Referral and Screening

Determining appropriateness of the individual for comprehensive medical rehabilitation occurs before admission (at the time of referral and again at pre-admission screening), after admission (in initial evaluation), and during treatment (in monitoring progress and continued appropriateness). This repeated process is intended to contain costs and to ensure the proper fit between patients and services. The process is not exclusively within the rehabilitation provider's control, however, which is one of the reasons the rehabilitation industry expends resources educating referral sources and regulators about the appropriate use of rehabilitation services. Referral and screening decisions, however, are not clear cut. Decisions may vary systematically by region and available resources, and must be factored into a multidimensional assessment of personal, environmental, and social resources that affect the appropriateness of one level of care over another.

Diagnosis and Assessment

Diagnosis commonly refers to the process of determining the status of disease or complaint and assigning the remedy. In rehabilitation, assessment is concerned with detailing the functional capacities of the patient, specifying those that are likely to benefit from treatment. It is at this functional level that the specific array of treatments are paired and sequenced with the individual patient or client's pattern of deficits.

It is ultimately a physician who makes a diagnosis and authorizes the treatment for a patient in a comprehensive medical rehabilitation program. Rehabilitation physicians have traditionally played a leadership role in the treatment team, organizing the information gathered from assessments and formulating a plan with the expert input of multiple clinical disciplines that make up the treatment team.

Team Treatment

In comprehensive, multidisciplinary rehabilitation settings, the assessment process is the first demanding test of the treatment team's ability to coordinate the scheduling of time for various assessments and to communicate its findings. It is usually at the initial team conference that information about the patient is exchanged and evaluated, culminating in a treatment plan that anticipates the patient's progress through the treatment stages.

The comprehensive multidisciplinary team model of treatment delivery served to distinguish rehabilitation from the rest of health care for many years. Reviews of research concluded that coordinated interdisciplinary team care was superior to general medical care or uncoordinated rehabilitation (Keith, 1991; Ottenbacher, & Jannell, 1993; Teasell, Foley, Bhogal, & Speechley, 2003). But research on team care outcomes is scarce, and results of some studies and reviews have been contradictory.

As mentioned earlier, there are serious challenges to the team concept. Using a full spectrum of specialists is expensive, particularly for an inpatient program. The prevailing philosophy among professions is still for team care. However, in recent years its form has been modified. The team has been attenuated in some instances by accommodating a continuum of levels of care with varying levels of therapy intensity and medical and nursing care. Acute inpatient rehabilitation is still governed by the multidisciplinary team. Skilled rehabilitation care or in-home services may reduce the team to its bare necessities to address specific functional and medical issues. Outpatient rehabilitation is frequently delivered by a single discipline. However, clinicians regularly provide feedback and recommendations for continued care to both the primary care physician and the patient.

Documentation, Progress Monitoring, and Communication

Rehabilitation is highly regulated by the government, voluntary accreditation organizations, and insurance payers. Like other tertiary care providers, rehabilitation sits downstream in a continuum of health care services and is dependent on referral sources for its flow of patients. Furthermore, it is responsible for handing patients back into the continuum of ongoing primary and specialty care services. In some instances, where managed care contracts put upstream providers at financial risk for tertiary services, rehabilitation providers are directly dependent on their referral sources for payment for services provided.

In this position of managing patient care both up- and downstream, documentation, monitoring patient progress, and communication become of paramount importance for both the quality of patient care and the financial success of rehabilitation providers.

As a result of these forces, rehabilitation providers spend an increasing amount of resources documenting patient's progress and what was done for the patient during the daily treatments. Some of this is necessary for clinical management, judging patient gains in relation to the treatment plan, and as a daily communication tool among the many clinicians who treat rehabilitation patients on a daily basis. But much documentation serves the benefit of third party payers, accreditation and regulatory standards that require detailed treatment justifications and documentation in permanent records.

Although much information is exchanged informally among team members as they go about day-to-day duties, the team conference is the place where formal communication is the focus. In this setting, reports from members are heard and information integrated and evaluated, with conclusions about progress and the direction of the therapeutic plan. Many teams choose to include the patient and family members in such deliberations at some point, because they are an integral part of the rehabilitation process and play an important role in understanding and carrying out the treatment plan both within the rehabilitation treatment setting and after returning to the community and the continuing network of primary and specialty health care providers.

Discharge Planning

When patients near the goals set in the treatment plan, or plateau in their progress towards those goals, the focus shifts more toward the setting in which the patients will continue to live. The plan may involve continued rehabilitation, long-term care, and reintegration into community life. The members of the rehabilitation team must understand as completely as possible the physical and social environment and create a discharge plan that accommodates the abilities and needs of patients and their support system. This is a complicated process, fraught with physical and social obstacles. With the trend for shortening inpatient length of stay, discharge planning must include preparing patients and family to manage home programs of exercise, unresolved medical and nursing issues, and an array of continuum of care services that the patient may be recommended to use.

Going forward in time, it is difficult to predict exactly where patients with serious physical impairments and disabilities will be receiving their rehabilitation services. It is likely that there will always be a continuum of post-acute rehabilitation settings. How these resources are allocated will be determined in part by policy and financial incentives, and partly by the force of evidence of the most effective application of the rehabilitation model.

RESEARCH AND EVALUATION ISSUES

R ESEARCH IN HEALTH care has two major functions: to test the effectiveness of current clinical practices and to identify promising new directions of assessment and treatment. Rehabilitation has an added dimension in its research activities, that of program evaluation. It is one of the few health care services that requires program evaluation for accreditation. The concern with program objectives, robust measures, and accountability has positioned the field to deal with the preoccupation with outcomes management more easily than many other sectors of health care. Evaluation addresses the social utility of a result, one step beyond the usual research orientation. It must be added, however, that evaluation has primarily influenced program management with few contributions to the scientific literature.

THEORETICAL AND CONCEPTUAL ISSUES

MOST FIELDS WITH a heavy practice orientation, such as medical rehabilitation, devote relatively little effort to examining the theoretical assumptions under which they operate or formulating new theories. As a social scientist observed many years ago, however, there is nothing so practical as a good theory. Theories are the blueprints to help understand what goes on in rehabilitation and to chart research directions for the future.

Disablement Theory

One of the earliest theories in rehabilitation, and the most familiar, concerns the consequences of disease and injury, that is, disablement. The World Health Organization (WHO) concepts of impairment, disability, and handicap (WHO, 1980) have been widely used in practice, research, and social policy. There have been a number of modifications to this theory, but its original form has remained the most influential. Impairments are deficiencies at the organ level, for example, paralysis resulting in loss of hand function. Disability is the performance deficit from such an injury, the inability to complete a meaningful task, such as dial a telephone. Finally, handicaps are losses as a result of social role functioning, the result of personal and social interactions, such as the inability to remain employed as a result of disability and social practices regarding who is employable.

There have been obvious deficiencies in this classification and for the past 10 years WHO officials have collaborated with health care investigators and practitioners in several countries on a revision, the International Classification of Functioning, Disability, and Health (ICF) (WHO, 2001). The new version incorporates some of the concerns of advocates of empowerment of the disabled by using more neutral terms. It has also been influenced by views of health status and quality of life (to be discussed later in this chapter). The term impairment has been retained, now to include problems in body structure or function. Disability has been discarded in favor of activities, which are an individual's performance of tasks or activities. Handicap has been losing favor as a term because of its pejorative connotation and has been replaced by participation, which is an individual's involvement in life situations, taking into account health conditions, body structures and functions, activities, and contextual factors. A new addition is contextual factors, which include environmental factors (physical, social, and attitudinal environments) and personal factors (gender, age, fitness, habits, etc.).

The ICF is considerably more ambitious than its predecessor and is intended to address health conditions for all populations, not just the disabled. Environmental factors, although important, are very difficult to catalog, including, for example, a span from physical geography to social support and relationships. Producing a coherent scheme to phenomena that vary widely by culture or social class is a daunting task. The ICF will go through a lengthy testing period to see how well the classifications can be used. A concise account of the development of the ICF can be found in Gray and Hendershot (2000), both of whom participated in the evolution of the scheme.

Treatment Theory

The drive to identify the most cost-effective treatment methods has brought about the realization that there must be a better understanding of the rationale of treatment. Most outcome research has not included detailed description of what treatment was given, so there has been little empirical basis on which to identify the elements of intervention that have the greatest effects.

The implicit assumption behind most rehabilitation is that greater exposure to treatment results in greater gains, but there is inconsistent evidence to support this assumption (Keith, 1997). A major paradox has been that discharge indicators for some conditions have remained at the same levels in the face of rapidly dropping lengths of stay. For example, over a 10-year period the length of stay for stroke in the UDS dropped from 32 days to 20 days, a decrease of 37%. At the same time, average admission and discharge FIM scores changed very little, as did the percentage of patients discharged home (Granger &

Hamilton, 1992; Fiedler, Granger, & Post, 2000). An important issue is what strategies therapists have used to deliver treatment in the face of such drastic reductions.

One of the goals of the Research and Training Center for Measuring Rehabilitation Outcomes, situated at Boston University, is to study detailed treatment methods and patient characteristics of individuals with stroke in eight facilities to determine how and to what degree various treatment components contribute to outcomes (Haley & Jette, 2000). A major first step is to begin a taxonomy of treatments to classify interventions.

Treatment strength has been advanced as a key ingredient in classifying and understanding the components of rehabilitation treatment (Keith, 1997). The formulations involved, taken from concepts in medicine and pharmacology and also used in program evaluation in the social sciences, include purity, specificity, dose, intensity, duration, timing, and the treaters and their organization. Review of both length of stay and intensity did not find consistent relations between greater gains and more therapy, although research designs varied greatly in explanatory power. Identifying the essential elements of comprehensive rehabilitation is made even more difficult, of course, with the use of the interdisciplinary team. Not only the effects of each disciplinary member must be studied, but also the manner in which the team is organized and deployed.

Measurement Issues

Although measurement has always had a central role in rehabilitation, the increased use of health status and health-related quality-of-life instruments has considerably widened its scope. In addition, technical developments in test construction and administration have brought new measurement directions.

Data Systems for Medical Rehabilitation
Uniform Data System. The greatest influence on patient assessment and data collection has been the Uniform Data System for Medical Rehabilitation (UDS), already mentioned. The system was designed with the recognition of the importance of having data elements and a functional status measure that would be used uniformly throughout a large number of facilities. The Functional Independence Measure (FIM), which was developed for the system, has become the most widely used functional status instrument in rehabilitation and has been used in dozens of research investigations. It is also a key ingredient in Medicare's current prospective payment system.

eRehabData. The American Medical Rehabilitation Providers Association, responding to the need for better financial data to accompany patient information, developed eRehabData, also already mentioned. It combines data elements from the UDS with detailed financial data for outcomes that are tailored for management.

Outpatient Data Systems. The two largest data services for outpatients, LifeWare (Granger, 1999) and FOTO (Focus on Therapeutic Outcomes) (Dobrzykowski & Nance, 1997), both have significant following, although neither has imposed the uniformity on outpatient services as has the UDS for hospitals. LifeWare is the evolution of several versions of brief outpatient assessment instruments developed by Granger and colleagues. There are currently versions for musculoskeletal, neurologic, and "complex" populations. It includes an amalgamation of physical skills related to everyday functioning, pain control, affect, well-being, and more specific items for various conditions. The FOTO system was created for providers of outpatient orthopedic rehabilitation, primarily physical therapy, but has evolved into a system that now includes forms for musculoskeletal, neuromuscular, cardiopulmonary, wound care, industrial, and pediatric patients. Patients answer questions from a pool of items in a computer-assisted testing format.

HEALTH STATUS, QUALITY OF LIFE, AND HEALTH-RELATED QUALITY OF LIFE

Health status measures are beginning to have a significant impact on the way rehabilitation outcomes are formulated and measured. Although rehabilitation, particularly inpatient treatment, has always regarded itself as providing comprehensive care, its outcome measures have had a narrow focus. The emphasis has been on functional status skills of the most basic kind, such as self-care and mobility. Generic health status instruments have a much broader scope. The SF-36, for example, the most widely used of such measures, has eight scales devoted to physical functioning, role limitations because of physical health problems, bodily pain, social functioning, general mental health, role limitations because of emotional problems, vitality (energy/fatigue), and general health perceptions (Ware & Sherbourne, 1992). Originally developed for health policy research with large populations, health status measures use a self-report questionnaire format, a significant departure from the tradition in rehabilitation of clinician observation and judgment of patient performance. Because of their generic nature, such scales can be used across clinical populations with a variety of diagnostic problems. An excellent review of the use of health status measures in disability outcomes research can be found in Andresen and Meyers (2000).

Quality of life (QOL) has been of interest in the social sciences for many years, although serious consideration by rehabilitation has been more recent as shown by a review by Dijkers (1997) and two supplements on the topic in the Archives of Physical Medicine and Rehabilitation (Tulsky, 2002). Rehabilitation medicine has traditionally been concerned with the remediation of functional deficits. Several forces in health care and in society at large have converged, however, to demand that attention be paid to the effects of treatment on everyday life as a legitimate aim of care. The mission of rehabilitation then becomes not only deficit reduction but life enhancement. Quality of life becomes a measurement issue, although there is no consensus about how it should be conceptualized or measured. Some authors have equated QOL with various health status scales, but no one instrument encompasses the domains involved.

Quality of life refers not only to one's satisfaction with life but also to a broad array of circumstances, such as housing, employment, social conditions, and the like, factors not related to health and for which health care providers are not responsible. To narrow the concept, the term health-related quality of life (HRQOL) has been devised. Patrick and Erickson (1993, p. 22) have defined HRQOL as "... the value assigned to duration of life as modified by the impairments, functional states, perceptions, and social opportunities that are influenced by disease, injury, treatment, or policy." Even with the narrower focus, there is no agreement about measuring HRQOL. Some generic measures, such as the SF-36 or the Sickness Impact Profile (Bergner, Bobbitt, Carter, & Gilson, 1981), sample several domains of activity and function that are affected by health. Others are more targeted, including disease-specific measures, such those concerning arthritis or spinal cord injury, and condition-specific instruments, such as those dealing with specific symptoms such as depression or pain. Authors often label measures at assessing HRQOL without providing any rationale. All these measures are self-report questionnaires with the assumption that the perceptions and judgments of patients are important in assessment. There is often no feasible alternative to self-report to determine the effect of treatment on the patient's ability to carry on a variety of life activities outside the clinical setting.

Although HRQOL measures are an attractive addition to rehabilitation's array of measures, as their use increases, many problems have been identified. Several authors have pointed out that health status measures often equate health with lack of disability (Hays, Hahn, & Marshall, 2002; Tate, Kalpakjian, & Forchheimer, 2002). For example, the SF-36 asks if work or other regular activities have been affected by physical health. An individual with spinal cord injury might have difficulty answering because his or her general state of health might be alright in spite of paralysis. Another problem is the often lack of relationship between an individual's objective condition and his or her perception of quality of life or satisfaction with life (Dijkers, 1997). It is also evident that individuals may recalibrate their expectations over time with fewer options for activities still bringing satisfaction with life (Schwartz & Sprangers, 2000). Tate and colleagues (2002) observe that this dynamic change in framework may threaten the foundations of our assumptions about the use of HRQOL measures to evaluate health care interventions.

The use of health status and HRQOL measures is rapidly increasing in rehabilitation. Their breadth of perspective and use of the patient's point of view are an important addition to outcome measures. There are many conceptual and methodological problems in use, however, that have to be addressed if these instruments are to have maximum utility for rehabilitation.

RESEARCH AND EVALUATION ISSUES

OUTCOMES RESEARCH

DETERMINING WHAT STRATEGIES will improve health while adhering to cost restraints is a continuing preoccupation of health care. Outcomes research is the term used to describe the search for cost-effective interventions. For outcomes research to have an impact on reducing costs and improving the quality of care, two conditions must be met. The research must be designed with sufficiently powerful research designs and measures to provide credible results. And second, such conclusions must be recognized and applied by health care providers and payers. Despite the resources devoted to outcomes research, there is scant evidence that the results have had much direct effect on health care policies and practices (Stryer, Tunis, Hubbard, & Clancy, 2000). This does not mean that outcomes research should be abandoned; only that expectations about its impact should be modest. A research topic that has had insufficient exploration is the extent to which managed care organizations and other funders pay attention to outcomes in their reimbursement policies. A useful discussion of the evidence needed for disability outcomes research can be found in Jette and Keysor (2002).

A major shift is occurring throughout health care in the goals of outcomes research, from a focus on clinical outcomes defined by professionals, to including the improvement of health and the patient's perspective on health (also discussed in the section on measurement). While the identification of effective interventions is important, administrators of managed care recognize that a major way to reduce health care costs is to encourage healthier life styles and reduce utilization of services. Health status and health-related quality-of-life measures are the major means to assess treatment outcomes related to these goals.

Commonly cited rehabilitation outcomes have included discharge to a home setting, improved functional status, reduction in the need for assistance or supervision, reduction of treatment costs, and improvement in productive activity (Keith, 1995). This list has been seen as narrow in light of the emphasis on patient perspectives and so additions such as satisfaction with services and treatment outcomes, improved sense of well-being, and improved life-satisfaction and other aspects of quality of life have been suggested. Granger (1998) has noted that improvements in functioning, the traditional aim of rehabilitation, must be demonstrated not only in the clinical setting but also in day-to-day activities. Although there is general agreement about the goals of rehabilitation, there is little consensus, beyond a core of basic indicators, about how such goals should be defined or measured.

EVIDENCE-BASED PRACTICE AND RANDOMIZED CLINICAL TRIALS

WITH RISING HEALTH care costs throughout the industrialized world has come the recognition of the importance of basing clinical procedures on firm scientific grounds. This has led to collaborative efforts to search the medical literature and establish uniform standards for judging the adequacy of research. The Cochrane Library, which archives the results of randomized clinical trials, is one example of this cooperation (http://www.cochrane.org/). In the U.S. the Agency for Health Care Policy and Research sponsored various centers to determine the best treatment procedures for many common medical conditions. One of the most well-known projects relevant to rehabilitation is clinical practice guidelines for poststroke rehabilitation (Gresham et al., 1995). This agency, now the Agency for Healthcare Research and Quality, funds Evidence-Based Practice Centers which develop evidence reports and technology assessments based on syntheses of the scientific literature. The Oregon Health and Science University, for example, has completed an exhaustive review of the literature on the effectiveness of interventions to rehabilitate individuals with traumatic brain injury (http://www.ahcpr.gov/).

Randomized clinical trials (RCTs) have long been recognized as the most powerful means of investigating research issues. In this research design subjects are randomly assigned to experimental or control groups, conditions for both groups are explicitly described, and the ultimate comparison has greater validity than other designs. For many years it was assumed that this methodology was most appropriate for drug trials or basic research. RCTs are expensive to conduct and there are often ethical issues about withholding treatment for a control group. In rehabilitation there is the added complication that most treatment is delivered by a team, which makes it difficult to identify which factors are responsible for improvement.

In spite of the barriers to implementation, there has been considerable interest in RCTs in rehabilitation; a recent supplement to the American Journal of Physical Medicine and Rehabilitation was devoted to the subject (Millis & Johnston, 2003). The perception has been that there have been few such applications in rehabilitation, but a review of the literature revealed a surprising 4,874 publications using RCTs (Johnston, 2003). Nearly two-thirds of the research was devoted to investigating pain, particularly back, neck, or joint pain. Only 10% involved patients with stroke; less than 4% included brain injury or spinal cord injury. So diagnoses of particular interest to medical rehabilitation have not had much study with RCTs.

Considerations in the deployment of RCTs will lead to better research whether or not that design is used. Whyte (2003) has outlined the important factors. First of all, there needs to be accurate characterization of research participants beyond the usual age and sex data. Second, treatment needs to be specified with sufficient detail to be able to identify what it is that affects the patient. It helps to have a treatment theory to guide formulations. Third, the outcomes of treatment must be measured in a reliable and valid manner with indexes that have clinical and social value.

CONSTRAINT-INDUCED MOVEMENT THERAPY

ONE OF THE MOST frustrating experiences of hemiplegia, whether from stroke or some other central nervous system damage, is the inability to use the affected upper extremity. Rehabilitation has commonly focused on lower limb restoration because of the greater gains, although patients value upper limb function more. Constraint-induced movement therapy (CIMT) is a promising method for improving upper arm function, reversing the assumption that there is usually little improvement. Edward Taub, a neuropsychologist at the University of Alabama, and colleagues initially worked on the training of monkeys with a deafferented limb, restricting use of the intact limb and using behavioral shaping techniques with very small steps to overcome what has been called learned nonuse (Taub, Crago, & Uswatte, 1998). In this state, the subject has aversive experiences in attempts to use the paretic limb and is positively reinforced for compensating with the intact limb. Taub was then able to apply the techniques from such research to chronic stroke patients with an upper extremity hemiparesis (Taub et al., 1993). The investigators found that individuals who agreed to wear a sling on their unaffected arm for 90% of waking hours for 14 days significantly improved on both laboratory tests and real-life skills. Other investigators have been able to duplicate the results of this research team.

COMPREHENSIVE REHABILITATION: PRESENT AND FUTURE

CURRENT STATUS

IN PREVIOUS EDITIONS of this chapter, mention was made of two potentially important directions of government policy regarding the disabled. Disability in America (Pope & Tarlov, 1991) was an Institute of Medicine report on the prevention of disability, reviewing the scope of disability and a new model for the disabling process from a social and public health perspective. The second publication, Enabling America (Brandt & Pope, 1997), was also an Institute of Medicine report, again reviewing conceptual models and examining research on assessment, health services research, the status of science and engineering, and the role of Federal research programs. Both of these works showed a lively interest in addressing the major problems of the disabled. In recent years, however, there have been few government policy initiatives regarding the disabled or rehabilitation The status of the economy and of health care has precluded many bold ventures.

For the last several years a dominant theme in rehabilitation has been the intense commercialization of the field which resulted in an explosion of expansion and reorganization. As in all of health care, the pressures to contain costs have continued the trend toward decreasing professional control over services. In addition, staff are asked to increase their work loads; individuals with lower qualifications are being used in treatment. Patients are often treated at a lower level of care than in previous practices. Many patients with strokes, for example, are now channeled to skilled nursing facilities for rehabilitation rather than to a hospital. It remains to be seen how well this situation serves health care needs.

Although the frenetic pace of acquisitions and mergers has subsided, the aftermath of overexpansion and instability continues, particularly with some of the large chains. A positive consequence of the restructuring has been an increase in the variety of facilities in which rehabilitation is carried on. Twenty years ago there were a few traditional settings that supported rehabilitation: inpatient hospitals, outpatient clinics, and private offices. Now there are organizations of physical, occupational, and speech therapists that do home visits; satellite clinics of hospitals; sports medicine facilities; and a variety of other organizational formats.

THE FUTURE

THE DELIVERY OF appropriate rehabilitation services to those who need and can profit from treatment rests, to a considerable extent, on reforms of the U.S. health care system. Despite heroic efforts to bring down costs through managed care and decreased payment by government agencies, the current trend, which threatens to continue, is for increasing expenditures for health care. Some 41 million individuals are without health insurance and those who are insured must struggle to maintain coverage. Physicians are limiting participation in government programs because of inadequate payment. The future of rehabilitation and of health care in general depends on changes.

On a brighter note, there are a number of developments that have furthered the rehabilitation cause. Keeping fit has become a national preoccupation, although the continuing increase in obesity shows that the preoccupation is not always translated into action. The distinction between exercise for fitness and for recovery during rehabilitation has become blurred, as it should be. Regular exercise is a cornerstone of physical medicine and is a key to the success of restorative treatment. Community hospitals are offering exercise classes that may target specific medical conditions. Some rehabilitation hospitals have formed partnerships with existing commercial health clubs to offer rehabilitation services within such clubs. Automobile manufacturers have added onsite rehabilitation centers for employees who are injured. In addition, many more individuals not previously disabled are becoming acquainted with rehabilitation routines after having arthroscopic surgery, hip replacements, or other types of surgery. Rehabilitation concepts and procedures are being used widely outside of traditional treatment facilities.

Advances in treatment and adaptive devices are occurring at a rapid pace because of miniaturization and digitalization of equipment. For example, wheelchairs had come in standard sizes, not all of which coincided with patient requirements. Now it is possible to build a wheelchair to fit individual specifications. For certain repetitive exercises, robots have been designed that take the patient through the movements involved and free up therapists' time. A major development will be the acceleration of innovative information technology with automated medical records, physicians having access to patients' records even at remote locations, and better organized systems of outcomes management. The Internet, already an important information source, will continue to grow in importance for accessing research data bases, exchange of data, teaching, and communication between facilities.

Although comprehensive rehabilitation has been diluted in recent years because of cost cutting, it is still the most appropriate model of care. If restorative treatment is to be effective, it is necessary to consider the patient's life in totality, not just the immediate physical deficits. Otherwise the gains realized during treatment may not endure once the patient returns home. And, as stated earlier, the mission of rehabilitation is to benefit the patient's everyday existence. Funders of care may find that if gains are not maintained, cost savings become illusory. Formulations about disablement, such as the International Classification of Functioning, Disability and Health (WHO, 2001), endorsed by the international health care community, have broadened the view of what health care should be concerned with. Likewise, the increasing use of health status and quality of life measures as legitimate outcomes also contributes to a wider perspective. The aging populations of all industrial nations, including the U.S., are producing inexorable pressures for restorative services. Comprehensive rehabilitation will prevail.

REFERENCES

Andresen, E. M., & Meyers, A. R. (2000). Health-related quality of life outcomes measures. Archives of Physical Medicine and Rehabilitation, 81(Suppl. 2), S30–S45.

Bergner, M., Bobbitt, R. A., Carter, W. B., & Gilson, B. S. (1981). The Sickness Impact Profile: Development and final revision of a health status measure. Medical Care, 19, 787–805.

Brandt, E. N., Jr., & Pope, A. M. (Eds.). (1997). Enabling America. Washington, DC: National Academy Press.

Centers for Medicare and Medicaid Services. (2002). Rehabilitation agencies and comprehensive outpatient rehabilitation facilities, by HCFA region, 2000. Report #10 from the Online Survey and Certification Reporting System. Retrieved November 17, 2003 from http://www.cms.hhs.gov/medlearn/therapy/sept02tab2.pdf

DeJong, G., Palsbo, S. E., Beatty, P. W., Jones, G. C., Kroll, T., & Neri, M. T. (2002). The organization and financing of health services for persons with disabilities. The Milbank Quarterly, 80, 261–301.

Deutsch, A., Fiedler, R. C., Granger, C. V., & Russell, C. F. (2002). The Uniform Data System for Medical Rehabilitation report of patients discharged from comprehensive medical rehabilitation programs in 1999. American Journal of Physical Medicine and Rehabilitation, 81, 133–142.

Dijkers, M. (1997). Measuring quality of life. In M. J. Fuhrer (Ed.), Assessing rehabilitation practices: The promise of outcomes research (pp. 153–179). Baltimore: Paul H. Brookes.

Dobrzykowski, E. A., & Nance, T. (1997). The Focus on Therapeutic Outcomes (FOTO) outpatient orthopedic rehabilitation database: Results of 1994–1996. Journal of Rehabilitation Outcomes Measurement, 1, 56–60.

Fiedler, R. C., Granger, C. V., & Post, L. A. (2000). The Uniform Data System for Medical Rehabilitation. Report of first admissions for 1998. American Journal of Physical Medicine and Rehabilitation, 79, 878–92.

Granger, C. V. (1998). The emerging science of functional assessment: Our tool for outcomes analysis. Archives of Physical Medicine and Rehabilitation, 79, 235–240.

Granger, C. V. (1999). Featured instrument. The LIFEware system. Journal of Rehabilitation Outcomes Measurement, 3, 63–69.

Granger, C. V., & Hamilton, B. B. (1992). UDS report. The Uniform Data System for Medical Rehabilitation report of first admissions for 1990. American Journal of Physical Medicine and Rehabilitation, 71, 108–113.

Gray, D. B., & Hendershot, G. E. (2000). The ICIDH-2: Developments for a new era of outcomes research. Archives of Physical Medicine and Rehabilitation, 81(Suppl. 2), S10–S14.

Gresham, G. E., Duncan, P. W., Stason, W. B., Adams, H. P., Adelman, A. M., Alexander, D. N., et al. (1995). Post-stroke rehabilitation. Clinical practice guideline. Rockville, MD: U.S. Department of Health and Human Services, Public Health Service, Agency for Health Care Policy and Research.

Gritzer, G., & Arluke, A. (1985). The making of rehabilitation. Berkeley, CA: University of California Press.

Haley, S. M., & Jette, A. M. (2000). RRTC for Measuring Rehabilitation Outcomes: Extending the frontier of rehabilitation outcome measurement and research. Journal of Rehabilitation Outcomes Measurement, 4(4), 31–41.

Hays, R. D., Hahn, H., & Marshall, G. (2002). Use of the SF-36 and other health-related quality of life measures to assess persons with disabilities. Archives of Physical Medicine and Rehabilitation, 83(Suppl. 2), S4–S9.

Health Care Financing Administration. (1982, September). Medicare hospital manual. Transmittal No. 313, U.S. Department of Health and Human Services, p 25:9–24m.2.

Institute of Medicine. (1989). Allied health services: Avoiding crises. Washington, DC: National Academy Press.

Jette, A. M., & Keysor, J. J. (2002). Uses of evidence in disability outcomes and effectiveness research. The Milbank Quarterly, 80, 325–345.

Johnston, M. V. (2003). Desiderata for clinical trials in medical rehabilitation. American Journal of Physical Medicine and Rehabilitation, 82(Suppl.), S5–S7.

Keith, R. A. (1991). The comprehensive treatment team in rehabilitation. Archives of Physical Medicine and Rehabilitation, 72, 269–274.

Keith, R. A. (1995). Conceptual basis of outcome measures. American Journal of Physical Medicine and Rehabilitation, 74, 73–80.

Keith, R. A. (1997). Treatment strength in rehabilitation. Archives of Physical Medicine and Rehabilitation, 78, 1298–1304.

Kramer, A. W., Steiner, J. F., Schlenker, R. E., Eilertsen, T. B., Hrincevich, C. A., Tropea, D. A., et al. (1997). Outcomes and costs after hip and stroke. A comparison of rehabilitation settings. Journal of the American Medical Association, 277, 396–404.

Liu, K., Gage, B., Harvell, J., Stevenson, D., & Brennan, N. (1999). Medicare's post-acute care benefit: Background, trends, and issues to be faced. Washington, DC: The Urban Institute. Retrieved November 17, 2003 from http://aspe.hhs.gov/daltcp/reports/mcapb.html

Millis, S., & Johnston, M. V. (Eds.). (2003). Clinical trials in medical rehabilitation: Enhancing rigor and relevance. American Journal of Physical Medicine and Rehabilitation, 82(Suppl).

Ottenbacher, K. J., & Jannell, S. (1993). The results of clinical trials in stroke rehabilitation research. Archives of Neurology, 50, 37–44.

Patrick, D. L., & Erickson, P. (1993). Health status and health policy. Allocating resources to health care. New York: Oxford University Press.

Pope, A. M., & Tarlov, A. R. (Eds.). (1991). Disability in America. Washington, DC: National Academy Press.

Schwartz, C. E., & Sprangers, M. A. G. (Eds.). (2000). Adaptation to changing health. Response shift in quality-of-life research. Washington, DC: American Psychological Association.

Stryer, D. S., Tunis, S., Hubbard, H., & Clancy, C. (2000). The outcomes of outcomes and effectiveness research: Impacts and lessons from the first decade. Health Services Research, 35, 977–993.

Tate, D. G., Kalpakjian, C. Z., & Forchheimer, M. B. (2002). Quality of life issues in individuals with spinal cord injury. Archives of Physical Medicine and Rehabilitation, 83(Suppl. 2), S18–S25.

Taub, E., Crago, J. E., & Uswatte, G. (1998). Constraint-induced movement therapy: A new approach to treatment in physical rehabilitation. Rehabilitation Psychology, 43, 152–170.

Taub, E., Miller, N. E., Novack, T. A., Cook, E. W. III, Fleming, W. D., Nepomuceno, C. S., et al. (1993). Technique to improve chronic motor deficit after stroke. Archives of Physical Medicine and Rehabilitation, 74, 347–354.

Teasell, R. W., Foley, N. C., Bhogal, S. K., & Speechley, M. R. (2003). An evidence-based review of stroke rehabilitation. Topics in Stroke Rehabilitation, 10, 29–58.

Tulsky, D. S. (2002). Quality of life measurement in rehabilitation medicine: Building an agenda for the future. Archives of Physical Medicine and Rehabilitation, 83(Suppl. 2), S1–S3.

Ware, J. E., Jr., & Sherbourne, C. D. (1992). The MOS 36-item short-form health survey (SF-36). I. Conceptual framework and item selection. Medical Care, 30, 473–483.

Wheatley, B., DeJong, G., & Sutton, J. (1998). Consolidation of the inpatient medical rehabilitation industry. Health Affairs, 17, 209–215.

Whyte, J. (2003). Clinical trials in rehabilitation: What are the obstacles? American Journal of Physical Medicine and Rehabilitation, 82(Suppl.), S16–S21.

World Health Organization (WHO). (1980). International classification of impairments, disabilities, and handicaps: A manual of classification relating to the consequences of disease. Geneva, Switzerland: Author.

World Health Organization (WHO). (2001). International classification of functioning, disability and health. Geneva, Switzerland: Author.

2

Body Systems: An Overview

Jung H. Ahn, MD

T**HE HUMAN BODY** consists of a complex combination of his-
toanatomical systems and biochemical materials (Clemente, 1985;
DeLisa & Stolov, 1981; Ganong, 1991). In this chapter, however, the
body is topographically divided for an adept understanding as follows:
the skin, the musculoskeletal system, the nervous system, the respiratory system, the cardiovascular system, the hematopoietic system, the
digestive system, the genitourinary system, the endocrine system, the
visual system, and the auditory and vestibular systems.

SKIN

T**HE MOST SUPERFICIAL** system of the body is the skin, which
consists of two parts: an epidermis and a dermis. The epidermis is
an outer, keratinized layer of the skin. The bottom layer of the epidermis is called the basal cell layer. The dermis is an inner, connective tissue layer containing nerve endings, tactile corpuscles, and blood vessels.
The sweat glands, sebaceous glands, and hair follicles are also contained
in the dermis, and they pass upward through the epidermis. The skin is
constantly exposed to external hazards, and therefore it is of utmost
importance to protect it from any disabling trauma.

MUSCULOSKELETAL SYSTEM

T HE MUSCULOSKELETAL SYSTEM includes bones, cartilages, ligaments, tendons, and muscles. It serves to provide mechanical support for the body, protect vital internal organs, store minerals, and
produce blood. The skeletal system also works as a lever system on which
muscles act across joints to result in body movements. The skeletal muscle is made of contractile muscle fibers (myofibrils) surrounded by the
sarcoplasmic reticulum and the T-system. The muscle fiber consists of
protein chains of actin and myosin. During muscle contraction the
strands of actin and myosin slide past each other (Figure 2.1) in the presence of Ca++ released from the sarcoplasmic reticulum via the T-system, thus shortening the fiber. The trigger to start this contraction comes
from the motor nerve attached to each muscle fiber. The attachment
occurs at the motor end plate, where acetylcholine (a neurotransmitter) is released at the moment an electrical impulse traveling in the motor
nerve reaches the muscle fiber.

Tendons attach the contracting part of the muscles to bones. They are
composed largely of parallel collagenous fibers that are closely bound into
fibrous bundles, forming tough cords. They include some elastic fibers.

Ligaments are also composed of collagenous fibers and some elastic

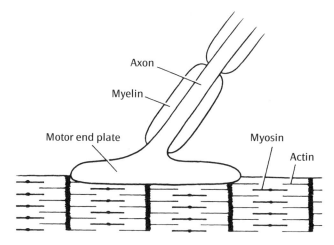

FIGURE 2.1 Very schematic representation of the terminal branch of a motor neuron
attaching to a muscle fiber via the motor end plate. When the nerve's electrical impulse
reaches the motor end plate, acetylcholine is released. The impulse then travels in both
directions along the fiber. During contraction, the strands of actin and myosin slide past
each other, thus shortening the fiber.

From DeLisa and Stolov: Significant Body Systems in Handbook of Severe Disability
edited by Stolov and Clowers, U.S. Department of Education, Rehabilitation Service
Administration, 1981.

fibers. They connect two or more bones and also stabilize joints. A ligamentous injury can be more problematic than a fracture and often requires prolonged immobilization. Congenital lax ligaments result in hypermobility of joints. Cartilage has a high content of collagen and proteoglycans combined with H2O, giving it a gel-like consistency. It has essentially no blood supply but receives nourishment by diffusion from nearby capillaries. Three kinds of cartilages are recognized: fibro- ,elastic, and hyaline. Fibrocartilage has a large concentration of less elastic collagen fibers and is dominant in intervertebral disks. Elastic cartilage has many elastic fibers, as is evident in the external ear. Hyaline cartilage contains few fibrils and is slightly elastic. It covers the opposing surfaces of movable joints such as the articular cartilage, which may wear out and become calcified with aging. Such changes are described as degenerative joint disease or osteoarthritis.

Joints are divided into the fibrous joint (immobile), the cartilaginous joint (slightly movable), and the synovial joint (movable). The fibrous joints are seen in the skull. Intervertebral disks are the cartilaginous joints. Limb joints are covered by the synovial membrane, which produces the viscous fluid in the joint space. The cartilaginous and synovial joints are susceptible to degenerative joint disease, and the synovial joint is prone to developing inflammation.

Bone is a hard, calcified connective tissue with 35% organic substance, 45% inorganic substance, and 20% water. Bone tissue consists of the matrix and the specialized cells of the bone, including osteoids (bone cells), osteoblasts (bone-forming cells), and osteoclasts (bone-destroying cells). The matrix contains mineral salts, mainly calcium phosphate. There are two major types of mature bone: sponge and compact. There are 206 bones in the adult human body; they can be divided into flat bones (e.g., skull), short bones (e.g., carpal bones), and long bones (e.g., humerus) or axial bones and appendicular bones (Figure 2.2., Table 2.1)

The gross structure of bones (Figure 2.3) is typically composed of the bone marrow, spongy bone, cortical bone, and periosteum. During growth, the red marrow, which manufactures the red blood cells in most bones, changes to the yellow marrow (fatty marrow) usually by about 6 years of age. The periosteum is a thick, fibrous membrane that covers the entire surface of a bone except its articular cartilage; it has two layers: an inner osteogenic layer and an outer connective tissue layer with blood vessels and nerve fibers.

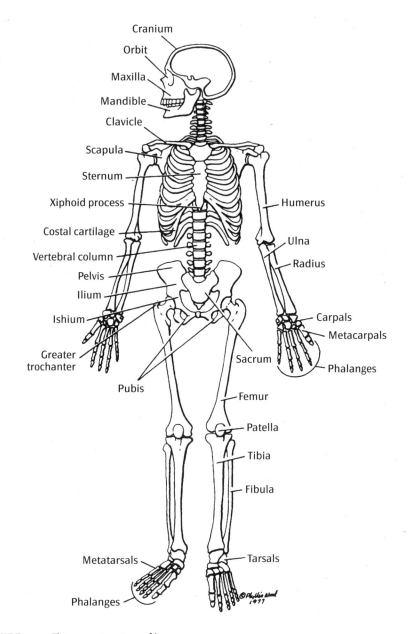

Cranium
Orbit
Maxilla
Mandible
Clavicle
Scapula
Sternum
Xiphoid process
Costal cartilage
Vertebral column
Pelvis
Ilium
Ishium
Greater
trochanter
Pubis
Humerus
Ulna
Radius
Carpals
Metacarpals
Phalanges
Sacrum
Femur
Patella
Tibia
Fibula
Metatarsals
Tarsals
Phalanges

FIGURE 2.2   The gross structure of bones.

TABLE 2.1   Human Bones

Axial bones		Appendicular bones	
Spine	26	Upper extremities	64
Skull	28	Lower extremities	62
Hyeid bone	1		126
Ribs & sternum	25		
	80		

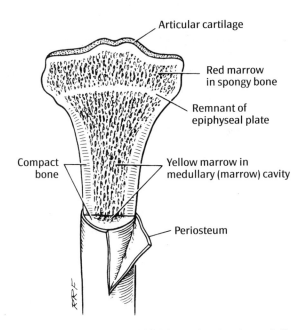

FIGURE 2.3   Cutaway section of an adult long bone showing the medullary cavity containing yellow marrow. In this section, only a residual line remains of the epiphyseal plate.

From DeLisa and Stolov: Significant Body Systems in Handbook of Severe Disability edited by Stolov and Clowers, U.S. Department of Education, Rehabilitation Service Administration, 1981.

NERVOUS SYSTEM

T**HE NERVOUS SYSTEM** is divided into the central nervous system (CNS) and the peripheral nervous system (PNS). The CNS includes the brain and the spinal cord. The PNS includes the cranial nerves, the spinal nerves, and the autonomic nervous system.

The basic functional unit of the nervous system is the neuron, and

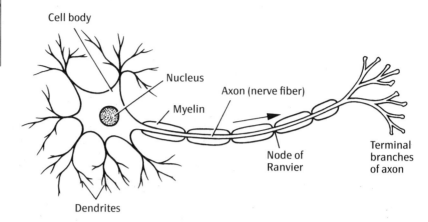

FIGURE 2.4 Basic myelinated nerve cell. Dendrites receive input from terminal branches of other axons. When sufficiently activated, the cell body transmits an electrical impulse down its axon. Myelin protects the axon and, together with the nodes of Ranvier, allows for very fast conduction. Nonmyelinated, slower-conduction axons also exist. Axon diameters range: 1–6 ¥10–4. Arrow indicates direction of impulse travel.

From DeLisa and Stolov: Significant Body Systems in Handbook of Severe Disability edited by Stolov and Clowers, U.S. Department of Education, Rehabilitation Service Administration, 1981.

there are about 1 trillion neurons in the human nervous system. The neuron consists of a cell body, dendrites, and an axon (Figure 2.4). The terms axon and nerve fiber are synonymous. Most axons are long and encased in a sheath called myelin, which acts as an insulator and aids the rapid transmission of conducting impulses away from the nerve cell body. The cell body is responsible for maintaining the functional and anatomical integrity of the axon. The length of the path traveled by afferent or efferent information is longer than any single axon. Therefore, chains of neurons are necessary to convey messages through the entire nervous system. The system for transfer from one neuron to the next is the synapse, in which a chemical neurotransmitter is released, triggering the next neuron into action.

CENTRAL NERVOUS SYSTEM

THE BRAIN AND spinal cord are covered by the meninges and surrounded by the cerebrospinal fluid (CSF). The brain is further protected by the skull, as the spinal cord is protected by the vertebral column. The meninges include the pia mater, arachnoid mater, and dura mater. The CSF, formed in the choroids plexuses around the cerebral vessels and along the ventricular walls, fills the subarachnoid space and cerebral ventricles and is absorbed through the arachnoid villi into the cerebral

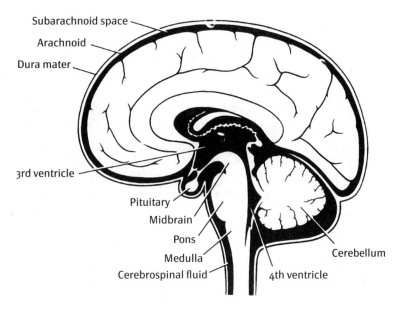

Subarachnoid space

Arachnoid

Dura mater

3rd ventricle

Pituitary

Midbrain

Pons

Medulla

Cerebrospinal fluid

Cerebellum

4th ventricle

FIGURE 2.5 Midline section through the cerebrum, cerebellum, and brain stem. This section passes through the third and fourth ventricles, both of which are midline structures. Note cerebral spinal fluid bathing the brain.

From DeLisa and Stolov: Significant Body Systems in Handbook of Severe Disability edited by Stolov and Clowers, U.S. Department of Education, Rehabilitation Service Administration, 1981.

venous sinuses. The fluid also serves as a medium through which nutrients and wastes can be exchanged between the blood and the CNS.

The brain is divided into the cerebrum, the cerebellum, and the brain stem (Figure 2.5). The cerebrum, consisting of left and right convoluted cerebral hemispheres, is the largest part of the brain. Its thin outer layer consists of gray matter (the cortex), and its interior portion consists of white matter. Each cerebral hemisphere is divided into the frontal, parietal, temporal, and occipital lobes.

The frontal lobe deals with emotions, abstract thinking, and judgment. The motor speech center (Broca's area) is also located in the frontal lobe. Essentially all right-handed individuals and about 85% of all left-handed individuals have the speech center on the left side. The frontal lobe and the parietal lobe are demarcated by the central sulcus. The motor cortex is in the precentral gyrus of the frontal lobe and is responsible for voluntary movements on the opposite side of the body. It is important to be aware that most motor fibers of the corticospinal tract cross the midline in the medulla. The primary olfactory cortex is contained in the base of the frontal lobe.

The parietal lobe is concerned with integrating sensations. The post-central gyrus is the major sensory receptive area (sensory cortex) for the highest integration and coordination of afferent information from the opposite side of the body, dealing with pain, temperature sense, proprioception, and fine touch. The sensory cortex is connected by the thalamic radiation from the thalamus, which is a sensory relay station. Nerve fibers mediating sensations via the spinal cord to the thalamus are the spinothalamic tracts and the dorsal columns.

The temporal lobe is located under the frontal and parietal lobes. Its cortex is the primary area where auditory stimuli are received. Wernicke's area for auditory comprehension is at the posterior end of the superior temporal gyrus. It is also one of the centers for dreams, memory, and emotions. The occipital lobe is located in the posterior part of each cerebral hemisphere, and its cortex is the primary area where visual stimuli are received.

The basal ganglia include the caudate nucleus, putamen, and globus pallidus. Close to the basal ganglia lies the internal capsule, which contains the important motor tracts (pyramidal tracts) descending from the motor cortex on their way to the spinal cord. The basal ganglia constitute part of the extrapyramidal system, which is made up of those areas in the CNS other than the pyramidal and cerebellar systems. They are concerned with the programming and initiation of movement and posture.

The hypothalamus is located below the thalamus and is intimately associated with the pituitary gland. It plays an important role in regulating the secretion of pituitary hormones. It also serves as a higher center for the autonomic nervous system and controls complex behavioral and emotional reactions, such as appetite, sexual behaviors, fear, and rage.

The limbic system consists of a rim of cortical tissue around the hilum of the cerebral hemisphere and a group of associated deep structures: the amygdale, the hippocampus, and the septal nuclei. It is directly concerned with smell and also with the control of feeding behavior, circadian rhythms, sexual behavior, rage, fear, and motivation.

The cerebellum can be found under the occipital lobe and is connected behind the brain stem. Like the cerebrum, it has right and left hemispheres, united by the vermis, and also has an outer layer of gray matter with numerous sulci and gyri. Almost all information to and from the cerebellum is transmitted by way of the midbrain. The cerebellum has three main functions: (1) maintenance of equilibrium and balance of the trunk, (2) regulation of muscle tension involved in the spinal nerve reflexes and posture and orientation of limbs, and (3) regulation of the coordination of fine limb movements.

The brain stem consists of the midbrain, the pons, and the medulla oblongata. Cranial nerves, except for the olfactory nerve and the optic nerve, originate in the brain stem. Cardiovascular and respiratory centers are located in the medulla. The reticular formation in the brain stem is generally associated with states of consciousness and alertness.

The spinal cord functions like a telephone cable between the brain and the PNS. Unlike the cerebrum and the cerebellum, the spinal cord consists of gray matter centrally and white matter peripherally. The zone of gray matter resembles a butterfly in cross section. Anterior projections of gray matter, termed anterior horns, are the site of the final synapse for efferent motor impulses leaving the cord. Poliomyelitis is a viral disease that affects this area. Posterior projections of gray matter, termed dorsal horns, convey afferent sensory information entering the cord from sensory organs. The peripheral zone of the cord consists of white matter and contains various ascending and descending tracts. For example, the spinothalamic tract carries pain and temperature impulses up to the thalamus, the posterior columns carry proprioceptive impulses up to the medulla, and the corticospinal tract delivers impulses downward from the motor cortex to initiate muscle activity.

The blood supply to the brain is derived from bilateral internal carotid and vertebral arteries, which are interconnected at the base of the brain at a vascular circuit known as the Circle of Willis. The middle cerebral artery supplies the lateral surface of most of the frontal lobe, nearly all of the parietal lobe, most of the temporal lobe, and part of the occipital lobe. The anterior cerebral artery supplies the medial surface of the frontal and parietal lobes. The precentral (motor) and postcentral (sensory) gyri representing the lower limbs lie within the distribution of this artery. The posterior cerebral artery supplies the upper pons, midbrain, much of the inferomedial aspect of the temporal lobe, and most of the occipital lobe. The blood supply to the brain stem and the cerebellum comes mostly from branches of the basilar artery, which is formed by bilateral vertebral arteries. The vertebral arteries also give rise to a single anterior spinal artery and two posterior spinal arteries, which run longitudinally along the spinal cord. This longitudinal arterial supply of the cord is further supplemented by radicular vessels at the cervicothoracic and thoracolumbar junctional areas.

Peripheral Nervous System

The cranial nerves (Table 2.2), with the exception of the olfactory and optic nerves, are defined as part of the PNS. At the spinal level, the PNS originates with the spinal nerves. Each spinal nerve has two roots: anterior (ventral) motor root and posterior (dorsal) sensory root. The anterior root contains the axons of the cell bodies in the anterior horn of the spinal cord. The posterior root has its cell bodies located in the sensory nerve ganglion outside but close to the cord. There are 31 pairs of spinal nerves (8 cervical, 12 thoracic, 5 lumbar, 5 sacral, and 1 coccygeal).

TABLE 2.2 Human Cranial Nerves

Name	Number	Motor	Sensory	Para-sympathetic
		Innervation		
Olfactory	I		Olfactory epithelium	
Optic	II		Retina	
Oculomotor	III	See Table 2.3 Levator palpebrae		Sphincter of iris Ciliary muscle
Trochlear	IV	See Table 2.3		
Trigeminal	V	Chewing muscles	Face	
Abducent	VI	See Table 2.3		
Facial	VII	Facial muscles orbicularis oculi	Ant. 2/3 of tongue	Salivary glands (submandibular and sublingual)
Vestibulocochlear	VIII		Inner ear	
Glossopharyngeal	IX	Swallowing muscle	Post. 1/3 of tongue Middle ear	Parotid gland
Vagus	X		Epiglottis External ear	Visceral organs Vocal cord
Accessory	XI	Sternocleidomastoid Trapezius		
Hypoglossal	XII	Tongue muscles		

The spinal cord ends at the upper level of the second lumbar vertebra. Because the spinal column is longer than the spinal cord itself, some of the spinal nerves, particularly at the lower levels, have to travel down a significant distance before actually leaving the bony canal. The very lower end of the cord is called the conus medullaris, and a bundle of spinal nerves passing downward within the aura mater below the first lumbar vertebra is referred to as the cauda equine. The phrenic nerve, which originates from the C3-5 spinal nerves, innervates the diaphragm.

All muscles in the upper extremities are controlled by the brachial plexus, which is a nerve complex formed by the C5-7-8-T1 spinal nerves. The main peripheral nerves of the brachial plexus include the axillary, musculocutaneous, median, ulnar, and radial nerves. These nerves contribute to both motor and sensation in the upper extremity.

The thoracic spinal nerves mainly innervate the thorax and abdomen, although the first and second thoracic nerves contribute partly to the upper extremities. All thoracic spinal and first and second lumbar spinal nerves contain sympathetic nerve fibers that innervate the viscera.

The lumbar and first and second sacral spinal nerves innervate the lower extremities in terms of motor control and sensory perception. The main peripheral nerves in the lower extremities include the femoral nerve, superior and inferior gluteal nerves, sciatic nerve, common peroneal nerve, and tibial nerve.

The pudendal nerve, originating from the S2-3-4, innervates the external genitalia, the perianal area, and the sphincter. The coccygeal nerve supplies the skin in the region of the coccyx. The autonomic nervous system (ANS) is divided into the sympathetic division and the parasympathetic division. The ANS regulates the activities of the viscera, such as the stomach and intestines, the heart, the smooth muscles of arteries, the sweat glands, the salivary glands, and the urinary bladder. The sympathetic preganglionic efferent nerve fibers, mostly myelinated, leave the spinal cord through the anterior roots of all of the thoracic spinal nerves and the upper lumbar spinal nerves. After exiting from the spinal canal, these nerve fibers branch off the spinal nerves to join a chain of ganglia that lies on either side of the spinal column, where they have their first synapse. The second sympathetic (postganglionic) fiber, mostly unmyelinated, then returns to the spinal nerves to be distributed to autonomic effectors in the areas supplied by these spinal nerves. Some postganglionic fibers may proceed directly to the viscera in the various sympathetic nerves rather than returning to the spinal nerve. Some preganglionic fibers pass through the paravertebral ganglion chain and end on the postganglionic neurons located in collateral ganglia close to the viscera.

The parasympathetic system is composed of cranial nerves III, VII, IX, and X, and the second, third, and fourth sacral spinal nerves. When the vagus (X) nerve is activated, the heart rate becomes slower, and the gastrointestinal tract becomes more active. The sacral parasympathetic nerves forming the pelvic nerve are important for contracting the detrusor muscle of the urinary bladder, for advancing the feces in the distal colon, and for erecting the penis.

RESPIRATORY SYSTEM

T**HE RESPIRATORY SYSTEM** includes the nose, nasal passages, nasopharynx, larynx, trachea, bronchi, and lungs. Each lung is covered by the pulmonary pleura, and the inner surface of the chest wall is lined by the parietal pleura. The potential space between these two pleurae is known as the pleural cavity. The right lung is divided into a superior lobe, a middle lobe, and an inferior lobe. The left lung is divided into a superior lobe and an inferior lobe. Nutrition to the tissue of the lungs is provided by the bronchial arteries. While the pulmonary arteries are delivering the venous blood to the lungs, the inspired air keeps traveling down to the alveoli (Figure 2.6), which are surrounded by pulmonary capillaries. There are 300 million alveoli in the human body, and the total area of the alveolar walls making contact with capillaries (Figure 2.7) in both lungs, to exchange carbon dioxide for oxygen, is about 70 m2. As oxygen diffuses into the blood, the hemoglobin molecule in the red blood cell immediately takes up oxygen, permitting more into the plasma.

Inspiration is an active process, primarily accomplished by contractions of the diaphragm, and expiration during quiet breathing results from the passive recoiling of the lungs. Inspiration can be aided by using neck muscles and external intercostals. For forcible expira-

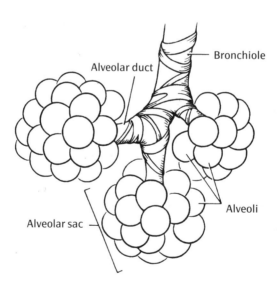

FIGURE 2.6 Schematic showing the structure of the alveolar ducts, alveolar sacs, and alveoli.

From DeLisa and Stolov: Significant Body Systems in Handbook of Severe Disability edited by Stolov and Clowers, U.S. Department of Education, Rehabilitation Service Administration, 1981.

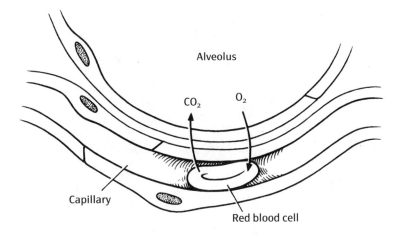

FIGURE 2.7 Schematic representation of the exchange of oxygen and carbon dioxide through the thin walls of the alveolus and a red blood cell of a capillary.

From DeLisa and Stolov: Significant Body Systems in Handbook of Severe Disability edited by Stolov and Clowers, U.S. Department of Education, Rehabilitation Service Administration, 1981.

tion, good strength of the abdominal muscles and the internal intercostals is necessary.

Besides gas exchange, the respiratory system secretes immunoglobulin to resist respiratory infections and has macrophages in the alveoli that serve to ingest inhaled bacteria and small particles. The hairs in the nostrils prevent large particles from entering the airway. Coughing and ciliary movements of the proximal airway with mucus are also capable of removing particles from the respiratory tract.

CARDIOVASCULAR SYSTEM

BLOOD CIRCULATION THROUGHOUT the body is accomplished by means of the cardiovascular system. The driving force for moving the blood is provided by the pumping action of the heart. The pulmonary circulation, driven by the right heart, delivers venous blood to the lungs, where the carbon dioxide is effectively removed and the oxygen is replenished. The systemic circulation, driven by the left heart, delivers oxygenated blood to active tissues of the body. The blood vessels leading from the heart are arteries, and the blood vessels returning the blood, containing increased carbon dioxide and decreased oxygen, to the heart are veins. The lymphatics take the extra fluid in the interstitial tissue and bring the fluid back into the blood, promoting turnover of tissue fluid.

The heart is about the size of a man's fist. Two thirds of it lies to the

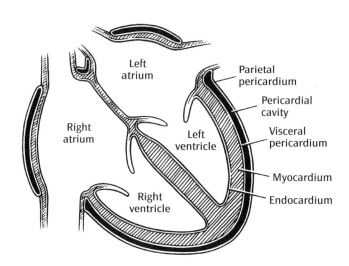

FIGURE 2.8 Schematic representation of the four chambers of the heart, the three layers of the heart wall, and the two layers of the pericardium.
  From DeLisa and Stolov: Significant Body Systems in Handbook of Severe Disability edited by Stolov and Clowers, U.S. Department of Education, Rehabilitation Service Administration, 1981.

left of the midline, within the chest cavity and between the lungs. The heart (Figure 2.8) is enclosed by a double-layered loose sac, the pericardium. A small amount of fluid between the two layers lubricates the surfaces to allow the heart to change its shape without much friction as it pumps. The wall of the heart has three distinct layers: the epicardium (outer thin membrane), the myocardium (thick middle layer of cardiac muscle), and the endocardium (inner layer). The pumping action is achieved by the myocardium, which is a special form of muscle, somewhat like skeletal muscle but not subject to the same type of voluntary control. The heart has four chambers: right atrium, right ventricle, left atrium, and left ventricle. Blood from the systemic circulation enters the right atrium through the inferior and superior vena cava. It passes through the tricuspid valve into the right ventricle. Right ventricular contraction propels the blood through the pulmonary semilunar valve into the pulmonary artery for pulmonary circulation. The blood from the lungs enters the left atrium through the pulmonary vein and passes through the mitral valve into the left ventricle. Left ventricular contraction propels the blood through the aortic semilunar valve into the aorta for systemic circulation. All valves—tricuspid, mitral, and semilunar—can pass blood in only one direction in the normal situation. The walls between the two ventricles and the two atria, the interventricular septum and the interatrial septum, block mixing of the two circulations in the normal condition.

Each cardiac cycle consists of two parts: diastolic and systolic. During diastole, all four chambers are relaxed, and both atria receive and fill with blood. Systole begins first with right and left atrial contraction, propelling blood through the tricuspid and mitral valves into the right and left ventricles, respectively. The myocardium of the atria is relatively thin, whereas the myocardium of the ventricles is thick. Ventricular systole, the main pumping action, forcefully propels blood into the pulmonary artery and aorta. When this contraction occurs, the tricuspid and mitral valves slam shut, thereby preventing the flow of blood back into the atria. The closures of these valves produce the first heart sound that can be heard with a stethoscope. The rush of blood out of the ventricles causes the pulse beat that can be felt at the wrist and other areas of the body where arteries are prominent. The rush of blood into the pulmonary artery and aorta distends the walls of these vessels. When ventricular contraction stops, the vessels recoil and the semilunar valves slam shut, thereby preventing the flow of blood back into the ventricles. The second heart sound is associated with the closure of the semilunar valves.

Cardiac murmurs are abnormal sounds heard over the heart and usually signify disease of the heart valves: stenosis or insufficiency. Abnormal sounds can also be heard outside the heart (e.g., carotid bruit when a carotid artery is partially occluded and thyroid bruit when a thyroid goiter is highly vascular).

Blood pressure recorded (usually in the arm) consists of two numbers that refer to the systolic pressure and the diastolic pressure. Pressures are recorded in millimeters of mercury (mmHg) and are written as systolic pressure over diastolic pressure (e.g.,120/80). The magnitudes of the pressure are dependent not only on the force produced by the thick myocardium of the ventricles but also by the resistance to flow produced by the progressively narrowing peripheral arterial vessels.

The heart has an inherent capacity to contract rhythmically. Each cycle originates in a special bundle of myocardial cells (sinoatrial node [SA node, or the pacemaker]) in the wall of the right atrium. These cells initiate electrical impulses at a regular interval without benefit of any external stimulation. The impulses travel in the walls of the atria, causing atrial contraction, and rapidly reach the atrioventricular (AV) node, which also lies in the right atrial wall near the interatrial septum. Impulses delay here slightly until atrial systole is completed. From the AV node, impulses travel down two bundles of special muscle fibers (bundle of His) on the right and left side of the interventricular septum. The two bundles branch out as Purkinje fibers and spread over both ventricles, causing ventricular contraction. The parasympathetic fibers from the vagus nerve cause the SA node to slow down, and the sympathetic nerve fibers from the upper thoracic cord are responsible for speeding up the

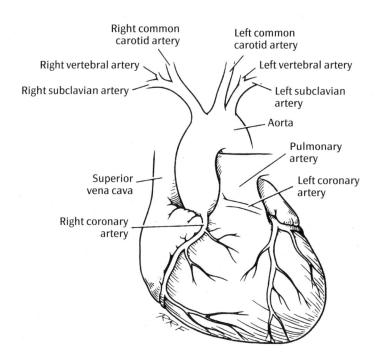

FIGURE 2.9 The two coronary arteries encircle the heart and supply blood to all portions of the myocardium. Each coronary artery can supply both atria and both ventricles, thus providing the heart with a safety factor in the event of disease in one of the coronary arteries. The vertebral and carotid arteries supply blood to the brain.
  From DeLisa and Stolov: Significant Body Systems in Handbook of Severe Disability edited by Stolov and Clowers, U.S. Department of Education, Rehabilitation Service Administration, 1981.

SA node. A number of chemicals and hormones, such as epinephrine and thyroxine, can accelerate the heart rate.

  The major branches of the aorta distribute blood to the head, abdomen, and extremities. The right and left coronary arteries (Figure 2.9), which also originate from the aorta, supply the heart itself. Some branches of these two coronary arteries anastomize (interconnect). Arterial walls are composed of three layers: the intima (inner layer with endothelial cells), the media (middle layer with smooth muscle and elastic connective tissue fibers), and the adventitia (outer fibrous layer). As these arteries branch further, they become progressively thinner-walled and smaller in diameter. The smallest divisions of the arteries are the arterioles, whose main component is smooth muscle. The diameter of the arterioles can be altered, even to the extent of closure, by sympathetic activation, hypertrophy of the arteriole smooth muscle, or arteriolosclerosis. The changes in the diameter of these vessels not only determine the quantity of blood delivered to capillaries but also influence the blood pressure.

The arteries lead into the microscopic capillaries that lie in close approximation to the fluid bathing the living cells (interstitial fluid). Capillary walls are very thin, consisting of only a thin lining of endothelial cells. This thin wall permits the passage of nutrients and oxygen into the interstitial fluid and also permits waste products and carbon dioxide from the cells to permeate into the venous system. The capillary walls, however, are relatively impermeable to the plasma proteins.

The venules are the smallest veins, yet larger than capillaries. They unite to form veins that return blood to the heart. The walls of veins have the same three layers as the arteries, but the media is much thinner. Many veins have valves to prevent the reflux of blood. The venous blood pressure is lower than the arterial blood pressure. The superior vena cava collects venous blood from the head, upper extremities, and thorax, and the inferior vena cava receives blood from the rest of the body. Although blood from all of the veins of the lower extremities is directly received by the inferior vena cava, visceral venous blood is first drained into the liver by the portal vein. In the liver the portal vein ends in sinusoids (capillary-like vessel in the liver) from which the blood is conveyed to the inferior vena cava. Both superior and inferior venae cavae open into the right atrium of the heart.

The lymphatic system is also an important vascular network, consisting of lymphatic capillaries, lymphatic collecting vessels, and lymph nodes through which the lymphatic fluid (lymph) recirculates from the tissue space of most organs into the venous system. Lymphatic capillaries allow the passage of extra-cellular fluids through their walls and reabsorb considerable amounts of proteins into the circulation. Unlike the capillary walls, the walls of the lymphatics are permeable to the macromolecules, and the proteins therefore are returned to the blood stream via the lymphatics. Two main lymphatic vessels are the thoracic duct, which ends in the left subclavian vein after draining the lymphatic fluid from most of the body, and the right lymphatic duct, which ends in the right subclavian vein after draining the fluid from the right side of the head and neck, the right upper extremity, the right side of the thorax, right lung, and right side of the heart. The lymph nodes manufacture lymphocytes, which have the ability to produce antibodies against many different foreign invaders (antigens). The main forces pushing lymph up toward the heart are skeletal muscle contractions, negative intrathoracic pressure during inspiration, the suction effect of high-velocity venous blood flow, and rhythmic contractions of the large lymphatic ducts.

HEMATOPOIETIC SYSTEM

BLOOD CELLS INCLUDE white blood cells (leukocytes), red blood cells (erythrocytes), and platelets. During fetal life, blood cells are formed not only in the bone marrow but in the liver and spleen as well. In addition, the thymus is a lymphocyte-producing organ. Shortly after birth, however, most of the blood cells are formed in the bone marrow, specifically the red marrow.

The white blood cells include granulocytes (neutrophils, eosinophils, and basophils), lymphocytes, and monocytes. There are normally 4,000 to 11,000 white blood cells per microliter of human blood. These provide powerful defenses for the body against tumors and infections (viral, bacterial, and parasitic).

The red blood cells carry hemoglobin, binding oxygen during circulation. They survive an average of 120 days, and their normal count is 5.4 million per microliter of blood in men and 4.8 million per microliter in women. Old red blood cells are destroyed by macrophages, and the hemoglobin of those is eventually converted into bilirubin. The formation of red blood cells (erythropoiesis) is controlled by a circulating glycoprotein hormone (erythropoietin) that is secreted primarily by the kidneys. Erythropoiesis is also stimulated by anemia or hypoxia and is inhibited by a rise in the circulating red blood cell level to supernormal values.

Platelets are smaller than the red blood cells and contain granules. Between 60% and 75% of platelets that have been extruded from the bone marrow are in the circulating blood, and the remainder are mostly in the spleen. Platelets play a significant role in the blood-clotting mechanism. They have a half-life of about 4 days.

Bone marrow is soft fatty tissue found in the medullary cavity of bones and consists of two types: red and yellow. Red marrow is a hematopoietic tissue producing granulocytes, red blood cells, and platelets. Some lymphocytes are formed in the bone marrow, but most are formed in the lymph nodes, thymus, and spleen from precursor cells that originated from bone marrow. Yellow marrow consists of fat cells for the most part and a few primitive blood cells. Red marrow is found in the flat and short bones.

The spleen is a highly vascular organ and is situated principally in the left hypochondriac region of the abdomen. It contains many platelets and macrophages and removes abnormal red blood cells. Additionally, the spleen plays a significant role in the immune system.

The thymus is situated between the sternum and great vessels. Although prominent in the infant, it is hardly recognizable in the adult. The thymus forms lymphocytes and is also believed to enable the body to produce the antibodies and to reject foreign tissue and cells.

DIGESTIVE SYSTEM

THE DIGESTIVE SYSTEM grossly consists of the mouth, teeth, tongue, salivary glands, throat, esophagus, stomach, duodenum, jejunum, ileum, cecum, colon, rectum, and anal sphincter, as well as the liver, gallbladder and pancreas. The salivary glands are present in the parotid, submandibular, and sublingual regions, secreting saliva into the mouth. The stomach secretes gastric acid (HCI) and various digestive enzymes that make the chewed food creamy, enabling further digestion by the intestine. The liver is the largest gland in the body, and is situated in the upper part of the abdomen, on the right side just under the diaphragm. It manufactures the plasma proteins concerned with blood clotting and detoxifies many drugs and toxins. It also converts sugars into glycogen, stores glycogen and blood, and secretes bile. The bile is concentrated in the gallbladder, a pear-shaped sac lodged on the liver. The bile is poured into the small intestine via the bile ducts. The pancreas is also a large gland, excreting the digestive pancreatic juice and secreting insulin; it is located transversely behind the stomach. The pancreatic duct opens into the duodenum. After chewing and swallowing of food, digestion and fluid absorption are major physiological events occurring in the gastrointestinal tract. Intestinal peristaltic movements then propel its contents down to the rectum, resulting in defecation.

GENITOURINARY SYSTEM

THE MALE REPRODUCTIVE organs include the testes, the epididymis, the vas deferns, the seminal vesicles, the ejaculatory duct, and the penis. The testes, consisting of convoluted seminiferous tubules, are suspended in the scrotum by the spermatic cords and produce the spermatozoa. The interstitial cells of the testes, which are nested between the tubules, secrete testosterone into the blood stream. Spermatozoa leaving the testes are not fully mobile but continue their maturation and acquire motility while they are passing through the epididymis. The vas deferens conveys spermatozoa to the ejaculatory duct. The seminal vesicles secrete a fluid that is added to the sperm. The ejaculatory duct begins at the base of the prostate, and the semen is propelled out of the urethra by contraction of the bulbocavernosus muscle. The penis is composed of the corpus spongiosum and the corpora cavernosa, with arterial, venous, and lymphatic vessels. Erection of the penis is basically due to engorgement of the elastic tissue when it is filled with blood.

The female genital organs include the ovaries, containing a number of immature ova, the uterine tubes, the uterus, and the vagina, along with the external genitalia. The uterus is composed of the endometrium (inner mucous membrane), the myometrium (middle muscular coat), and the perimetrium (external serous coat). After puberty, the uterine endometrium develops periodic changes, under hormonal influence, that manifest menstrual bleeding. The changes in the uterus are closely correlated with cyclic changes in the ovary. The length of the cycle is usually 28 days. During the menstrual cycle there are also cyclic changes in the breasts, with distention of the mammary ducts, hyperemia, and edema of the interstitial tissue affected by estrogen and progesterone. At about the 14th day of the menstrual cycle, only one matured ovum is extruded from the ovary into the abdominal cavity (ovulation). The ovum is taken up by the fimbriated end of the uterine tube and is conveyed to the uterus. Fertilization of the ovum by the sperm usually occurs in the midportion of the tube. When one sperm cell fuses to the ovum, embryonic development begins. The developing embryo then moves down the tube into the uterus. Without fertilization, the ovum is passed out through the vagina.

The urinary organs include the kidneys, the ureters, the urinary bladder, and the urethra. The kidney is grossly composed of the outer cortex, the inner medulla, and the renal pelvis. In the kidneys, the glomerular capillaries filter a fluid resembling the blood plasma into the renal tubules (glomerular filtration). The tubules then reabsorb glucose and some of the water and solutes (tubular reabsorption) and secrete some electrolytes (tubular secretion) to the tubular fluid. In this manner physiological levels of blood electrolytes are maintained. Finally, the urine is formed and is conveyed from the renal pelvis via the ureters down to the urinary bladder. The detrusor muscle of the bladder contracts to expel the urine out through the urethra and relaxes to act as a reservoir for the urine until the next voiding becomes necessary. In addition to their excretory function, the kidneys work as endocrine organs, secreting erythropoietin to enhance the formation of red blood cells in the bone marrow and rennin to maintain the blood pressure.

ENDOCRINE SYSTEM

THE MAJOR ENDOCRINE glands are the thyroid gland, the parathyroid glands, the pituitary gland, the adrenal glands, and the pancreas.

The thyroid gland is located in the anterior neck and secretes thyroxine (an oxygen-consumption-stimulating hormone) and calcitonin (a calcium-lowering hormone). The secretion of thyroxine is regulated by thyroid-stimulating hormone (TSH), which is one of the anterior pituitary hormones. The parathyroid glands are situated on the thyroid gland, two on each side, and produce parathormone for calcium metabolism.

The pituitary gland is seated in the sella turcica of the spheroid bone and is composed of anterior, intermediate (rudimentary), and posterior lobes. The anterior lobe, which is under hypothalamic control, secretes growth hormone (GH), TSH, adrenocorticotropic hormone (ACTH), follicle-stimulating hormone (FSH), luteinizing hormone (LH), and prolactin. FSH and LH act on the ovaries and control the function of the testes. Prolactin stimulates lactation. The posterior lobe secretes oxytocin, for uterine contractions at term and ejection of milk during lactation, and vasopressin (antidiuretic hormone [ADH]) for inhibition of renal diuresis.

The adrenal glands are situated at the upper pole of each kidney and are therefore sometimes referred to as the supradrenal glands. The adrenal gland is composed of the outer cortex and the inner medulla. The adrenal cortex elaborates steroid hormones, which are derivatives of cholesterol. The function of the adrenal cortex is regulated by pituitary ACTH. The adrenal medulla synthesizes the catecholamines, including epinephrine, norepinephrine, and dopamine.

As an endocrine organ, the pancreas secretes insulin and glucagons for the metabolism of carbohydrates, proteins, and fats.

VISUAL SYSTEM

THE OCULAR SYSTEM is situated peripherally in orbit. The eyeball (Figure 2.10) is composed anteriorly of the cornea, an avascular transparent structure, but mostly of the opaque posterior segment, which consists of an outer thick layer (sclera), a middle vascular layer (choroid), and an inner neural layer (retina). In addition, the anterior part of the sclera is covered by the conjunctival membrane. This iris, which is a circular, colored disk suspended in the aqueous humor, contains circular and radial muscle fibers that, respectively, constrict and dilate the pupil. A space between the cornea and the iris is called the anterior chamber. The crystalline lens is located immediately behind the iris. The lens is encircled by the ciliary processes, which produce the aqueous humor in the posterior chamber (a small space between the iris and the lens). The aqueous humor then flows into the chamber via the pupil. Posterior to the lens there is a large cavity containing a transparent semigelatinous material that is known as the vitreous body. The vitreous body is surrounded posteriorly by the retina, which consists of an outer pigmented layer and an inner neural wall (retina proper). The retina proper is further microscopically divided into 10 layers, which contain visual receptors (rods and cones) and nerve cells. However, a small area in the retina, where the optic nerve leaves the eye, has no visual receptors and is known as the blind spot. This region is also known as the optic disk.

Generally speaking, visual images are formed in the retina and con-

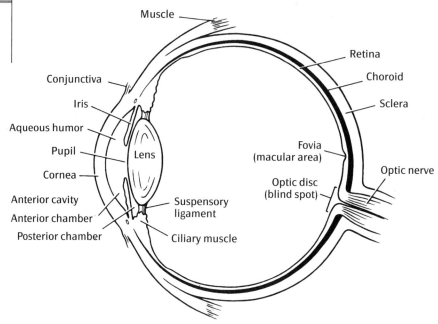

FIGURE 2.10   Schematic section of the human eye. The lens, the suspensory ligament, and the ciliary muscle divide the eye into anterior and posterior cavities. The iris further divides the anterior cavity into anterior and posterior chambers. Note the two extraocular muscles attached to the sclera.

From DeLisa and Stolov: Significant Body Systems in Handbook of Severe Disability edited by Stolov and Clowers, U.S. Department of Education, Rehabilitation Service Administration, 1981.

TABLE 2.3   Extraocular Muscles

Name	Innervation cranial nerve	Eye movement
Superior rectus	III	Elevation/intorsion
Inferior rectus	III	Depression/extorsion
Medial rectus	III	Adduction
Lateral rectus	VI	Abduction
Superior oblique	IV	Intorsion/depression
Inferior oblique	III	Extorsion/elevation

veyed to the occipital lobes of the brain via the optic nerves. For details, the visual field of each eye is divisible into the temporal field and the nasal field. Images from the temporal field are formed in the nasal portion of the retina, and images from the nasal field are formed in the temporal portion of the retina. The nerve fibers of the retina then convey visual impulses, which are transmitted by the optic nerve. However, the fibers from the nasal portion of the retina cross over in the optic chiasm, and the fibers from the temporal portion of the retina continue on the same side. These fibers combine (half from the nasal portion of one retina and half from the temporal portion of the other retina) to form the optic tract. Impulses are conveyed via the optic tract and end in the lateral geniculate body, where the fibers synapse on the cells, whose axons form the geniculocalcarine tract (the tract that finally conveys visual impulses to the occipital lobe of the cerebral cortex) (Figure 2.11).

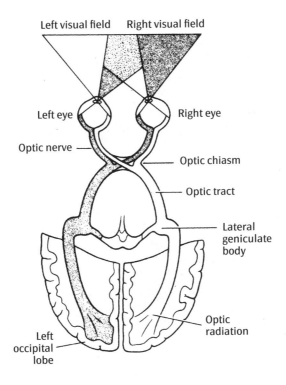

FIGURE 2.11 Note the crossover of optic nerve fibers from both nasal retinas at the optic chiasma, with the result that the right visual field can project onto the left occipital cortex, and vice versa.

From DeLisa and Stolov: Significant Body Systems in Handbook of Severe Disability edited by Stolov and Clowers, U.S. Department of Education, Rehabilitation Service Administration, 1981.

AUDITORY AND VESTIBULAR SYSTEM

THE RECEPTORS OF hearing and equilibrium are located in the inner ears. The ear is divisible into the external ear, the middle ear (tympanic cavity), and the inner ear (labyrinth). The external ear includes the auricular, which collects sound, and the external auditory canal extending to the eardrum.

The middle ear is an air-filled space in the temporal bone that opens into the nasopharynx via the eustachian tube. This tube is usually closed, but it opens during chewing, swallowing, and yawning and thereby maintains the equality of air pressure on both sides of the eardrum. There are three movable auditory ossicles: the malleus, the incus, and the stapes, whose leverlike linkage serves to amplify the pressure of the sound. Sound waves passed through the external ear, eardrum, and ossicles are transformed into movements of the stapes, which set up fluid waves in the inner ear (Figure 2.12). There are also two small skeletal muscles: the tensor tympani and the stapedius. Their role is to reduce the oscillations of the ossicles to protect the inner ear from acoustic injury during a loud noise.

The inner ear is located in the petrous portion of the temporal bone and is divided into the bony labyrinth and the membranous labyrinth. The bony labyrinth consists of the cochlea, the vestibule, and the semicircular canals and contains a clear fluid, the perilymph. The perilymph surrounds most parts of the membranous labyrinth, which also con-

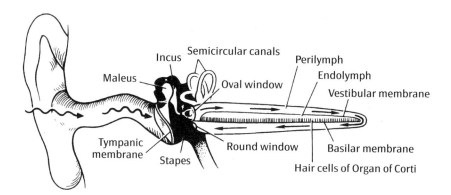

FIGURE 2.12 Schematic drawing of sound wave transmission. Sound wave vibrates the tympanic membrane, which in turn oscillates the malleus, incus, and stapes. Stapes vibrating in oval window agitates perilymph, which transmits vibration to vestibular membrane and then to endolymph to reach the hair cells of the organ of Corti. Wave dissipates at the round window. Note the two muscles anchoring the malleus and incus.

From DeLisa and Stolov: Significant Body Systems in Handbook of Severe Disability edited by Stolov and Clowers, U.S. Department of Education, Rehabilitation Service Administration, 1981.

tains a fluid, the endolymph. The cochlea, resembling a snail shell, contains the organ of Corti in its basal turn. This organ contains hair cells, innervated by the cochlear (auditory) division of the eighth cranial nerve, which function as auditory receptors. Auditory impulses then pass through the medial geniculate body in the thalamus and ultimately reach the auditory cortex of the temporal lobe.

In contrast, the vestibule and semicircular canals of the inner ear serve to maintain body equilibrium. There are two membranous sacs, called the utricle and the saccule, in the vestibular portion of the membranous labyrinth. These contain hair cells, as do the semicircular canals, that are innervated by the vestibular division of the eighth cranial nerve. Depending on body position, they are stimulated by otoliths in the maculae of the utricle and saccule and by the endolymph in the ampula of the semicircular canals. However, the anatomical pathways within the brain underlying vestibular function are yet to be clearly unveiled.

REFERENCES

Clemente, C. A. (1985). Gray's anatomy (30th American ed.). Philadelphia: Lea and Febiger.

DeLisa, J., & Stolov, W. A. (1981). Significant body systems. In W. A. Stolov & M. R. Clowers (Eds.), Handbook of severe disabilities (pp. 19–54). Washington, DC: U.S. Department of Education, Rehabilitation Services Administration.

Ganong, W. A. (1991). Review of medical physiology (15th ed.). Los Altos, CA: Lange Medical Publications.

Part II

Disabling Conditions and Disorders

3

Acquired Immune Deficiency Syndrome and Human Immunodeficiency Virus

JAMES SATRIANO, PhD, ALAN BERKMAN, MD,
AND ROBERT H. REMIEN, PhD

SINCE THE FIRST case descriptions of what is now known as acquired immune deficiency syndrome (AIDS) appeared in the literature in the early 1980s (Centers for Disease Control [CDC], 1981), much has been learned about the disease. The causative agent of the disease, the human immunodeficiency virus (HIV), belongs to a family of viruses that have RNA as their core genetic material and are known as retroviruses. They are known as retroviruses because the process of converting RNA into DNA is the reverse of the normal cellular process. For HIV to infect a host cell, the viral RNA must be converted into DNA, which can then be integrated into the host cell's DNA. Reverse transcriptase is the enzyme responsible for this conversion process. Once incorporated into the host cell, the viral genetic material causes the cell to produce more viral particles, which then bud from the host to infect other cells. Essentially, HIV converts healthy cells into virus factories.

HIV does not attack all of the cells of the body but has a special affinity for cells known as lymphocytes and phagocytes. These are a class of white blood cells that circulate in the blood stream and are present in blood-forming organs of the body. These cells represent our major defense against foreign materials that have gained entry into the body.

IMMUNE FUNCTIONING

THE FUNCTIONING OF an intact immune system is a well-orchestrated interplay of many factors (see Siegal, 1987, for a detailed explanation). Immune system cells are created in the bone marrow and consist of phagocytes (of which a macrophage is a special type) and two kinds of lymphocytes (T cells and B cells). When the body detects an invading organism, the phagocytes are the first line of defense. Macrophages will attack the invading virus and break off and display a piece of its surface protein, known as an antigen, so that other immune cells can identify the invader as a threat. The macrophages displaying the viral antigen muster the T cells into action. There are four different types of T cells (helper, killer, suppressor, and memory) created in the thymus. The antigen-carrying macrophage first activates helper T cells (also known as CD4+ lymphocytes) that are specific to the antigen being displayed. There are millions of types of helper T cells, each responsive to a different kind of antigen. The antigen fits the specific T-cell receptor like a key into a lock. The activated helper T cells travel to the spleen and lymph nodes, where they stimulate the production of killer T cells that are also specific to the antigen displayed by the macrophage. The killer T cells migrate to the site of the invading organism and, through a chemical process, kill the invader and any infected cells. The antigen-displaying macrophage also activates the production of another type of immune system weapon, known as the B cell. The B cells are the immune system cells responsible for the production of antibodies. Antibodies are protein molecules made by the B cells and are, like the helper and killer T cells, specific to the antigen displayed by the macrophage. Antibodies can act against an invader in several ways. They destroy invading cells indirectly, by stimulating chemical reactions against them. They bind to the surface of the invaders, thereby causing them to clump together into aggregates and thus becoming more attractive targets to the phagocytes. Also, by binding to the surface of invading viruses, antibodies prevent the virus from binding with and thus infecting other cells.

When the battle is won and invading viral particles and infected cells have been destroyed, the suppressor T cells come into play. These cells, as their name implies, release a chemical that subdues the activated B and T cells and brings the production of new lymphatic cells to a halt. In the aftermath, memory B and T cells remain, giving the individual immunity to that specific strain of virus. However, very similar viruses can bear antigens with subtle differences, and immunity to one strain may not provide protection from another.

HIV VIROLOGY

HIV IS A PARTICULARLY insidious virus in that its major targets are the very cells of the immune system designed to protect against viral assault. HIV enters the body via blood or body fluids and is probably concealed in infected phagocytes or lymphocytes. The envelope protein of HIV (gp120) has a high affinity for the CD4 protein found on the surface of T cells and macrophages. Once these molecules fuse, the viral RNA is released into the cell. The viral enzyme reverse transcriptase converts the viral RNA into DNA, which is then integrated into the host cell's genome. The viral genetic components replicate within the host cell, and new viral particles are assembled and bud from the host cell to infect other cells (Shaw, Wong-Staal, & Gallo, 1988).

The reason that HIV damages the immune system is that it infects the very cells designed to fight off invading organisms, the macrophages and T cells. By infecting T cells and converting them into viral factories whose progeny can infect other cells, HIV slowly disables the immune system. As the number of healthy T cells drops, the immune system is made less effective in defending against other invading organisms, and the person becomes susceptible to opportunistic infections (Koenig & Fauci, 1988).

EPIDEMIOLOGY

THE HIV INFECTION in the United States was first noted among homosexual men in New York and California in 1981, as clusters of rare protozoal pneumonia, Pneumocystis carinii pneumonia (PCP), and rare skin cancer, Kaposi's sarcoma (KS), began to be reported. At that time it was unclear how these diseases came about, and it was several years before a blood/body fluid-borne virus was discovered as the etiological agent. By that time, well-delineated disease clusters were established (Kaslow & Francis, 1989). Infection rates among homosexual men continued to rise. Also noted were escalating infection rates among intravenous drug users and blood transfusion recipients, especially hemophiliacs who received frequent transfusions of blood products.

By the mid-1980s it was well established that HIV was transmitted through sexual contact, blood, and blood products, but at that time the disease in this country was largely confined to males. Soon reports of women infected by sexual partners began to emerge. These women were, by and large, the sexual partners of bisexual men or men who used intravenous drugs. As the rates of infected women began to rise, the virus was discovered to infect some of their children. A percentage of infants become infected either in utero, during the birth process, or following birth through breast feeding. Smaller but news-making cases of transmission have occurred from health care workers to patients, from patients to health care workers, and through organ or tissue transplantation.

Although in the U.S., HIV infection continues to be mainly a disease of men, with about 70% of new cases occurring in males, globally, the dominant mode of HIV transmission has been and remains heterosexual sex. Outside the United States and Europe, the ratio of infected men to women is 1:1. During the middle and latter part of the 1990s, the epidemiological pattern in large urban areas of the United States increasingly resembled that of Africa, Asia, and Latin America, with a growing proportion of new HIV infection occurring in young women with unprotected heterosexual sex as their primary risk factor (CDC, 1997).

According to the Centers for Disease Control and Prevention (CDC, 2004):

* Approximately 40,000 new HIV infections occur each year in the United States.
* There are estimated to be between 800,000 and 900,000 people currently living with HIV in the U.S.
* More than half of all new infections in the U.S. occur among blacks.
* Blacks make up 54% of new infections despite being only 13% of the total U.S. population.

According to the World Health Organization (WHO, 2004):

* There are approximately 40 million people living with HIV infection worldwide.
* About 5 million new cases of infection occur annually.
* It is estimated that about 3 million deaths occur annually from HIV infection worldwide.

FUNCTIONAL PRESENTATION OF MEDICAL CONDITION/DISABILITY

COURSE OF ILLNESS

INFECTION WITH HIV can occur when contaminated blood or body fluids (especially sperm or vaginal fluids) come into contact with the bloodstream or mucosal tissue. The most common modes of transmission are sexual (unprotected anal, vaginal, or oral intercourse), blood-borne (transfusion or contaminated blood or blood products, needle stick injuries, the use of "dirty" IV drug injection equipment), or from mother to child (either perinatally or through breast feeding). It should be noted that the course of illness described below does not hold for all individuals infected with HIV. Also, it should be stressed that the time of progression from HIV infection to AIDS may be considerable (more than 10 years), and it is still not clear if all HIV-infected individuals will develop AIDS.

Following contact with fluids contaminated with a sufficient number of viral particles, acute HIV infection may occur. The initial reaction to infection with HIV may be a constellation of flu-like symptoms that can include fever, headache, and sore throat. These symptoms may last from a few days to a few weeks before dissipating (Yarchoan & Pluda, 1988). The immune system develops antibodies to HIV indicating an immunological response, albeit an ineffective one. The development of antibodies to HIV usually occurs within 2 to 6 months after initial infection. The currently licensed HIV tests (ELISA and Western Blot) are tests for viral antibodies, not direct tests of the virus itself. There now exists an HIV RNA viral load assay that provides a direct measure of circulating virus per unit of blood (Ho, 1996). This measure can show the presence of HIV infection, even in the absence of a positive antibody test. Thus, one could be infected with HIV and able to transmit it to others and still test HIV-negative, by Western Blot, if one had not yet developed viral antibodies.

Following infection, patients generally enter a phase of asymptomatic HIV infection (Yarchoan & Pluda, 1988). During this phase of the illness patients may look and feel well. As noted above, this phase can last more than 10 years, and some HIV-infected individuals may never develop AIDS; we don't yet know. This period is known as the asymptomatic phase of the disease. CD4+ cell counts are over 500 (normal is considered 800 or higher) at this point. When CD4+ cell counts drop below 500, HIV infected persons may develop non-life-threatening infection like shingles or thrush. The development of these conditions is due to the moderate immune deficiency caused by HIV and their treatment is complicated by the virus.

As the immune system continues to deteriorate and the CD+ cells fall below 200, AIDS-defining opportunistic infections are common. A list of AIDS-defining conditions can be found in Table 3.1.

FUNCTIONAL PRESENTATION OF DISABILITY

PRIOR TO THE development of severe immune-deficiency, the HIV-infected individual may have no disabling condition at all. However, later in the course of the disease, many of the opportunistic infections described above can have a protracted course and may lead to prolonged

TABLE 3.1   List of AIDS-Defining Conditions

Candidiasis of bronchi, trachea, or lungs

Candidiasis, esophageal

Cervical cancer, invasive

Coccidioidomycosis, disseminated or extrapulmonary

Cryptococcosis, extrapulmonary

Cryptosporidiosis, chronic intestinal (> 1 month duration)

Cytomegalovirus disease (other than liver, spleen, or nodes),

Cytomegalovirus retinitis (with loss of vision)

HIV encephalopathy

Herpes simplex: chronic ulcers (> 1 month duration); or bronchitis, pneumonitis or esophagitis

Histoplasmosis, disseminated or extrapulmonary

Isosporiasis, chronic intestinal (> 1 month duration)

Kaposi's sarcoma

Lymphoma, Berkett's

Lymphoma, immunoblastic

Lymphoma, primary in brain

Mycrobacterium avium complex or M. Kansasii, disseminated or extrapulmonary

Mycrobacterium tuberculosis, any site (pulmonary or extrapulmonary)

Mycrobacterium, other species or unidentified species, disseminated or extrapulmonary

Pneumocystis carinii pneumonia

Pneumonia, recurrent

Progressive multi-focal leukoencephalopathy

Salmonella septicemia, recurrent

Toxoplasmosis of brain

Wasting syndrome due to HIV

Source: Centers for Disease Control (1992).

periods of illness and hospitalization. Generally, the onset of the symptoms of AIDS is considered to be a disabling condition.

Aside from the physical disability caused by opportunistic infection, HIV is neurotropic. That is, it directly infects the central nervous system (CNS) and can result in a progressive dementing illness. Although the HIV-associated dementia (HAD) is estimated to affect about 15% of asymptomatic HIV-infected people, about 30% of patients may show some signs of neurological impairment (McArthur et al., 1989). These symptoms may be as subtle as a slightly disturbed gait or very elusive memory complaints. Early manifestations of HAD include: impaired concentration, memory loss, depressed mood, unsteady gait, motor weakness, and ataxia. Late stage symptoms include: global cognitive dysfunction, amnesic- like features, mutism, organic hallucinations and parkinson-like symptoms. It is important to note that some opportunistic infections may result in altered mental states that mimic HAD but respond well to medical treatment. Therefore, all patients showing changes in mental status should be referred for a medical workup.In patients with end-stage HAD, organic psychotic symptoms may be present; they most commonly involve hallucinations and/or delirium. It should also be noted that as the dementia progresses, the patient will require increasing amounts of assistance in activities of daily living. For example, moderately demented patients may require supervision in taking medication and preparing food. End-stage patients typically require 24-hour nursing care and supervision in all activities.

TREATMENT AND PROGNOSIS

THE INTRODUCTION OF effective drug therapy for HIV must be seen as one of the most dramatic episodes in the history of modern medicine. Prior to the development of highly active antiretroviral therapy (HAART) in 1996, the natural history of untreated HIV infection was progressive destruction of the immune system until infection, inanition or cancer resulted in death. While untreated individuals progressed from primary infection to death at widely varying rates based on a number of known and unknown host and viral factors, it seemed inescapable that all HIV-infected individuals would eventually succumb to the infection. Improvement in the diagnosis and treatment of HIV-related conditions throughout the 1980s, and particularly the introduction of prophylaxis for PCP in the late 1980s and early 1990s, lengthened the average length of life after an AIDS diagnosis from 24 months to greater than 36 months. AZT and a variety of other nucleosides (DDI, DDC, D4T, 3TC) caused some improvement when used alone or in combinations of two in patients with advanced disease, but there was no significant improvement in survival. The introduction in 1995 of a new class of anti-retrovirals, protease inhibitors, and their use in combination with two nucleosides (commonly referred to as a "cocktail") resulted in marked clinical improvement for many patients with advanced disease (Egger, May et al., 2002; Hammer, Squires, et al., 1997). Patients and clinicians alike were euphoric, and there was an upsurge in optimism that a cure would quickly be achieved.

Those hopes were not fully realized. While HAART did suppress viral replication and allow the immune system to heal, it soon became clear that there were significant obstacles to its use (Autran, Carcelaint, et al., 1998). Some patients could not tolerate the immediate side-effects that accompany these powerful drug combinations and had to stop them. Many, if not most patients, had difficulty in adhering to the complex dosing regimens that early HAART therapy required, and it soon became clear that drug resistance and clinical deterioration could rapidly ensue if adherence was not optimal. Patients who had been on mono or dual therapy with the earlier nucleosides were more likely to develop resist-ant virus and had to anxiously wait for newer drugs with different resist-ance profiles to be developed and approved. But those who were able to take these medications effectively could look forward to several, if not many years of relative good health (Chun, Fauci, 1999; Chun, Davey, et al., 2000).

It soon became clear that effective treatment would not result in a cure. Clinical researchers enrolled patients with early HIV infection into trials in which they were immediately placed on HAART. Using a poly-merase chain reaction (PCR) assay, researchers verified that the amount of virus (viral load) in these subjects was reduced below the level of detection of the assay. Even after 24–36 months of uninterrupted viral suppression, patients experienced a rapid increase in their viral load when HAART was stopped. HIV remained protected from antiretrovi-rals in a number of "sanctuary" sites. Mathematical modeling suggests that it would take more than 60 years of uninterrupted treatment with the current generation of antiretrovirals to eradicate these sanctuaries, if it is possible at all (Chun, Fauci, 1999).

The treatment of HIV-positive patients increasingly resembles the management of other complex chronic illnesses requiring polyphar-macy and frequent clinical follow-up. Individuals with risk factors for HIV infection are encouraged to have HIV testing as part of routine care, the goal being to identify infection before significant damage is done to the immune system. Initial assessment includes staging the infection through a combination of CD4 testing, medical history and physical examination. Viral load levels offers additional information, with higher viral loads suggesting a more rapid progression of illness; it is now rec-ommended that viral resistance testing also be included as part of the initial evaluation because of the growing frequency with which new patients are found to have been infected with virus resistant to one or more of the antiretrovirals (Hammer 2002).

The baseline evaluation allows for clinical decisions regarding the need for prophylaxis and antiretroviral therapy. It also affords the opportunity to initiate patient education about HIV and to begin the process of discussing treatment readiness and adherence support. A complete sexual and substance abuse risk history should be part of the baseline assessment and become the basis for discussions with the patient about his or her role in preventing transmission of the virus to sexual and needle-sharing partners. For all patients, but for women of childbearing age in particular, there is a need to discuss the complex issue of family planning.

When to initiate antiretroviral therapy is not easily decided. Guidelines developed by the U.S. Department of Health and Human Services and by the U.S. chapter of the International AIDS Society are regularly revised as the understanding of HIV pathogenesis and the complexity of treatment deepen. In the early HAART era, the expert consensus was to "hit early, hit hard". In practice, this meant that treatment was recommended for essentially all patients with CD4 cell counts under 500 in the hopes that the immune system would be protected from permanent damage and that mutations leading to drug resistance would be avoided. This approach to treatment initiation was brought into question by a combination of factors that included: 1) many patients (see above) had difficulty with adherence and this led to viral resistance, 2) as data on long-term use of HAART accumulated, it appeared that initiation of therapy above a CD4 cell count of 350 rarely resulted in improved clinical outcomes, and 3) moderate to severe metabolic complications frequently accompany long-term therapy. More recent versions of these guidelines now strongly urge treatment of symptomatic patients and of those asymptomatic patients with CD4 counts under 200; it is suggested that practitioners begin discussion of starting HAART with asymptomatic patients with CD4 counts between 350 and 200 (DHHS, 2003). HAART is additionally recommended for HIV+ pregnant women and for those patients seen shortly after primary infection.

Treatment guidelines are helpful, but the decision to initiate HAART requires a dialogue between the practitioner and the patient. The subject of that discussion is the patient's readiness for treatment. Certainly, the patient's willingness to start treatment is crucial, and that willingness must be based on a good understanding of the risks, benefits and rigors of HAART as explained by healthcare personnel. In addition, the practitioner must assess if the patient's expressed willingness has been reflected in the patient's behavior . . . keeping appointments, getting recommended laboratory tests, adhering to prophylactic medications.

Problems in these areas indicate a likelihood of difficulty adhering to HAART and should be directly and respectfully addressed by the practitioner. Adherence to therapy is the most powerful determinant of successful treatment (Stone, 2001).

The overarching goal of therapy is to maintain or return the patient to a state of clinical wellness, prevent opportunistic infections, improve immune function and prevent the emergence of viral resistance for as long as possible. To accomplish this goal, viral load should be lowered below the limit of detection of the ultrasensitive viral load assays currently available. This is frequently achievable with initial and even second regimens, but is less frequently achieved with so-called "salvage" regimens used when treating multiple drug resistant virus. Drug resistance can now be ascertained by commercially available genotypic or phenotypic assays.

Therapeutic options have increased dramatically since the introduction of HAART. Early HAART therapy combined nucleoside reverse transcriptase inhibitors (NRTIs) and protease inhibitors (PIs). The number of drugs in each of these two classes is now much greater and there are new classes of drugs, including powerful non-nucleoside reverse transcriptase inhibitors (NNRTIs), a nucleotide RTI and a new class of fusion inhibitors. Unfortunately, cross-resistance within classes limits the number of effective combinations, and active research continues into the development of new classes of antiretrovirals and to new drugs within existent classes that are effective against resistant virus.

Effective suppression of viral replication is usually accompanied by restoration of significant parts of the immune system and is reflected in a rise of the CD4 count. Clinically, patients whose CD4 counts rise above 200 for three months or more regain the capacity to fight many of the opportunistic infections associated with AIDS, and prophylaxis against common OIs, such as PCP, toxoplasmosis and Mycobacterium avium intracellulare can be stopped (Kirk, Reiss, et al., 2002; El Sadr, Burman, 2000). The use of HAART in combination with other indicated treatment has been demonstrated to improve the prognosis of other HIV-associated conditions, including cervical neoplasia, tuberculosis, Kaposi's sarcoma, CMV retinitis, HIV-associated dementia and primary brain lymphoma (USPHS, 2001).

Epidemiologically, there has been a dramatic reduction in both morbidity and mortality associated with HIV infection, although these improvements were most marked in the first few years after the introduction of HAART and have now plateaued (CDC, 2002). For the cohort of ARV-naïve patients started on HAART since 1996, it is not yet possible to calculate the average lifespan after an AIDS diagnosis because of the relatively small proportion of deaths as of the time of the writing of this chapter in mid-2003.

The improved treatment of HIV and its associated conditions has allowed other underlying medical conditions to emerge as leading causes of death among people living with AIDS. Hepatitis C, for example, is almost universal among those patients with a history of injection drug use and not uncommon among others with a history of multiple sexual partners. Patients coinfected with hepatitis C and HIV are more likely than those with hepatitis C alone to develop end-stage liver disease, and they do so at a more rapid rate. Once cirrhosis is established, treatment with HAART cannot reverse the scarring that has already occurred, and it is unclear if patients with low CD4 counts will respond to current therapy for hepatitis C (Sulkowski, Thomas, 2003). Further complicating the treatment of the two infections is the potential for ARVs to cause inflammation of an already damaged liver. Much more clinical research remains to be done.

Metabolic complications of HAART have become a cause of morbidity, and perhaps mortality, among patients on long-term therapy. Fat redistribution (lipodystrophy) had been noted occasionally in the pre-HAART era, but the widespread use of PI-based regimens after 1996 focused attention on what was commonly called "protease paunch" . . . truncal obesity accompanied by loss of fat from the extremities, face and buttocks. In women, significant enlargement of the breasts was often noted, and in both men and women, deposition of fat at the base of the neck (buffalo hump) was sometimes seen. Considerable and occasionally heated debate then ensued about the frequency and cause of this fat redistribution with a particular focus on whether lipodystrophy resulted from a specific drug class (e.g., protease inhibitors) or perhaps from the effective suppression of HIV itself (Martinez, Mocroft, et al., 2001; Max, Sherer, 2000).

There have been few definitive answers to questions concerning the metabolic consequences of HAART. It is now known that NRTIs cause mitochondrial dysfunction that underlies the observed problems with peripheral neuropathy, liver disease and pancreatitis in some patients; mild, and occasionally fatal lactic acidosis is now recognized as a complication of nucleosides, with some drugs more likely to cause problems than others. Protease inhibitors are associated with glucose intolerance and frank diabetes in some patients, and may result in a significant rise in lipids, including low-density lipoproteins and triglycerides associated with cardiovascular disease (Morris, Benson, et al., 2002).

The polypharmacy required to control HIV not only has its own complications but can also complicate the management of other medical disorders. Considerable attention has been focused on the dangers of drug/drug interactions between various ARVs and a range of medications metabolized by the liver's P450 cytochrome system. Drugs commonly used to treat conditions such as epilepsy, tuberculosis, opiate addiction, a number of psychiatric conditions and hypercholesterolemia have their blood levels raised or lowered by protease inhibitors and non-nucleoside reverse transcriptase inhibitors. Perhaps more important are the pharmacodynamic interactions between ARVs and many other medications; the side-effects caused by ARVs on the liver, pancreas, bone marrow and other organ systems can have an additive or synergistic impact on the effects of other medications on these same organs, resulting in serious or even life-threatening complications. Avoiding such problems requires that each healthcare practitioner caring for a patient with HIV be aware of all medications that the patient is taking and that all practitioners involved communicate with each other when initiating, changing or stopping a drug.

The introduction of HAART dramatically changed the lives of people with advanced HIV and brought a new series of psychosocial issues to the fore. In the pre-HAART era, an AIDS diagnosis frequently dictated a period of progressive poor health that led to loss of job, loss of income, occasionally loss of friends and frequently loss of self-esteem. Social workers spent much of their energy on helping patients secure adequate health and income benefits while working on the depression that accompanied the diagnosis. Since 1996, there have been a series of new psychosocial issues, including decisions about patients returning to work and giving up Medicaid benefits. For patients with a history of substance abuse, a return to health was frequently accompanied by a return to drug use if the substance abuse issues were not adequately addressed. Active drug use can lead to poor adherence to care and treatment, the emergence of resistant virus and clinical deterioration.

Adherence to treatment has emerged as the strongest predictor of clinical outcome for patients on HAART (Stone, 2001). More than one-third of drug-naïve patients fail their regimen within one year of initiation, and inadequate adherence is usually the underlying explanation. While earlier regimens required frequent dosing and numerous pills, most new medications can be taken on a once or twice a day basis and frequently with no dietary conditions. These improvements are important but psychological and social problems underlie the difficulty with adherence that many patients continue to have. These are best addressed directly and on an individual basis, and adherence support is a critical aspect and a profound challenge of AIDS care.

Prolonging the life and improving the health of people with HIV is a wonderful medical achievement, but it has also precipitated a crisis for HIV prevention efforts. While death rates from HIV plummeted after 1996, the number of new infections remained steady at approximately 40,000 per year; the net result is an increasing number of people living with HIV. This increases the pool of people who can potentially transmit HIV to others, and as more patients on HAART develop drug-resistant virus, there is a corresponding increase in the number of primary (new) infections with virus already resistant to one or more antiretrovirals. This is a serious public health threat that has already impacted on the clinical management of HIV. The CDC has responded by refocusing prevention efforts on people who are positive, and clinicians caring for those with HIV are strongly encouraged to engage their patients in discussion about their role in preventing further spread of HIV.

The pace of change of our understanding of HIV and of its clinical management has been impressive. Our capacity to change the human behavior that drives its spread or that which leads to poor adherence is not nearly as impressive. HIV continues to pose profound challenges to both science and society.

PSYCHOLOGICAL AND VOCATIONAL IMPLICATIONS

THE INTRODUCTION OF HAART dramatically changed the lives of people with advanced HIV and brought a new series of psychosocial issues to the fore. In the pre-HAART era, an AIDS diagnosis frequently dictated a period of progressive poor health that led to loss of job, loss of income, occasionally loss of friends, and frequently loss of self-esteem. Social workers spent much of their energy on helping patients secure adequate healthcare and income benefits while working on the depression that accompanied the diagnosis. Since 1996, there have been a series of new psychosocial issues, including decisions about patients returning to work and giving up Medicaid benefits. For patients with a history of substance abuse, a return to health was frequently accompanied by a return to drug use if the substance abuse issues were not adequately addressed. Active drug use can lead to poor adherence to care and treatment, the emergence of resistant virus, and clinical deterioration.

Adherence to treatment has emerged as the strongest predictor of clinical outcome for patients on HAART. More than one third of drug-naïve patients fail their regimen within 1 year of initiation, and inadequate adherence is usually the underlying explanation. While earlier regimens required frequent dosing and numerous pills, most new medications can be taken on a once or twice a day basis and frequently with no dietary conditions. These improvements are important but psychological and social problems underlie the difficulty with adherence that many patients continue to have. These are best addressed directly and on an individual basis, and adherence support is a critical aspect and a profound challenge of AIDS care.

Prolonging the life and improving the health of people with HIV is a wonderful medical achievement, but it has also precipitated a crisis for HIV prevention efforts. Although death rates from HIV plummeted after 1996, the number of new infections remained steady at approximately 40,000 per year; the net result is an increasing number of people living with HIV. This increases the pool of people who can potentially transmit HIV to others, especially when people living with HIV are feeling better and have a renewed interest in relationships and sexual activity. And although findings are mixed, some evidence indicates that increased optimism associated with treatment advances are leading to increases in transmission risk behaviors among some groups (Dilley, Woods, & McFarland, 1997; Kalichman, Nachimson, Cherry, & Williams, 1998; Kelly, Hoffman, Rompa, & Gray, 1998; Ostrow et al., 2002; Remien, Wagner, Carballo-Dieguez, & Dolezal, 1998). Further, as more patients on HAART develop drug-resistant virus, there is a corresponding increase in the number of primary (new) infections with virus already resistant to one or more antiretrovirals. This is a serious public health threat that has already impacted on the clinical management of HIV. The CDC has responded by refocusing prevention efforts on people who are positive, and clinicians caring for those with HIV are strongly encouraged to engage their patients in discussion about their role in preventing further spread of HIV.

The pace of change of our understanding of HIV and of its clinical management has been impressive. Our capacity to change the human behavior that drives its spread or that which leads to poor adherence is not nearly as impressive. HIV continues to pose profound challenges to both science and society.

It has become increasingly clear that psychologists and other mental health workers can and do play a primary role in the overall management and care of HIV-infected people and people living with AIDS. Both research and clinical experience show us that adverse social and psychological consequences are associated with various stages of the HIV illness spectrum. Notable time points that often require mental health intervention include initial knowledge of one's antibody status, onset of physical symptoms, receiving an AIDS-defining diagnosis, and entering the terminal phase of the illness. Significant psychological reactions can occur during any and all of these phases of HIV illness. Such reactions include psychological distress, typically depression, despair, hopelessness, anxiety, and panic reactions, and psychiatric disorders, usually depressive, anxiety, or adjustment disorders. Vegetative symptoms often include sleep and appetite disturbances, headaches, and fatigue. It is important to note that the stigma associated with this disease is an additional psychological burden to those infected and affected by HIV. Some studies have indicated significantly higher rates of suicide and suicidal ideation (e.g., Marzuk et al., 1988).

Conversely, some studies have shown that there can be remarkable psychological resilience in HIV-infected persons in both asymptomatic (Williams, Rabkin, Remien, Gorman, & Ehrhardt, 1991) and symptomatic stages. Research has consistently shown there to be an association between lower psychological distress and good social supports, active coping strategies, and an optimistic attitude in people living with chronic and life-threatening illnesses (Namir, Wolcott, Fawzy, & Alumbaugh, 1987). The goals of psychological intervention include addressing these factors, namely, reducing isolation, facilitating good social supports, teaching and enhancing positive coping strategies, and helping to maintain hope (Chesney, Folkman, & Chambers, 1996). A psychological study of long-term survivors with AIDS found low rates of clinical depression and a positive quality of life, even in the context of profound illness (Remien, Rabkin, Katoff, & Williams, 1992). Participants in this study were all connected to a community-based service organization, and a majority of them had received individual psychotherapy since their AIDS diagnosis. Additionally, they were active in the medical management of their disease and worked hard to obtain what they felt was optimal medical care. As new treatment options are made available it becomes increasingly complicated for patients to make treatment decisions regarding when to initiate and/or change medication regimens and which combination therapies to use. It is equally as challenging to initiate and maintain strict adherence to complicated dosing schedules. The counselor can play a role in facilitating optimal medical management of this disease and assisting in overcoming barriers to adherence.

Because persons with HIV infection and AIDS may experience a range of mental health needs, it is important that a range of mental health services be available to them (Remien & Rabkin, 2002). These include the following:

1. *Crisis intervention.* Interventions should be designed to enhance adaptive and integrative functioning through past and newly acquired coping skills. Whenever possible, having crisis services available in medical or community settings can provide early intervention and possibly prevent further crisis.
2. *Individual therapy.* A wide range of individual therapies can be helpful for the person with HIV infection and AIDS, including supportive, cognitive-behavioral, and insight-oriented approaches. It is important to address the patient's ability to manage distress and crises, deal with the ramifications of perceived loss, recognize and resolve grief, enhance support systems, maintain hopefulness, and maximize decision-making skills.
3. *Family interventions.* The overall goals of family intervention include

enhancing the family members' ability to support each other, to focus on the immediate crisis and environmental situation, to facilitate the grieving process, and to encourage the use of community social supports and resources. Case management, couples counseling, family therapy, home visits, and multiple family group interventions can be used to address these goals.

4. *Support groups.* Support groups can be extremely useful for people coping with HIV infection and AIDS because they allow for the enhancement of social support. A range of modalities may be useful, including cognitive-behavioral groups, therapy groups, and self-help groups. Both short-term and long-term closed groups can provide predictable consistency and ongoing social support. Drop-in groups can be especially useful for persons requiring immediate support.

5. *Substance abuse treatment.* Treatment of substance use problems associated with HIV infection is important for several reasons, including the prevention of further HIV transmission, health concerns for the infected individual, and the effect of psychoactive substance use on decision-making capability. Relapse in substance use is common following significant stressors such as knowledge of a seropositive antibody status, the onset of medical symptoms, or receiving an AIDS-defining diagnosis.

There are also prevention issues that the counselor can address with HIV-infected persons. Once an individual knows the test result to be positive, he or she shoulders a significant responsibility for preventing further transmission. As many years of intervention research have shown, the initiation and, more importantly, the maintenance of safer sexual practices is not easily accomplished, even for the most committed. HIV-infected individuals also need psychological counseling to facilitate frank discussions of sex behavior and honest disclosure to sex partners. Some studies show that individuals who changed their sexual behavior to lessen the risk of transmission were more distressed than those who maintained high-risk behaviors. To forestall recidivism, the psychological cost of changing sexual behavior needs to be acknowledged, and mental health supportive services should be made available to assist those individuals in making and maintaining behavior changes.

It is important for mental health workers to educate themselves about all aspects of HIV illness, including medical aspects and treatment strategies, which continue to evolve over time. It is also essential that counselors be familiar with information, medical, social, and legal resources available in the community to which they can refer patients and their significant others.

REFERENCES

Autran, B., Carcelaint, G., Li, T. S., Gorochov, G., Blanc, C., et al. (1998). Restoration of the immune system with antiretroviral therapy. *Immunology Letters, 66*, 207–211.

CDC National Center for HIV, STD and TB Prevention, Divisions of HIV/AIDS Prevention. (2002). HIV/AIDS Surveillance Report 2002. Retrieved from http://www.cdc.gov/hiv/stats/hasrlink.htm.

Centers for Disease Control. (1981). Pneumosystis pneumonia—Los Angeles. Morbidity and Mortality Weekly Report, 30(21), 1–3.

Centers for Disease Control. (1993). From the Centers for Disease Control and Prevention. 1993 revised classification system for HIV infection and expanded AIDS surveillance case definition for adolescents and adults. Journal of the American Medical Association, 269, 129–730.

Centers for Disease Control. (1997). Update: Trends in AIDS incidence, deaths, and prevalence—United States, 1996. Morbidity and Mortality Weekly Report, 46(8), 165–173.

Centers for Disease Control. (2004). Estimated numbers of persons living with HIV/AIDS by year and selected characteristics. Retrieved from http://www.cdc.gov/hiv/stats

Chesney, M., Folkman, S., & Chambers, D. (1996). Coping effectiveness training for men living with HIV: Preliminary findings. International Journal of STD & AIDS, 7(2), 75–82.

Chun T. W., Davey, R. T. Jr, Ostrowski, M., Shawn Justement, J, Engel, D., et al. (2000). Relationship between pre-existing viral reservoirs and the re-emergence of plasma viremia after discontinuation of highly active anti-retroviral therapy. *Nature Medicine,* 6(7):757–761.

Chun, T. W., & Fauci, A. S. (1999, September 28). Latent reservoirs of HIV: obstacles to the eradication of the virus. *Proceedings of the National Academy of Sciences of the United States of America, 96*(20), 10958–10961.

Department of Health and Human Services (DHHS). Panel on Clinical Practices for Treatment of HIV Infection convened by the Department of Health and Human Services (DHHS). (2003, November 10). *Guidelines for the use of antiretroviral agents in HIV-1-infected adults and adolescents*. Retrieved from http://aidsinfo.nih.gov/guidelines/adult/AA_111003.pdf.

Dilley, J. W., Woods, W. J., & McFarland, W. (1997). Are advances in treatment changing views about high-risk sex? New England Journal of Medicine, 337, 501–502.

Egger, M., May, M., Chene, G., Phillips, A., Ledergerber B., et al. (2002). Prognosis of HIV-1-infected patients starting highly active antiretroviral therapy: a collaborative analysis of prospective studies. *The Lancet, 360,* 119–129.

El Sadr, W. M., Burman, W.J., Grant, L. B., Matts, P., Hafner, R., et al. for the Terry Beirn Community Programs for Clinical Research on AIDS. (2000). Discontinuation of Mycobacterium avium complex disease in HIV-infected patients who have a response to antiretroviral therapy. *New England Journal of Medicine, 342,*1085–1192.

Hammer, S. M. (2002). HIV Drug Resistance: Implications for Management. *Topics in HIV Medicine, 10*(5),10–15.

Hammer, S. M., Squires, K. E., Hughes, M. D., Grimers, J. M., Demeter, L. M., et al. for the AIDS Clinical Trials Groups 320 Study Team. (1997). A controlled trial of two nucleoside analogues plus indinavir in persons with human immunodeficiency virus infection and CD4 cell counts of 200 per cubic millimeter or less. *New England Journal of Medicine, 337*(11), 725–733.

Ho, D. D. (1996, May 24). Viral counts count in HIV infection. Science, 272, 1124–1125.

Kalichman, S. C., Nachimson, D., Cherry, C., & Williams, E. (1998). AIDS treatment advances and behavioral prevention setbacks: Preliminary assessment of reduced perceived threat of HIV/AIDS. Health Psychology, 17, 546–550.

Kaslow, R. A., & Francis, D. P. (1989). The epidemiology of AIDS. New York: Oxford University Press.

Kelly, J. A., Hoffman, R. G., Rompa, D., & Gray, M. (1998). Protease inhibitor combination therapies and perceptions of gay men regarding AIDS severity and the need to maintain safer sex. AIDS, 12, 91–95.

Kirk O, Reiss P, Uberti-Foppa, C, Bickel, M., Gerstoft, J., et al. (2002). Safe interruption of maintenance therapy against previous infection with four common HIV-associated opportunistic pathogens during potent antiviral therapy. *Annals of Internal Medicine, 137,* 239–250.

Koenig, S., & Fauci, A. (1988). AIDS: Immunopathogenesis and immune response to the human immune-deficiency virus. In V. DeVita, S. Hellman, & S. Rosenberg (Eds.), AIDS etiology, diagnosis, treatment and prevention. Philadelphia: J. B. Lippincott.

Martinez, E., Mocroft, A., Garcia-Viejo, M. A., Perez-Cuevas, J. B., Blanco, J. L., et al. (2001). Risk of lipodystrophy in HIV-1-infected patients treated with protease inhibitors: A prospective cohort study. *Lancet, 357,* 592–598.

Marzuk, P., Tierney, H., Tardiff, K., Gross, E., Morgan, E., Hsu, M., et al. (1988). Increased risk of suicide in persons with AIDS. Journal of the American Medical Association, 259, 1333–1337.

Max, B., & Sherer, R. (2000). Management of adverse effects of antiretroviral therapy and medication adherence. *Clinical Infectious Diseases, 30*(Suppl 2):S96-S116.

McArthur, J. C., Cohen, B. A., Selnes, O. A., Kumer, A. J., Cooper, K., McArthur, J. H., et al. (1989). Low prevalence of neurological and neuropsychological abnormalities in otherwise healthy HIV-I-infected individuals: Results from the multicenter AIDS cohort study. Annals of Neurology, 26, 601–611.

Morris, S., Benson, C. A., Carr, A., Currier, J.S., Dubé, M. P., et al. (2002). Management of metabolic complications associated with antiretroviral therapy for HIV-1 infection: Recommendations of an International AIDS

Society-USA panel. *Journal of Acquired Immune Deficiency Syndromes, 31,* 257–275.

Namir, S., Wolcott, D. L., Fawzy, F., & Alumbaugh, M. (1987). Coping with AIDS: Psychological and health implications. Journal of Applied Social Psychology, 17, 309–328.

Ostrow, D. E., Fox, K. J., Chimel, J. S., Silvestre, A., Visscher, B. R., Vanable, P. A., et al. (2002). Attitudes towards highly active antiretroviral therapy are associated with sexual risk taking among HIV-infected and uninfected homosexual men. AIDS, 16, 775–780.

Remien, R. H., & Rabkin, J. G. (2002), Managing chronic disease: Individual counseling with medically ill patients. In M.A. Chesney & M. Antoni (Eds.), Health psychology innovations: New target populations for prevention and care. Health Psychology Book Series, American Psychological Association, 117–139.

Remien, R. H., Rabkin, J. G., Katoff, L., & Williams, J. B. W. (1992). Coping strategies and health beliefs of AIDS longterm survivors. Psychology and Health: An International Journal, 6, 335–345.

Remien, R. H., Wagner, G., Carballo-Dieguez, A., & Dolezal, C. (1998). Who may be engaging in high-risk sex due to medical treatment advances? AIDS, 12, 1560–1561.

Shaw, G. M., Wong-Staal, F., & Gallo, R. C. (1988). Etiology of AIDS: Virology, molecular biology, and evolution of human immune-deficiency viruses. In V. DeVita, S. Hellman, & S. Rosenberg (Eds.), AIDS etiology, diagnosis, treatment and prevention. Philadelphia: J. B. Lippincott.

Siegal, F. P. (1987). The immune deficiency in AIDS. In G. Wormser, R. Stahl, & E. Bottone (Eds.), AIDS and other manifestations of HIV infection. Park Ridge, NJ: Noyes Publications.

Stone, V. E. (2001). Strategies for optimizing adherence to highly active anti-retroviral therapy: Lessons from research and clinical practice. *Clinical Infectious Diseases, 33,* 865–872.

Sulkowski, M. S., & Thomas, D. L. (2003). Hepatitis C in the HIV-Infected Person. *Annals of Internal Medicine, 138,* 197–207.

U.S. Public Health Service (USPHS) and Infectious Diseases Society of America (IDSA). USPHS/IDSA Prevention of Opportunistic Infections Working Group. (2001). 2001 USPHS/IDSA guidelines for the prevention of opportunistic infections in persons infected with Human Immunodeficiency Virus. Retrieved from http://aidsinfo.nih.gov/guidelines/op_infections/OI_112801.pdf.

Williams, I. B. W., Rabkin, J. G., Remien, R. H., Gorman, I. M., & Ehrhardt, A. A. (1991). Multidisciplinary baseline assessment of homosexual men with and without human immune-deficiency virus infection. Archives of General Psychiatry, 48, 124–130.

World Health Organization. (2004). Global summary of the HIV/AIDS epidemic

December 2003. Retrieved from http://www.unaids.org/wad/2003/
Epiupdate2003_en/Epi03_02_en.htm

Yarchoan, R., & Pluda, J. M. (1988). Clinical aspects of infection with AIDS retro-
virus: Acute HIV infection, persistent generalized lymphadenopathy, and
AIDS-related complex. In V. DeVita, S. Hellman, & S. Rosenberg (Eds.),
AIDS etiology, diagnosis, treatment and prevention. Philadelphia: J. B.
Lippincott.

4

Alzheimer's Disease

BARRY REISBERG, MD, ALI JAVED, MD, SUNNIE
KENOWSKY, DVM, AND STEFANIE R. AUER, PHD

EVIDENCE SUGGESTS THAT approximately 10% to 15% of
community-residing elderly persons in the United States may be
afflicted with Alzheimer's disease (AD) or closely related dementing illnesses of late life (Evans et al., 1989; Katzman, 1986). Consequently,
it is estimated that in the United States more than 4 million persons
may have AD (Herbert et al., 2003; Small et al., 1997). AD is the fourth
leading cause of death in the elderly, after heart disease, cancer, and
stroke, and is the single major cause of institutionalization of aged people in the United States and in many other industrialized nations in the
world. Studies have indicated that a large majority of the more than 1.5
million residents in nursing homes in the United States manifest a
dementia syndrome generally associated with AD (Chandler & Chandler,
1988; Rovner, Kafonek, Filipp, Lucas, & Folstein, 1986). The dimensions
of the institutional burden associated with AD are even more striking
when it is noted that well under 1 million persons are in U.S. hospitals
at any particular time.

The course of AD has been described in increasing detail over the
past several years. The cognitive, functional, and behavioral concomitants at each stage of the illness can presently be described in detail. The
clinically observable symptomatology of AD dramatically changes in
form from the earliest manifest deficits to the most severe stage; therefore, recognition and differentiation of the stages of this illness is imper-

ative for proper diagnosis, prognosis, management, and treatment. Progressive cognitive changes that occur are manifest in concentration, recent memory, past memory, orientation, functioning and self-care, language, praxis ability, and calculation, among other areas (Reisberg, London, et al., 1983; Reisberg, Schneck, Ferris, Schwartz, & de Leon, 1983). Characteristic behavioral symptoms are also a frequent component of AD (Kumar, Koss, Metzler, Moore, & Friedland, 1988; Reisberg, Franssen, Sclan, Kluger, & Ferris, 1989; Rubin, Morris, Storandt, & Berg, 1987). These behavioral symptoms peak in occurrence at various points in the course of AD and subsequently recede in magnitude and frequency with the progression of the disease. A comprehensive view of the nature and progression of these cognitive, functional, and behavioral changes is critical for the optimization of residual capacity and the identification and management of excess disability in these patients.

An outline of global cognitive, functional, and behavioral changes in normal aging and progressive AD is provided in the Global Deterioration Scale (Reisberg, Ferris, de Leon, & Crook, 1982), outlined in Table 4.1 and described in greater detail in the text that follows.

GLOBAL DESCRIPTION OF NORMAL BRAIN AGING AND AD

SEVEN MAJOR, CLINICALLY distinguishable, global stages from normality to most severe AD have been described (Reisberg et al., 1982). These stages and their implications are as follows:

Stage 1: No cognitive decline. Diagnosis: Normal. No objective or subjective evidence of cognitive decrement is seen. A significant proportion, although possibly only a minority, of elderly persons fall within this category (Lane & Snowdon, 1989; Lowenthal et al., 1967; Reinikainen et al., 1990; Sluss, Rabins, & Gruenberg, 1980). The prognosis is excellent for continued adequate cognitive functioning (Geerlings, Jonker, Bouter, Ader, & Schmand, 1999; Kluger, Ferris, Golomb, Mittelman, & Reisberg, 1999).

Stage 2: Subjective cognitive decline only. Diagnosis: Age-associated memory impairment. Many persons over age 65 have subjective complaints of cognitive decrement such as a subjective perception of forgetting names of people they know well or of forgetting where they placed particular objects such as keys or jewelry. These subjective complaints may be elicited by comparing the person's perceived abilities with their perceptions of their performance 5 to 10 years previously.

Complaints of cognitive impairment may also occur with other, much more serious conditions common in the elderly, notably dementia and depression. Persons with the comparatively benign complaints

TABLE 4.1 Global Deterioration Scale (GDS) for Age-Associated Cognitive Decline and Alzheimer's Disease

GDS stage	Clinical Characteristics	Diagnosis
1	No subjective complaints of memory deficit. No memory deficit evident on clinical interview.	Normal
2	Subjective complaints of memory deficit, most frequently in following areas: (a) forgetting where one has placed familiar objects. (b) forgetting names one formerly knew well. No objective evidence of memory deficit on clinical interview. No objective deficit in employment or social situations. Appropriate concern with respect to symptomatology.	Age-associated memory impairment
3	Earliest subtle deficits. Manifestations in more than one of the following areas: (a) patient may have gotten lost when traveling to an unfamiliar location. (b) co-workers become aware of patient's relatively poor performance. (c) word- and/or name-finding deficit becomes evident to intimates. (d) patient may read a passage or book and retain relatively little material. (e) patient may demonstrate decreased facility remembering names upon introduction to new people. (f) Patient may have lost or misplaced an object of value. (g) concentration deficit may be evident on clinical testing. Objective evidence of memory deficit obtained only with an intensive interview. Decreased performance in demanding employment and social settings. Denial begins to become manifest in patient. Mild to moderate anxiety frequently accompanies symptoms.	Mild cognitive impairment

(Continued)

TABLE 4.1 Global Deterioration Scale *(Continued)*

GDS stage	Clinical Characteristics	Diagnosis
4	Clear-cut deficit on careful clinical interview. Deficit manifest in following areas: (a) decreased knowledge of current and recent events. (b) may exhibit some deficit in memory of one's personal history. (c) concentration deficit elicited on serial subtractions. (d) decreased ability to travel, handle finances, etc. Frequently no deficit in following areas: (a) orientation to time and place. (b) recognition of familiar persons and faces. (c) ability to travel to familiar locations. Inability to perform complex tasks. Denial is dominant defense mechanism. Flattening of affect and withdrawal from challenging situations occur.	Mild Alzheimer's disease
5	Patient can no longer survive without some assistance. Patient is unable during interview to recall a major relevant aspect of their current life, e.g.: (a) their address or telephone number of many years. (b) the names of close members of their family (such as grandchildren). (c) the name of the high school or college from which they graduated. Frequently some disorientation to time (date, day of the week, season, etc.) or to place. An educated person may have difficulty counting back from 40 by 4s or from 20 by 2s. Persons at this stage retain knowledge of many major facts regarding themselves and others. They invariably know their own names and generally know their spouse's and children's names. They require no assistance with toileting or eating, but may have difficulty choosing the proper clothing to wear.	Moderate Alzheimer's disease

(Continued)

TABLE 4.1   Global Deterioration Scale *(Continued)*

GDS stage	Clinical Characteristics	Diagnosis
6	May occasionally forget the name of the spouse upon whom they are entirely dependent for survival. Will be largely unaware of all recent events and experiences in their lives. Retain some knowledge of their surroundings; the year, the season, etc. May have difficulty counting by 1s from 10, both backward and sometimes forward. Will require some assistance with activities of daily living. (a) may become incontinent. (b) will require travel assistance but occasionally will be able to travel to familiar locations. Diurnal rhythm frequently disturbed. Almost always recall their own name. Frequently continue to be able to distinguish familiar from unfamiliar persons in their environment. Personality and emotional changes occur. These are quite variable and include: (a) delusional behavior, e.g., patients may accuse their spouse of being an imposter; may talk to imaginary figures in the environment, or to their own reflection in the mirror. (b) obsessive symptoms, e.g., person may continually repeat simple cleaning activities. (c) anxiety symptoms, agitation, and even previously non-existent violent behavior may occur. (d) cognitive abulia, e.g., loss of willpower because an individual cannot carry a thought long enough to determine a purposeful course of action.	Moderately severe Alzheimer's disease

(Continued)

TABLE 4.1 Global Deterioration Scale *(Continued)*

GDS stage	Clinical Characteristics	Diagnosis
7	All verbal abilities are lost over the course of this stage. Early in this stage words and phrases are spoken but speech is very circumscribed Later there is no speech at all—only babbling. Incontinent of urine; requires assistance toileting and feeding. Basic psychomotor skills (e.g. ability to walk) are lost with the progression of this stage. The brain appears to no longer be able to tell the body what to do. Generalized and cortical neurologic signs and symptoms are frequently present.	Severe Alzheimer's disease

associated with this stage can usually recall the names of two or more primary school teachers, classmates, or friends and are oriented to the time of day, date, day of week, month, season, and year (although, of course, occasional minor errors may occur). They also display normal recall when queried about recent events and normal concentration and calculation abilities, for example when asked to perform serial subtractions of sevens from one hundred. The terminology "age-associated memory impairment" has been suggested for this condition (Crook et al., 1986; Reisberg, Ferris, Franssen, Kluger, & Borenstein, 1986). The American Psychiatric Association's *Diagnostic and Statistical Manual of Mental Disorders, 4th edition*, refers to this condition under the more inclusive category of "age-related cognitive decline" (American Psychiatric Association, 1994). Clinical interview reveals no objective evidence of memory deficit, and there are no deficits in employment or social situations.

Current data from prospective longitudinal study indicates that these subjective impairments are in most cases a harbinger of subsequently manifest cognitive impairments after an average of about 7.5 years (Reisberg et al., 2004). Therefore the total duration of this stage has been estimated to be an average of about 15 years prior to the onset of more overtly manifest impairments such as those associated with mild cognitive impairment (Reisberg, 1986; Reisberg, Ferris, Oo, & Franssen, 2003). Although medications and nostrums are frequently taken for these perceived deficits, largely in order to prevent further decline, there is no convincing evidence of their efficacy in treating the symptoms of this stage at the present time.

Stage 3: *Mild cognitive decline. Diagnosis: Mild cognitive impairment (MCI).* Subtle evidence of objective decrement in complex occupational or social tasks may become evident in various ways. For example, the person may become confused or hopelessly lost when traveling to an unfamiliar location; relatively poorer performance may be noted by co-workers in a demanding occupation; persons may display overt word- and name-finding deficits; concentration deficits may be evident to family members and upon clinical testing; relatively little material may be retained after reading a passage from a book or newspaper; and/or an overt tendency to forget what has just been said and to repeat oneself may be manifest. A teacher who had routinely recalled the names of all of the students in his class by the end of a semester now may have difficulty recalling the names of any students. This same teacher may, for the first time, begin to miss important appointments. Similarly, a professional who had previously completed hundreds, perhaps thousands, of reports in the course of her lifetime now, for the first time, may be unable to accurately complete a single report. The person may lose or misplace objects of value. Mild to moderate anxiety is frequently observed and is an appropriate reaction to the awareness of impairment.

The prognosis associated with these subtle but objectively identifiable symptoms varies. In some cases, these symptoms are the result of brain insults, such as small strokes, which may not be evident from the clinical history, neurological examination, or neuroimaging findings. In other cases, symptoms are due to subtle and perhaps not clearly identifiable psychiatric, medical, and neurological disorders of diverse etiology. These symptoms are benign in many of the subjects who report them. However, in most cases where other conditions have been ruled out in terms of etiology, these symptoms do represent the earliest symptoms of subsequently manifest AD. The mean true duration of this stage has been estimated to be approximately 7 years. However, subjects commonly present with these MCI symptoms well into this stage and mild AD frequently becomes manifest after a much briefer temporal interval (Bowen et al., 1997; Daly et al., 2000; Devanand, Folz, Gorlyn, Moesller, & Stern, 1997; Flicker, Ferris, & Reisberg, 1991; Kluger et al., 1999; Morris et al., 2001; Petersen et al., 1999; Tierney et al., 1996). Presently, no pharmacologic agents have demonstrated convincing efficacy in preventing further decline or in treating cognitive impairments in MCI.

Stage 4: *Moderate cognitive decline. Diagnosis: Mild AD.* Clinical interview reveals clearly manifest deficits in various areas, such as concentration, recent and past memory, orientation, calculation, and functional capacity. Concentration deficit may be of sufficient magnitude that patients may have difficulty subtracting serial 4s from 40. Recent memory may be affected to the degree that some major events of the previous week are not recalled, and there may be superficial or scanty knowledge of current events and activities. Detailed questioning may reveal that the spouse's knowledge of the patient's past is superior to the patient's own recall of his or her personal history, and the patient may confuse the chronology of past life events. The patient may mistake the date by 10 days or more but generally knows the year and the season. The patient may manifest decreased ability to handle such routine activities as marketing or managing personal and household finances.

Psychiatric features that may be prominent in this stage include decreased interest in personal and social activities, accompanied by a flattening of affect and emotional withdrawal. These behavioral changes are related to the person's decreased cognitive abilities rather than to depressed mood. However, they are frequently mistaken for depression. True depressive symptoms may also be noted but are generally mild, requiring no specific treatment. In cases where depressive symptoms are of sufficient severity to warrant treatment, a low dose of an antidepressant is frequently effective in reducing affective symptoms. At this stage patients are still capable of independent community survival if assistance is provided with complex but essential activities such as bill paying and managing the patient's bank account. Denial is the dominant defense mechanism protecting the patient from the devastating consequences of awareness of dementing illness.

The diagnosis of probable AD can be arrived at with confidence in this stage. It is possible to follow patients through the course of this stage, whose mean duration has been estimated to be approximately 2 years (Reisberg, 1986; Reisberg, Ferris, Franssen, et al., 1996). The cholinesterase inhibitors (donepazil, galantamine, and rivastigmine) have been approved for treating the symptoms of AD in this stage and appear to slow cognitive decline.

Stage 5: *Moderately severe cognitive decline. Diagnosis: Moderate AD.* Cognitive and functional deficits are of sufficient magnitude that patients can no longer survive without assistance.

Patients at this stage can no longer recall major relevant aspects of their lives. They may not recall the name of the current president, their correct current address or telephone number, or the names of schools they attended. Patients at this stage frequently do not recall the current year and may be unsure of the weather or season. Concentration and calculation deficits are generally of sufficient magnitude as to create difficulty in subtracting serial 4s from 40 and possibly even serial 2s from 20. Patients at this stage retain knowledge of many major facts regarding themselves and others and generally require no assistance with toileting or eating, but they may have difficulty choosing the appropriate clothing to wear for the season or the occasion and may begin to forget to bathe regularly unless reminded.

Psychiatric symptoms in this stage of moderate AD are in many ways similar, although generally more overt, than those noted in mild AD. The patient's denial and flattening of affect tend to be more evident. True depressive symptoms, with mild to moderate mood dysphoria, may occur. Anger and other more overt behavioral symptoms of AD, such as anxieties, paranoia, and sleep disturbances, are frequently evident. Paranoid and delusional ideation peak in occurrence at this stage, with almost 75% of patients exhibiting one or more delusions. Such delusions as people stealing the patient's belongings or money, that one's house is not one's home, or that one's spouse is an impostor, are common. Aggressivity may include verbal outbursts, physical threats and violence, or a general agitation. Depending on the nature and magnitude of the psychiatric symptomatology, treatment with an antidepressant or an antipsychotic medication may be indicated. When the latter is used, the dictum for the treatment of psychosis in the elderly applies: "Start low and go slow."

Patients who are living alone in the community at this stage require at least part-time assistance for continued community survival. When additional community assistance, such as day care or home health aides, is not feasible or available, institutionalization or a more protective environment such as an assisted living facility may be required. Patients who are residing with a spouse frequently resist additional assistance at this stage as an invasion of their home. The duration of this stage is approximately a year and a half (Reisberg, 1986; Reisberg, Ferris, Franssen, et al., 1996). The cholinesterase inhibitor medications have been approved for the treatment of AD symptoms at this stage. Another class of pharmacologic treatment which has recently been shown to be efficacious in slowing the course of AD in this stage is glutamatergic antagonist treatment. Memantine, the first medication in this new class of agents, is believed to reduce the glutamate-induced excitotoxicity caused by presynaptic neuronal injury. Memantine reduces glutamate transmission postsynaptically at the NMDA receptor through its function as an uncompetitive NMDA-receptor antagonist. A pivotal study has indicated that memantine slowed the progression of AD in this stage and the subsequent stage by about 50% in terms of cognitive and functional outcomes (Reisberg, Doody, et al., 2003). A subsequent study has indicated that the effects of memantine remain robust and may even be enhanced when memantine is given in combination with the cholinesterase inhibitor donepezil (Tariot et al., 2004).

Stage 6: Severe cognitive decline. Diagnosis: Moderately severe AD. Cognitive and functional deficits are of sufficient magnitude as to require assistance with basic activities of daily living.

Recent and remote memory are increasingly affected. Patients at this stage frequently have no idea of the date and may occasionally forget the name of the spouse upon whom they are dependent for survival but usually continue to be able to distinguish familiar from unfamiliar persons in their environments. Patients know their own names but frequently do not know their correct address, although they may be able to recall some important aspects of their domicile, such as the street or town. Patients have generally forgotten the schools they attended but recall some aspect of their early lives, such as their birthplace, their former occupation, or one or both of their parents' names. Concentration and calculation deficits are of such magnitude that patients with moderately severe AD frequently have difficulty counting backward from 10 by ones and may even begin to count forward during this task.

Agitation and even violence frequently occur in this stage. Language ability declines progressively so that by the end of this stage speaking is impaired in obvious ways. At this point in the late sixth stage, stuttering and word repetition are common; patients who learned a second language in adulthood sometimes revert to a varying degree to their childhood language; other patients may use neologisms, or nonsense words, interspersed to a varying degree in the course of their speech.

In this stage, emotional and behavioral problems generally become most manifest and disturbing, with 90% of patients exhibiting one or more behavioral symptoms (Reisberg, Franssen, Sclan, et al., 1989). A fear of being left alone or abandoned is frequently exhibited. Agitation, anger, sleep disturbances, physical violence, and negativity are examples of symptoms that commonly require treatment at this point in the illness. Low doses of so-called atypical antipsychotics may be useful for many patients. Side effects can be avoided if the medication is titrated upward with intervals of weeks between dosage adjustments. Present efficacy data on the treatment of these symptoms is most compelling for the atypical antipsychotic risperidone (Brodaty et al., 2003; De Deyn et al., 1999; Katz et al., 1999).

The magnitude of cognitive and functional decline, combined with disturbed behavior and affect, make caregiving especially burdensome to spouses or other family members at this stage. They literally must devote their lives to helping patients who often can no longer even recall their names, much less appreciate in all the ways which may be desired the kindness and care being provided. The caregivers' burden may be alleviated, for example, through regular participation in a dementia caregiver's support group, utilization of day care and respite centers for patients, or utilization of home health aides, either part-time or full-time. Clinical experience suggests that if behavioral disturbances are not successfully managed, they become the primary reason for institutionalization, and successful management of the disturbances can postpone this need. The mean duration of this stage is approximately 2.5 years (Reisberg, 1986; Reisberg, Ferris, Franssen, et al., 1996). Memantine has been approved for treatment of AD in this stage and does appear to be useful in slowing the progression of cognitive and functional decline (Reisberg, Doody, et al., 2003; Tariot et al., 2004; Winblad & Poritis, 1999). Although cholinesterase inhibitors have not been approved for treating symptoms in this stage, there is some evidence for their utility (Feldman et al., 2001).

Stage 7: Very severe cognitive decline. Diagnosis: Severe AD. A succession of functional losses in this stage results in the need for continuous assistance in all aspects of daily living. Verbal abilities are severely limited early in this stage, to approximately a half dozen different intelligible words during the course of an average day, frequently interspersed with unintelligible babbling. Eventually, only a single word remains: commonly "yes," "no," or "OK." Subsequently, the ability to speak even this final single word is largely lost, although the patient may utter seemingly forgotten words and phrases in response to various circumstances for years after meaningful, volitional speech is lost. It is important to recognize that although the patient may no longer be capable of speaking, thinking capacity remains. Test measures originally developed for infants are able to demonstrate continuing thinking capacities of the patient (Auer, Sclan, Yaffee, & Reisberg, 1994). Although agitation can be a problem for some patients at this stage, psychotropic medication can generally be reduced as this stage progresses and it can be ultimately discontinued. Memantine has been approved for treating the symptoms (cognitive and functional) of AD patients in this stage. However, only one published memantine study has included these patients. That study (Winblad & Poritis, 1999) did investigate memantine's efficacy in institutionalized, primarily nursing home residing patients. However, very few of the patients in the Winblad and Poritis study were in this final, severe AD stage. Therefore, there is very little current information regarding the role of memantine, or any other medication, in this final stage of the disease.

Nursing homes or similar care facilities may be better equipped than spouses for the management of patients in this stage. If family members maintain the patient at home, round-the-clock health care assistance may be necessary to manage incontinence and basic activities of daily living such as bathing and feeding. Human contact continues to make a great difference in the quality of life of a patient, whether in the home or in an institution. A loving voice, attention, and touch are important for the patient's emotional and physical well-being. As described subsequently, movement and physical activity are particularly important.

AD patients who survive until some point in the severe stage generally die from pneumonia, traumatic or decubital ulceration, or a less specific failure in the central regulation of vital functions. Although approximately half of all patients who reach this stage are dead within 2 to 3 years, patients may potentially survive for 7 years or longer in this final stage.

FUNCTIONAL CHANGES IN AD

UNDERSTANDING THE PROGRESSION of AD from the standpoint of change and deterioration in functional abilities is of great importance to both clinicians and families. In terms of a primary diagnosis, as well as differential diagnosis, it is useful to determine whether the nature of the dementia is consistent with uncomplicated senile dementia of the Alzheimer type, because dementing processes associated with other causes frequently proceed differently from those of AD. Knowledge of the functional progression of AD can assist in this differential diagnostic process and, additionally, in identifying possible remediable complications of the illness. Furthermore, even the most severe AD patients can be assessed in terms of a functional level when all traditional mental status and psychometric assessment measures produce uniform bottom (zero) scores (Reisberg, Franssen, Bobinski, et al., 1996). Functional assessment is presently capable of producing a detailed, meaningful map of the entire course of AD and, from the standpoint of physical rehabilitation, is extremely important in describing the AD patient's level of incapacity and areas of residual capacity.

Requirements for the management of AD fall into two categories: those relating to the patient and those relating to the primary caregiver. It is essential for the benefit of both that management advice be appropriate to each stage of the illness.

FUNCTIONAL DESCRIPTION OF AD

A PRACTICAL DIAGNOSTIC AND assessment tool, the Functional Assessment Staging of Alzheimer's Disease (FAST) (Reisberg, 1988; Sclan & Reisberg, 1992) permits identification of the stages of characteristic decline in functional activities in AD and their estimated duration (outlined in Table 4.2). Because of their utility, these FAST stages of AD are mandated for usage for certain purposes by the Center for Medicare Services in the U.S., as well as in certain international jurisdictions (Health Care Financing Administration, 1998). These stages of functional deterioration in AD correspond optimally with the Global Deterioration Scale (GDS) stages described above. Table 4.2 indicates the approximate corresponding mean Mini-Mental State Examination

TABLE 4.2 Functional Assessment Stages(FAST) and Time Course of
Functional Loss in Normal Aging and Alzheimer's Disease

Fast stage	Clinical characteristics	Clinical Diagnosis	Estimated duration in AD[a]	Mean MMSE[b]
1	No decrement	Normal adult		29–30
2	Subjective deficit in word finding or recalling location of objects	Age-associated memory impairment		29
3	Deficits noted in demanding employment settings	Mild cognitive impairment	7 years	24–27
4	Requires assistance in complex tasks, e.g., handling finances, planning dinner party	Mild AD	2 years	19–20
5	Requires assistance in choosing proper attire	Moderate AD	18 months	15
6a	Requires assistance in dressing	Moderately severe AD	5 months	9
6b	Requires assistance in bathing properly		5 months	8
6c	Requires assistance with mechanics of toileting (such as flushing, wiping)		5 months	5
6d	Urinary incontinence		4 months	3
6e	Fecal incontinence		10 months	1
7a	Speech ability limited to about a half-dozen words	Severe AD	12 months	0
7b	Intelligible vocabulary limited to a single word		18 months	0
7c	Ambulatory ability lost		12 months	0
7d	Ability to sit up lost		12 months	0
7e	Ability to smile lost		18 months	0
7f	Ability to hold head up lost		12 months or longer	0

[a]In subjects without other complicating illnesses who survive and progress to the subsequent deterioration stage.
[b]MMSE = Mini-Mental State Examination score (Folstein et al., 1975). Estimates based in part on published data summarized in Reisberg, Ferris, de Leon, et al., 1989 and in Reisberg, Ferris, Torossian, et al., 1992.
Adapted from Reisberg (1986). Copyright © 1984 by Barry Reisberg, MD.

(MMSE) scores for each of the FAST stages and substages (Folstein, Folstein, & McHugh, 1975). Research has indicated strong relationships between progressive functional deterioration assessed on the FAST and progressive cognitive deterioration in AD (e.g., Pearson correlation coefficients of ~0.8 or greater between MMSE and FAST scores have been reported [Reisberg, Ferris, Anand, et al., 1984; Sclan & Reisberg, 1992]). Therefore, the relationships shown between FAST and MMSE scores are approximations of likely findings in individual patients, although there is variability. Functionally, the late stages of AD can be subdivided into stages 6a-e and stages 7a-f. Consequently, a total of 16 functioning stages can be recognized that describe in detail the characteristic changes with the progression of AD. In uncomplicated dementia of the Alzheimer's type, progression through each of the functional stages described below occurs in a generally ordinal (sequential) pattern (Sclan & Reisberg, 1992).

Stage 1: No objective or subjective functional decrement. The aged subject's objective and subjective functional abilities in occupational, social, and other settings remain intact compared with prior performance. The prognosis is excellent for continued adequate cognitive functioning.

Stage 2: Subjective functional decrement but no objective evidence of decreased performance in complex occupational or social activities. The most common age-related functional complaints are forgetting names and locations of objects or decreased ability to recall appointments. Subjective decrements are generally not noted by intimates or co-workers, and complex occupational and social functioning is not compromised.

When affective disorders, anxiety states, or other remediable conditions have been excluded, the elderly person with these symptoms can be reassured with respect to the relatively benign prognosis for persons with these subjective symptoms.

Stage 3: Objective functional decrement of sufficient severity to interfere with complex occupational and social tasks. This is the stage at which persons may begin to forget important appointments, seemingly for the first time in their lives. Functional decrements may become manifest in complex psychomotor tasks, such as ability to travel to new locations. Persons at this stage have no difficulty with routine tasks such as shopping, handling finances, or traveling to familiar locations, but they may stop participating in demanding occupational and social settings. These symptoms, although subtle clinically, can considerably alter lifestyle. When psychiatric, neurological, and medical concomitants apart from AD have been excluded, the clinician may advise withdrawal from complex, anxiety-provoking situations. Because patients at this stage can still perform all basic activities of daily living satisfactorily, withdrawing from demanding activities may result in complete symptom amelioration for a period of years.

Stage 4: *Deficient performance in the complex tasks of daily life.* Aspects of decreased functioning from former levels are apparent. At this stage, shopping for adequate or appropriate food and other items is noticeably impaired. The patient may return with incorrect items or inappropriate amounts of a certain item. The individual may have difficulty preparing meals for family dinners and may display similar deficits in the ability to manage complex occupational and social tasks. Family members may note that the patient no longer is able to balance the checkbook, no longer remembers to pay bills properly, and may make significant financial errors. Persons who are still able to travel independently to and from work may not recall names of clients or details of their employment duties. Because choosing clothing, dressing, bathing, and traveling to familiar locations can be adequately performed at this stage, patients may still function independently in the community, although supervision is often useful.

Maximizing the patient's functioning at this stage is the goal of the family and health professionals. Financial supervision and structured or supervised travel should be arranged. Identification bracelets or clothing labels with a name, address, and telephone number may be useful for unusually stressful situations where anxiety or other factors further impair the patient's capacities.

Stage 5: *Incipient deficit in performance in basic tasks of daily life.* At this stage patients can no longer satisfactorily function independently in the community. The patient not only requires assistance in managing financial affairs and marketing but also begins to require help in choosing the appropriate clothing for the season and the occasion. The patient may wear obviously incongruous clothing combinations or wear the same clothing day after day unless supervision is provided.

At this stage, some patients develop anxieties and fears about bathing. Another functional deficit that frequently becomes manifest at this stage is difficulty in driving an automobile. The patient may slow down or speed up the vehicle inappropriately or may go through a stop sign or traffic light. Occasionally, the patient may have a collision with another vehicle for the first time in many years. The patient may be sufficiently alarmed by these deficits to voluntarily discontinue driving. Sometimes, however, intervention and coercion are necessary from family members or even from the patient's physician or licensing authorities. A useful strategy for the physician is to arrange for an automobile driving retest.

It is important that functional abilities be maximized. Patients are still capable of putting on their clothing with minimal guidance once it has been selected for them. They are also capable of bathing and washing themselves, even though they may have to be cajoled into performing these activities. A supportive environment that provides adequate stimulation, in addition to adequate protection, is desirable. It is important that the patient continue to engage in and practice skills in which they remain capable.

Stage 6: *Decreased ability to dress, bathe, and toilet independently.* Throughout the course of stage 6, which lasts for approximately 2.5 years and encompasses five substages, increasing deficits in dressing and bathing occur. In addition to not being able to choose the proper clothing, early stage 6 patients develop difficulties in putting on their clothing properly (stage 6a). Other dressing difficulties include putting on street clothing over night clothing, putting clothing on backward or inside out, and putting on multiple and inappropriate layers of clothing. The patient may also have difficulty zippering or buttoning their clothing or tying their shoelaces. More overt dressing difficulties develop as this stage progresses and the patient requires increasing assistance in dressing.

A bathing difficulty that becomes apparent at this stage is a decreased ability to adjust the temperature of bath or shower water (stage 6b). Subsequently, taking a bath or shower without assistance becomes increasingly problematic, with difficulty getting into and out of the bath and washing properly. Fear of bathing may develop, combined with resistance to bathing. This fear of bathing sometimes precedes actual difficulties in handling the mechanics of bathing.

Later in the course of this stage, patients begin to have difficulties with the mechanics of toileting: initially, they may forget to flush the toilet, dispose of toilet tissue improperly, and clean themselves inadequately (stage 6c). Subsequently, urinary incontinence begins (stage 6d), followed by fecal incontinence (stage 6e), both of which appear to be the result of decreased cognitive capacity to respond appropriately to urinary or fecal urgency. Assisting the patient to use the toilet often helps to forestall and remediate incontinence. Anxieties regarding toileting are frequently noted in stage 6c prior to the actual development of incontinence. Patients may go to the toilet repeatedly even in the absence of a true need for elimination.

Motor capacity deficits also become notable during stage 6. Walking becomes more halting and steps generally become smaller and slower, but the ability to ambulate is still maintained. Because orientation in space is affected, patients may approach a chair and sit down with greater difficulty. Patients may also require assistance in walking up and down a staircase.

Full-time home health care is frequently useful at this time, and it may be appropriate or necessary to discuss nursing home placement with the caregiver and family members. Management strategies and supportive techniques must be developed to assist the patient in bathing, dressing, and toileting, as well as in minimizing the emotional stress of the caregiver.

Stage 7: *Loss of speech and locomotion.* This final stage of AD is marked by decreased vocabulary and speech abilities. Speech becomes increasingly limited, from a vocabulary of a half-dozen different words (stage 7a), to a single distinguishable word that may be uttered repeatedly (stage 7b). Eventually, speech becomes limited to only babbling, unintelligible utterances, and crying out.

Prior to the loss of ambulatory ability, patients may exhibit a twisted gait, take progressively smaller and slower steps, or lean forward, backward, or sideways while walking. Eventually, the ability to walk unassisted is lost with the progression of AD (stage 7c). Approximately a year after ambulatory ability is lost, the ability to sit up without assistance (such as lateral chair rests) is also lost (stage 7d). Subsequently, the ability to smile (stage 7e) and to hold up the head independently (stage 7f) are also lost. At this point, babbling and grasping may still be observed, and patients can still move their eyes, although familiar persons or objects are apparently no longer recognized. Approximately 3 to 4 years after the onset of stage 7, generally after the loss of ambulatory ability, many patients die. However, some patients survive in this stage for 7 years or longer. Pneumonia, which is often associated with aspiration, is a frequent cause of death.

Full-time assistance at home or in an institution is a necessity at this stage, and as AD patients are increasingly well cared for, it is likely that more will survive to these final substages of the illness.

FEEDING CONCOMITANTS OF AD

PROGRESSIVE CHANGES IN the ability to prepare meals and in feeding skills have been observed in AD patients and enumerated in accordance with the corresponding GDS and FAST stages (Reisberg et al., 1990). These "Feeding Concomitants of Alzheimer's Disease" are outlined in Table 4.3. The progression of these disturbances in meal preparation and self-feeding, as with the progression of deterioration in cognitive and functional abilities, appears to be characteristic of AD.

BALANCE AND COORDINATION

ALTHOUGH IT IS clear from the preceding description of functional losses in AD that balance and coordination are eventually lost with the progression of the illness process, these aspects are actually very early changes, coincident with the advent of MCI and mild AD. For example, a detailed study indicated that tandem walking, foot tapping speed, hand pronation and supination speed, and finger to thumb

TABLE 4.3 Feeding Concomitants of Alzheimer's Disease

Stage	Clinical characteristics
1-2	No objective or subjective decrement in the ability to adequately prepare meals, order food and beverages in a restaurant setting, or in table etiquette
4	Decreased facility in preparing and/or serving relatively complex meals, and/or decreased facility in ordering food and beverages in restaurant setting
5	Decreased ability in preparing simple foods or beverages (e.g., coffee or tea); may occasionally make mistakes in eating food (e.g., improper use of seasoning or condiments)
6	(a) Occasional difficulty with proper manipulation or choice of eating utensils. (b) Meat and similar foods must be cut up for the patient (c) No longer trusted to use a knife; may also eat foods that would have formerly been refused (d) No longer trusted to properly use a knife and decreased ability to use a fork, but can still properly use a spoon; may also display occasional misrecognition of dietary substances (pica) (e) Capable of going to the refrigerator or cupboard but has difficulty discerning and choosing food, may have difficulty chewing hard food
7	(a) Capable of picking up spoon or fork; will occasionally drop food or misutilize silverware (e.g., may attempt to drink soup or other liquids with a fork); capable of reaching for a cup when desirous of fluid (b) Must be assisted in actual feeding; generally, patients are not permitted to handle a knife or fork; may not be able to properly lift a cup (c) Can reach for and pick up food with hands; cannot properly pick up a fork or a spoon but can grasp a spoon or other utensil; must be spoon-fed, but can chew. (d) Cannot distinguish foods from nondietary substances; will reach out for objects, including food.

*Stages have been enumerated to be optimally concordant with the corresponding global deterioration scale (GDS) and functional assessment staging (FAST) stages in Alzheimer's disease.
Copyright © 1988 by Barry Reisberg, M.D. From Reisberg, Pattschull-Furlan, Franssen, et al., 1990.

apposition speed, all decreased significantly in MCI subjects in comparison with normal elderly controls (Franssen, Souren, Torossian & Reisberg, 1999). Additional decrements were noted in mild AD subjects.

Another study has demonstrated that complex motor and fine motor measures can be just as robust markers of MCI and mild AD as a cognitive psychometric battery (Kluger et al., 1997). These observations of motor and equilibrium changes in MCI and AD are consistent with neuropathologic observations of robust clinicopathologic correlations with cerebellar atrophy in AD (Wegiel et al., 1999).

RIGIDITY AND CONTRACTURES

IN THE LATTER stages of AD, rigidity becomes increasingly manifest (Franssen, Reisberg, Kluger, Sinaiko, & Boja, 1991; Franssen, Kluger, Torossian, & Reisberg, 1993). Initially, this rigidity is of a paratonic type, i.e., elicited in response to an irregular motion of an extremity, such as an irregular movement of an elbow. Later, the rigidity becomes increasingly evident. Figure 4.1 depicts the emergence of paratonic rigidity in AD. Although infrequently manifest in patients with mild AD (i.e., GDS stage 4), approximately 50% of patients with moderate AD (GDS stage 5), 75% of patients with moderately severe AD (GDS stage 6), and virtually all patients with severe AD (GDS stage 7) manifest at least a mildly detectable form of paratonic rigidity.

One probable result of this increasing rigidity is the development of contractures. Contractures are irreversible deformities of joints, limiting range of motion. In a study of Souren et al. (Souren, Franssen, & Reisberg, 1995), a contracture was defined as a limitation of 50% or more

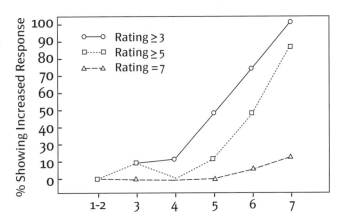

FIGURE 4.1 Percentage of subjects with increased paratonic rigidity in normal aging and Alzheimer's disease of progressively increasing severity.

The graph depicts the percentages of subjects showing paratonia as a function of the Global Deterioration Scale (GDS) stage, using three different ratings of activity. Paratonic rigidity, defined as stiffening of a limb in response to contact with the examiner's hand and an involuntary resistance to passive changes in position and posture, was graded according to the amount of passive force necessary to elicit it. A rating of 1 denotes an absence of paratonic rigidity, whereas a rating of 7 indicates that minimal passive force is required for elicitation of the sequence.

Further detail regarding the scoring procedure can be found in Franssen, E., "Neurologic signs in ageing and dementia," in *Aging and Dementia, a Methodological Approach,* edited by Burns, A., London, Edward Arnold, 1993, pp. 144–174. Data and figure are from Franssen et al., (1991), "Cognition-independent neurologic symptoms in normal aging and probable Alzheimer's disease," *Archives of Neurology, 48,* 148–154.

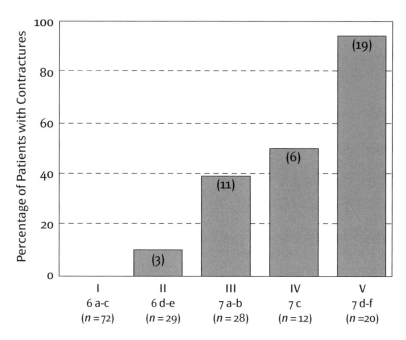

FIGURE 4.2 Percentages of patients with contractures in FAST stage 6 and stage 7 AD.
All subjects fulfilled criteria for probable AD. FAST (Functional Assessment Staging
[Reisberg, 1988]) categories are as follows: *I*, ADL (activities of daily life) deficient, 6a, b,
and c; *II*, incipient incontinence, 6d and e; *III*, incipient nonverbal, 7a and b; incipient
nonambulatory, 7c; and *V*, immobile, 7d, e, and f. The numbers in parentheses indicate
the number of patients with contractures in the functional categories. The significance
of change in the prevalence of contractures from the preceding functional categories is
as follows: between functional categories I and II: $p < .01$; between functional categories II and III: $p < .05$; between functional categories III and IV: not significant; and
between functional categories IV and V: $p < .01$.
Across the five functional categories, there are significant differences in the proportions of patients with contractures ($X^2 = 88.4$, $df = 4$, $p < .001$). The prevalence of contractures was highly correlated with FAST staging levels ($r = 0.70$, $p < .001$).
Data and figure are adapted from Souren et al. (1995).

of the passive range of motion of a joint, secondary to permanent muscle shortening, ankylosis, or both. Souren and associates found that contractures meeting this definition were present in 10% of moderately
severe AD patients with incipient incontinence (i.e., AD patients at FAST
stages 6d and 6e) (Figure 4.2). In severe AD, contractures are very common. Forty percent of incipient averbal AD patients (FAST stages 7a and
7b) manifested contractures and 50% of incipient non-ambulatory AD
patients (FAST stage 7c) manifested these deformities. By late stage 7,
i.e., in immobile patients (FAST stages 7d to f), 95% of AD patients manifested these deformities. Furthermore, at all stages, when contractures

occurred, they tended to be present in more than one extremity. There is anecdotal evidence based upon patient observations that contractures may be prevented until very late in the course of AD by maintenance of patient activities and movements.

TREATMENT IMPLICATIONS

COGNITIVE AND FUNCTIONAL deficits in patients with AD characteristically follow the progression outlined in the preceding sections. However, other disorders frequently associated with the presence of dementia do not necessarily follow this characteristic pattern. It has been observed that the characteristic pattern of functional loss in AD is useful in differential diagnosis (Reisberg, 1986; Reisberg, Ferris, & Franssen, 1985). Common functional presentations of non-AD dementing disorders are outlined in Table 4.4. For example, normal-pressure hydrocephalus (NPH) commonly presents with gait disturbance as the earliest symptom, antedating any overt cognitive disturbance. In NPH this ambulatory disturbance is commonly followed by urinary incontinence. Only subsequently, after the advent of ambulatory disturbance and urinary incontinence in NPH, may cognitive disturbances become manifest. As summarized in Table 4.2, the sequence of functional loss in AD is very different. In AD overt cognitive disturbance precedes urinary incontinence, which in turn precedes ambulatory loss.

Creutzfeldt-Jacob disease is a rare form of rapidly progressive dementia that presents with ambulatory disturbance as the earliest symptom in approximately one third of cases. In AD, the ambulatory disturbance is a much later event. The two conditions also may be distinguished temporally. The course of AD extends over many years, as outlined in Table 4.2, and is frequently much slower than the relatively rapid course of the acute and subacute forms of Creutzfeldt-Jacob disease.

Multi-infarct dementia, or dementia associated with an overt, large infarction, may produce speech disturbance as the only symptom. Alternatively, the infarction may produce urinary incontinence as the major overt manifestation. Commonly, ambulatory loss may be the major sequela of a stroke. Clearly, the evolution of functional losses in AD follows a very different and much more stereotyped pattern (as outlined in Tables 4.2). As shown in Table 4.4, the evolution of functional disturbance in dementia associated with multiple infarctions may follow a very different course from that which is characteristic of AD.

Depression is a psychiatric disturbance associated with mood dysphoria and other symptoms. Among these other symptoms are negativity and subjective complaints of cognitive impairment. Occasionally, the depression produces a dementia-like syndrome that is potentially

TABLE 4.4 Functional Loss in Non-Alzheimer Disorders Associated with Progressive or Gradual Onset of Dementia and FAST Characteristics in AD

	Functional loss in non-Alzheimer disorders			FAST AD distinctions	
Disorder	**Pathology or presumed etiology**	**Functional loss in non-AD disorder[a]**	**Equivalent FAST stage**	**Functional loss in AD per FAST**	**FAST stages in AD**
Normal pressure hydrocephalus	Dilated cerebral ventricles	1. Gait disturbance 2. Urinary incontinence 3. Loss of ability to perform complex tasks	7c 6d 4	1. Loss of ability to perform complex tasks 2. Urinary incontinence 3. Ambulatory (gait) disturbance	4 6d 7c
Creutzfeldt-Jakob disease	Prion	1. Gait disturbance 2. Loss of ability to perform complex tasks	7c 4	1. Loss of ability to perform complex tasks 2. Ambulatory (gait) disturbance	4 7c
Multi-infarct dementia	Multiple cerebral infarctions	1. Loss of speech 2. Loss of urinary continence 3. Loss of ability to put on clothing 4. Loss of ability to bathe without assistance 5. Loss of ambulatory capacity 6. Loss of ability to perform complex tasks 7. Loss of ability to pick out clothing 8. Fecal incontinence	7a-7b 6d 6a 6b 7c 4 5 6e	1. Loss of ability to perform complex tasks 2. Loss of ability to pick out clothing properly 3. Loss of ability to put on clothing without assistance 4. Loss of ability to bathe without assistance 5. Loss of urinary continence 6. Loss of fecal continence 7. Loss of speech 8. Loss of ambulatory capacity	4 5 6a 6b 6c 6d 6e 7a-7b

Condition	Etiology	Sequence (example 1)	Stage	Sequence (example 2)	Stage
Dementia Syndrome of Depression ("Pseudo-dementia")	Affective disorder associated with neurotransmitter imbalance	1. Loss of ability to perform complex tasks	4	1. Loss of ability to perform complex tasks	4
		2. Refusal to put on clothing (associated with negativity)	6a	2. Inability to pick out clothing properly	5
		3. Refusal to bathe (associated with negativity)	6b	3. Inability to put on clothing without assistance.	6a
		4. Loss of ability to pick out clothing properly	5	4. Inability to bathe without assistance	6b
Dementia associated with hyponatremia	Electrolyte disturbance	1. Loss of ability to perform complex tasks	4	1. Loss of ability to perform complex tasks	4
		2. Loss of ability to pick out clothing properly	5	2. Loss of ability to pick out clothing properly	5
		3. Loss of ability to dress, bathe, and toilet independently	6a-6c	3. Loss of ability to dress, bathe, and toilet independently	6a-6c
		4. Loss of ambulation capacity	7c	4. Loss of urinary and fecal continence	6d-6e
		5. Loss of urinary and fecal continence	6d-6e	5. Loss of speech	7a-7b
		6. Loss of speech	7a-7b	6. Loss of ambulatory capacity	7c
Dementia associated with diffuse CNS metastasis	Neoplastic diffuse cerebral trauma	1. Loss of ability to perform complex tasks	4	1. Loss of ability to perform complex tasks	4
		2. Loss of ability to dress, bathe, and toilet independently	6a-6c	2. Loss of ability to dress, bathe, and toilet independently	6a-6c
		3. Loss of ambulation capacity	7c	3. Loss of urinary and fecal continence	6d-6e
		4. Loss of urinary and fecal continence	6d-6e	4. Loss of speech	7a-7b
		5. Loss of speech	7a-7b	5. Loss of ambulatory capacity	7c

a The sequences of functional loss shown are typical for normal pressure hydrocephalus and Creutzfeldt-Jakob disease; the sequence for multi-infarct dementia is one of various common presentations; the sequences in the dementia syndrome of depression, dementia associated with hyponatremia, and dementia associated with diffuse CNS metastasis are previously observed examples of the presentation of these dementias. It should be noted that in some of the non-AD disorders, particularly multi-infarct dementia, the "sequence" described may appear abruptly, rather than over an extended time interval.

Note: From Reisberg, Pattschull-Furlan, et al. (1990).

reversible when the underlying mood disturbance is treated. This potentially reversible dementia syndrome of depression, formerly called pseudodementia, does not necessarily follow the functional course outlined in Table 4.2. For example, as outlined in Table 4.4, depression may be accompanied by a refusal to dress and bathe as a result of the patient's negativity. However, the patient may be able to point to exactly the clothes he or she wishes to wear. In AD, the loss of ability to pick out clothing properly precedes the loss of ability to put on one's clothing properly.

As outlined in Table 4.4, dementia associated with hyponatremia or other electrolyte disturbances, CNS metastases, and other conditions all may follow a course markedly at variance with the course of AD as outlined in the FAST.

In a patient with AD, a variety of coexisting conditions may result in functional disturbances that may occur prematurely or nonordinally (i.e., out of sequence) in terms of the FAST predictions. Examples of conditions that may be associated with premature (i.e., nonordinal) functional losses in an AD patient are outlined in Table 4.5. For example, if an AD patient is at GDS stage 5 and FAST stage 5 and develops urinary incontinence, this incontinence may, at this early point in AD, be a remediable complication, perhaps secondary to a urinary tract infection.

Similarly, if a patient with AD at GDS stage 5 and FAST stage 5 develops loss of independent ambulation, this may be the result of a stroke or possibly of a variety of potentially treatable conditions common in the elderly, such as medication-induced Parkinsonian symptoms, arthritis, a fracture, and so on. Table 4.5 provides an extensive list of causes of premature functional losses in an AD patient, many of which are potentially remediable.

The relationship between the FAST and the GDS or the FAST and the MMSE is also useful in the identification of excess functional disability that may be remediable. Specifically, if an AD patient is notably more impaired functionally in comparison with the magnitude of the cognitive impairment (e.g., a GDS stage 5 patient who is at stage 6d on the FAST), this is an indication of the likely presence of excess functional disability. For example, the patient may have coexisting arthritis and AD. As a result of the combination of arthritis and dementia, in addition to not being able to handle finances and to pick out clothing without assistance (deficits that occur only because of the patient's AD), the patient may be unable to dress, bathe, and toilet without assistance, the latter resulting in occasional urinary incontinence. The arthritis may or may not be remediable. Similarly, the excess functional disability may or may not be remediable. Interestingly, when excess functional disability occurs in AD patients, it tends to occur "along the lines of the FAST." It appears that AD predisposes to functional losses outlined on the FAST.

TABLE 4.5   Differential Diagnostic Considerations in Cases of Deviations from FAST

Stage	FAST characteristics	Differential diagnostic considerations (particularly if FAST stage occurs prematurely in the evolution of dementia)
1	No functional decrement, either subjectively or objectively, manifest	
2	Complains of forgetting location of objects; subjective work difficulties	Anxiety, neurosis, depression
3	Decreased functioning in demanding employment settings evident to co-workers, difficulty in traveling to new locations	Depression, subtle manifestations of medical pathology
4	Decreased ability to perform complex tasks such as planning dinner for guests, handling finances, and marketing	Depression, psychosis, focal cerebral process (e.g., Gerstmann's syndrome)
5	Requires assistance in choosing proper clothing, may require coaxing to bathe properly	Depression
6	(a) Difficulty putting on clothing properly	(a) Arthritis, sensory deficit, stroke, depression
	(b) Requires assistance in bathing, may develop fear of bathing	(b) Arthritis, sensory deficit, stroke, depression
	(c) Inability to handle mechanics of toileting	(c) Arthritis, sensory deficit, stroke, depression
	(d) Urinary incontinence	(d) Urinary tract infection, other causes of urinary incontinence
	(e) Fecal incontinence	(e) Infection, malabsorption syndrome, other causes of fecal incontinence
7	(a) Ability to speak limited to one to five words	(a) Stroke, other dementing disorder (e.g., diffuse space-occupying lesions)
	(b) Intelligible vocabulary lost	(b) Stroke, other dementing disorder (e.g., diffuse space occupying lesions)
	(c) Ambulatory ability lost	(c) Parkinsonism, neuroleptic-induced or other secondary extrapyramidal syndrome, Creutzfeldt-Jakob disease, normal pressure hydrocephalus, hyponatremic dementia, stroke, hip fracture, arthritis, overmedication
	(d) Ability to sit up independently lost	(d) Arthritis, contractures
	(e) Ability to smile lost	(e) Stroke
	(f) Ability to hold up head lost	(f) Head trauma, metabolic abnormality, other medical abnormality, overmedication, encephalitis, other causes

Note. From Reisberg (1986).

When an insult occurs, the closer the AD patient is to the inevitable point of loss of a functional ability on the FAST, the more predisposed the AD patient is to the premature loss of that capacity on the FAST. Not only illnesses but psychological stressors may also produce these premature losses. For example, if an AD patient at GDS stage 6 and FAST stage 6c is moved to an unfamiliar environment, the patient may develop urinary and fecal incontinence that remits when the patient is returned to familiar surroundings. Subsequently, these capacities will, tragically, be lost with the advance of AD.

Knowledge of the FAST progression of AD, in conjunction with the global concomitants, feeding concomitants, and other aspects, also provides invaluable information on the potential for treatment of disability, even in AD, that is uncomplicated by the presence of additional pathology. For example, strategies for forestalling incontinence can be contemplated in FAST stage 6c. In FAST stage 6d or 6e, treatment of incontinence requires different strategies, such as frequent toileting. With the advance of deficits in FAST stage 7, strategies and goals for the management of incontinence need to be modified.

Other symptoms in AD, notably symptoms associated with the behavioral syndrome as outlined in Table 4.6, also require treatment. These symptoms are commonly treated with neuroleptics or other psychotropic medications. It should be noted that treatment of these symptoms may also be related to the treatment of functional disabilities. For example, it has been observed that AD patients with excess functional disability in relation to the magnitude of their cognitive disturbances may frequently have particularly marked behavioral disturbances. Conversely, marked behavioral disturbances may be associated with excess functional disability. This excess functional disability may be remediated in part by successful treatment of the behavioral symptoms.

OVERALL MANAGEMENT SCIENCE

As SHOWN IN Table 4.7, a very interesting and important aspect of the functional progression of AD is that the order of losses on the FAST is a precise reversal of the order of acquisition of the same functions in normal human development (Reisberg, 1986; Reisberg, Ferris, & Franssen, 1986). Subsequent work has indicated that AD also reverses normal development in terms of other functional parameters (Reisberg, Pattschull-Furlan, et al., 1990), as well as cognitively (Auer et al., 1994; Ouvrier, Goldsmith, Ouvrier, & Williams, 1993; Sclan, Foster, Reisberg, Franssen, & Welkowitz, 1990; Shimada et al., 2003). Table 4.7 illustrates that the FAST stages of AD can be expressed in terms of developmental ages (DAs). Remarkably, so-called developmental infantile reflexes appear

TABLE 4.6   Behavioral and Psychological Pathologic Symptomatology in
Alzheimer's Disease*

Paranoid and Delusional Ideation

The "people are stealing things" delusion.   Alzheimer's patients can no longer recall
the precise whereabouts of household objects. This is probably the psychological explanation
for what apparently is the most common delusion of AD patients—that someone is hiding
or stealing objects. More severe manifestations of this delusion include the belief that
persons are actually speaking with or listening to the intruders.

The "house is not one's home" delusion.   As a result of their cognitive deficits, AD
patients may no longer recognize their home. This appears to account, in part, for the
common conviction of the AD patient that the place in which they are residing is not their
home. Consequently, while actually at home, AD patients commonly request that their
caregiver "take me home." They may also pack their bags for their return home. More disturbing to the caregiver, and of great potential danger to the patient, are actual attempts
to leave the house to go "home." Occasionally attempts to prevent the patient's departure may result in anger or even violence toward the caregiver, which is extremely upset-
ting to the spouse caregiver.

The "spouse (or other caregiver) is an imposter" delusion.   As cognitive deficit progresses, AD patients recognize their caregivers less well. Perhaps for this reason, a frequent delusion of the AD patient is that persons are imposters. In some instances anger and
even violence may result from this conviction.

The delusion of "abandonment."   With the progression of intellectual deficit in AD,
patients retain a degree of insight into their condition. Although AD patients are largely aware
of their cognitive deficits, denial protects them from their awareness. Similarly, they may
be aware of the burden they have become. These insights are probably related to common delusions of abandonment, institutionalization, or of conspiracy or plot to institu-
tionalize the patient.

The "delusion of infidelity."   The insecurities described above are also related to the AD
patient's occasional conviction that the spouse is unfaithful, sexually or otherwise. This conviction of infidelity may also apply to other caregivers.

Other suspicions, paranoid ideation, or delusions.   Although the above specific delusions are the ones most commonly observed in AD, others may also be present, e.g., phantom boarder (strangers are living in the home); delusions that one still carries on activities
in which one actually no longer participates (e.g., working, traveling); delusions about
former family members or the present status of family members (e.g., father is still alive;
daughter is still a child); delusions of doubles (e.g., there are two of the same person).
Suspicion and paranoid ideation may occur regarding strangers, people staring, people plot-
ting to do harm, and so forth.

Hallucinations

Visual hallucinations.   These can be vague or clearly defined. Commonly, AD patients
see intruders or dead relatives at home or have similar hallucinatory experiences.

Auditory hallucinations.   Occasionally, in the presence or absence of visual hallucinations, AD patients may hear dead relatives, intruders, or others whispering or speaking
to them; sometimes voices are only heard when caregivers are not present.

Other hallucinations.   Less commonly other forms of hallucinations may be observed
in AD patients (e.g., smelling a fire or something burning; the patient perceiving imaginary objects, such as piece of paper, which they offer the caregiver).

(Continued)

TABLE 4.6   *(Continued)*

Activity Disturbances

The decreased cognitive capacity of AD patients renders them less capable of channeling their energies in socially productive ways. Since motor abilities are not severely compromised until the final stage of illness, the patient may develop various psychological/motoric solutions for the need to channel their energies. A few of the most common examples are the following:

Wandering.   For a variety of reasons including inability to channel energies, anxieties, delusions such as those described above, and the decreased cognitive abilities per se, AD patients frequently wander away from the home or caregiver. Restraints may be necessary and this, in turn, may provoke anger or violence in the patient.

Purposeless activity (cognitive abulia).   As the condition advances, the AD patient loses the ability to complete or to carry out many of the activities in which they formerly engaged. This may be the basis in part of a variety of purposeless, frequently repetitive activities including: opening and closing a purse or pocketbook; packing and unpacking clothing; putting on and removing clothing; opening and closing drawers; incessant repetition of demands or questions; or simply pacing. In the absence of more productive, structured activities, these purposeless activities provide a means for the patient to channel their energies and their need for movement. Among the most severe manifestations of this syndrome is repetitive self-abrading.

Inappropriate activities.   These occur primarily as a result of decreased cognitive capacities, increased anxieties and suspiciousness, and excess physical energies. They include storing and hiding objects in inappropriate places (e.g., throwing clothing in the wastebasket, putting empty plates in the oven). Attempts by the caregiver to prevent these inappropriate activities may be met by anger or even violence.

Aggressivity

Verbal outbursts.   As already noted, these may occur in association with many of the behavioral symptoms already described. They can also occur as isolated phenomena. For example, an AD patient may begin to use unaccustomed foul and abrasive language with intimates and/or with strangers.

Physical outbursts.   These also may occur as a part of aforementioned syndromes or as an isolated manifestation. The AD patient may, in response to frustration or seemingly without cause, strike out at the spouse or caregiver.

Other agitation.   This includes anger which is expressed non-verbally, for example, the patient's "stewing." Also common is negativity manifested by the patient's resistance to bathing, dressing, toileting, walking, or participating in other activities. Agitation may also be expressed as continuous and seemingly incessant talking (i.e., pressured speech), by panting (hyperventilation), banging, or in other ways.

Diurnal Rhythm Disturbance

Sleep problems are a frequent and significant part of the behavioral syndrome of AD. They may, in part, be the result of decreased cognition (which upsets habitual and other diurnal cues), the energy and motoric changes occurring in the illness, and the neurochemical processes predisposing to agitation and false beliefs.

Day/night disturbance.   The most common sleep problem in AD patients is multiple

(Continued)

TABLE 4.6   *(Continued)*

awakenings in the course of the evening. These can occur in the context of an overall decrease in sleep or in association with increased daytime napping.

Affective Disturbance

The depressive syndrome of AD is primarily reactive in nature; it tends to frequently become manifest somewhat earlier in the course of AD than many of other symptoms described above and may be related to the pattern of insight and denial in the patient.

Tearfulness.   This predominant depressive manifestation generally occurs in brief periods. If queried as to the reason for the tearfulness, the patient might respond that they are crying because "the person I once was is gone," or "of what is happening to me," or "I forgot the reason." This tearfulness frequently may be a precursor of more severe behavioral symptomatology.

Other depressive manifestations.   A depressive syndrome may coexist with early AD just as other illnesses may coexist with AD. The most common affective symptom in AD is the patient saying "I wish I were dead," or uttering a similar phrase, frequently in a repetitive and manneristic fashion. These pessimistic commentaries of the patient are not accompanied by any more overt suicidal ideation or gestures.

Anxieties and Phobias

These may be related to the previously described behavioral manifestations of AD or may occur independently.

Anxiety regarding upcoming events (Godot syndrome).   This common symptom appears to result from decreased cognition and, more specifically, memory disabilities in AD patients, and from the inability to channel remaining thinking capacity productively. Consequently, the patient will repeatedly query with respect to an upcoming event. These queries may be so incessant and persistent as to become intolerable to family and caregiver.

Other anxieties.   Patients commonly express previously non-manifest anxieties regarding their finances, future, health (including memory), and previously non-stressful activities, such as being away from home.

Fear of being left alone.   This is the most commonly observed phobia in AD, but as a phobic phenomenon, it is out of proportion to any real danger. For example, the anxieties may become apparent as soon as the spouse goes into another room. Less dramatically the patient may simply request of the spouse or caregiver, "don't leave me alone."

Other phobias. Patients with AD sometimes develop a fear of crowds, travel, the dark, or activities such as bathing.

*Source: Reisberg, B., Borenstein, J., Franssen, E., Shulman, E., Steinberg, G., and Ferris, S.H. (1986). Potentially remediable behavioral symptomatology in Alzheimer's disease. *Hospital and Community Psychiatry*, 37, 1199–1201. Also adapted from "Behavioral Pathology in Alzheimer's Disease (BEHAVE-AD)" copyright © 1986 by Barry Reisberg, M.D. All rights reserved. Published in: Reisberg, B., Borenstein, J., Salob, S. P., Ferris, S. H., Franssen, E., and Georgotas, A. (1987). Behavioral symptoms in Alzheimer's disease: Phenomenology and treatment. *Journal of Clinical Psychiatry*, 48(5, suppl), 9–15.

TABLE 4.7 Functional Landmarks in Normal Human Development and Alzheimer's Disease (AD)

	Normal Development — Approximate Total Duration: 20 Years			Alzheimer's Degeneration — Approximate Total Duration: 20 Years			
Approximate age	Approximate duration in development	Acquired abilities	Lost abilities	Alzheimer stage	Approximate duration in AD	Developmental age of AD	
Adolescence	13–19 years	7 years	Hold a job	Hold a job	3—Incipient	7 years	19–13 years: Adolescence
Late Childhood	8–12 years	5 years	Handle simple finances	Handle simple finances	4—Mild	2 years	12–8 years: Late Childhood
Middle Childhood	5–7 years	2.5 years	Select proper clothing	Select proper clothing	5—Moderate	1.5 years	7–5 years: Middle Childhood
Early Childhood	5 years	4 years	Put on clothes unaided	Put on clothes unaided	6a—Moderately Severe	2.5 years	5–2 years: Early Childhood
	4 years	Shower unaided	Shower unaided		6b		
	4 years	Toilet unaided	Toilet unaided		6c		
	3 years	Control urine	Control urine		6d		
	2–3 years	Control bowels	Control bowels		6e		
Infancy	15 months	1.5 years	Speak 5–6 words	Speak 5–6 words	7a—Severe	7 years or longer	15 months to birth: Infancy
	1 year	Speak 1 word	Speak 1 word		7b		
	1 year	Walk	Walk		7c		
	6–10 months	Sit up	Sit up		7d		
	2–4 months	Smile	Smile		7e		
	1–3 months	Hold up head	Hold up head		7f		

to be equally good markers of the emergence of the stage of severe AD, corresponding to a DA of infancy, as the same reflexes are in marking the emergence from infancy in normal development (Franssen, Souren, Torossian, & Reisberg, 1997). This process, by which the degenerative changes in AD, and to some extent other dementias, reverse the order of acquisition of capacities and processes in normal development, has been termed retrogenesis (Reisberg, Franssen, Hasan, et al., 1999).

Interestingly, the retrogenesis process can explain many of the other symptoms and findings in AD, such as the nature of patient behavioral disturbances (Reisberg, Auer, Monteiro, Franssen, & Kenowsky, 1998) and the kind of symptoms which are progressively and invariably lost, in comparison with the kind of symptoms which are more variable (Reisberg, Franssen, Souren, Auer, & Kenowsky, 1998). Most importantly, the retrogenic process provides a rapid appreciation of the general care and management needs of the AD patient at each stage of the disease (Reisberg, Kenowsky, Franssen, Auer, & Souren, 1999) (Table 4.8).

An understanding of the retrogenic process in AD also provides the basis for a detailed management science (Reisberg, Franssen, Souren, Auer, Akram, & Kenowsky, 2002). This science includes care axioms, care postulates, and care caveats. The care axioms apply to all human beings and to AD patients at all stages (Table 4.9). The postulates are testable hypotheses of AD patient care based on the DA retrogenesis model (Table 4.10). Finally the caveats are based upon acknowledged differences between AD patients and their DA peers (Table 4.11). The combination of these care axioms, postulates, and caveats forms the nascent science of AD management.

CONCLUSIONS

AD IS A very common condition in elderly persons, marked by a characteristic cognitive and functional course of disability. Knowledge of this characteristic course is essential for the identification and treatment of excess functional disability and for many other aspects of patient management and care. Proper management and care can alleviate, indeed, even eliminate suffering in the patient and reduce burden in the caregivers of AD victims.

TABLE 4.8 Stages of Aging and Alzheimer's Disease (AD) and Corresponding Developmental Ages (DAs): Care Needs and Care Recommendations

GDS stage	Diagnosis	Developmental age (DA)	Care needs	Care recommendations
1	Normal	Adult	None	None.
2	Age-associated memory impairment	Aged adult	None	Reassurance with respect to relatively benign prognosis.
3	Mild cognitive impairment	Adolescence	None	"Tactical" withdrawal from situations that have become, by virtue of their complexity, anxiety provoking.
4	Mild AD	Late childhood	Independent survival still attainable	Assistance towards goal of maximum independence with financial supervision; structured or supervised travel; identification bracelets and labels may be useful.
5	Moderate AD	Middle childhood	Patient can no longer survive in the community without assistance; needs supervision with respect to travel and social behavior.	Part-time home health care assistance can be very useful in assisting the patient's caregiver. Driving becomes hazardous and should be discontinued at some point over the course of this stage. Family may require guidance in handling patient's emotional outbursts.
6	Moderately severe AD	Early childhood	Patient requires assistance with basic activities of daily life. Early in this stage, assistance with dressing and bathing is required. Subsequently, assistance with continence becomes necessary as well.	Full-time home health care assistance is frequently very useful in assisting the patient's caregiver. Strategies for assistance with bathing, toileting, and in the management of incontinence should be discussed with the family. Emotional stress in the caregiver should be minimized with supportive techniques.
7	Severe AD	Infancy	Early in this stage assistance with feeding as well as dressing, bathing, and toileting is required. Subsequently, assistance with ambulation and purposeful movement becomes necessary. Prevention of decubiti, aspiration, and contractures is a major issue in care.	Full-time assistance in the community home residence or institutional setting is a necessity. Strategies for maintaining locomotion should be explored. The need for psychopharmacological intervention for behavioral disturbances decreases. Soft food or liquid diet is generally tolerated. Patients must be fed and instructed/encouraged to maintain chewing and basic eating skills.

TABLE 4.9 Alzheimer's Disease Care Axioms

Axiom I	All human beings avoid trauma and humiliation
Axiom II	All human beings seek a sense of accomplishment
Axiom III	All human beings seek a sense of dignity and self-worth
Axiom IV	All human beings are social organisms
Axiom V	All human beings seek praise and acceptance
Axiom VI	All human beings have the capacity to learn
Axiom VII	All human beings require love
Axiom VIII	All human beings have the capacity for happiness if basic needs are fulfilled
Axiom IX	All human beings have the need for physical movement
Axiom X	All human beings have the capacity to remember
Axiom XI	All human beings have the capacity to think
Axiom XII	All human beings seek to influence their environment
Axiom XIII	All human beings have a sense of "taste," i.e., likes and dislikes

TABLE 4.10 Alzheimer's Disease (AD) Care Postulates

Postulate I	The magnitude of care and supervision required by an AD patient, at a developmental age (DA), is mirrored by the amount of care and supervision required by a child or infant at the corresponding DA.
Postulate II	The kinds of activities enjoyed by an AD patient, at a particular DA, are mirrored by the kinds of activities enjoyed by children at a corresponding DA.
Postulate III	The capacity of an AD patient to perform in an area of residual expertise is dependent on the patient's DA.
Postulate IV	Previous experiences may determine the kinds of activities enjoyed by an AD patient.
Postulate V	The emotional level of the AD patient is dependent on the DA.
Postulate VI	Life experiences appropriate to the DA become most relevant for AD patients at any particular stage.
Postulate VII	Socialization of the AD patient is dependent on the DA.
Postulate VIII	Diversity in children's and infants' activities and interests is mirrored in diversity in AD patient's interests and activities at a corresponding DA.
Postulate IX	The emotional changes that occur in AD at a DA are mirrored by the emotional changes observed in children at a corresponding DA.
Postulate X	Care settings appropriate to AD patients at a DA are mirrored by care settings appropriate to children at the corresponding DA.
Postulate XI	Vulnerability (emotional, physical, and cognitive) of the AD patient at a DA is mirrored by the vulnerability of children at the corresponding DA.

(Continued)

TABLE 4.10   Alzheimer's Disease (AD) Care Postulates *(Continued)*

Postulate XII	The need of an AD patient for physical movement is mirrored by the corresponding DA.
Postulate XIII	Just as one judges development in an infant or child by what the infant or child can do and has achieved, not by what the infant or child cannot do, the AD patient at any particular DA should be assessed in terms of his or her residual skills and accomplishments, what they have learned and relearned, not by what they cannot do.
Postulate XIV	The developmental analogy is sufficiently strong to trigger DA-appropriate childhood memories, beliefs, and anxieties in the AD patient.
Postulate XV	The language changes of the AD patient are mirrored by the DA.

TABLE 4.11   Alzheimer's Disease (AD) Care Caveats

Caveat I	Development in infants and children is accompanied by increasing expectations, whereas AD at all stages is accompanied by progressively diminished expectations.
Caveat II	AD patients experience developmentally analogous brain changes; however, they do not undergo developmentally analogous physical changes.
Caveat III	AD patients can, to some extent, draw upon previously mastered skills, whereas infants and children may not have access to these skills.
Caveat IV	AD patients can, to some extent, draw upon previously mastered knowledge, whereas infants and children may not have access to this knowledge.
Caveat V	AD patients are older than their developmental age (DA) peers, and old age predisposes to various physical disabilities that influence the life and experience of an AD patient.
Caveat VI	AD patients appear to be more prone to rigidity than their DA peers.
Caveat VII	AD patients can potentially concentrate on a task longer than infants or children at a corresponding DA.
Caveat VIII	AD patients appear to be less fascinated by the world and less inquisitive than infants and children at a corresponding DA.

ACKNOWLEDGMENT

THIS WORK WAS supported in part by: U.S. Department of Health and Human Services (DHHS) grants AG03051, AG08051, AG09127, and AG11505 from the National Institute on Aging of the U.S. National Institutes of Health; grants 90AZ2791, 90AR2160 and 90AM2552 from the U.S. DHHS Administration on Aging; grant NCRR M01 RR00096 from the General Clinical Research Center Program of the National Center for Disease Research Resources of the U.S. National Institutes of Health; the Fisher Center for Alzheimer's Disease Research Foundation; and grants from Mr. William Silberstein and Mr. Leonard Litwin.

REFERENCES

American Psychiatric Association. (1994). *Diagnostic and Statistical Manual of Mental Disorders* (4th ed.). Washington, DC: Author.

Auer, S. R., Sclan, S. G., Yaffee, R. A., & Reisberg, B. (1994). The neglected half of Alzheimer's disease: Cognitive and functional concomitants of severe dementia. *Journal of the America Geriatrics Society, 42,* 1266–1272.

Bowen, J., Teri, L., Kukull, W., McCormick, W., McCurry, S. M., & Larson, E. B. (1997). Progression to dementia in patients with isolated memory loss. *Lancet, 349,* 763–765.

Brodaty, H., Ames, D., Snowdon, J., Woodward, M., Kirwan, J., Clarnette, R., et al. (2003). A randomized placebo-controlled trial of risperidone for the treatment of aggression, agitation, and psychosis of dementia. *Journal of Clinical Psychiatry, 64,* 134–143.

Chandler, J. D., & Chandler, J. E. (1988). The prevalence of neuropsychiatric disorder in a nursing home population. *Journal of Geriatric Psychiatry and Neurology, 1,* 71–76.

Crook, T., Bartus, R. T., Ferris, S. H., Whitehouse, P., Cohen, G. D., & Gershon, S. (1986). Age-associated memory impairment: Proposed diagnostic criteria and measures of clinical change—report of a NIMH work group. *Developmental Neuropsychology, 2,* 261–276.

Daly, E., Zaitchik, D., Copeland, M., Schmahmann, J., Gunther, J., & Albert, M. (2000). Predicting conversion to Alzheimer disease using standardized clinical information. *Archives of Neurology, 57,* 675–680.

De Deyn, P. P., Rabheru, K., Rasmussen, A., Bocksberger, J. P., Dautzenberg, P. L., Eriksson, S., et al. (1999). A randomized trial of risperidone, placebo, and haloperidol for behavioral symptoms of dementia. *Neurology, 53,* 946–955.

Devanand, D. P., Folz, M., Gorlyn, M., Moesller, J. R., & Stern, Y. (1997). Questionable dementia: Clinical course and predictors of outcome. *Journal of the American Geriatrics Society, 45,* 321–328.

Evans, V. A., Funkenstein, H., Albert, M. S., Soherr, P. A., Cook, N. R., Chown, M.

J., et al. (1989). Prevalence of Alzheimer's disease in a community population of older persons. *Journal of the American Medical Association, 262*,
2551–2556.

Feldman, H., Gauthier, S., Hecker, J., Vellas, B., Subbiah, P. W. E., & Donepezil
MSAD Study Investigators Group. (2001). A 24-week, randomized, double-
blind study of donepezil in moderate to severe Alzheimer's disease.
Neurology, 57, 613–620.

Flicker, C., Ferris, S. H., & Reisberg, B. (1991). Mild cognitive impairment in the
elderly: Predictors of dementia. *Neurology, 41*, 1006–1009.

Folstein, M. F., Folstein, S. E., & McHugh, P. R. (1975). Mini-mental state: A practical method for grading the cognitive state of patients for the clinician.
Journal of Psychiatry Research, 12, 189–198.

Franssen, E. H., Kluger, A., Torossian, C. L., & Reisberg, B. (1993). The neurologic
syndrome of severe Alzheimer's disease: Relationship to functional
decline. *Archives of Neurology, 50*, 1029–1039.

Franssen, E. H., Reisberg, B., Kluger, A., Sinaiko, E., & Boja, C. (1991) Cognition
independent neurologic symptoms in normal aging and probable
Alzheimer's disease. *Archives of Neurology, 48*, 148–154.

Franssen, E. H., Souren, L. E. M., Torossian, C. L., & Reisberg, B. (1997). Utility of
developmental reflexes in the differential diagnosis and prognosis of
incontinence in Alzheimer's disease. *Journal of Geriatric Psychiatry and
Neurology, 10*, 22–28.

Franssen, E. H., Souren, L. E. M., Torossian, C. L., & Reisberg, B. (1999). Equilibrium
and limb coordination in mild cognitive impairment and mild Alzheimer's
disease. *Journal of the American Geriatrics Society, 47*, 463–499.

Geerlings, M. I., Jonker, C., Bouter, L. M., Ader, H. J., & Schmand, B. (1999).
Association between memory complaints and incident Alzheimer's disease in elderly people with normal baseline cognition. *American Journal
of Psychiatry, 156*, 531–537.

Health Care Financing Administration (HCFA). (1998). Hospice-determining terminal status in non-cancer diagnoses-dementia. *Medicare News
Brief/Empire Medical Services, (MNB-98-7)*, 45–47.

Herbert, L. E., Scherr, P. A., Bienias, J. L., Bennett, D. A., & Evans, D. A. (2003).
Alzheimer disease in the U.S. population: Prevalence estimates using the
2000 census. *Archives of Neurology, 60*, 1119–1122.

Katz, I. R., Jeste, D., Mintzer, J. E., Clyde, C., Napolitano, J., & Brecher, M. (1999).
Comparison of Risperidone and placebo for psychosis and behavioral
disturbances associated with dementia: A randomized, double-blind trial.
Journal of Clinical Psychiatry, 60, 107–115.

Katzman, R. (1986). Alzheimer's disease. *New England Journal of Medicine, 314*,
964–973.

Kluger, A., Ferris, S. H., Golomb, J., Mittelman, M. S., & Reisberg, B. (1999).

Neuropsychological prediction of decline to dementia in nondemented elderly. *Journal of Geriatric Psychiatry and Neurology, 12,* 168–179.

Kluger, A., Gianutsos, J. G., Golomb, J., Ferris, S. H., George, A. E., Franssen, E., et al. (1997). Patterns of motor impairment in normal aging, mild cognitive decline and early Alzheimer's disease. *Journal of Gerontology: Psychological Sciences, 52B,* P28–P39.

Kumar, A., Koss, E., Metzler, D., Moore, A., & Friedland, R. (1988). Behavioral symptomatology in dementia of the Alzheimer's type. *Alzheimer Disease and Associated Disorders, 2,* 363–365.

Lane, F., & Snowdon, J. (1989). Memory and dementia: A longitudinal survey of suburban elderly. In P. Lovibond & P. Wilson (Eds.), *Clinical and abnormal psychology* (pp. 365–376). North-Holland: Elsevier Science Publishers B. V.

Lowenthal, P. M., Berkman, P. L., Buehler, J. A., Pierce, R. C., Robinson, B. C., & Trier, M. L. (1967). *Aging and Mental Disorder in San Francisco: A Social Psychiatric Study.* San Francisco: Jossey Bass.

Morris, J. C., Storandt, M., Miller, P., McKeel, D. W., Price, J. L., Rubin, E. H., et al. (2001). Mild cognitive impairment represents early-stage Alzheimer disease. *Neurology, 58,* 397–405.

Ouvrier, R. A., Goldsmith, R. F., Ovrier, S., & Williams, I. C. (1993). The value of the mini-mental state examination in childhood: A preliminary study. *Journal of Child Neurology, 8*(2), 145–148.

Petersen, R. C., Smith, G. E., Waring, S. C., Ivnik, R. J., Tangalos, E. G., & Kokmen, E. (1999). Mild cognitive impairment: Clinical characterization and outcome. *Archives of Neurology, 56,* 303–308.

Reinikainen, K. J., Koivisto, K., Mykkänen, L., Hanninen, T., Laakso, M., Pyorala, K., et al. (1990). Age-associated memory impairment in aged population: An epidemiological study. *Neurology, 40,* 177.

Reisberg, B. (1986). Dementia: A systematic approach to identifying reversible causes. *Geriatrics, 41,* 30–46.

Reisberg, B. (1988). Functional assessment staging (FAST). *Psychopharmacology Bulletin, 24,* 653–659.

Reisberg, B., Auer, S. R., Monteiro, I., Franssen, E., & Kenowsky, S. (1998). A rational psychological approach to the treatment of behavioral disturbances and symptomatology in Alzheimer's disease based upon recognition of the developmental age. *International Academy for Biomedical and Drug Research, 13,* 102–109.

Reisberg, B., Doody, R., Stöffler, A., Schmitt, F., Ferris, S., Möbius, H.-J., for the Memantine Study Group. (2003). Memantine in moderate-to-severe Alzheimer's disease. *New England Journal of Medicine, 348,* 1333–1341.

Reisberg, B., Ferris, S. H., Anand, R., de Leon, M. J., Schneck, M. K., Buttinger, C., et al. (1984). Functional staging of dementia of the Alzheimer's type. *Annals of the New York Academy of Sciences, 435,* 481–483.

Reisberg, B., Ferris, S. H., de Leon, M. J., & Crook, T. (1982). The global deterioration scale for assessment of primary degenerative dementia. *American Journal of Psychiatry, 139,* 1136–1139.

Reisberg, B., Ferris, S. H., de Leon, M. J., Kluger, A., Franssen, E., Borenstein, J., et al. (1989). The stage specific temporal course of Alzheimer's disease: Functional and behavioral concomitants based upon cross-sectional and longitudinal observation. In K. Iqbal, H. M. Wisniewski, & B. Winblad (Eds.), *Alzheimer's disease and related disorders: Progress in clinical and biological research* (vol. 317, pp. 23–41). New York: Alan R. Liss.

Reisberg, B., Ferris, S. H., & Franssen, E. (1985). An ordinal functional assessment tool for Alzheimer's-type dementia. *Hospital and Community Psychiatry, 36,* 593–595.

Reisberg, B., Ferris, S. H., & Franssen, E. (1986). Functional degenerative stages in dementia of the Alzheimer's type appear to reverse normal human development. In C. Shagass, R. Josiassen, W. H. Bridger, K. Weiss, D. Stoff, & G. M. Simpson (Eds.), *Biological psychiatry* (Vol. 7, pp. 1319–1321). New York: Elsevier.

Reisberg, B., Ferris, S. H., Franssen, E. H., Kluger, A., & Borenstein, J. (1986). Age-associated memory impairment: The clinical syndrome. *Developmental Neuropsychology, 2,* 401–412.

Reisberg, B., Ferris, S. H., Franssen, E., Shulman, E., Monteiro, I., Sclan, S. G., et al. (1996). Mortality and temporal course of probable Alzheimer's disease: A five-year prospective study. *International Psychogeriatrics, 8,* 291–311.

Reisberg, B., Ferris, S. H., Oo, T., & Franssen, E. (2003). Staging: Relevance for trial design in vascular burden of the brain. *International Psychogeriatrics, 15*(Supp. 1), 231–239.

Reisberg, B., Ferris, S. H., Torossian, C., Kluger, A., Monteiro, I. (1992). Pharmacologic treatment of Alzheimer's disease: A methodologic critique based upon current knowledge of symptomatology and relevance for drug trials. *International Psychogeriatrics, 4*(Suppl. 1), 9–42.

Reisberg, B., Franssen, E., Bobinski, M., Auer, S., Monteiro, I, Boksay, I., et al. (1996). Overview of methodologic issues for pharmacologic trials in mild, moderate, and severe Alzheimer's disease. *International Psychogeriatrics, 8,* 159–193.

Reisberg, B., Franssen, E. H., Hasan, S. M., Monteiro, I., Boksay, I., Souren, L. E. M., et al. (1999). Retrogenesis: Clinical, physiologic and pathologic mechanisms in brain aging, Alzheimer's and other dementing processes. *European Archives of Psychiatry and Clinical Neuroscience, 249*(Suppl. 3), 28–36.

Reisberg, B., Franssen, E., Sclan, S. G., Kluger, A., & Ferris, S. H. (1989). Stage specific incidence of potentially remediable behavioral symptoms in aging and Alzheimer's disease: A study of 120 patients using the BEHAVE-AD. *Bulletin of Clinical Neuroscience, 54,* 95–112.

Reisberg, B., Franssen, E. H., Souren, L. E. M., Auer, S. R., Akram, I., & Kenowsky, S. (2002). Evidence and mechanisms of retrogenesis in Alzheimer's and other dementias: Management and treatment import. *American Journal of Alzheimer's Disease, 17,* 202–212.

Reisberg, B., Franssen, E. H., Souren, L. E. M., Auer, S., & Kenowsky, S. (1998). Progression of Alzheimer's disease: Variability and consistency: Ontogenic models, their applicability and relevance. *Journal of Neural Transmission, 54*(Suppl.), 9–20.

Reisberg, B., Kenowsky, S., Franssen, E. H., Auer, S. R., & Souren, L. E. M. (1999). President's Report: Towards a science of Alzheimer's disease management: A model based upon current knowledge of retrogenesis. *International Psychogeriatrics, 11,* 7–23.

Reisberg, B., Laska, E., Monteiro, I., Boksay, I., Torossian, C, Javed, A., et al. (2004). Predicting MCI and dementia in elderly subjects with subjective complaints. *Neurobiology of Aging, 25,* s26.

Reisberg, B., London, E., Ferris, S. H., Borenstein, J., Scheier, L., & de Leon, M. J. (1983). The Brief Cognitive Rating Scale: Language, motoric, and mood concomitants in primary degenerative dementia. *Psychopharmacology Bulletin, 19,* 702–708.

Reisberg, B., Pattschull-Furlan, A., Franssen, E., Sclan, S. G., Kluger, A., Dingcong, L., et al. (1990). Cognition related functional, praxis and feeding changes in CNS aging and Alzheimer's disease and their developmental analogies. In K. Beyreuther & G. Schettler (Eds.), *Molecular mechanisms of aging* (pp. 18–40). Berlin: Springer-Verlag.

Reisberg, B., Schneck, M. K., Ferris, S. H., Schwartz, G. E., & de Leon, M. J. (1983). The brief cognitive rating scale (BCRS): Findings in primary degenerative dementia (PDD). *Psychopharmacology Bulletin, 19,* 47–50.

Rovner, B. W., Kafonek, S., Filipp, L., Lucas, M. J., & Folstein, M. F. (1986). Prevalence of mental illness in a community nursing home. *American Journal of Psychiatry, 143,* 1446–1449.

Rubin, E., Morris, J., Storandt, M., & Berg, L. (1987). Behavioral changes in patients with mild senile dementia of the Alzheimer's type. *Psychiatry Research, 21,* 55–61.

Sclan, S. G., Foster, J. R., Reisberg, B., Franssen, E., & Welkowitz, J. (1990). Application of Piagetian measures of cognition in severe Alzheimer's disease. *Psychiatric Journal of the University of Ottawa, 15,* 221–226.

Sclan, S. G., & Reisberg, B. (1992). Functional assessment staging (FAST) in Alzheimer's disease: Reliability, validity and ordinality. *International Psychogeriatrics, 4,* 55–69.

Shimada, M., Hayat, J., Meguro, K., Oo, T., Jafri, S., Yamadori, A., et al. (2003). Correlation between functional assessment staging and the `Basic Age' by the Binet scale supports the retrogenesis model of Alzheimer's disease: A preliminary study. *Psychogeriatrics, 3,* 82–87.

Sluss, T. K., Rabins, P., & Gruenberg, E. M. (1980). Memory complaints in community residing men. *Gerontologist, 20,* 201.

Small, G. W., Rabins, P. V., Barry, P. P., Buckholtz, N. S., DeKosky, S. T., Ferris, S. H., et al., (1997). Diagnosis and treatment of Alzheimer's disease and related disorders. Consensus statement of the American Association for Geriatric Psychiatry, the Alzheimer's Association, and the American Geriatrics Society. *Journal of the American Medical Association, 278,* 1363–1371.

Souren, L. E. M., Franssen, E. M., & Reisberg, B. (1995). Contractures and loss of function in patients with Alzheimer's disease. *Journal of the American Geriatrics Society, 43,* 650–655.

Tariot, P. N., Farlow, M., Grossberg, G. T., Graham, S. M., McDonald, S., Gergel, I., for the Memantine Study Group. (2004). Memantine treatment in patients with moderate to severe Alzheimer Disease already receiving Donepezil. *Journal of the American Medical Association, 3,* 317–324.

Tierney, M. C., Szalai, J. P., Snow, W. G., Fisher, R. H., Nores, A., Nadon, G., et al. (1996). Prediction of probable Alzheimer's disease in memory-impaired patients: A prospective longitudinal study. *Neurology, 46,* 661–665.

Wegiel, J., Wisniewski, H. M., Dziewiatkowski, J., Badmajew, E., Tarnawski, M., Reisberg, B., et al. (1999). Cerebellar atrophy in Alzheimer's disease—clinicopathological correlations. *Brain Research, 819,* 41–50.

Winblad, B., & Poritis, N. (1999). Memantine in severe dementia: Results of the M-BEST Study (Benefit and efficacy in severely demented patients during treatment with memantine). *International Journal of Geriatric Psychiatry, 14,* 135–146.

5

Traumatic Brain Injury

THOMAS M. DIXON, PhD, BARRY S. LAYTON, PhD,
AND ROSE MARY SHAW

BRAIN INJURIES RESULTING from trauma constitute a major
source of neurological disability throughout the world. Acquired
damage to the brain affects the biological substrate that underlies fundamental functional capacities such as motor control, sensation, perception, cognition, memory, personality, and emotion. The
physical and neurobehavioral sequelae of brain impairment often produce devastating consequences involving the ability to live independently, maintain competitive employment, sustain intimate relationships,
and generally to establish a meaningful existence. Thus, the rehabilitation of brain injuries poses a vital challenge to survivors, families, and
professionals.

For the purposes of this discussion, the term "traumatic brain injury"
(TBI) refers to the disruption of brain structure and/or function from
the sudden application of physical force, usually involving a blow to
the head or penetration of the skull by a foreign object. Other descriptions applied to this phenomenon are head injury, concussion, cranio-
cerebral trauma, and posttraumatic encephalopathy. The term TBI, rather
than head injury, is preferred because it correctly indicates the focus
of damage.

The social and personal costs of TBI have received national recogni-
tion in the past 20 years. The National Institute on Disability and
Rehabilitation Research initiated the Traumatic Brain Injury Model
Systems of Care (TBIMS) in 1987. The TBIMS currently consists of 17

rehabilitation centers in urban areas, with the mission of providing comprehensive care and conducting studies that document and enhance outcomes (Bushnik, 2003). In 1996, the United States Congress passed Public Law 104-166, the Traumatic Brain Injury Act, which mandates coordinated public policy and research on TBI.

DISTINCTIVE CHARACTERISTICS OF DISABILITY FROM TBI

TBI POSSESSES AT least three distinctive characteristics as a disability. First, in many other disabling conditions, the cognitive and emotional characteristics of the individual remain intact, allowing the deployment of the full range of preinjury intellectual and affective resources to compensate for lost function. However, brain injury almost always disrupts intellect and emotion, limiting available resources for coping. Cognitive and emotional impairments, therefore, not only become a focus for feelings of loss but may also interfere with psychological adaptation.

Second, the psychosocial impact of TBI is different from that of developmental cognitive disabilities. Intellectual difficulties beginning early in life (e.g., mental retardation) create limited expectations for productivity and social integration. TBI, on the other hand, often abruptly changes the social and vocational roles of individuals who have achieved a stable lifestyle or who anticipate doing so at a level determined by preinjury abilities that have been lost.

A third distinguishing feature of TBI as a disability is that it may seem invisible. Observers casually notice problems associated with physical losses such as paraplegia or limb amputation, but casual inspection often does not reveal the cognitive disorders that form the core of disability as a result of brain injury. TBI without visible physical changes may become a burden that other people do not fully appreciate. The Brain Injury Association, a longstanding consumer advocacy group, calls TBI "the silent epidemic" to describe this lack of societal awareness.

EPIDEMIOLOGY

THE RATE OF survival from TBI has increased over the past 20 years due to advances in emergency medicine, neurosurgery, and intensive care. As a result, the cumulative number of people with TBI is increasing. Many individuals who formerly would have died as a result of accidents or assaults now are saved in the acute period following injury. The decrease in fatality, in combination with the overrepresen-

TABLE 5.1 Causes of Traumatic Brain Injury

Cause	Percentage
Motor vehicle crashes	48.9
Falls	25.8
Firearms	9.7
Other assaults	7.5
Other/Unknown	8.0

From CDC (1999).

tation of TBI among young people, creates a population with chronic disability because those who survive acute hospitalization may have a normal lifespan. TBI is a major public health problem, outnumbering many other forms of neurological disability, including spinal cord injury, multiple sclerosis, Parkinson's disease, Guillain-Barre syndrome, motor neuron disease, and myasthenia gravis (Alexander, 1995). The primary cause of hospitalization due to TBI is motor vehicle crashes, while violence involving firearms is the leading cause of TBI-related death (Centers for Disease Control and Prevention [CDC], 1999). Table 5.1 shows recent data on percentages of TBI by cause.

INCIDENCE AND PREVALENCE

THE CDC ESTIMATES that approximately 1.5 million people sustain a TBI each year in the United States, with 230,000 needing hospitalization (CDC, 1999). Population studies reveal an incidence rate of approximately 175–200 TBIs per 100,000 people (Kraus & MacArthur, 1999). Estimates of incidence vary based on the region of the United States under survey and the criteria used to define TBI. For injuries involving a visit to the emergency room or hospital admission, roughly 80% are classified as mild, 10% as moderate, and 10% as severe (Kraus & Sorenson, 1994). Incidence data may not reflect many cases of mild TBI that are either undiagnosed or treated outside of hospitals. TBI is associated with substantial loss of life, with 50,000 deaths annually. Mortality has declined substantially since 1980, in part due to preventive measures such as use of helmets and seatbelts (CDC, 1999).

Prevalence of persisting disability related to TBI is difficult to document because the majority of injuries are mild and not disabling. In addition, no database exists to record the number of people who receive rehabilitation or disability payments for TBI. According to CDC estimates, around 5.3 million people in the U.S. have TBI-related disabilities, and TBI causes 80,000 new disabilities per year.

RISK FACTORS

CERTAIN SEGMENTS OF the population face increased risk of sustaining TBI. With respect to age, people between the ages of 15 and 24 have a relatively high rate of injury. Risk gradually declines through the middle-age years and then rises sharply after age 75 (CDC, 1999). Older adults have increased TBI incidence and mortality, especially due to falls, with generally poorer neuropsychological recovery, compared to younger people. With respect to gender, TBI occurs 2 to 2.8 times more frequently in males than in females. In addition, males are 3.5 times more likely to die as a result of TBI than females, presumably because of greater exposure to high-risk activities and violence. Additional demographic correlates of TBI include low income, ethnic minority status, and inner city residence (Kraus & McArthur, 1999).

Alcohol intoxication represents another major risk factor. Corrigan (1995) examined the available studies and found a 36% to 51% incidence of intoxication at time of injury.

ECONOMIC IMPACT

TBI RESULTS IN an enormous economic cost to society in the form of medical expenses, rehabilitation services, lost productivity, and disability payments. Medical care in the United States alone for new cases of TBI costs $9–10 billion (NIH Consensus Development Panel, 1999). Max, MacKenzie, and Rice (1991) estimated the annual total cost to society for TBI in 1985 at $37.8 billion.

MECHANISMS OF INJURY AND PATHOPHYSIOLOGY

THE TYPE AND magnitude of physical force to the brain determine the nature, location, and extent of trauma. Levin, Benton, and Grossman (1982) and Lishman (1998) summarize the physical mechanisms of TBI in detail. Brain injuries are commonly classified as closed or open, depending on whether the skull remains intact or is penetrated by a bullet or other object. Closed head trauma occurs when the head undergoes a sudden change in momentum through acceleration or deceleration. Consider the prototypical case of an automobile collision. The vehicle traveling at a high rate of speed collides with a fixed object, such as a telephone pole. The occupant suffers rapid deceleration as the head hits the dashboard or windshield, followed by acceleration as the head whips back in an arc. These blows cause the brain to move within the skull, thereby generating rotational forces—an abnormal twisting or swirling of neural tissue. The brain also may come into forcible contact with bony prominences of the skull, such as the orbital ridges that form a shelf supporting the frontal lobes; or recoil from one side of the skull to the other, causing what is referred to as coup/countrecoup injury.

The physical mechanisms outlined above cause a variety of pathological changes in the nervous system. Shear-strain forces during rotational acceleration of the head can produce diffuse axonal injury (DAI)—that is, stretching, swelling, or shearing of axons resulting in multiple, small, focal lesions scattered throughout the white matter, particularly in the brain stem, corpus callosum, and junctions between the gray and white matter of the cerebral cortex (Meythaler, Peduzzi, Eleftheriou, & Novack, 2001). Damage to long axons in the brain stem produce a period of unconsciousness of variable duration and impairment of vital functions (Adams, Graham, & Gennarelli, 1985). Injury to connecting axons may impair communication between the two cerebral hemispheres and between cortical and subcortical structures. As a result of DAI, various areas of the brain function with less efficiency because they have been deprived of input from other cerebral regions or are less able to convey their output to control behavior.

Another primary form of damage resulting from TBI consists of laceration and focal cortical contusion, or bruising of brain tissue. The frontal and anterior temporal lobes are especially vulnerable to contusion because they sit within the skull's jagged inner surface. In injuries that do not entail high-speed acceleration/ deceleration (e.g., falls, blunt blows to the head with an object, penetrating missile wounds), focal cerebral contusions may occur in the absence of underlying DAI.

Following the moment of injury, numerous secondary complications can develop that affect survival and ultimate outcome. For example, cerebral swelling or edema may increase tissue volume within the rigid cranial vault, creating an elevation in intracranial pressure and associated conditions of reduced blood flow (ischemia) and loss of oxygen (hypoxia). Leakage from ruptured blood vessels may produce space-occupying blood clots, known as hematomas that compress the brain tissue and necessitate neurosurgery for evacuation.

Microvascular bleeding and stretching of axons from the initial injury initiates a secondary cascade of adverse advents at the cellular level (Stein, Glasier, & Hoffman, 1994). Gradual destruction of neurons occurs through excessive release of neurotransmitters, overexcitation due to influx of calcium ions into cells, and degradation of membranes by lipid peroxidation. Various pharmacologic agents have been investigated to minimize cellular damage, but none of the neuroprotective drugs tested so far has proven effective (Doppenberg, Choi, & Bullock, 2004).

Medical complications and associated injuries in the early stage of TBI may add to impairment. For example, people in motor vehicle crashes frequently sustain bone fractures or other internal injuries besides brain trauma. Common acute medical complications of TBI include hypertension, electrolyte imbalances, pulmonary dysfunction, and seizures (Hammond & McDeavitt, 1999)

FUNCTIONAL PRESENTATION OF TBI

BRAIN INJURIES LEAD to distinctive physical, cognitive, and behavioral syndromes corresponding to the nature and extent of neuroanatomical damage. Diffuse axonal injury produces areas of neuronal fallout throughout the brain and tends to result in generalized loss of cognitive efficiency and adaptive capacity. In addition, TBI often results in focal injury that affects circumscribed areas of the brain and generates specific symptoms according to location. Focal damage also may have nonspecific consequences because disparate regions of the brain operate together in functional systems; therefore, suppressing the activity in one area alters the operation of the whole system. Virtually any behavioral or neurocognitive syndrome can result from TBI, depending on the specific site(s) of injury. However, the prototypical acceleration/deceleration TBI comprises some degree of DAI, accompanied by frontotemporal cerebral contusions.

The manifestations of TBI vary not only in relation to lesion type but also as a function of unique attributes of the injured person. Considering the relationship between personality style and coping with TBI, one early observer concisely stated: "It is not only the kind of head injury that matters but the kind of head" (Symonds, 1937). Individual differences in age, education, intelligence, family support, social context, and psychological adjustment interact with neurological deficits, giving rise to heterogeneity in the functional impact of a given impairment. For example, a mild brain injury in a business executive or air traffic controller might have disastrous consequences, whereas, at least in some vocational situations, a more severe injury may not interfere with effective functioning.

NATURE OF IMPAIRMENTS AFTER TBI

THIS SECTION PROVIDES a brief, selective overview of neuropsychological syndromes following TBI. Common signs and symptoms of brain impairment include disturbances of motor and sensory abilities, language and communication, visual-perceptual skills, attention, memory, executive functions, personality, and awareness. The interested reader will wish to explore basic texts by Lezak (1995), Lishman (1998), Prigatano (1999), and Walsh and Darby (1999) to gain a greater appreciation of this complex topic.

MOTOR AND SENSORY IMPAIRMENTS

DAMAGE TO THE precentral gyrus or motor strip of the cerebral cortex produces paralysis (hemiplegia) or weakness (hemiparesis) on the side of the body contralateral to the affected hemisphere. Thus, left-sided weakness of the upper and lower extremities usually signals right brain damage, and vice versa. Damage to other components of the motor system may cause not only paralysis but also tremor, incoordination of movements (ataxia), and loss of dexterity. Motor impairments interfere with mobility as well as performance of self-care and other skilled tasks. In a study of people with moderate to severe TBI, 3 to 5 years post injury, roughly 45% reported difficulties with ambulation and 30% indicated trouble with personal care activities such as toileting, grooming, and bathing (Dikmen, Machamer, Powell, & Temkin, 2003). Deficits in fine motor speed, which may only become apparent on formal tests of finger tapping, appear to correlate with injury severity (Prigatano & Borgaro, 2003).

Sensory impairments such as hemianesthesia or heminanopsia (blindness in one visual field) occur as a result of damage contralateral to the affected limb or visual field. Any sensory function (olfactory, tactile, auditory, etc.) may be diminished as a result of damage to a specific site in the brain or cranial nerves.

LANGUAGE AND COMMUNICATION IMPAIRMENTS

DISORDERS OF THE oral–motor musculature produce speech articulation difficulties called dysarthria. Impairment of expressive or receptive language, or aphasia, usually is a sign of damage to the left frontal and/or temporal lobes. Depending on the location of injury, aphasia may result in disorders of the ability to name, to use the grammatical structure of language, to comprehend speech, to read (dyslexia), or to write (dysgraphia). One study found that around 11% of people with TBI have pure aphasic syndromes similar to those observed in left hemisphere stroke (Gil, Cohen, Korn, & Grosswater, 1996).

Apart from gross aphasia, other forms of communicative dysfunction likely contribute to social isolation following TBI. Many people experience conversational problems in connection with subtle naming difficulties and diminished ability to rapidly process complex verbal information (Prigatano, 1999). Other communication barriers revolve around the qualitative aspects of conversation, such as staying on track, understanding the listener's perspective, and reading nonverbal social cues. For example, research has shown that people with TBI have difficulties with emotion recognition and detection of deception (Stuss, Gallup, & Alexander, 2001; Turkstra, McDonald, & DePompei, 2001).

VISUAL–PERCEPTUAL IMPAIRMENTS

VISUAL PERCEPTION INCLUDES the ability to recognize objects visually, to appreciate relationships among objects in space, and to organize elements in three dimensions. These abilities depend largely on the integrity of the right hemisphere, particularly the inferior temporal and parietal lobes (Lezak, 1995). When deficits occur, as in cases of right hemisphere contusion or bullet wounds, they often result in restrictions on activity. One disabling form of perceptual disturbance is left neglect, which refers to an inability to attend to stimuli in the left half of visual space even though vision is normal. Functionally, visuospatial deficits may affect dressing, finding one's way around, meal preparation, interpretation of maps or drawings, and driving.

ATTENTIONAL IMPAIRMENTS

ATTENTIONAL FUNCTIONS HAVE multiple aspects: maintaining optimal levels of arousal and alertness, registering new information as it is presented, manipulating information held in mind (referred to as working memory), filtering out distractions, sustaining vigilance to tasks over time, and keeping track of multiple stimuli simultaneously. DAI and more focal lesions to the reticular activating system of the brain stem and frontal lobes contribute to attentional impairment (Mateer & Mapou, 1996; Whyte, 1992).

Severe deficits in basic arousal and alertness stemming from DAI may produce a temporary lack of conscious awareness or even a permanent vegetative state. Moderate to severe TBI typically produces slowing of reaction times and processing speed. Milder injuries result in higher level attentional impairments, impacting on ability to perform complex tasks (Gronwall, 1989). Deficits in the capacity to handle two or more sources of information simultaneously—in other words, divided attention—may interfere with performing tasks in the in the presence of distractions or doing more than one thing at a time, such as listening and taking notes in school. Inadequate processing of material to be learned probably accounts in part for memory difficulty following TBI.

Attentional problems are among the core complaints reported by persons with TBI and their family members, endorsed in 33–74% of cases (McKinlay & Watkiss, 1999). A large body of research shows that people with TBI perform significantly worse than normal controls on various neuropsychological measures of attention.

Memory Impairments

Memory impairments constitute a defining characteristic of TBI (Levin et al., 1982). After regaining consciousness, the person with TBI passes through a period of disorientation and confusion during which ongoing events are not encoded into memory. This severe impairment of new learning capacity is a form of anterograde amnesia called posttraumatic amnesia (PTA). Focal brain injury from penetrating missile wounds may not produce PTA, but diffuse TBI almost always does to some extent. A period of retrograde amnesia (RA)—that is, inability to recall events that predate the injury—often accompanies anterograde amnesia. Figure 5.1 illustrates the temporal relationship of PTA and RA to the time of injury. During recovery, RA usually shrinks so that preinjury memories are restored up until the minutes or hours immediately preceding the time of impact. PTA, however, is a permanent gap in memory from the moment of injury until the consistent return of the ability to recall daily events. Agitation, restlessness, and other signs of delirium often characterize the period of acute amnesia. Ideally, PTA is evaluated by daily administration of a standardized measure such as the Galveston Orientation and Amnesia Test (Levin, O'Donnell, & Grossman, 1979). As will be discussed, the duration of PTA reflects the severity of TBI.

TBI usually entails chronic memory impairment following the resolution of PTA. In fact, trouble in remembering things is the most common problem noted by people with TBI and their relatives (McKinlay & Watkiss, 1999). Several factors play a role in chronic memory disturbance associated with TBI. Diffuse axonal injury, which affects registration and processing of new material, and damage to the deep structures of the temporal lobes, which form the cerebral substrate for storing memories, contribute to the high frequency of memory disorders. TBI also produces deficits in the ability to organize new information; organizational problems may interfere with understanding the gist of information or with using strategies to cluster information in ways to facilitate retrieval. According to Levin (1997), approximately 40% of people with

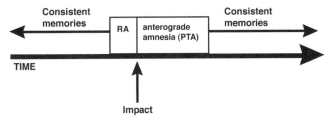

FIGURE 5.1 Temporal relationship between posttraumatic amnesia and retrograde amnesia (RA) following traumatic brain injury.

moderate to severe TBI recover normal functioning on general intellectual measures but still show disproportionately poor memory skills. From a practical standpoint, memory disorders undermine the continuity of day-to-day events and induce confusion as the injured person struggles to recall previous conversations, task instructions, things to do, schedules, and the location of lost objects.

EXECUTIVE FUNCTION IMPAIRMENTS

EXECUTIVE FUNCTIONS REFER to a group of skills that enable self-regulation of behavior. Activities like pursuing personal goals, resisting impulses, controlling one's temper, working in spite of boredom, or adhering to rules reflect the executive functions of personality (Tangney, Baumeister, & Boone, 2004). Cognitive abilities typically associated with executive functions include reasoning, planning, concept formation, and mental flexibility (McDonald, Flashman, & Saykin, 2002). Extensive research indicates that the frontal lobes are the neurological substrate for executive functioning. Frontal systems allow the formation of plans and intentions, the integration and deployment of the skills required to carry out those plans, and monitoring of behavior to maintain effectiveness (Stuss & Levine, 2002). Clinical observations suggest that people with frontal and/or diffuse cerebral impairment due to TBI may demonstrate seemingly intact cognition in structured situations, such as the hospital or psychological testing room, leading to optimistic predictions of outcome. However, the same individuals often decompensate in complex, unstructured situations because of self-regulatory failures. Executive dysfunction may create long-term reliance on others for supervision and day-to-day guidance as well as a lack of efficacy and productivity, even with retention of the individual components of intelligence.

PERSONALITY AND EMOTIONAL CONSEQUENCES

PERSONALITY DISTURBANCES REPRESENT a common consequence of TBI, often comprising part of a larger pattern of impaired executive function. Thomsen (1984) reported that 80% of relatives who were interviewed 2.5 years after injury described their family member with a severe TBI as "another person," a finding that several other studies have replicated (McKinlay & Watkiss, 1999). Using traditional psychiatric criteria for personality disorder, Hibbard, Uysal, et al. (2000) estimated that around one quarter of their TBI group had personality disorder characteristics prior to injury but that after injury over 60% showed such characteristics. Table 5.2 lists common behavioral disturbances documented by Prigatano (1992) in his comprehensive review of literature. Insufficient

TABLE 5.2   Emotional and Motivational Disturbances Associated with TBI

Active types	Passive types
Irritability	Aspontaneity
Agitation	Sluggishness
Belligerence/anger	Loss of interest in environment
Impulsiveness	Loss of drive or initiative
Impatience	Tires easily
Restlessness	Depression
Inappropriate social responses	
Emotional lability	
Sensitivity to noise or distress	
Anxiety	
Suspiciousness or mistrust of others	
Delusional beliefs	
Paranoia	
Mania or manic-like states	

Note. From Prigatano (1992).

control of impulses and behavioral excesses versus lack of drive or inertia appear as themes in clinical observation.

Prigatano distinguishes between the direct and reactive emotional changes that result from TBI. Some difficulties such as impulsivity or loss of initiation may flow directly from the frontal/diffuse neuropathology of TBI, whereas problems such as irritability and depression may signify a psychological reaction to catastrophic loss and repeated failure in day-to-day life. Understanding the distinction between direct and reactive emotional effects is clinically important because reactive emotional problems may be more amenable to psychotherapeutic treatment than neurologically-based behavioral impairments, which may respond to pharmacological therapy.

UNAWARENESS OF DEFICITS

A SIGNIFICANT PROPORTION of persons with TBI who present with clearcut cognitive and behavioral difficulties report that they have nothing wrong with them or that whatever problems they do have will not interfere with their participation in life. This impaired recognition of deficits is called anosognosia. The capacity for self-awareness, which fundamentally involves the comparison of self against relevant standards, has been described as the superordinate function of the frontal lobes (Stuss, 1991). In research investigations, unawareness may be measured by comparing self-ratings of ability with ratings made by family members or rehabilitation staff. People with TBI have a tendency to minimize cognitive and behavioral impairments (Prigatano & Altman, 1990; Sherer et al., 1998). Clinically, unawareness may result in choosing a level of work that is beyond actual abilities or failure to recognize the negative impact of behavior on others. Providing gentle confrontation or performance feedback about deficits to a person with unawareness may create temporary confusion or disbelief, without changing insight or behavior (Prigatano, 1991). The proportion of unawareness that is neurologically-based varies among individuals, depending on their coping style. Self-protective psychological denial, activated by the painful feelings of loss associated with trauma, may interfere with insight as well. Unawareness is the bane of rehabilitation, for people are less likely to cooperate with remediation of problems that, from their perspective, do not exist.

CONTINUUM OF OUTCOME AND MEASUREMENT OF SEVERITY OF TBI

TBI PRODUCES A wide continuum of outcomes, ranging from death to return of normal function, with varying degrees of disability in between. Criteria for assessing outcome include rating scales for specific functional abilities, neuropsychological tests, productivity and employment status, living arrangements after rehabilitation, social and emotional functioning, length of hospitalization, and cost of care (Hall & Johnston, 1994).

One widely accepted measure for classifying global outcome following TBI is the Glasgow Outcome Scale (GOS), which classifies outcome as follows: (a) death, (b) persistent vegetative state (i.e., no conscious awareness or purposeful activity), (c) severe disability (conscious but physically or cognitively dependent on others for daily care), (d) moderate disability (disabled but independent in self-care and basic access to community), and (e) good recovery (mild, persistent residual sequelae but capable of normal social life) (Jennett & Bond, 1975); an extended version of the scale has been developed to provide additional gradations within outcome categories (Wilson, Pettigrew, & Teasdale, 1998). The GOS has received criticism for its relative crudeness and insensitivity to higher-level cognitive and emotional problems (Lezak, 1995). However, use of the GOS has been invaluable in understanding the relationship between severity of TBI and long-term outcome.

Although many personal and environmental variables may affect brain injury recovery, the initial severity of TBI, as determined by objective measures, is one of the most important predictors of eventual out-come. Several objective methods exist for grading the severity of TBI, including duration and depth of unconsciousness, length of posttrau-matic amnesia, and radiologic findings.

LEVEL OF COMA

THE GLASGOW COMA Scale (GCS; Table 5.3) is the most widely used clinical indicator of initial severity of TBI (Teasdale & Jennett, 1974). The GCS measures level of consciousness based on eye opening, capacity for purposeful movement, and verbalization.

GCS scores vary from 3 (profound coma) to 15 (normal awareness and orientation). By definition, GCS ratings in the range of 3–8 denote severe TBI; 9–12, moderate TBI; and 13–15, mild TBI. In a review of nine large-scale studies, severe TBI (defined by GCS of 8 or lower at 6 hours or more postinjury) resulted in the following GOS classifications at 6 months: dead, 42%; vegetative, 3%; severe disability, 10%; moderate disability, 13%; and good recovery, 33% (Eisenberg, 1985). In general, lower initial GCS scores are associated with greater mortality (Jennett et al., 1979).

For persons served by the TBI Model Systems, the average lowest GCS

TABLE 5.3   Glasgow Coma Scale

Eye opening (E)
Spontaneous	4
To speech	3
To pain	2
Nil	1

Best motor response (M)
Obeys	6
Localizes	5
Withdraws	4
Abnormal flexion	3
Extensor response	2
Nil	1

Verbal response (V)
Oriented	5
Confused conversation	4
Inappropriate words	3
Incomprehensible sounds	2
Nil	1

Coma score (E + M + V) = 3 to 15.

Note. From Teasdale and Jennett (1974).

score is 7. Outcomes are fairly divided among severe, moderate, and good recovery, with approximately 30% in each category, suggesting heterogeneity of outcome even at severe levels of injury (Millis, 2004).

DURATION OF COMA

ANOTHER IMPORTANT OUTCOME predictor, duration of coma, may be defined as the number of days between the onset of injury and consistent ability to follow commands based on the motor subscale of the GCS. In a series of studies, Dikmen and her colleagues have shown that coma duration measured by time to follow commands (TFC) predicts GOS classification, functional abilities, cognitive status at one year, and likelihood of return to work (Dikmen, Machamer, Winn, & Temkin, 1995; Dikmen, Temkin, et al., 1994; Whyte, Cifu, Dikmen, & Temkin, 2001). People with TFC of less than 1 hour performed at the same level as controls on a neuropsychological test battery, but as TFC increased, so did cognitive impairment. Individuals with 1–13 days of coma showed selective impairments of cognitive functioning, whereas coma of 14 days or more predicted pervasive deficits and lower probability of return to work. The chances of good recovery clearly decrease with coma duration of 1 month or longer. A review of 434 TBI cases with more than one month of coma found that only 7% eventually reached the good recovery classification on the GOS (Multi-Society Task Force on PVS, 1994).

DURATION OF PTA

Russell (1932) proposed the classic scheme for classifying severity of TBI according to duration of PTA:

PTA < 1 hour = mild brain injury
PTA 1–24 hours = moderate injury
PTA 1–7 days = severe injury
PTA > 7 days = very severe injury

Table 5.4 shows the relationship between PTA and outcome, illustrating that longer PTA corresponds with increased frequency of severe disability (Wilson, Pettigrew, & Teasdale, 2000).

RADIOLOGICAL FINDINGS

Radiologic procedures such as computed tomography (CT) scanning and magnetic resonance imaging (MRI) provide information about severity, particularly in the acute stage of medical care. CT reveals structural injuries such as skull fractures as well as the presence of hemorrhage,

TABLE 5.4 Duration of Posttraumatic Amnesia (PTA) and Glasgow Outcome Scale (GOS) Classification During the First Year Following TBI

Duration of PTA	N	Severe disability (%)	Moderate disability (%)	Good recovery (%)
<1 hr	13	0	23	77
1–2 hrs	15	0	20	80
1–7 days	46	22	37	41
>7 days	61	48	34	18

Note. From Wilson, Pettigrew and Teasdale (2000).

hematomas, and cerebral edema. Severe brain injury, as measured by GCS, results in abnormal head CT scan findings in 95% of cases, whereas moderate TBI produces abnormal CT findings in only 25% of cases. Mild TBI rarely is disclosed by CT (Levin, Amparo, et al., 1987). Acute abnormalities on CT increase the long-term probability of restrictions in mobility, activities of daily living, and ability to live without supervision (Englander, Cifu, Wright, & Black, 2003).

MRI appears superior in detecting nonhemorrhagic white matter lesions in TBI and thus may have greater sensitivity to diffuse injuries that do not involve bleeding contusions or hematomas. MRI with T2-weighted imaging has detected DAI in some people with mild TBI whose CT findings were normal (Mittl et al., 1994). The severity of DAI, estimated radiologically by determining the volume of fluid space within the brain or the surface area of specific structures, correlates fairly well with cognitive outcome (Bigler, 2001). For example, one study showed that the size of the fornix, a white matter bundle in the deep temporal region, relates to cognitive performance; individuals with the smallest fornix size obtained the lowest scores on tests of memory (Gale, Johnson, Bigler, & Blatter, 1995).

LIMITATIONS OF SEVERITY RATINGS

THE GENERALLY POSITIVE statistical relationship between early measures of TBI severity and later outcome still is far from perfect. The terms mild, moderate, and severe applied at or near the time of the trauma are not intended to characterize subsequent disability in a simplistic, one-to-one manner. Indicators of severe brain injury—say, an initial GCS of 5 and PTA of 3 weeks—do not preclude the possibility of a favorable outcome in an individual case. By the same token, a mild brain injury may result in a poor outcome for a given person. Confusing initial severity with outcome may cause misconceptions in the study of milder injuries, where clinicians minimize or even reject the likelihood of complicated recovery (Dikmen & Levin, 1993).

MULTIVARIATE MODELS OF OUTCOME PREDICTION

TBI OUTCOME HAS numerous physical, cognitive, and social aspects, subject to influence by a variety of factors besides severity of injury. Thus, researchers in the TBI Model Systems have increasingly used multivariate statistical models to weigh the effects of multiple variables on outcome (Bush et al., 2003; Novack, Bush, Meythaler, & Canupp, 2001). Table 5.5 shows factors included in a contemporary predictive model of outcome at one year. Empirical tests of the model indicate complex relationships among the variables. For instance, injury severity does not appear determine outcome directly; instead, severity is associated with cognitive and functional status, which then predicts outcome. Premorbid factors such as level of education and substance abuse relate to initial severity and outcome, implying that people that people with more effective preinjury functioning tend to have less severe injuries and better outcomes. Strong links in the model between outcome and cogni-

TABLE 5.5   A Multivariate Model for Predicting TBI Outcome

Predictor variables	Outcomes
Premorbid factors	Disability
Age	Self-care activities
Education	Dependence on others
Employment	
Social difficulties	Community integration
Injury severity	Home integration
GCS	Social integration
PTA	Productive activities
CT scan results	
Cognitive status	
Memory	
Processing speed	
Visual problem-solving	
Functional status	
Mobility	
Speech	
Feeding self	

Note. From Bush et al. (2003).

tive/functional status suggest that improved rehabilitation of these impairments has the potential to improve global outcome (Bush et al.).

COURSE AND MECHANISMS OF RECOVERY AFTER TBI

T HE NATURAL HISTORY of TBI includes sudden onset, a variable length of unconsciousness and PTA, a period of recovery, and residual sequelae. The course of recovery generally follows a negatively accelerating curve, as depicted in Figure 5.2. People often make marked gains in the first several months after trauma, followed by a longer period of slowly tapering improvement (Levin, 1985). In general, the less severe the injury, the closer recovery may approximate pre-injury functioning. For severe TBI, the phase of rapid improvement contains dramatic gains in basic attention, day-to-day memory, ambulation, and performance of basic activities of daily living. A longer stage follows that centers on reacquisition of complex cognitive and interpersonal skills. Table 5.6 shows the Rancho Los Amigos Level of Cognitive Functioning Scale, a classification scheme that describes the phases of recovery often evident during acute recovery (Center for Outcome Measurement in Brain Injury, 2000).

Research reveals varying estimates for the time frame of recovery. For example, studies using the GCS have shown that 90% of people with TBI attain their ultimate outcome classification within 6 months. In contrast, more sensitive neuropsychological studies have documented functional improvement over 2 or 3 years (Levin, 1985). Thomsen (1984, 1990) followed a group of 40 persons with very severe brain injuries over a

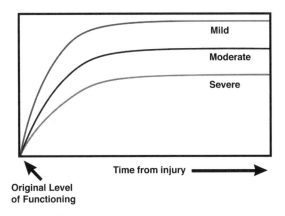

FIGURE 5.2   Negatively accelerating course of recovery following brain injury.

TABLE 5.6   Rancho Level of Cognitive Functioning Scale

Level I	No response to stimuli
Level II	Generalized response to stimuli
Level III	Localized response to stimuli
Level IV	Confused, agitated response
Level V	Confused, inappropriate, nonagitated response
Level VI	Confused, appropriate response
Level VII	Automatic, appropriate response
Level VIII	Purposeful, appropriate response

10–15-year period, finding that a mixture of both positive and negative functional changes occurred during that time. Recent TBIMS studies reveal a variable pattern of recovery among individuals between one and five years post injury, but the majority do not improve. Using a standardized neuropsychological test battery, Millis et al. (2001) found 62.6% of people were unchanged between 1 and 5 years, 22.2% improved, and 15.2% declined. Ratings of ability to live independently and employability mirrored neuropsychological findings, with 76%–79% of people remaining the same and less than 20% improving (Hammond et al., 2004).

Neuroscience is beginning to unravel the mechanisms by which the brain heals itself following injury (Stein, Brailowsky, & Will, 1995; Turkstra, Holland, & Bays, 2003). As evidenced by the many instances of remarkable recovery after TBI, the brain possesses resilience and plasticity. One theory of recovery is based on the construct of "brain reserve capacity" (Satz, 1993). This theory holds that the brain has latent or redundant pathways, permitting some neuronal injury to occur without necessarily impairing function. Once brain reserves are exhausted, then impairments become manifest. In TBIs, individuals with severe injury who have excellent recovery probably are drawing on strong neuronal reserves.

Research in animals has demonstrated that nerve cells may form new connections after injury by collateral sprouting of dendrites and thereby restore some lost function. Another recovery mechanism involves increased sensitivity of receptor sites so that neural circuits can work despite the absence of some neurons. Environmental context plays a role in these mechanisms because better recovery takes place in enriched environments than in deprived ones. The stimulation and challenge of rehabilitation activities after TBI likely facilitates neurological recovery, however incomplete. In the future, the "cure" for TBI may center on the recruitment of restoration processes by means of pharmacological and environmental interventions.

OBSERVATIONS ON MILD TBI

W E WISH TO include a separate section on mild TBI because this disorder possesses unique features not covered by our previous discussion. Mild TBI is defined by (a) application of force to the head, (b) loss of consciousness for less than 30 minutes or simply dazed consciousness, (c) PTA not more than 24 hours, and (d) initial GCS of 13–15 within 30 minutes of injury (Evans, 1992). Commonly recognized early symptoms of mild TBI include headache, dizziness, fatigue, insomnia, memory difficulties, impaired concentration, ringing in the ears, sensitivity to lights and noises, depression, anxiety, and irritability (Lishman, 1998).

Mild TBI recently has attracted considerable interest (Alexander, 1995; Rees, 2003; Satz, Alfano, et al., 1999). Prospective clinical studies reveal that 85%–90% of individuals with mild TBI return to normal functioning with little or no intervention (Levin, Mattis, et al., 1987).

A vigorous and sometimes partisan debate revolves around the topic of why certain people fail to recover function after mild TBI. At issue is the relative contribution of neuropathology versus psychological factors such as posttraumatic stress, somatization, and impaired motivation in connection with pending personal injury litigation. The controversy is not merely an academic one, because if we assume that 80% of all TBI are mild in degree and that mild TBI results in disability even 10% of the time, then thousands of people may suffer disabling mild injuries each year (Kraus & Sorenson, 1994).

From our perspective, "minor" brain trauma is like minor surgery: it's only minor if it happens to somebody else. The etiology of mild TBI symptoms probably has both neurological and psychological components, and for each individual, multiple factors interact to produce dysfunction.

Three lines of evidence implicate a neurological component for sequelae of mild TBI (Alexander, 1995). First, animal research models and human autopsy studies demonstrate that observable, permanent damage occurs to brain structure after "mild" trauma (Jane, Steward, & Gennarelli, 1985). Second, various forms of physical stress can unmask symptoms in otherwise asymptomatic cases (see Gronwall, 1989, for a review). For example, one study showed that college students who had sustained mild TBI and appeared to recover were abnormally prone to mental inefficiency when physiologically stressed by hypoxic conditions. Third, studies of collegiate athletes who sustain concussion in sports indicate specific impairments in cognition and balance on repeated examinations. Although symptoms typically resolve within 2 to 7 days, the presence of these acute neuropsychological and physical deficits is compatible with neurological injury (Macciocchi, Barth, Alves, Rimel, & Jane, 1996; McCrea et al., 2003).

Effects of mild TBI that begin as neurological symptoms may be maintained by psychological variables long after the physical injury has resolved. Psychogenic factors contributing to mild TBI symptoms include preinjury personality and reactive emotional distress in connection with cognitive deficits. Individuals prone to somatization—that is, the expression of psychological stress in the form of physical symptoms—may be particularly vulnerable to chronic impairment. The symptoms of mild TBI are found among individuals who have been exposed to stressors but have never had a blow to the head. Accordingly, examination of mild TBI requires consideration of sources for complaint other than brain injury. Rees (2003) argues that post-concussion syndrome primarily reflects nonspecific posttraumatic stress.

A relationship exists between involvement in litigation and symptom severity insofar as litigants are much more likely than nonlitigants to report persisting problems. Interestingly, the settlement of litigation generally does not improve symptoms, so simple desire for financial gain does not entirely account for symptom formation (Rutherford, 1989). Nevertheless, because financial incentives are associated with successful litigation involving brain damage, a certain proportion of individuals who have been involved in an accident or assault may contrive or exaggerate deficits that they either never suffered or that have resolved to a greater extent than expressed at the time of clinical examination. Specialized techniques have been developed to detect malingering. Numerous research investigations indicate poorer performance by litigating mild TBI patients than by nonlitigating patients with severe brain injuries (Binder, 1997; Larrabee, 1997).

PSYCHOLOGICAL AND VOCATIONAL IMPLICATIONS OF TBI

IN TBI MODELS Systems, more than 90% of people with moderate to severe TBI eventually leave hospital or residential care and return to live in their home communities on a long-term basis (Millis, 2004). Although the high percentage of individuals living at home marks a desirable and impressive outcome, numerous investigations have clearly shown that people with TBI confront enormous challenges in psychosocial functioning and that cognitive and behavioral disorders impair adaptation to a greater extent than physical problems do. This section provides an overview of psychosocial sequelae of TBI, including problems with psychological adjustment, community integration, impact on families, and vocational issues.

Psychological Adjustment

Prigatano (1994) uses the metaphor of life's journey to describe psychological adjustment after brain injury. A person who is progressing along a certain path through life and who suddenly has a TBI may wish to continue along the same road, even though this is no longer possible. Finding a new path (or failing to find one) defines the struggle of living with a brain injury. Prigatano also observes that people with TBI repeatedly confront three existential questions: (I) "Why did this happen to me?" (2) "Will I ever be normal again?" (3) "Is life worth living after brain injury?" (pp. 174–175). He believes that individuals with the internal resources to come to grips with their impairments and redefine themselves tend to become productive again.

The empirical literature on psychosocial outcome following TBI suggests that many people have trouble adapting successfully. Dikmen and her colleagues (2003) found that 45–60% of people in their long-term outcome study reported restrictions in major activity (work or school) social integration, and recreation. Similarly, another study showed that in comparison to nondisabled peers, people with TBI experience lower quality of life in several areas, including satisfaction of basic needs, independence, social support, productivity at home, employability, and use of leisure time (Gordon, Hibbard, Brown, Flanagan, & Campbell, 1999).

The theme of loneliness and isolation emerges in studies of psychosocial sequelae. People with TBI face a high risk of loss of relationships and social support, as evidenced by decreased number of friends, fewer social contacts, and recreational activity in the community (Morton & Wehman, 1995). Individuals with more severe injuries may tend to become more isolated because they may lack access to the community (e.g., not driving) and have more noticeable alteration in interpersonal skills. Jacobs (1988) noted that people who are single at the time of TBI tend to remain single. Negative changes in sexual behavior occur commonly, including physiological difficulties and body image concerns (Hibbard, Gordon, Flanagan, Haddad, & Labinsky, 2000).

Not surprisingly, a parallel psychosocial theme is the development of emotional disorders such as anxiety and depression. Clinical studies suggest that people with TBI have increased risk for depression, with up to 30 to 40% meeting diagnostic criteria for major depressive disorder in the post-acute phase (Deb, Lyons, Koutzoukis, Ali, & McCarthy, 1999; Hibbard, Uysal, Kepler, Bogdany, & Silver, 1998; Jorge et al., 2004; Kreutzer, Seel, & Gourley, 2001; Seel & Kruetzer, 2003). Neurobehavioral symptoms frequently reported by TBI patients include frustration, restlessness, rumination, boredom, and sadness (Seel & Kreutzer, 2003). Prolonged depressive episodes may interfere with recovery, as evidenced by deceased functional status at one year (Jorge, Robinson, Starkstein, & Arndt, 1994).

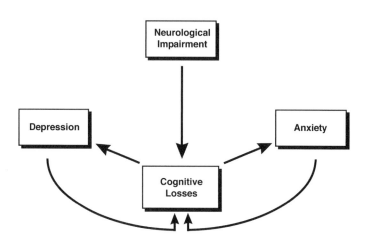

FIGURE 5.3 Relationship between neurocognitive losses and emotional functioning after brain injury.

Anxiety disorders such as generalized anxiety, panic disorder, and post-traumatic stress disorder (PTSD) also have been associated with TBI (Hiott & Labatte, 2002). For example, one study found that 18% of a community sample of individuals with severe TBI endorsed moderate-to-severe PTSD symptoms (Williams, Evans, Wilson, & Needham, 2002).

The cognitive and emotional disorders following TBI may interact with each other in a vicious cycle, as depicted in Figure 5.3. For example, the slowing, decreased concentration and poor initiative that characterize depression may intensify cognitive losses resulting from brain damage. The intensified cognitive losses, in turn, serve as a focus for increased self-depreciation, depression, and anxiety.

IMPACT OF TBI ON FAMILIES

TBI PRESENTS A challenge not only to the person who is injured but for the entire family (Dikmen, Machamer, Savoie, & Temkin, 1996; Kreutzer, Marwitz, & Kepler, 1992). Relatives typically experience stress and a sense of burden, beginning with the initial catastrophe of the injury and acute hospitalization and continuing long afterward. In cases of severe TBI, families often hear initial medical reports that their loved one may not live; great relief ensues when the person survives, followed by a long period of gradual understanding of residual problems.

Research consistently has found that a significant proportion of family members report stress, anxiety, and depression. Some studies suggest that the perceived burden of caring for the person disabled by TBI increases over time. The caregiver distress caused by physical impairments appears to be relatively short lived, decreasing within the first year postinjury, while neurobehavioral and cognitive problems have a greater and more persistent impact (Marsh, Kersel, Havill, & Sleigh 2002). Social support appears to buffer the distress experienced by families. Ergh, Hanks, Rapport, and Coleman (2003) showed that cognitive dysfunction increases caregiver dissatisfaction, but only in people with low perceived social support.

Family functioning prior to the injury probably affects post injury adjustment. In a study of three TBI Model Systems centers, Sander et al. (2003) found that 25%–33% of caregivers reported unhealthy family functioning in the month before the injury. Preinjury family conflicts may increase vulnerability to distress.

Financial drain from the costs of TBI represents another stressor. For example, Jacobs (1988) found that 34% of families reported mild to moderate financial drain and that some family members had to give up working in order to care for the individual with TBI or spend substantial sums on professional caregivers.

Return to Work After TBI

ALTHOUGH POSTINJURY EMPLOYMENT rates vary from sample to sample, research invariably shows that TBI results in an increase in unemployment (Sander, Kreutzer, Rosenthal, Delmonico, & Young, 1996). Two widely cited studies found that 80% of persons with severe TBI were employed prior to injury but only 30% were able to resume working (Brooks, McKinlay, Symington, Beattie, & Campsie, 1987; Jacobs, 1988). The TBI Models Systems reports a decrease in competitive employment from approximately 61% preinjury to 30% postinjury at the time of 5- and 10-year follow-ups (Millis, 2004). Demographic groups at risk for unemployment consist of minority group members, people who did not complete high school, and unmarried people (Kreutzer et al., 2003). In addition, a preinjury history of substance abuse dramatically reduces the likelihood of employment (Sherer, Bergloff, High, & Nick, 1999). Many people with TBI who are able to return to work may have to change jobs in order to accommodate impaired abilities; job changes of this nature entail reductions in pay and status, perhaps engendering resistance, anger, and feelings of loss.

The severity of TBI and associated neurobehavioral impairments have predictive value in determining the probability vocational success. As problems with cognitive and interpersonal problems increase, the chances of successful employment generally decrease (Dikmen et al., 1994; Yasuda, Wehman, Targett, Cifu, & West, 2001). A review of by Sherer et al. (2002) found considerable support for the use of early neuropsychological assessment to predict employment outcome. However, other factors, such as level of job availability, employer attitudes toward disability, access to rehabilitation services, and driving play a role in employment. Intensive neuropsychological rehabilitation and supported employment have shown some success in enhancing employment outcomes for people with TBI (Klonoff, Lamb, & Henderson, 2000; Yasuda et al., 2001). In many respects, vocational struggles exemplify the complex physical, cognitive, and interpersonal effects of brain injury on the efficacy of the individual.

REFERENCES

Adams, J. H., Graham, D. I., & Gennarelli, T. A. (1985). Contemporary neuropathological considerations regarding brain damage in head injury. In D. P. Becker & J. T. Povlishock (Eds.), *Central nervous system trauma status report* (pp. 65–77). Bethesda, MD: National Institutes of Health.

Alexander, M. P. (1995). Mild traumatic brain injury: Pathophysiology, natural history, and clinical management. *Neurology, 45,* 1253–1260.

Bigler, E. D. (2001). Quantitative magnetic resonance imaging in traumatic brain injury. *Journal of Head Trauma Rehabilitation, 16,* 117–34.

Binder, L. M. (1997). A review of mild head trauma. Part 2. Clinical implications. *Journal of Clinical and Experimental Neuropsychology, 19,* 433–458.

Brooks, N., McKinlay, W., Symington, C., Beattie, A., & Campsie, L. (1987). Return to work within the first seven years of severe head injury. *Brain Injury, 1,* 5–19.

Bush, B. A., Novack, T. A., Malec, J. F., Stringer, A. Y., Millis, S. R., & Madan, A. (2003). Validation of a model for evaluating outcome after traumatic brain injury. *Archives of Physical Medicine and Rehabilitation, 84,* 1803–1807.

Bushnik, T. (2003). Introduction: The Traumatic Brain Injury Model Systems of Care. *Archives of Physical Medicine and Rehabilitation, 84,* 151–152.

Center for Outcome Measurement in Brain Injury. (2000, March). *Level of Cognitive Functioning Scale.* Retrieved on May 18, 2004, from http://www.tbims.org/combi/lcfs/index.html

Centers for Disease Control and Prevention. (1999, December). *Traumatic brain injury in the United States: A report to Congress.* Retrieved on May 5, 2004, from http://www.cdc.gov/doc.do/id/0900f3ec8001012b.

Corrigan, J. D. (1995). Substance abuse as a mediating factor in outcome from traumatic brain injury. *Archives of Physical Medicine and Rehabilitation, 76,* 302–309.

Deb, S., Lyons, I., Koutzoukis, C., Ali, I., & McCarthy, G. (1999). Rate of psychiatric illness 1 year after traumatic brain injury. *American Journal of Psychiatry, 156,* 374–378.

Dikmen, S., & Levin, H. S. (1993). Methodological issues in the study of mild head injury. *Journal of Head Trauma Rehabilitation, 8,* 30–37.

Dikmen, S. S., Machamer, J. E., Powell, J. M., & Temkin, N. R. (2003). Outcome 3 to 5 years after moderate to severe traumatic brain injury. *Archives of Physical Medicine and Rehabilitation, 84,* 1449–1457.

Dikmen, S., Machamer, J., Savoie, T., & Temkin, N. (1996). Life quality outcome in head injury. In I. Grant & K. M. Adams (Eds.), *Neuropsychological assessment of neuropsychiatric disorders* (2nd ed., pp. 552–576). New York: Oxford University Press.

Dikmen, S., Machamer, J. E., Winn, H. R., & Temkin, N. R. (1995). Neuropsychological outcome at 1-year post head injury. *Neuropsychology, 9,* 80–90.

Dikmen, S. S., Temkin, N. R., Machamer, J. E., Holubkov, A. L., Fraser, R. T., & Winn, H. R. (1994). Employment following traumatic head injuries. *Archives of Neurology, 51,* 177–186.

Dijkers, M. P. (2004). Quality of life after traumatic brain injury: A review of research approach and findings. *Archives of Physical Medicine and Rehabilitation, 85,* S21–35.

Doppenberg, E. M., Choi, S. C., & Bullock, R. (2004). Clinical trails in traumatic brain injury: Lessons for the future. *Journal of Neurosurgical Anesthesiology, 16,* 87–94.

Eisenberg, H. M. (1985). Outcome after head injury: Part 1. General considerations. In D. P. Becker & J. T. Povlishock (Eds.), *Central nervous system trauma status report* (pp. 271–280). Bethesda, MD: National Institutes of Health.

Englander, J. Cifu, D. X., Wright, J. M., & Black, K. (2003). The association of early computed tomography scan findings and ambulation, self-care, and supervision needs at rehabilitation discharge and at 1 year after traumatic brain injury. *Archives of Physical Medicine and Rehabilitation, 84,* 14–20.

Ergh, T. C., Hanks, R. A., Rapport, L. J., & Coleman, R. D. (2003). Social support moderates caregiver life satisfaction following traumatic brain injury. *Journal of Clinical Experimental Neuropsychology, 25,* 1090–1101.

Evans, R. W. (1992). Mild traumatic brain injury. *Physical Medicine and Rehabilitation Clinics of North America, 3,* 427–439.

Gale, S. D., Johnson, S. C., Bigler, E. D., & Blatter, D. D. (1995). Nonspecific white matter degeneration following traumatic brain injury. *Journal of the International Neuropsychological Society, 1,* 17–28.

Gil, M., Cohen, M., Korn, C., & Grosswater, Z. (1996). Vocational outcome of aphasic patients following severe traumatic brain injury. *Brain Injury, 10,* 39–45.

Gordon, W. A., Hibbard, M. R., Brown, M., Flanagan, S., & Kloves, M. C. (1999). Community integration and quality of life of individuals with traumatic brain injury. In M. Rosenthal, J. S. Kreutzer, E. R. Griffith, & B. Pentland (Eds.), *Rehabilitation of the adult and child with traumatic brain injury* (3rd ed., pp. 312–325). Philadelphia: F. A. Davis.

Gronwall, D. (1989). Cumulative and persisting effects of concussion on attention and cognition. In H. S. Levin, H. M. Eisenberg, & A. L. Benton (Eds.), *Mild head injury* (pp. 153–163). New York: Oxford University Press.

Hall, K. M., & Johnston, M. V. (1994). Outcomes evaluation in TBI rehabilitation. Part 2. Measurement tools for a nationwide data system. *Archives of Physical Medicine and Rehabilitation, 75*, SC10–SC18.

Hammond, F. M., Grattan, K. D., Sasser, H., Corrogan, J. D., Rosenthal, M., Bushnik, T., et al. (2004). Five years after traumatic brain injury: A study of individual outcomes and predictors of change in function. *NeuroRehabilitation, 19*, 25–35.

Hammond, F. M., & McDeavitt, J. T. (1999). Medical and orthopedic complications. In M. Rosenthal, J. S. Kreutzer, E. R. Griffith, & B. Pentland (Eds.), *Rehabilitation of the adult and child with traumatic brain injury* (3rd ed., pp. 53–73). Philadelphia: F. A. Davis.

Hibbard, M. R., Gordon, W. A., Flanagan, S., Haddad, L., & Labinsky, E. (2000). Sexual dysfunction after traumatic brain injury. *NeuroRehabilitation, 15*, 107–120.

Hibbard, M. R., Uysal, S., Kepler, K., Bogdany, J., & Silver, J. (1998). Axis I psychopathology in individuals with traumatic brain injury. *Journal of Head Trauma Rehabilitation, 13*, 24–39.

Hibbard, M. R., Uysal, S., Kepler, K., Bogdany, J., Silver, J. M., Gordon, W. A., et al. (2000). Axis II psychopathology in individuals with traumatic brain injury. *Brain Injury, 14*, 45–61.

Hiott, D. W., & Labbate, L. (2002). Anxiety disorders associated with traumatic brain injuries. *NeuroRehabilitation, 17*, 345–355.

Jacobs, H. E. (1988). The Los Angeles Head Injury Survey: Procedures and initial findings. *Archives of Physical Medicine and Rehabilitation, 69*, 425–431.

Jane, J. A., Steward, o., & Gennarelli, T. (1985). Axonal degeneration induced by experimental noninvasive minor head injury. *Journal of Neurosurgery, 62*, 96–100.

Jennett, B., & Bond, M. (1975). Assessment of outcome after severe brain damage: A practical scale. *Lancet, 1*, 480–484.

Jennett, B., Teasdale, B., Braakman, R., Minderhoud, J., Heiden, J., & Kurze, T. (1979). Prognosis of patients with severe head injury. *Neurosurgery, 4*, 283–289.

Jorge, R. E., Robinson, R. G., Moser, D., Tateno, A., Crespo-Facorro, B., & Arndt, S. (2004). Major depression following traumatic brain injury. *Archives of General Psychiatry, 61*, 42–50.

Jorge, R. E., Robinson, R. G., Starkstein, S. E., & Arndt, S. V. (1994). Influence of major depression on 1-year outcome in patients with traumatic brain injury. *Journal of Neurosurgery, 81*, 726–733.

Klonoff, P. S., Lamb, D. G., & Henderson, S. W. (2000). Milieu-based neurorehabilitation in patients with traumatic brain injury: Outcome at up to 11 years postdischarge. *Archives of Physical Medicine and Rehabilitation, 81*, 1535–1537.

Kraus, J. F., & McArthur, D. L. (1999). Incidence and prevalence of, and costs associated with, traumatic brain injury. In M. Rosenthal, J. S. Kreutzer, E. R.

Griffith, & B. Pentland (Eds.), *Rehabilitation of the adult and child with traumatic brain injury* (3rd ed., pp. 3–18). Philadelphia: F. A. Davis.

Kraus, J. F., & Sorenson, S. B. (1994). Epidemiology. In J. M. Silver, S. C. Yudofsky, & R. E. Hales (Eds.), *Neuropsychiatry of traumatic brain injury* (pp. 3–41). Washington, DC: American Psychiatric Press.

Kreutzer, J. S., Marwitz, J. H., & Kepler, K. (1992). Traumatic brain injury: Family response and outcome. *Archives of Physical Medicine and Rehabilitation, 73,* 771–778.

Kreutzer, J. S., Marwitz, J. H., Walker, W., Sander, A., Sherer, M., Bogner, J., et al. (2003). Moderating factors in return to work and job stability after traumatic brain injury. *Journal of Head Trauma Rehabilitation, 18,* 128–138.

Kreutzer, J. S., Seel, R. T., & Gourley, E. (2001). The prevalence and symptom rates of depression after traumatic brain injury: A comprehensive examination. *Brain Injury, 15*(7), 563–576.

Larrabee, G. J. (1997). Neuropsychological outcome, post concussion symptoms, and forensic considerations in mild closed head trauma. *Seminars in Clinical Neuropsychiatry, 2,* 196–206.

Levin, H. S. (1985). Outcome after head injury: Part 2. Neurobehavioral recovery. In D. P. Becker & J. T. Povlishock (Eds.), *Central nervous system trauma status report*(pp. 281–303). Bethesda, MD: National Institutes of Health, NINCDS.

Levin, H. S. (1997). Memory dysfunction after head injury. In T. E. Feinberg & M. J. Farah (Eds.), *Behavioral neurology and neuropsychology* (pp. 479–489). New York: McGraw-Hill.

Levin, H. S., Amparo, E. G., Eisenberg, H. M., Williams, D. H., High, W. M., McArdle, C. B., et al. (1987). Magnetic resonance imaging and computerized tomography in relation to neurobehavioral sequelae of mild and moderate head injury. *Journal of Neurosurgery, 66,* 706–713.

Levin, H. S., Benton, A. L., & Grossman, R. O. (1982). *Neurobehavioral consequences of closed head injury.* New York: Oxford University Press.

Levin, H. S., Mattis, S. M., Ruff, R. M., Eisenberg, H. M., Marshall, L. F., Tabbador, K., et al. (1987). Neurobehavioral outcome following minor head injury: A three center study. *Journal of Neurosurgery, 66,* 234–243.

Levin, H. S., O'Donnell, V. M., & Grossman, R. G. (1979). The Galveston Orientation and Amnesia Test: A practical scale to assess cognition after head injury. *Journal of Nervous and Mental Disease, 167,* 675–684.

Lezak, M.D. (1995). *Neuropsychological assessment* (3rd ed.). New York: Oxford University Press.

Lishman, W. A. (1998). *Organic psychiatry: The psychological consequences of cerebral disorder* (3rd ed.) Oxford: Blackwell.

Macciocchi, S. N., Barth, J. T., Alves, W., Rimel, R. W., & Jane, J. A. (1996). Neuropsychological functioning and recovery after mild head injury in collegiate athletes. *Neurosurgery, 39,* 510–514.

Marsh, N. V., Kersel, D. A., Havill, J. A., & Sleigh, J. W. (2002). Caregiver burden during the years following severe traumatic brain injury. *Journal of Clinical Experimental Neuropsychology, 24*(4), 434–447.

Mateer, C. A., & Mapou, R. L. (1996). Understanding, evaluating, and managing attention disorders following traumatic brain injury. *Journal of Head Trauma Rehabilitation, 11*, 1–16.

Max, W., MacKenzie, E. J., & Rice, D. P. (1991). Head injuries: Costs and consequences. *Journal of Head Trauma Rehabilitation, 6*, 76–87.

McCrea, M., Guskiewicz, K. M., Marshall, S. W., Barr, W., Randolph, C., Cant, R. C., et al. (2003). Acute effect of recovery time following concussion in collegiate football players: The NCAA Concussion Study. *Journal of the American Medical Association, 290*, 2556–2563.

McDonald, B. C., Flashman, L. A., & Saykin, A. J. (2002). Executive dysfunction following traumatic brain injury: Neural substrates and treatment strategies. *NeuroRehabilitation, 2002, 17*, 333–344.

McKinlay, W. W., & Watkiss, A. J. (1999). Cognitive and behavioral effects of brain injury. In M. Rosenthal, J. S. Kreutzer, E. R. Griffith, & B Pentland (Eds.), *Rehabilitation of the adult and child with traumatic brain injury* (3rd ed., pp. 74–86). Philadelphia: F. A. Davis.

Meythaler, J. M., Peduzzi, J. D., Eleftheriou, E., & Novack, T. A. (2001). Current concepts: Diffuse axonal injury-associated traumatic brain injury. *Archives of Physical Medicine and Rehabilitation, 82*, 1461–1471.

Millis, S. R. (2004). Database update. *Traumatic Brain Injury Facts and Figures, 10*(1), 8–10. Retrieved May 15, 2004 from http://www.tbindc.org/registry/pdf/ff_winter2004.pdf

Millis, S. R., Rosenthal, M., Novack, T. A., Sherer, M., Nick, T. G., et al. (2001). Long-term neuropsychological outcome after traumatic brain injury. *Journal of Head Trauma Rehabilitation, 16*, 343–355.

Mittl, R. L., Grossman, R. I., Hiehle, J. F., Hurst, R. W., Kauder, D. R., Gennarelli, T. A., et al. (1994). Prevalence of MR evidence of diffuse axonal injury in patients with mild head injury and normal head CT findings. *American Journal of Neuroradiology, 15*, 1583–1589.

Morton, M. V., & Wehman, P. (1995). Psychosocial and emotional sequelae of individuals with traumatic brain injury: A literature review and recommendations. *Brain Injury, 9*, 81–92.

Multi-Society Task Force on PVS. (1994). Medical aspects of the persistent vegetative state. *New England Journal of Medicine, 330*, 1572–1579.

NIH Consensus Development Panel. (1999). Consensus conference. Rehabilitation of persons with traumatic brain injury. *Journal of the American Medical Association, 282*, 974–983.

Novack, T. A., Bush, B. A., Meythaler, J. M., & Canupp, K. (2001). Outcome after traumatic brain injury: Pathway analysis of contributions from premorbid, injury severity, and recovery variables. *Archives of Physical Medicine and Rehabilitation, 82*, 300–305.

Prigatano, G. P. (1991). Disturbances of self-awareness of deficit after traumatic brain injury. In G. P. Prigatano & D. L. Schacter (Eds.), *Awareness of deficit after brain injury: Clinical and theoretical issues* (pp. 111–126). New York: Oxford University Press.

Prigatano, G. P. (1992). Personality disturbances associated with traumatic brain injury. *Journal of Consulting and Clinical Psychology, 60,* 360–368.

Prigatano, G. P. (1994). Individuality, lesion location, and psychotherapy after brain injury. In A. L. Christensen & B. P. Uzzell (Eds.), *Brain injury and neuropsychological rehabilitation: International perspectives* (pp. 173–186). Hillsdale, NJ: Lawrence Erlbaum Associates.

Prigatano, G. P. (1999). *Principles of neuropsychological rehabilitation.* New York: Oxford University Press.

Prigatano, G. P., & Altman, I. M. (1990). Impaired awareness of behavioral limitations after traumatic brain injury. *Archives of Physical Medicine and Rehabilitation, 71,* 1058–1064.

Prigatano, G. P., & Borgaro, S. R. (2003). Qualitative features of finger movement during the Halstead finger oscillation test following traumatic brain injury. *Journal of the International Neuropsychological Society, 9,* 128–133.

Rees, P. M. (2003). Contemporary issues in mild traumatic brain injury. *Archives of Physical Medicine Rehabilitation, 84,* 1885–1894.

Russell, W. R. (1932). Cerebral involvement in head injury. *Brain, 55,* 549–603.

Rutherford, W. H. (1989). Concussion symptoms: Relationship to acute neurological indices, individual differences, and circumstances of injury. In H. S. Levin, H. M. Eisenberg, & A. L. Benton (Eds.), *Mild head injury* (pp. 217–228). New York: Oxford University Press.

Sander, A. M., Kreutzer, J. S., Rosenthal, M., Delmonico, R., & Young, M. E. (1996). A multicenter longitudinal investigation of return to work and community integration following traumatic brain injury. *Journal of Head Trauma Rehabilitation, 11,* 70–84.

Sander, A. M., Sherer, M., Malec, J. F., High, W. M., Thompson, R. N., Moessner, A. M., et al. (2003). Preinjury emotional and family functioning in caregivers of persons with traumatic brain injury. *Archives of Physical Medicine Rehabilitation, 84,* 197–203.

Satz, P. (1993). Brain reserve capacity on symptom onset after brain injury: A formulation and review of evidence for threshold theory. *Neuropsychology, 7,* 273–295

Satz, P. S., Alfano, M. S., Light, R. F., Morgenstern, H. F., Zaucha, K. F., Asarnow, R. F., et al. (1999). Persistent post-concussive syndrome: A proposed methodology and literature review to determine the effects, if any, of mild head and other bodily injury. *Journal of Clinical and Experimental Neuropsychology, 21,* 620–628.

Seel, R. T., & Kreutzer, J. S. (2003). Depression assessment after traumatic brain injury: An empirically based classification method. *Archives of Physical Medicine Rehabilitation, 84,* 1621–1628.

Sherer, M., Boake, C., Levin, E., Silver, B. V., Ringholz, G., & High, W. M. (1998).

Characteristics of impaired awareness after traumatic brain injury. *Journal of the International Neuropsychological Society, 4,* 380–387.

Sherer, M., Bergloff, P., High, W., Jr., & Nick, T. G. (1999). Contributions of functional ratings to prediction of longterm employment outcomes after traumatic brain injury. *Brain Injury, 13,* 973–981.

Sherer, M., Novack, T. A., Sander, A. M., Struchen, M. A., Alderson, A., & Thompson, R. N. (2002). Neuropsychological assessment and employment outcomes after traumatic brain injury: A review. *Clinical Neuropsychologist, 16,* 157–178.

Stein, D. G., Brailowsky, S., & Will, B. (1995). *Brain repair.* New York: Oxford University Press.

Stein, D. G., Glasier, M. M., & Hoffman, S. W. (1994). Pharmacological treatments for brain injury repair: Progress and prognosis. In A. L. Christensen & B. P. Uzzell (Eds.), *Brain injury and neuropsychological rehabilitation: International perspectives* (pp. 17–39). Hillsdale, NJ: Lawrence Erlbaum Associates.

Stuss, D. T. (1991). Disturbances of self-awareness after frontal system damage. In G. P. Prigatano & D. L. Schacter (Eds.), *Awareness of deficit after brain injury: Clinical and theoretical issues* (pp. 63–83). New York: Oxford University Press.

Stuss, D. T., Gallup, G. G., & Alexander, M. P. (2001). The frontal lobes are necessary for `theory of mind'. *Brain, 124,* 279–286.

Stuss, D. T., & Levine, B. (2002). Adult clinical neuropsychology: Lessons from studies of the frontal lobes. *Annual Review of Psychology, 53,* 401–433.

Symonds, C. P. (1937). Mental disorder following bead injury. *Proceedings of the Royal Society of Medicine, 30,* 1081–1092.

Tangney, J. P., Baumeister, R. F., & Boone, A. L. (2004). High self-control predicts good adjustment, less pathology, better grades, and interpersonal success. *Journal of Personality, 72,* 271–324.

Teasdale, G., & Jennett, B. (1974). Assessment of coma and impaired consciousness. *Lancet, 2,* 81–84.

Thomsen, I. V. (1984). Late outcome of very severe blunt head trauma: A 10–15 year follow-up. *Journal of Neurology, Neurosurgery, and Psychiatry, 47,* 250–268.

Thomsen, I. V. (1990). Recognizing the development of behavior disorders. In R. L. I. Wood (Ed.), *Neurobehavioural sequelae of traumatic brain injury* (pp. 52–68). New York: Taylor & Francis.

Turkstra, L. S., Holland, A. L., & Bays, G. A. (2003). The neuroscience of recovery and rehabilitation: what have we learned from animal research? *Archives of Physical Medicine Rehabilitation, 84,* 604–612.

Turkstra, L. S., McDonald, S., & DePompei, R. (2001). Social information processing in adolescents: data from normally developing adolescents and preliminary data from their peers with traumatic brain injury. *Journal of Head Trauma Rehabilitation, 16,* 469–483.

Walsh, K., & Darby, D. (1999). *Neuropsychology: A clinical approach* (4th ed.). Edinburgh, Scotland: Churchill Livingstone.

Williams, W. H., Evans, J. J., Wilson, B. A., & Needham, P. (2002). Brief report: prevalence of post-traumatic stress disorder symptoms after severe traumatic brain injury in a representational community sample. *Brain Injury, 16*(8), 673–679.

Wilson, J. T. L., Pettigrew, L. E. L., & Teasdale, G. M. (1998). Structured interviews for the Glasgow Outcome Scale and extended Glasgow Outcome Scale: Guidelines for their use. *Journal of Neurotrauma, 15*, 573–585.

Wilson, J. T. L., Pettigrew, L. E. L., & Teasdale, G. M. (2000). Emotional and cognitive consequences of head injury in relation to the Glasgow Outcome Scale. *Journal of Neurology, Neurosurgery, and Psychiatry, 69*, 204–209.

Whyte, J. (1992). Attention and arousal: Basic science aspects. *Archives of Physical Medicine and Rehabilitation, 73*, 940–949.

Whyte, J., Cifu, D., Dikmen, S., & Temkin, N. (2001). Prediction of functional outcomes after traumatic brain injury: A comparison of two measures of duration of unconsciousness. *Archives of Physical Medicine Rehabilitation, 82*, 1355–1359.

Yasuda, S., Wehamn, P., Targett, P, Cifu, D., & West, M. (2001). Return to work for persons with traumatic brain injury. *American Journal of Physical Medicine and Rehabilitation, 80*, 852–864.

6

Burn Injuries

EDWIN F. RICHTER III, MD

OVER 1 MILLION burn injuries occur in the United States per year. Fire is the most common cause of burn injuries, but contact with extreme cold (frostbite), electricity, chemicals, or radiation can cause burns as well. About 4,500 burn-related deaths occur per year. Death rates have dropped despite population growth, suggesting that improved acute care may generate more survivors who will need rehabilitation services. Approximately 45,000 hospitalizations for burns annually are divided almost evenly between the nation's 125 specialized burn centers, which average 200 burn admissions per year, and other hospitals (averaging 5 burn admissions per year). Patients admitted to a burn center on average have 14% of their total body surface area (TBSA) involved, but 4% of the patients have over 60% of TBSA involved (American Burn Association, 2000).

The skin is the largest organ of the body, and the most frequently injured structure in burns. The outer layer, which is typically first to be injured, is called the epidermis. This contains four layers (five at the hands and feet). The innermost layer houses collections of cells called keratocytes that migrate toward the surface and create a protective layer of the protein keratin at the surface. A pigment called melanin determines skin color. Other important appendages of the epidermis are hair follicles, sebaceous glands (providing sebum to moisturize skin), and sweat glands. The sweat glands are of great importance in regulating body temperature.

Beneath the epidermis lies the dermis. This layer provides nutrition and structural support. Elastic fibers allow the skin to tolerate pressure and shearing forces. Under the dermis is a layer of subcutaneous fat and connective tissue.

There are many nerve endings in the skin, which allow us to feel pain and temperature, light touch, pressure, and vibration. Burn injuries may jeopardize all of these functions.

FUNCTIONAL PRESENTATION

SEVERAL KEY FACTORS are considered when evaluating burn injuries. The depth or thickness of the injury is considered very important. Strata include superficial (epidermis), superficial partial (extending into dermis), deep partial (epidermis and most of dermis, with impaired healing and high risk of scarring), and full thickness (not expected to heal).

Percentage of total body surface area (TBSA) involved is also critical. The "Rule of 9s" allocates 9% to the head and each upper extremity, 18% to anterior trunk, posterior trunk, and each lower extremity, and 1% to the perineum.

Cause of burn is also considered. Electrical burns are considered particularly worrisome because of the risk of deeper injuries not evident on initial inspection. Concurrent smoke inhalation injury, other significant injuries, or comorbidities are also considered. Presence of any of these factors leads to categorization as a major burn in the American Burn Association classification system, as does involvement of > 25% TBSA partial-thickness (> 20% in children), > 10% full thickness, or involvement of face, eyes, ears, feet, or perineum. Moderate burns involve 15–25% TBSA (10–20% in children) partial or 2–10% full thickness burns. Less extensive burns are classified as minor (American Burn Association, 1990).

Other organ systems may be injured during burns and associated trauma. Respiratory involvement after inhalation of smoke or fumes may be the most critical. Damage to the gastrointestinal tract may hinder the critical process of providing nutritional support to allow healing. Electrical injuries may cause cardiac damage.

Nerve injuries are of particular importance. Nerve endings may be damaged in partial thickness burns, causing neuropathic pain while reducing useful sensation. Full thickness injuries destroy nerves, taking away protective sensation. Electrical injuries, burns covering over 15% TBSA, and stays over 20 days in intensive care are associated with a particularly high risk of neuropathy (Kowalske, Holavanahalli, & Helm, 2001).

There are also general systemic processes at work after acute burns. Loss of fluids can occur from bleeding and from loss of the skin's function as a barrier to loss of water. Fluid volume replacement is an important aspect of critical care. Protein is also lost at a time when the body's needs are high.

Loss of the skin's barrier function also creates significant risk for infection. Wound care must be performed with great care to reduce this risk. Hydrotherapy, used to remove dead tissue, must be performed with precautions to avoid transmission of infections via shared equipment.

Partial thickness burns heal by repair of dermis and growth of epithelium in from the borders of the wound. Even after the wound is covered, a maturation process goes on. As scar forms, there is the risk of excessive scarring and tightness, which may reduce joint mobility.

Full thickness and deeper partial thickness burns require skin grafts. Most commonly, a split-thickness autograft takes skin (epidermis and some dermis) from the patient's own body, and the donor site heals like a superficial partial thickness burn. More recently, bioengineered skin substitutes have been employed with some success (Boyce & Warden, 2002).

Mobilizing the patient is a priority. Range of motion (ROM) exercises are done regularly to prevent joint contracture. When feasible, ambulation is encouraged.

Edema (accumulation of fluid in soft tissues with swelling) may be significant. Use of elastic dressings, elevation, and mobilization may be employed for edema control. In severe cases involving burns around the circumference of a limb, nerves may be injured and flow through blood vessels may be compromised, even to a degree leading to amputation. Compartment syndrome may require surgical intervention.

Pressure garments are commonly used on grafted burns or those that take longer than 14 days to heal. These are intended to reduce hypertrophic (overgrown) scarring, perhaps by reducing rates of blood flow to the scar, although efficacy of this treatment has been questioned (Chang, Laubenthal, & Lewis, 1995). They are supposed to be worn at all times except for wound care and hygiene.

Sheets of silicone are sometimes applied to wounds. The treatment may work by changing wound temperature or by increasing hydration of scar tissue.

Splinting is a standard procedure to preserve range of motion or protect a healing wound. In this population, custom-made orthotics are often required. Lightweight plastic materials are popular. The clinical challenge is to provide a device that will achieve goals of protecting range of motion and preserving joint function without causing undue discomfort to the patient. The use of orthotics is part of the larger issue of preventing contracture. Typically patients are more comfortable in flexed positions, but best practices usually require positioning in extension to minimize risk of contracture (Cromes & Helm, 1999). This might even include discouraging use of pillows if there are burns on the anterior neck and chest.

Pain management is a critical part of patient care. Patients with poorly controlled pain will have difficulty complying with the rigors of acute care and rehabilitation. Nerve endings that were painfully stimulated in the initial injury may be further stimulated by inflammatory processes, and by mechanical stresses during wound care and therapies. Resulting pain syndromes can be associated with significant functional and psychological morbidity (Gallagher, Rae, & Kinsella, 2000). As nerve endings heal, severe pruritis (itching) also becomes a common problem.

Heterotopic ossification is a process in which bone is created in inappropriate tissue locations outside of bones. About 3% of burn patients are affected by this condition, particularly under areas of full-thickness burns (Peterson, Mani, & Crawford, 1989). Range of motion may be significantly reduced. Treatment may include surgical resection and administration of medications (indomethacin or etidronate) or radiation to reduce the risk of recurrence.

Involuntary weight loss, including reduced lean body mass, is a common significant complication of burns. A diet high in calories and protein is usually offered while physical therapists encourage exercise, although physical discomfort and emotional distress may limit the effectiveness of these interventions. Treatment with anabolic steroids may prove beneficial in some cases (Demling & DeSanti, 1997).

When the burn patient is discharged from the inpatient setting, some wounds are often not completely healed. Wound care is a major focus of outpatient rehabilitation. Hydrotherapy, debridement, and dressing changes are performed as needed. When healing has progressed to where a few spotty areas remain, hydrotherapy is stopped. Appropriate lubricants are applied frequently to treat skin dryness. The new skin and scar tissue may benefit from massage to reduce sensitivity and improve flexibility (Cromes & Helm, 1999).

Contracture control is another major focus of outpatient care. The physical or occupational therapist stretches the involved joints. Patients may fail to achieve the same extent of stretch because of pain, but are encouraged to try. The joint or extremity can be packed in paraffin prior to stretching, and there is evidence that greater range of motion can be achieved with this modality (Head & Helm, 1977). This process continues until the skin is mature and loss of range of motion no longer occurs between therapy appointments or overnight.

After formal treatment is completed, patients may need to follow careful skin care precautions, including avoidance of excessive exposure to ultraviolet light, such as direct sunlight. When significant TBSA is burned, reduced ability to sweat may limit ability to regulate temperature in hot environments.

PSYCHOLOGICAL AND VOCATIONAL IMPLICATIONS

RECOVERY FROM MODERATE to major burns can be very stressful. Depression and post-traumatic stress disorders (PTSD) are common sequellae. Literature review has yielded reported PTSD rates of 8–45% (Yu & Dimsdale, 1999). Burn patients have reported higher rates of depression and anxiety than other trauma patients (Wisely & Tarrier, 2001). Counseling, referral to support groups, and psychopharmacologic interventions may be considered.

Monitoring for development or exacerbation of PTSD after discharge is recommended. One should also be aware of potential anxiety about leaving the hospital, which may lead to ambivalence about discharge (Cromes & Helm, 1999).

Cognitive distortions in patients who have recovered from burns have been reported (Willebrand et al., 2002). When asked to perform the "emotional Stroop" task, these patients had longer latencies to burn-related words, as well as slight cognitive slowness as compared to controls.

Reports of quality of life after burns have been varied. Significant rates of emotional issues have been reported after burns (Cobb, Maxwell, & Silverstein, 1990; Cromes, Voege, Kowalske, & Helm, 1997). However, children who survived burns over more than 70% of TBSA have reported quality of life similar to that of peers (Sheridan et al., 2000). The Revised Burn-Specific Health Scale (Blalock, Bunker, & DeVellis, 1994) has been developed to quantify quality of life issues, measuring domains of functional activities, work, body image, interpersonal relationships, affect, heat sensitivity, and treatment regimens. It has proven valid and reliable. Quality of life has been shown to improve with lower pain levels at 2 months and 6 months after discharge, better community reentry at 6 and 12 months, and less emotional distress at 2, 6, and 12 months (Cromes, Holvanahalli, & Helm, 2002).

Return to work may be challenging. Less than half of patients who sustained major burn injuries return to the same job and employer without accommodations, and mean time off from work for those who returned to work by 24 months was 17 weeks. Psychiatric history, extremity burns, and increased percentage of TBSA reduced probability of return to work (Brych et al., 2001). Prior employment status is a strong predictor of ability to return to work (Fauerbach et al., 2001), with prior unemployment being associated with higher rates of substance abuse and prior physical disability.

Return to vocational and avocational roles may be affected by emotional issues, including those of the patient and those of other individuals reacting to the cosmetic impact of burns. Sensitivity to heat, cold, and exposure to ultraviolet light may limit options. Reduced joint mobility may create significant physical limitations. Location of the burn may be critical. Presence of hand burns (Helm, Walker, & Peyton, 1986) and TBSA involved (Helm & Walker, 1992) have been cited as factors that may influence amount of time missed from work.

Despite the problems noted previously, most people who are employed when they sustain burns do manage to return to work. Comprehensive evaluation by a specialist expert in the treatment of patients with burns is advised when questions arise about possible return to work (Cromes & Helm, 1999). Obtaining the best clinical and functional outcomes often requires the efforts of clinicians from several different disciplines, creating opportunities for team collaboration and enhancement of patient care.

REFERENCES

American Burn Association. (1990). Hospital and pre-hospital resources for optimal care of patients with burn injury. *Journal of Burn Care and Rehabilitation, 11*, 98–104.

American Burn Association. (2000). *Burn Incidence Fact Sheet.*

Blalock, S. J., Bunker, B. J., & DeVellis, R. F. (1994). Measuring health status among survivors of burn injury: Revisions of the Burn Specific Health Scale. *Journal of Trauma, 36*, 508–515.

Boyce, S. T. & Warden, G. T. (2002). Principles and practices for treatment of cutaneous wounds with cultured skin substitutes. *American Journal of Surgery, 183*, 445–456.

Brych, S. B., Engrav, L. H., Rivara, F. P., Ptacek, J. T., Lezotte, D. C., Esselman, P. C., et al. (2001). *Journal of Burn Care and Rehabilitation, 22*(6), 401–405.

Chang, P., Laubenthal, K. N., & Lewis, R. W. (1995). Prospective randomized study of the efficacy of pressure garment therapy in patients with burns. *Journal of Burn Care and Rehabilitation, 16*, 473–480.

Cobb, N., Maxwell, G., & Silverstein, P. (1990). Patient perception of quality of life after burn injury: Results of an eleven-year study. *Journal of Burn Care and Rehabilitation, 10*, 251–257.

Cromes, G. F., & Helm, P. A. (1999). Burn injuries. In M. G. Eisenberg, R. L. Glueckauf, & H. H. Zaretsky (Eds.), *Medical aspects of disability: A handbook for the rehabilitation professional* (pp. 121–136). New York: Springer Publishing Co.

Cromes, G. F., Holavanahalli, R., Kowalske, K. J., & Helm, P.A. (2002). Predictors of quality of life as measured by the Burn Specific Health Scale in persons with major burn injury. *Journal of Burn Care and Rehabilitation, 23*(3), 229–234.

Cromes, G. F., Voege, J., Kowalske, K. J., & Helm, P.A. (1997). Prospective changes in psychological, functional, and community integration measures at discharge and 2, 6, and 12 months of persons with major burn injury. *Journal of Burn Care and Rehabilitation, 18*(3), 595.

Demling, R. H., & DeSanti, L. (1997) Oxandrolone, an anabolic steroid, significantly increases the rate of weight gain in the recovery phase after major burns. *Journal of Trauma, 43*, 47–51.

Fauerbach, J. A., Engrav, L., Kowalske, K., Brych, S., Bryant, A., Lawrence, J., et al. (2001). *Journal of Burn Care and Rehabilitation, 22*, 24–26.

Gallagher, G., Rae, C. P., & Kinsella, J. (2000). Treatment of pain in severe burns. *American Journal of Clinical Dermatology, 1*(6), 329–335.

Head, M. D., & Helm, P. A. (1977). Paraffin and sustained stretching in the treatment of burn contractures. *Burns, 4*, 136–139.

Helm, P. A., & Walker, S. C. (1992). Return to work after burn injury. *Journal of Burn Care and Rehabilitation, 13*, 53–57.

Helm, P. A., Walker, S. C., & Peyton, S. A. (1986). Return to work following hand burns. *Archives of Physical Medicine and Rehabilitation, 67*, 297–298.

Kowalske, K., Holavanahalli, R., & Helm, P. (2001). Neuropathy after burn injury. *Journal of Burn Care and Rehabilitation, 22*, 353–357.

Peterson, S. L., Mani, M. M., & Crawford, C. M. (1989). Post-burn heterotopic ossification: Insights for management decision-making. *Journal of Trauma, 29*, 365–377.

Sheridan, R. L., Hinson, M.I., Liang, M. H., Nackel, A. F., Schoenfeld, D. A., Ryan, C. M., et al. (2000). *Journal of the American Medical Association, 283*, 69–73.

Willebrand, M., Norlund, F., Kildal, M., Gerdin, B., Ekselius, L., & Andersson, G. (2002). Cognitive distortions in recovered burn patients: The emotional Stroop task and autobiographical memory test. *Burns, 28*, 465–471.

Wisely, J. A., & Tarrier, N. (2001). A survey of the need for psychological input in a follow-up service for adult burn-injured patients. *Burns, 27*, 801–807.

Yu, B. H., & Dimsdale, J. E. (1999). Posttraumatic stress disorder in patients with burn injuries. *Journal of Burn Care and Rehabilitation, 20*, 426–433.

7

Cancers

INGRID FREIDENBERGS, PhD,
ILANA GRUNWALD, PhD, AND ESIN KAPLAN, MD

PSYCHOLOGICALLY, PHYSICALLY, AND economically, the impact of cancer in the United States is staggering. New malignancies will develop in an estimated 1,368,030 individuals in 2004. This number does not include carcinoma in situ of any site except urinary bladder, and it does not include basal and squamous cell cancers, which will total over one million cases. The 2004 estimated cancer incidence by site and sex indicates that the most frequent site will be the breast (32%) in women and the prostate (33%) in men. Lung cancer will be by far the leading cause of cancer deaths in men (32%). In 2004 the leading cause of cancer death for women will also be lung cancer (25%), surpassing even breast cancer (15%). In 2001, cancer was the second most common cause of death following heart disease; 553,768 Americans died of cancer (American Cancer Society, 2004).

Cancer is not only a major problem in terms of the number of people afflicted, but it is a very complex management problem as well. Complicating matters is the fact that the etiology of cancer remains generally unknown, the prognosis often uncertain, and cancer is not even considered a single disease but rather a group of more than 100 different diseases.

The word "cancer" continues to evoke high levels of anxiety and fear. Why is this so? In our lifetime medicine's central promise has been that all diseases can be cured. Cancer, however, still remains a disease that is not readily understood and is therefore mysterious, and it has even come to be used as a metaphor for what is socially or morally wrong (Susan Sontag, 1979). In addition, because cancer is so prevalent, all of us know someone with the disease, which may call forth many personal associations that can interfere with our role as "objective" helpers. Given the profound impact even the mere use of the word "cancer" holds for so many, it is imperative that the counselor has a clear understanding of both the physical nature and the emotional sequellae of the disease. Only in this manner can the myths surrounding the disease be dispelled and the patients helped to adjust.

DESCRIPTION OF MEDICAL CONDITION

THERE ARE MORE than 100 forms of neoplastic disease, with different biological and clinical manifestations. A neoplasm is defined as the growth of new cells proliferating without control and serving no useful function. Abnormal growth of a cell, with local tissue invasion and spread to other organ systems via the blood system or lymphatic channels, is typical for malignancies. The spread to other body parts is termed metastasis. Under the microscope, the actual cells may be classified as either well differentiated or undifferentiated. This distinction is important because well-differentiated cells offer a better prognosis than do undifferentiated ones. Cancers are further specified in terms of the type of tissue of origin: carcinoma (those tissues arising from epithelial cells), sarcoma (cancers arising from connective and supportive tissue), lymphoma (malignancies of lymphatic tissue), and leukemia (malignant transformation of white blood cells).

Because of the variety of cancers, it is most unlikely that a single causative factor will be identified. In fact, more than one factor most likely will be found that will convert a normal cell into a "cancerous" one. Epidemiological studies have shown environmental hazards, social practices, and heritable factors to play a part in the etiology of the various cancers. For example, smoking has been linked to lung cancer, alcohol and tobacco consumption to head and neck cancer, x-ray therapy to thyroid cancer, family history to breast cancer, diet to colon cancer, and the sun to melanoma and other skin cancers. Genetic as well as immunological factors may predispose one to acquiring cancer. Viruses, especially the DNA viruses, also play a role. Public awareness/education is a major contribution for early detection and diagnosis of those diseases.

Cancer can develop at any age, in any tissue of any organ system. If it is detected at an early stage, it is potentially curable. About 40% of the cancer population is clinically cured with surgical treatment. Fifteen percent of the remaining 60% will survive at least another 15 years. The cancer warning signs include change in bowel or bladder habits, a sore that does not heal, unusual bleeding or discharge, a thickening or lump in breast tissue or elsewhere, indigestion or difficulty swallowing, an obvious change in a wart or mole, a nagging cough, and persistent fevers, sweats, pain, fatigue, or weight loss.

A detailed careful history and physical exam of all patients is essential. Screening tests for cancer detection include the routine use of the Pap smear, which has led to a significant decrease in mortality from cervical cancer. Breast self-examination, mammography, and ultrasound of the breast may contribute to an early diagnosis and reduce mortality from breast cancer. Stool testing for occult blood and periodic colonoscopy may lead to an early diagnosis of colon cancer. Chest x-rays, CT scans, and a sputum exam are helpful in lung cancer diagnosis, especially for those with a history of heavy smoking and exposure to well-known carcinogenic agents. Biopsy techniques include incisional biopsy, excisional biopsy, fine-needle biopsy, bronchial washes, and others. To determine the stage of the malignant process, diagnostic tests such as liver, spleen, bone, and brain scans are used. Magnetic resonance imaging is helpful for early metastatic detection in the various organ systems. The elevation of certain blood serum enzymes or chemistries is very specific for certain malignancies. Relatively recent tests include the CEA (carcinoembryonic antigen) for colon cancer, CA-125 for ovarian cancer, alpha-fetaprotein or beta human chorionic gonadotropin testing for testicular cancer, and serum immunoglobulins for multiple myeloma. Occasionally, the diagnosis of ametastatic cancer is made by biopsy without the presence of a primary site.

Age has a significant impact on both incidence and mortality. For example, certain cancers, such as prostate, stomach, or colon, reach a peak at ages 60–80, whereas others, such as acute lymphoma or acute lymphoblastic leukemia, peak at infancy to 10 years. Thus, if a mediastinal mass is found in a 20-year-old patient, the differential diagnosis would include Hodgkin's disease or non-Hodgkin's lymphoma, but the same mass in a 50-year-old would include lung cancer, non-Hodgkin's lymphoma, or thymoma (a malignancy of the thymus gland).

Treatment for cancer is directed at eradicating the primary tumor and any metastatic areas. The basic treatment modalities include surgery and radiation for regional control of disease and chemotherapy for systemic control. Other treatment modalities include immunotherapy, hormonal therapy, and hyperthermia.

Surgery is the oldest and still one of the most effective forms of cancer therapy. Cancers curable in the early stages with surgery alone include cancers of the oral cavity, larynx, lung, colon, prostate, kidney, testis, bladder, ovary, endometrium, cervix, and breast. Recently, laser beam techniques have been used in place of surgery to control regional disease.

Radiation therapy uses ionizing radiation, with radioactive cobalt usually being the source. Radiation generates a large amount of energy, which eradicates the localized population of neoplastic cells; the cell content is directly affected by changing the DNA structure. Radiation treatment is very effective with the non-Hodgkin's lymphomas and cancers of the testis, prostate, larynx, nasopharynx, cervix, and lung. Side effects may be systemic (e.g., nausea, vomiting, fatigue, bone marrow suppression) or local (e.g., skin or mucosal irritation). Long-term effects may include peripheral or central nervous system degeneration or the development of another malignancy.

Chemotherapy has become a powerful tool in reducing or controlling tumor activity. During recent years it has become more apparent that a combination of chemotherapy agents may potentiate a therapeutic effect. Chemotherapy agents include the alkylating agents, antimetabolites, plant alkaloids, antitumor antibodies, and enzymes. These agents affect cancer cell growth at various stages. Antineoplastic chemotherapy is considered curative of certain tumors, such as testicular tumors, acute leukemia, Burkitt's lymphoma, Hodgkin and non-Hodgkin's lymphoma, and certain childhood tumors. Because all of the currently available antitumor drugs act on similar structures and metabolic pathways in both normal and neoplastic cells, the use of these agents is limited because of the toxic effect on normal tissue, such as bone marrow, liver, kidney, and the nervous system. In addition, many chemotherapeutic agents are carcinogenic as well. Side effects may include nausea, vomiting, bone marrow suppression, hair loss, mouth sores, and peripheral neuropathy or myopathy (Body, Lossignol, & Ronson, 1997; Colvin & Owens, 1988).

Cancer carries risks to the patient that extend over many years. Even though the primary disease may be cured, the patient may have functional or physical difficulties as a result of the medical treatments. When evaluating the functional status of patients, it is essential to determine the region of anatomical structure of the body that is affected, the type of tumor, the course the disease has taken, and the individual variables the patient presents. Because rehabilitation requires a holistic and comprehensive approach, the combined expertise of a multidisciplinary team is necessary. The following are examples of rehabilitation issues facing cancer patients (Kaplan & Gumport, 1988).

In treating tumors of the head and neck, functional and cosmetic deformities are frequently encountered. Because it has been noted that a history of alcohol and tobacco consumption is present in about 85% of patients, rehabilitation efforts are often made more difficult. Ninety percent of head and neck cancers are of the squamous cell type, the most common site being the larynx, followed by the tonsils and hypopharynx. The salivary glands, thyroid, and sinuses are less often involved. Depending on the source of the tumor and the extent of the disease, either surgical or radiation treatments, or both, are chosen. Many patients who have been treated for these tumors have had neck dissections. Physical limitation may include difficulties in opening the mouth, chewing or swallowing, speaking, or even breathing. Prostheses may be made to replace a lost body part. Head and neck prostheses include eyes, ears, nose, and even the palate.

The types of surgical treatments available for breast cancer include radical and modified-radical mastectomies and partial breast resection with axillary node and sentinel node dissections (Golshan, Martin, & Dowlatshahi, 2003). During recent years immediate breast reconstructions have been more commonly performed, but these may be done at a later date as well. Depending on the extent of the disease, either radiation (which is mostly given to patients who undergo partial breast resection) or chemotherapy is the choice of treatment.

Currently, the use of the hormone tamoxifen is advocated as a treatment, especially in women with estrogen-receptor cells. After a mastectomy, instructions about postoperative arm positioning, exercises, and arm care are essential for the prevention of "frozen shoulder," pain syndromes, and lymphedema (swelling of the arm and hand). The prevention of lymphedema includes avoidance of obesity and minimizing any trauma, infection, or sunburn to the arm.

Soft-tissue tumors include those of connective tissue, blood and lymphatic vessels, smooth and striated muscles, fat fascia, and synovial structures. Treatment may range from a simple excision to amputation. Rehabilitation depends on the extent of the operative procedure as well as whether chemotherapy or radiation therapy is required. Adequate treatment of soft-tissue tumors may require removal of a large amount of muscle tissue. Splinting or supporting of major joints might be necessary to permit early resumption of daily living activities and ambulation. If amputation is to be done, preoperative consideration should be given to the level of amputation, type of prosthesis, and type of training that will make the postoperative transition easier.

Primary malignant tumors of the skeleton account for less than 1% of all tumors, with the greatest incidence found in children and young adults. Treatment may require amputation or limb-sparing procedures. Metastatic bone tumors stemming from the lung, breast, prostate, kidney, and thyroid gland are the most common malignancies affecting bones. The spine, pelvis, and long bones are the most common metastatic sites. General management includes steroids in high doses, radiation, surgical decompression, and stabilization. Appropriate external support is provided with braces and assistive devices to improve the patient's mobility, safety, and independence.

The most common primary malignant tumors of the central nervous system (CNS) are gliomas, which represent 45% of intracranial tumors. Malignant tumors of the CNS do not metastasize to other organ systems of the body, but they do spread within the CNS itself. Ten percent of CNS tumors are metastatic from other parts of the body. The most common site of the primary neoplasm is typically the lung. Almost any part of the brain may be involved in a metastatic process. The functional aftermath of CNS tumors includes paralysis, paresthesias, aphasia, memory impairment, confusion, and any other of the usual sequellae of brain damage.

PSYCHOLOGICAL IMPACT OF CANCER

IT IS SAFE to say that cancer may interfere with many daily activities and that the patient may react with anxiety, depression, loss of self-esteem, post-traumatic stress and a disruption of defense mechanisms. Many different types of fears can be activated: fears of loss of control, loss of independence, loss of privacy, loss of normal bodily functions, mutilation, isolation from family and friends, loss of income, pain, and death. However, it has been difficult to measure the actual psychosocial impact of the disease because study results vary according to such factors as site and histological type of cancer, staging of the disease, type of medical treatment administered, clinical course, functional impairment, cosmetic impairment, or the time interval separating cancer diagnosis and psychosocial assessment. Individual variables, such as the patient's age, gender, religion, race, socioeconomic status, living arrangements, prior exposure to trauma, and premorbid personality, also enter into consideration in determining one's response to cancer. Finally, the availability of rehabilitation services and psychological management by the medical team play important roles in influencing the impact of this disease. When research on the actual emotional impact of cancer has been conducted, dysphoric reactions have been reported in roughly 4.5% to 50% of patients (Spiegel, 1996). For example, when the emotional status of 112 women with breast cancer was assessed, 50% admitted being either anxious or depressed. Derogatis et al. (1983) studied the prevalence of psychiatric disorders in 215 patients with cancer (varying sites) and found that 47% had some psychiatric disorders meeting DSM-III-R criteria, such as anxiety or adjustment disorder (*Diagnostic and Statistical Manual of Mental Disorders*, 3rd ed., rev.; APA, 1991). Of the total number of patients, only 11% had psychiatric problems prior to their illness. The remaining 36% exhibited disorders that were reactions to the disease or its treatment. Pasacreta and Massie (1990), in their study of 475 patients, found that 55% were perceived as having symptoms that required psychiatric consultation, situation depression and anxiety being the most common. Hopwood and Stephens (2000) examined rates of depression by self-report in 322 patients. They found that 33% of patients met classification for depression before treatment and that this persisted in more than 50% of these patients. Recent studies have shown that anxiety is also extremely prevalent among cancer patients. Stark et al. (2002) found that 48% of their subjects reported heightened anxiety and 18% met ICD 10 criteria for an anxiety disorder. Even after successful treatment, fear of recurrence causes some patients to continue to suffer from affective disorders, particularly anxiety, despite the absence of disease (Thomas, Glynn-Jones, Chait, & Marks, 1997). According to the National Cancer Institute (NCI), cancer patients are at an increased risk for post-traumatic stress disorder (PTSD). The trauma of the diagnosis, the disease, and its treatment can all contribute to PTSD symptoms. These results indicate that, by and large, cancer patients do not suffer from psychiatric conditions other than those posed by the stresses of the disease and/or its medical treatments. Research does suggest that cancer patients are more likely to seek out mental health services when compared to individuals without a self-reported history of cancer (Hewitt & Rowland, 2002). Research studies have also centered on the impact of medical treatments on the cancer patient. For example, Peck and Boland (1972) used psychiatric interviews to study the affective reactions of patients undergoing radiation therapy. The most common affective responses were anxiety (98% of patients) and depression (75% of patients). Evans and Connis (1995) showed that both cognitive-behavioral and social support therapies resulted in fewer psychiatric symptoms and reduced maladaptive interpersonal relations in patients undergoing radiation therapy. When the effects of chemotherapy were examined, Carey and Burish (1988) noted that approximately 45% of adult cancer patients experience psychological side-effects in the 24-hour period preceding treatment. These researchers state that such negative psychological symptoms are the product of both associative learning and the stress associated with chemotherapy and that those side-effects can be ameliorated with psychological techniques. Chen (2003) studied factors associated with hope in cancer patients. The author found a relationship between patient's perceptions of treatment effect and hope but not between disease stage and hope.

Research also suggests that many cancer treatments may result in cognitive changes to the patient. Ahles et al. (2002) administered neuropsychological test batteries to breast and lung cancer patients who had undergone chemotherapy and met criteria of "survivors" (i.e., 5 years post-diagnosis and currently disease-free). They found that chemotherapy patients had significantly lower scores than patients treated only with local therapy on the battery of tests administered. The results were most pronounced in the cognitive domains of memory and psychomotor functioning. Armstrong et al. (2002) also looked at long-term changes in cognitive functioning in cancer survivors. They found cognitive decline, especially in the domain of memory, in some patients' post-radiation therapy. They concluded that patients who did not have risk factors for vascular damage did not evidence significant cognitive changes. Brown et al. (2003) assessed cognitive function in patients who had undergone radiotherapy to treat low-grade gliomas. Median time post-treatment was 7.4 years. They concluded that most patients did not evidence significant cognitive decline. Several groups of authors (Klein & Heimans, 2004; Meyers & Wefel, 2003) have expressed concerns that the instrument administered to these patients was not sensitive enough to detect most cognitive deterioration and that the Brown et al. findings may represent a significant underestimate of actual cognitive deficits post cancer treatment. Cancer patients have historically received a low priority for vocational rehabilitation services. Much has been written in the popular press about the prejudices that exist toward cancer patients when they apply for new job positions or when they return to work. The rate at which patients return to work varies by study from 44% to 100% (Verbeek, Spelten, Kamneijer, & Sprangers, 2003). In a study of 100 recovered cancer patients, the findings indicted that 13% perceived some form of job-related discrimination, and 11% were excluded from group health benefits or had their previous benefits reduced (Feldman, 1978).Confirming such discrimination, a study of 422 cancer patients showed that although 76% of the respondents indicated that they were working at the time of diagnosis, only 56% were working at the time of the study. However, 82% stated that they wanted to work full- or part-time (Rothstein, Kennedy, Ritchie, & Pyle, 1995). Indeed, one of the most widespread consequences of having had cancer is the tendency to be locked into pre-existing jobs; losing insurance coverage is too great a risk for patients to take.

Another area that is affected by cancer is sexuality. Cancer and its treatment can potentially damage sexual response by affecting emotions, central or peripheral components of the nervous system, the pelvic vascular system, and the hypothalamic-pituitary-gonadal axis (Lederberg, Holland, & Massie, 1989). Site of cancer has been found to be an important variable affecting sexual response, even in patients of comparable prognosis and treatment. For example, when patients with testicular cancer were compared to those with Hodgkin's disease, the former exhibited a greater degree of sexual dysfunction, as well as greater difficulty in their resolution of their sexual difficulties (Johnstone et al., 1989).The psychosocial impact of cancer changes over time. Some researchers are of the opinion that there is a specific time-related pattern of patient response to the disease in which the emotional reactions of persons who have cancer evolve through the stages of denial, anxiety, regression, depression, and finally, realistic adaptation (Kubler-Ross, 1969). It is our experience that although these are generally typical behavioral responses of cancer patients, the sequence of such response is not so neatly predictable. Even in the space of a single psychotherapy session, the patient's feelings may fluctuate among several different "stages." Furthermore, the disease is not static; there are certain crisis or transition points that exacerbate emotional upheaval. For example, the start of primary treatment, changing treatment modalities, and relapse are all points of stress at which one's response is often unpredictable. Cancer can thus be seen as a series of traumas rather than as a single traumatic event (Hopwood & Stephens, 2000). In a prospective study, Gordon et al. (1980) interviewed 308 patients over a 6-month period and noted that upon hospitalization the most frequent problems fell in the area of worry about disease. Immediately upon discharge, problems fell into the area of negative affect. Six months after discharge, problems were found to be more broadly distributed in the areas of physical discomfort, concern about medical treatment, dissatisfaction with health care services, mobility, financial concerns, family problems, social problems, worry about disease, experience of negative affect, and body image. When gender differences in response to the disease were investigated in a group of advanced cancer patients, Leiber, Plumb, Gerstenzang, and Holland (1976) noted that women patients were more depressed than their husbands, male patients, or the spouses of male patients. On the other hand, when Baider, Perez, and De-Nour (1989) studied 39 couples in which one partner had cancer of the colon, it was found that although male patients adjusted better than female patients did, male spouses adjusted far worse than female spouses and even worse than male patients. And in a study of the role of psychological variables in a group of 100 melanoma patients, Baider and her colleague's note that on all adjustment measures women did not do as well as men (Baider et al., 1997). Stark et al. (2002) found that women were more likely than men to suffer from anxiety-related disorders. Such findings suggest that more studies must be conducted on cultural, social, or intrapsychic factors that might influence differing gender responses to the disease and its ramifications.

One must consider age when evaluating the impact of the disease on the patient. Mages and Mendelsohn (1979) note that for young adults the experience of cancer tends to impede the development of self-sufficiency and results in delay and disruption in the establishment of adult roles. For mid-life adults the occurrence of cancer threatens to disrupt roles and important life tasks yet to be carried out. For older adults, cancer leads to an acceleration of the aging process and results in more rapid disengagement from work and social and leisure activities and a greater dependency on others. If the patient is a long-term survivor, as is often now the case due to improved medical treatments, difficulties in adjustment occur in that there is a fear of recurrence and often a permanent sense of physical vulnerability that may diminish self-assurance and confidence. Once cancer has been diagnosed, are some patients more likely than others to develop psychological problems? Vulnerability factors, such as prior psychiatric problems, alcohol or drug abuse, depression, and chronic anxiety, are said to be strong predictors for poor adjustment (Lederberg et al., 1989). Morris, Greer, and White (1977) found that at-risk patients were those who were clinically depressed prior to surgery and who were emotionally labile as well. Craig and Abeloff (1974) divided a sample of 30 primary leukemia and lymphoma patients into high- and low-psychiatric symptom sub-groups. Patients in the high-symptom sub-group were younger, were more likely to be White females, were of higher socioeconomic level, had a higher degree of physical impairment, and had a poorer prognosis than did patients in the low-symptom group. Whether cancer patients represent an increased risk for suicide compared to other patients also has been addressed. Recent studies have suggested that although relatively few cancer patients actually commit suicide, they are nonetheless at greater risk (Breitbart, 1987). High suicide potential exists when the following factors are present: emotional stress, severe depression with feelings of hopelessness, anxiety, mood swings, low tolerance for pain and discomfort, chronic and poorly controlled pain, history of alcoholism or substance abuse, feeling of lack of support from family or medical team, and prior suicide threats or attempts.

Another area investigated is the patient's style of coping with cancer. Coping is seen as an extremely important variable in the patient's response to disease. For example, it has been noted that it is not exposure to a stressor per se but the ability to cope with it effectively that is most likely to influence even the course of the disease itself. When 53 cancer patients who dropped out of chemotherapy were compared to a group who completed their treatment, it was found that those who dropped out had more adjustment problems on every measure that was used (Gilbar & De-Nour, 1989). Weisman and Worden (1977) discuss coping strategies and state that coping and vulnerability have a reciprocal relationship. Vulnerability is an index of distress, whereas coping is what one does about the disease and its ramifications. They found that good copers face facts, find something favorable, and then confidently comply with their doctors' recommendations. In contrast, poor copers use suppression, passivity, and stoic submission. Nezu, Nezu, Felgoise, McClarke, and Houts (2003) investigated the impact of problem-solving therapy (PST) in adults with cancer. They found that subjects who participated in PST evinced less psychological distress and reported higher levels of quality of life (QOL). The findings of this and many other studies suggest that psychological interventions should be considered a regular part of treatment for cancer. Prior to the 1980s a common research topic involved the role of premorbid personality factors in the development of cancer. These early studies did not yield consistent results, and the quest for a cancer-prone personality diminished. There was then a shift in interest to consideration of the role that psychosocial factors play in the outcome of disease. For example, in a study conducted by Achterberg, Lawlis, Simonton, and Mathews-Simonton (1977), factors such as denial, a view of one's body as having little ability to fight disease, and a significant dependency on others proved to be predictors of poor prognosis. On the other hand, when testing the degree to which certain psychosocial factors predict survival and relapse, Cassileth, Lusk, Miller, Brown, and Miller (1985) reported contradictory findings. Three hundred fifty-one patients were investigated, using variables such as social ties, marital history, job satisfaction, use of psychotropic drugs, general life evaluation/satisfaction, degree of hopelessness/helplessness, subjective view of adult health, and subjective view of the amount of adjustment required to cope with the new diagnosis. The results indicated that none of these variables predicted longevity or survival. This well-designed study shows that in many cases the biology of the disease is the major factor determining the prognosis, "overriding the potentially mitigating influence of psychosocial factors" (p. 1555). Richardson, Zarnegar, Bismo, and Levine (1990) examined 139 patients as to the effect on survival of depression, coping style, and locus of control. Again, none of these variables was found to be significantly related to survival. However, these same researchers have shown that factors such as compliance and the number of appointments kept are important predictors of survival. It is clear that many further studies are needed to answer adequately the question of the link between psychosocial status and outcome of disease.

An expanding field of research has centered on the connection between psychological events, endocrine secretion, and modulation of immunity (Kripke & Morison, 1984). A number of studies have shown that various stressors can adversely affect immune function and that there exists the possibility of a reciprocal relationship—the enhancement of immune function through psychological interventions (Kiecolt-Glaser & Glaser, 1992). When the effects of a structured group intervention program for patients with melanoma were studied, researchers found reduced psychological distress and significant immunological improvement in the control group (Fawzy et al., 1993). Similar effects were reported by Spiegel (1996), who studied the effects of group intervention in women with metastatic breast cancer. However, when Gellert, Maxwell, and Siegel (1993) followed up on the survival of breast cancer patients 10 years after they had received adjunctive psychosocial support, the results indicated that these patients did not live longer, on average, than did a comparable group of nonparticipants. Whether interventions that produce relatively small immunological changes can actually affect the incidence, severity, or duration of cancer is simply not yet known. Kiecolt-Glaser and Glaser suggest that the answer may depend on the type and intensity of the psychological intervention, degree of immune modulation, and the individual's own prior health status. Although the effectiveness of psychological intervention on the outcome of disease is still in question, most researchers agree that, at minimum, adjunctive psychological interventions improve mood and enhance quality of life (Andersen, 1992; Cunningham & Edmonds, 1996). What is left to study are the classic questions of psychotherapy research, that is, what type of treatment should be administered and to whom, when should it occur, by whom should it be administered, and under what set of circumstances should it be conducted. A variety of professionals (e.g., psychologists, social workers, psychiatrists, nurses, and a more recent category of helpers named "psycho-oncologists") are involved in the psychosocial management of cancer patients. There are obviously separate areas of expertise that these professionals provide, but an overlapping of functions does exist. Therefore, team members must work closely and noncompetitively with each other. Self-help groups have become a modality for helping patients, with or without a professional facilitator. Such groups provide emotional support, a feeling of belonging, and even stress management and coping skills (Freidenbergs, 1997). More recently, patients have been receiving help by participating in Internet support groups. This innovation allows patients to partake of psychological help without leaving home and with the option of remaining anonymous (Weinberg, Schmale, Uken, & Wessel, 1996). Estimates of the use of medical information obtained on the Internet increase daily. Oncologists view Internet information as having both positive and negative effects in clinical encounters. Further research will be needed to determine the effects of patient use of the Internet to obtain cancer information and support. In assessing the patient's reactions to cancer, the counselor should be well versed in both the physical and emotional consequences of the disease. Education is required to differentiate "normal" from "pathological" responses. When is a patient's negative response self-limited and when has it become pathological? For example, if depression is noted, is the depression reactive to the knowledge that one has cancer or is it a result of the toxin released by the disease itself? Is it a consequence of fatigue, or is it caused by a metabolic imbalance, nutritional deficiency, or infection? Is it a result of the medical treatment administered, or is it a result of the assault on body image? Or does it have nothing to do with the above but rather is caused by either a premorbid depressive pattern or some current interpersonal stress? Further, as Kubler-Ross (1969) has pointed out, there are two different depressive processes to consider: one, a reactive process involving mourning what has been lost, and the other, preparatory depression involving what is going to be lost. It is up to the counselor to determine what the cause of the patient's distress may be. In certain cases it is appropriate to allow patients to mourn their losses, whereas in other situations it might be advisable for the counselor to attempt amelioration of the distress through the counselor's own efforts or via referral to another resource. Does the psychotherapy offered to cancer patients differ from the therapy offered to other types of patients? Although general principles of clinical psychotherapy remain the same, there are variations in approach that are necessary in treating the cancer patient. First, it is imperative to deal with physical issues relating to the disease and its various medical treatments.

Table 7.1 contains a list of psychosocial intervention principles developed by the author and her colleagues (Freidenbergs, Gordon, Hibbard, & Diller, 1980). As can be seen from this list, great emphasis is placed on educating patients, both about their medical condition and about the emotional reactions one may have in response to the disease. Another variation in psychotherapeutic principles involves the timing of interventions. In some cases psychological interpretation must be hastened; in other cases, delayed. Although counter-transference is present in all clinical work, the cancer patient may pose even more challenges to the counselor. One should be especially sensitive to emotional fatigue and burnout and seek help quickly if one notices such feelings in oneself.

When working with cancer patients, counselors must allow them to express their feelings about their illness. One has to explore with patients what they think their cancer may signify, what they have been told of the nature of their disease by other medical personnel, and what impact they believe the disease may have on their lives. Patients' efforts at coping should be viewed in the context of their personal backgrounds, experiences, strivings, guilt, fears, and antecedent personalities. Because patients tend to engage in medical "role modeling" (i.e., comparing themselves with other people who have had similar diseases), it is advisable to ask if any family members or friends have had cancer, what kind it was, what course it took, how it was managed medically, and how the condition was coped with. In reporting on research suggesting that psychological attitudes affect the development, course, and outcome of cancer, the popular media has contributed to many patients' feeling that they have brought on their own disease because of their "negative personality" or that they can improve their prognosis by improving their "mental outlook." It is the counselor's role to make clear that self-blame is counterproductive and at times even clinically harmful. The counselor needs to stress that at this point we still do not know what the relationship between psychological factors and the course of the disease may be, and we do not know whether stress is necessarily always harmful (Freidenbergs, 1991).

TABLE 7.1   Psychosocial Intervention Principles

Educational

(Ed 1)   Clarifying/giving information about the medical system—e.g., explaining hospital procedures, teaching patients' rights, informing patients of existing outpatient services.

(Ed 2)   Clarifying the patient's own medical condition—e.g., what type of cancer the patient has, the meaning of test results.

(Ed 3)   Teaching about cancer and its side effects—e.g., the side effects to be expected from treatment, what the norms are regarding resumption of activities.

(Ed 4)   Teaching what to do to relieve physical discomfort, emotional discomfort, etc.—e.g., relaxation training, self-hypnosis.

(Ed 5)   Reinforcing what other medical personnel have said—i.e., helping patients comply with prescribed medical regimen—e.g., reinforcing the necessity of medical treatment, reinforcing MD statement about the medical condition or treatment.

(Ed 6)   Teaching about the emotional reactions to cancer—e.g., what emotional responses can be expected by the patient himself/herself, what reactions can he/she expect from others.

Counseling

(C1)   Allowing or encouraging the patient to vent feelings.

(C2)   Offering the patient reassurance or verbal support.

(C3)   Helping the patient clarify own feelings and interpreting thoughts, feelings, and behavior in more psychodynamic terms to patient.

(C4)   Encouraging the patient to act on his/her environment—e.g., urging patient to speak to medical personnel and to family, urging patient to ask questions.

(C5)   Exploring the patient's past and/or current situation.

(C6)   Offering indirect support—e.g., by listening to patient, chatting with patient about events unrelated to medical condition.

Environmental

(Ev 1)   Speaking with health care personnel about the patient.

(Ev 2)   Making a formal health service referral.

When viewing the coping strategies patients' use, the counselor needs to focus not on whether the strategy is "good" or "bad" but rather whether or not it is appropriate to the situation. For example, active attempts to deal with cancer, such as seeking information about the illness, can reinforce a patient's sense of control while reducing feelings of helplessness. However, delaying needed treatment because one is continuously seeking information is obviously inappropriate. Denial may be an adaptive defense in temporarily rescuing patients from overwhelming anxiety, or it can be pathological in that it prevents the patient from being alert to possible symptoms of recurrence. Being aware of both the positive and negative effects of psychological defenses can thus be critical in treating the cancer patient. Genetic counselors for hereditary cancer should also be made aware of the psychological impact of available options. Close monitoring of patients' emotional well-being is critical and the importance of adapting information to the person's coping style in order to reduce unnecessary psychological distress cannot be underestimated (Nordin, Liden, Hansson, Rosenquit, & Berglund, 2002).

SOME SPECIFIC THERAPEUTIC ISSUES

CANCER MAY ASSAULT body image in a multitude of ways. Amputation of limbs may result from osteosarcoma; mastectomies and lymphoedema from breast carcinoma; wide and deep scars from malignant melanoma; and loss of parts of the face from skin tumors. Chemotherapy may cause alopecia, mouth sores, and weight loss or gain. Radiation may cause skin changes such as puckering and hardening in addition to a blistering redness. The disease may also cause a generalized weakening of muscles, a premature aged look, bloating of the stomach, and a host of other bodily assaults. It is the task of the counselor to assess the psychological effect that such assaults may cause and to provide support throughout the many physical changes the patient may undergo. It must be kept in mind that there is a process of readjustment to any change in one's appearance. Each change, however minor, may provoke disturbance in the body image equilibrium. Equipped with the knowledge that any change in appearance (for better or for worse) will require a period of adjustment, the counselor may then be more able to sensitively assist the patient (Freidenbergs, 1991).Surgical procedures such as mastectomies, breast reconstruction, oophorectomies, laryngectomies, thyroidectomies, or colostomies are common in the treatment of cancer. When patients face such surgeries, many fears are encountered (e.g., fear of loss of control, of the unknown, or even of death). The counselor may help by encouraging the verbalization of these fears, by exploring any personal experiences the patient may have had with surgery, and by providing objective information and emotional support. Realistic anticipation of results should be addressed, especially in light of newer breast conservation and breast reconstruction techniques. Second opinions, which are now an established part of health care, can also put a strain on the patient and communication needs to be eased between the helpers. Mental rehearsal of upcoming medical procedures may be particularly helpful in alleviating anxiety. Some common postsurgical reactions, such as shock followed by emotional numbness and a feeling of derealization, should be discussed. It should also be noted that patients may experience mood swings and difficulty in concentrating, sleeping, or eating. It should be explained that these symptoms are temporary and usually subside quickly. If there is any residual discomfort following surgical intervention, it should be explored in depth. Furthermore, the approach the patient is taking to alleviate this discomfort, as well as whether or not it is effective, also should be discussed. Counselors must clarify the misunderstanding, confusion, and fear of the unknown that patients often feel when facing radiation therapy. This is especially true given the context of the public's long-held fear of radiation's harmful effects. The effect of radiation is often progressive, and side effects such as fatigue may increase as the cumulative dose of radiation is increased. Patients, therefore, should be advised about the changing nature of the treatment. Knowing that even after the radiation treatments have stopped there may be a worsening of side effects prior to resolution also may help patients. When patients are undergoing chemotherapy, they often have to balance toxicity against benefits. Patients are now often asked to participate in clinical trials. Open communication with oncologists should be encouraged so that patients can make psychologically sound decisions. It is extremely important that patients be made aware that all chemotherapies are not the same and that it is not helpful to compare oneself to others. Even if the chemotherapy protocols are the same, the "host"—namely, the patient—differs biologically from all other patients and therefore may respond in a different manner. In addition to reassuring the patient regarding anticipated nausea and vomiting, preparing the patient for hair loss is critical. This bodily change may provoke a severe psychological reaction in both male and female patients. This reaction is not abnormal as it occurs too regularly in too many patients to be considered as such. Therefore, much reassurance before, during, and after chemotherapy is required. As hair does not often grow back for many weeks following the last chemotherapy treatment, the counselor should be giving support throughout what may appear to be an endless period for the patient. Finally, some patients may experience completion of chemotherapy as a mixed blessing in that stopping treatment might imply the regrowth and relapse of disease.

Much attention has been focused on the terminally ill patient, and in-depth discussions can be found by Burge, Lawson, and Johnston (2003), Chochinova and Holland (1989), and Osterweis, Solomon, and Green (1984). Open discussion of reactions to approaching death may allow for less emotional distress. Grief also may be tolerated better when the loss is expected and there has been some psychological preparation. However, as with all issues, individual differences predominate, and the counselor must be sensitive to just how much reality can be absorbed by patients and family members at any time. Duration of grieving when a family member dies also varies tremendously. A close, trusting, and supportive relationship with caregivers is important at whatever stage grief is encountered.

REFERENCES

Achterberg, J., Lawlis, G. F., Simonton, O. C., & Mathews-Simonton, S. (1977). Psychological factors and blood chemistries as disease outcome predictors for cancer patients. *Multivariate Experimental Clinical Research, 3,* 107–122.

American Cancer Society. (2004). *Cancer facts and figures.*

Ahles, T. A., Saykin, A. J., Furstenberg, C. T., Cole, B., Mott, L. A., Skalla, K., et al. (2002). *Journal of Clinical Oncology, 20*(2), 485–493.

American Psychiatric Association. (1991). *Diagnostic and statistical manual of mental disorders* (3rd ed., rev.). Washington, DC: American Psychiatric Press.

Andersen, B. L. (1992). Psychological interventions for cancer patients to enhance the quality of life. *Journal of Consulting and Clinical Psychology, 60,* 552–568.

Armstrong, L. L., Hunter, J. V., Ledakis, G. E., Cohen, B., Tallent E. M., Tocher, Z., et al. (2002). Late cognitive and radiographic changes related to radiotherapy. *Neurology, 59,* 40–48.

Baider, L., Perez, T., & De-Nour, A. T. (1989). Gender and adjustment to chronic disease: A study of couples with colon cancer. *General Hospital Psychiatry, 60,* 552–568.

Baider, L., Perry, S., Sison, A., Holland, J., Usiely, B., & De-Noor, A. K. (1997). The role of psychological variables in a group of melanoma patients. *Psychosomatics, 38,* 45–53.

Body, J., Lossignol, D., & Ronson, A. (1997). The concept of rehabilitation of cancer patients. *Current Opinion in Oncology, 9,* 332–340.

Breitbart, W. (1987). Suicide in cancer patients. *Current Opinion in Oncology, 1,* 49–54.

Brown, P. D., Buckner, J. C., O'Fallon, J. R., Iturria, N. L., Brown C. A., O'Neill, B. D., et al. (2003). Effects of radiotherapy on cognitive functioning in patients with low-grade glioma measured by the Folstein Mini-Mental State Examination. *Journal of Clinical Oncology, 21,* 2519–2524.

Burse, F., Lawson, B., & Johnston, G. (2003). Trends in the place of death of cancer patients 1992–1997. *Canadian Medical Association Journal, 168,* 265–270.

Carey, M. P., & Burish, T. G. (1988). Etiology and treatment of the psychological side effects associated with cancer chemotherapy: A critical review and discussion. *Psychological Bulletin, 104,* 307–325.

Cassileth, B. R., Lusk, E. J., Miller, D. S., Brown, L. L., & Miller, C. (1985). Psychosocial correlates of survival in advanced malignant disease. *New England Journal of Medicine, 312,* 1551–1555.

Chen, M. L. (2003). Pain and hope in patients with cancer: A role for cognition. *Cancer Nursing, 26*(1), 61–67.

Chochinovar, H., & Holland, J. C. (1989). Bereavement: A special issue in oncology. In J. C. Holland & J. H. Rowland (Eds.), *Handbook of psychooncology* (pp. 612–627). New York: Oxford University Press.

Colvin, M., & Owens, A. H. (1988). Neoplastic diseases. In A. M. Harvey, R. J. Johns, V. A. McKusick, A. H. Owens, & R. S. Ross (Eds.), *The principles and practices of medicine* (pp. 384–449). East Norwalk, CT: Appleton & Lange.

Craig, T. J., & Abeloff, M. D. (1974). Psychiatric symptomatology among hospitalized hospital patients. *American Journal of Psychiatry, 131,* 1323–1327.

Cunningham, A. J., & Edmonds, C. V. (1996). Group psychological therapy for cancer patients: A point of view and discussion of the hierarchy of options. *International Journal of Psychiatry in Medicine, 26,* 51–82.

Derogatis, L. R., Morrow, G. R., Fetting, J., Penman, D., Piasetsky, S., Schmale, M., et al. (1983). The prevalence of psychiatric disorders among cancer patients. *Journal of the American Medical Association, 249,* 751–757.

Evans, R. L., & Connis, R. T. (1995). Comparison of brief group therapies for depressed cancer patients receiving radiation treatment. *Public Health Reports, 110,* 306–311.

Fawzy, F. I., Fawzy, N. W., Hyun, C., Elashoff, R., Guthrie, D., Fahey, J. L., et al. (1993). Malignant melanoma: Effects of an early structured psychiatric intervention, coping, and affective state on recurrence and survival 6 years later. *Archives of General Psychiatry, 50,* 681–689.

Feldman, F. L. (1978). *Work and cancer related histories.* New York: American Cancer Society.

Freidenbergs, I. (1991). Psychological understanding and management of the skin cancer patient. In R. J. Friedman, D. S. Rigel, A. W. Kopf, M. N. Harris, & D. Baker (Eds.), *Cancer of the skin* (pp. 580–588). Philadelphia: W. B. Saunders.

Freidenbergs, I. (1997). How support groups benefit melanoma patients. *Skin Cancer Foundation Journal, 15,* 43–44.

Freidenbergs, I., Gordon, W., Hibbard, M. R., & Diller, L. (1980). Assessment and treatment of psychosocial problems of the cancer patient: A case study. *Cancer Nursing, 3,* 111–119.

Gellert, G. A., Maxwell, R. M., & Siegel, B. S. (1993). Survival of breast cancer patients receiving adjunctive psychosocial support therapy: A 10-year follow-up study. *Journal of Clinical Oncology, 11,* 66–69.

Gilbar, O., & De-Nour, A. K. (1989). Adjustment to illness and dropout of chemotherapy. *Journal of Psychosomatic Research, 33,* 1–5.

Golshan, M., Martin, W. J., & Dowlatshahi, K. (2003). Sentinel lymph node biopsy lowers the rate of lymphedema when compared with standard axillary lymph node dissection. *American Surgeon, 669*(3), 209–211.

Gordon, W. A., Freidenbergs, I., Diller, L., Hibbard, M., Wolf, C., Levine, L., et al. (1980). Efficacy of psychosocial intervention with cancer patients. *Journal of Consulting and Clinical Psychology, 48,* 743–759.

Hewitt, M., & Rowland, J. H. (2002). Mental health service use among adult cancer survivors: Analysis of the National Health Interview Survey. *Journal of Clinical Oncology, 20,* 4581–4590.

Hopwood, P., & Stephens, R. J. (2000). Depression in patients with lung cancer: Prevalence and risk factors derived from quality of life date. *Journal of Clinical Oncology, 18*(4).

Johnstone, B. G., Silberfeld, M., Chapman, J., Phoenix, C., Sturgeon, J., Till, J. E., et al. (1989). Heterogeneity in responses to cancer: Part 2. Sexual responses. *Canadian Journal of Psychiatry, 36,* 182–185.

Kaplan, E., & Gumport, S. L. (1988). Cancer rehabilitation. In J. Goodgold (Ed.), *Rehabilitation medicine* (pp. 285–297). St. Louis, MO: C. V. Mosby.

Kiecolt-Glaser, J. K., & Glaser, R. (1992). Psychoneuroimmunology: Can psychological interventions modulate immunity? *Journal of Consulting and Clinical Psychology, 60,* 569–575.

Klein, M., & Heimans, J. J. (2002). Patients after radiotherapy: The measurement of cognitive functioning in low-grade glioma patients after radiotherapy. *Journal of Clinical Oncology, 22,* 966–967.

Klein, M., & Heimans, J. J. (2004). The measurement of cognitive functioning in low-grade glioma patients after radiotherapy. *Journal of Clinical Oncology, 22,* 966–967.

Kripke, M. L., & Morison, W. L. (1984). Immunology of skin cancer. In R. Fleishmajor (Ed.), *Progress in diseases of the skin* (pp. 31–51). New York: Grune and Stratton.

Kübler-Ross, E. (1969). *On death and dying.* New York: Macmillan.

Landis, S. H., Murray, T., Bolden, S., & Wingo, P. A. (1998). Cancer statistics, 1998. *CA: A Cancer Journal for Clinicians, 48*(1), 6–30.

Lederberg, M. S., Holland, J. C., & Massie, M. (1989). Psychological aspects of patients with cancer. In V. T. De Vita (Ed.), *Cancer: Principles and practice of oncology* (pp. 2191–2204). Philadelphia: J. B. Lippincott.

Leiber, L., Plumb, M. M., Gerstenzang, M. L., & Holland, J. (1976). The communication of affection between cancer patients and their spouses. *Journal of Psychosomatic Medicine, 38,* 379–389.

Mendelsohn, G. A., & Mages, L. L. (1979). Effects of cancer on patients' lives: A personological approach. In E. C. Stone & N. E. Adler (Eds.), *Health psychology* (pp. 755–784). San Francisco: Jossey-Bass.

Meyers, C. A., & Wefel, J. S. (2002). Examination to assess cognitive functioning in cancer trails. No ifs, ands, buts, or sensitivity. *Journal of Clinical Oncology, 21*(19), 3557–3558.

Morris, T., Greer, H. S., & White, P. W. (1977). Psychological and social adjustment to mastectomy. *Cancer, 40,* 2381–2387.

National Cancer Institute. (2004). U.S. National Institutes of Health. Posttraumatic stress disorder. Available: www.cancer.gov/cancertopics/pdg/supportive care/post-traumatic-stress/Healthprof.

Nezu, A. M., Nezu, C. M., Felgoise, S. H., McClarke, K. S., & Houts, P. S. (2003). Project genesis: Assessing the efficacy of problem-solving therapy for distressed adult cancer patients. *Journal of Consulting and Clinical Psychology, 71*(6), 1036–1042.

Nordin, K., Liden, A., Hansson, M., Rosenquit R., & Berglund, G. (2002). Coping style, psychological distress, risk perception, and satisfaction in subjects attending genetic counseling for hereditary cancer. *Journal of Medical Genetics, 39*, 689–694.

Osterweis, M., Solomon, F., & Green, M. (Eds.). (1984). *Bereavement reactions, consequences and care*. Washington, DC: National Academy Press.

Pasacreta, J. V., & Massie, M. (1990). Nurses' reports of psychiatric complications in patients with cancer. *Oncology Nursing Forum, 17*, 347–354.

Peck, A., & Boland, L. (1972). Emotional reaction to having cancer. *American Journal of Roentgenology, Radiation Therapy and Nuclear Medicine, 114*, 591–599.

Richardson, J. L., Zarnegar, Z., Bismo, B., & Levine, A. (1990). Psychosocial status at initiation of cancer treatment and survival. *Journal of Psychosomatic Research, 34*, 189–201.

Rothstein, M. A., Kennedy, K., Ritchie, K. J., & Pyle, K. (1995). Are cancer patients subject to employment discrimination? *Oncology, 9*, 1303–1306.

Sontag, S. (1979). *Illness as metaphor*. New York: Vintage Books.

Spiegel, D. (1996). Cancer and depression. *British Journal of Psychiatry, 168*(30), 109–116.

Stark, D., Kiely, M., Smith, A., Velikous, G., House, A., & Selby, P. (2002). Anxiety disorders in cancer patients. Their nature, associations, and relation to quality of life. *Journal of Clinical Oncology, 20*(14), 1337–1348.

Thomas, S. F., Glynn-Jones, R., Chait, I., & Marks, D. F. (1997). Anxiety in long-term cancer survivors influences the acceptability of planned discharge from follow-up. *Psycho-Oncology, 6*, 190–196.

Verbeek, J., Spelten, E., Kamneijer, M., & Sprangers, M. (2003). Return to work of cancer survivors. A prospective cohort study into the quality of rehabilitation by occupational physicians. *Occupational and Environmental Medicine, 60*(5), 352–357.

Weinberg, N., Schmale, J., Uken, J., & Wessel, K. (1996). Online help: Cancer patients participate in a computer-mediated support group. *Health and Social Work, 21*(1), 24–29.

Weisman, A. D., & Worden, J. W. (1977). *Coping and vulnerability in cancer patients* (research report). Washington, DC: National Cancer Institute.

8

Cardiovascular Disorders

Mariano J. Rey, MD

CARDIOVASCULAR DISEASES REPRESENT the major health epidemic of the 20th century. In the United States and in most other industrialized countries nearly two thirds of all deaths are caused by cardiovascular disorders. One person dies every minute from cardiovascular disease in the United States. In countries of the developing world, cardiovascular disease accounts for a quarter of all deaths, and this fraction increases with increasing economic development. It is estimated that cardiovascular disease will be the major killer in the world by the year 2025 as infectious diseases are brought under better control and as the unhealthy lifestyles of Western society spread across the globe.

Cardiovascular diseases also represent the most common cause of disability in the United States. It is estimate that in 1990 alone about 1 million Americans survived an acute, discrete, major cardiac event or intervention (500,000 Americans suffered heart attacks, about 250,000 underwent coronary artery bypass surgery, and another 250,000 underwent coronary artery angioplasty). In addition, at any given time there are about 6 million Americans with symptoms of cardiovascular disease. The prevalence of chronic atrial fibrillation is on the rise as the average age of the American population increases and a greater number of individuals live beyond the age of 80 years. During this decade congestive heart failure became the most common diagnosis on discharge from United States hospitals. Such is the magnitude of the cardiac disease epidemic that it is rare to find an American family that is not affected by its mortality and morbidity.

Cardiovascular disease constitutes the major health challenge to all providers of medical, psychological, rehabilitative, and vocational services. A comprehensive review of the cardiovascular system and its diseases is therefore imperative for all health professionals.

DISEASES OF THE HEART

CARDIOVASCULAR DISEASES ARE those that affect the heart and the vascular system. By structural and functional criteria (or by anatomy and physiology) the heart has five components: the coronary arteries, the pericardium, the myocardium, the endocardium, and the electrical conduction system.

THE CORONARY ARTERIES

THE CORONARY ARTERIES can be deemed to be the most important blood vessels in the body—for they supply the heart itself. Without normal coronary blood flow the heart cannot carry out its function of supplying blood to the rest of the body. There are two coronary arteries: the left coronary artery and the right coronary artery. The left coronary vessel, after a short main segment, bifurcates into two branches. One branch is the left anterior descending coronary artery, which brings blood to the spectrum (the muscle between the two ventricles) and to the anterior wall of the left ventricle; the other branch is the circumflex coronary artery, the vessel that supplies blood to the right ventricle and to the inferior wall of the left ventricle. In any individual, the blood supply to the posterior wall of the left ventricle can originate from either the circumflex or the right coronary artery, or from both.

Disabling Conditions and Disorders

The cause of coronary heart disease can be best described as biopsychosocial failure. It is a complex constellation of biological, psychological, and social factors that have resulted in the epidemic of coronary heart disease. The risk factors for coronary atherosclerosis are elevated blood cholesterol, high blood pressure, cigarette smoking, diabetes, and a sedentary but stressful life style. These risk factors, alone or in several combinations, create the initial lesion of coronary heart disease, the atherosclerotic plaque, or atheroma. The pathophysiological process is one in which the endothelium, the single-cell thick lining of the inner surface of the coronary arteries, becomes structurally or functionally damaged. The injury to the endothelial cell is directly or indirectly caused by one of the risk factors for atherosclerosis. Once this endothelial barrier is broken, there is deposition of cells, fats, calcium, and amorphous debris inside the arterial wall. Eventually, the atherosclerotic plaques create rigid arterial walls and lead to progressive narrowing of the arteries—which is termed coronary stenosis. Once the coronary vessel has a 70% stenosis, the reduced blood flow may still meet the metabolic needs of the heart when the individual is at a state of rest. Such a narrowing can no longer allow an increase in blood flow to meet the tissue's increased metabolic and oxygen needs during a state of exercise, however. Such an imbalance between oxygen demand and supply, which results in metabolic derangement of heart cells, is called myocardial ischemia. Coronary artery disease is therefore also known as ischemic heart disease.

Furthermore, the atherosclerotic plaque is an unstable structure that can easily become damaged. At the site of such an ulcerated or fissured plaque there is a tendency to form a clot, or thrombus, and to have arterial spasm. Alone or in combination, thrombus and spasm lead to more severe stenosis and at times to a total, or 100%, occlusion of the artery, with complete cessation of all blood flow to the segment of heart muscle supplied by that artery. The understanding of the clinical presentations of coronary heart disease must be based on this understanding of atheroma pathophysiology.

Ischemic chest pain, or angina pectoris, is the only cardiac symptom in the relatively fortunate group of cardiac patients who have stable atheromas that result in coronary narrowing greater than 70% but in less than a total occlusion. Angina pectoris is described as a visceral pain because it is usually felt deeply, rather than superficially, in the chest. The angina sufferer describes the discomfort as squeezing, pressing, or crushing, or as heaviness or a dull ache. Angina is usually felt in the midchest or sternal area. It often radiates to the left arm or the jaw. It is brought on by physical exertion or by mental stress. It is relieved by the cessation of the activity that caused it. Angina usually lasts less than 5 minutes. Patients with this typical pattern are said to have the clinical syndrome of stable angina. It is estimated that at any given time there are about 5 million Americans with stable angina pectoris.

Angina that occurs at rest, without obvious provocation, or with less effort than usual, is unstable angina. This syndrome is usually a manifestation of an unstable atheroma, which has a superimposed thrombus and spasm that has caused further acute stenosis of the coronary artery. When such unstable angina is severe in intensity or sustained in duration, it is termed pre-infarction angina. It may be an indication that a 100% coronary artery occlusion is taking place.

If there is total blood flow cessation for 30 minutes or more the usual consequence is death to the segment of heart muscle supplied by the occluded artery. This muscle death is a myocardial infarction, popularly known as a heart attack. The main presenting symptom of an acute myocardial infarction is angina that is much more severe in intensity and that lasts for a much longer time than the typical episode of stable angina syndrome. The pain often occurs in the context of generalized symptoms such as weakness, sweating, and anxiety. Many have a sense of impending doom—they feel they are going to die. Contrary to popular misinformation, myocardial infarctions are seldom a result of physical activity. They nearly always strike at rest and often during the early morning hours, shortly after awakening. The timing of the event reflects its pathophysiology. Myocardial infarctions are not a consequence of myocardial demand of exercise outstripping a compromised blood supply, but are caused by the sudden thrombus formation on an unstable atheroma, which then totally occludes the atherosclerotic coronary artery.

Over the last decade, aggressive treatment of hospitalized myocardial infarction patients, with acute thrombolytic (clot-dissolving) therapy and with beta receptor blockers, has drastically reduced both the in-hospital death rate and the 1-year death rate to less than 10% for treated patients. Unfortunately, about 60% of all deaths from an acute infarction occur within 1 hour after the onset of symptoms. Half of all individuals die before they reach the hospital and before they can receive the benefits of these new therapies. Yearly, about 500,000 Americans have myocardial infarctions, and in spite of all recent advances, these acute myocardial infarctions still cause 25% of all deaths in the United States every year.

Sudden cardiac death is best defined as an unexpected demise with a lack of warning symptoms or prodrome. About 80% of victims of sudden death have coronary heart disease. Sudden death is usually the result of a lethal ventricular rhythm disturbance that has its origin in the unstable electrical milieu of heart muscle cells that are affected by ischemia or that are adjacent to an area of scar caused by a prior myocardial infarction. Some persons are fortunate to have the benefit of prompt cardiopulmonary resuscitation within a few minutes of being stricken. They are said to be sudden-death survivors. Their long-term prognosis is poor, with a chance of about 50% of a subsequent fatal event within a year or 2. It is estimated that there are about 300,000 sudden cardiac deaths in the United States yearly. They account for about 50% of all the deaths from cardiovascular disease.

Two recent developments may help decrease the frequency of sudden electrical cardiac death. One is the creation of small defribillators (about the size of the better known pacemakers) that can be permanently implanted within the chest wall of survivors of sudden death (or of those deemed susceptible to such a tragic event). These devices can deliver a resuscitative electric shock to the heart whenever a potentially lethal arrhythmia occurs. The other development is the more extensive availability of external defibrillators in public places such as airports and train and bus stations—so that victims of severe arrhythmias can be quickly brought back to stable rhythms and to life itself.

The concept of silent myocardial ischemia is relatively new. It is based on the observation that the cardiac muscle can be ischemic (or even infarcted) without any symptoms. Such silent ischemia has been detected by electrocardiogram (ECG) changes in 24-hour ambulatory recordings by Holter monitors and described in the findings of the Framingham Study and other investigations that show that as many as 25% of all myocardial infarctions can be silent. Such individuals with silent ischemia and infarction can have as their first presentation sudden cardiac death. They can also present with an ischemic cardiomyopathy, a heart that has suffered small multiple silent infarctions and has become boggy and dilated. Their symptoms will be those of congestive heart failure.

Every year in the United States about 1 million men in the total male population older than 30 years of age manifest symptomatic coronary heart disease for the first time. About 40% present with angina pectoris; another 40% with an acute myocardial infarction; and another 10% have sudden death as their first, last, and only symptom. In the remaining 10%, the first symptoms are those of heart failure, palpitations, or syncope, the sudden loss of consciousness. One should not adopt the common misconception that coronary heart disease afflicts only men. Coronary atherosclerosis and its clinical syndromes affect just as many women as men. On average, however, women experience their clinical coronary heart disease 10 years later than men do. For example, women in their 60s have an incidence of coronary syndromes similar to that of men in their 50s. This is because of the loss of the protective effect of the female hormones, mainly estrogens, whose production is greatly decreased at the onset of menopause.

Function and Disability

The major determinant of impaired function and disability in coronary heart disease is angina. Coronary artery atherosclerosis is not a stable condition. For a myriad of reasons, the tonicity of the muscles in the vessel wall varies during any given time interval and so does the severity of coronary artery stenosis. Thus, an individual patient's angina pattern may have minor weekly, and even daily, variations in severity, frequency, and the level of exertion needed to provoke it. Nonetheless, the typical patient with a typical stable angina syndrome usually has a predictable functional impairment. That is, a similar number of blocks walked on a level surface or on an incline, a similar number of flights of stairs climbed, a similar weight that he lifted or carried, will reproducibly, time after time, result in the same intensity and duration of angina pectoris. The functional impairment and disability can be best determined based on a careful history, which is unique for each individual. Based on this unique individual history medical therapy can be instituted, referral to surgical intervention can be made, and rehabilitation protocols can be carried out.

The estimated functional capacity and subsequent disability of an individual with angina can be confirmed by exercise stress testing. Exercise tests, whether performed on a treadmill or on a bicycle, approximate the exertion of normal activities of daily living. The goal of all stress testing is to increase the work of the heart and its muscle oxygen demand by increasing the exerciser's heart rate and systolic blood pressure. The age-adjusted target heart rate is roughly the number 220 minus the patient's age. For example, the exercise target heart rate of a 40-year-old is 180 beats per minute; that of a 60-year-old, 160 beats per minute. The systolic blood pressure should rise about 60 mm from the rest level to the peak exercise level, and the diastolic blood pressure should drop slightly or remain unchanged. The increasing heart rates and blood pressures are achieved by increasing the workload. On a treadmill, workload is increased by a progressively faster speed and higher incline and on a bicycle, by gradual greater pedal resistance.

The most widely used treadmill protocol for establishing functional capacity, as well as diagnosis and prognosis, is the Bruce protocol. For patients who are undergoing evaluation before or after a program of cardiac rehabilitation and for individuals in whom gas-exchange metabolic evaluation is also being performed, we prefer to use the Bensen protocol at our institution. This is a gentler protocol of 2-minute stages, in which energy expenditure increases in each stage by only 25% over the prior stage. By comparison, the Bruce protocol elicits more demanding increases of 50% in work with each successive stage.

Heart-imaging techniques with exercise, such as with Thallium or the newer Technetium myocardial perfusion agents, nuclear ventriculograms, and echocardiography, have independent value in establishing diagnosis and prognosis and give insightful understanding of the anatomical and physiological basis for an individual's exercise tolerance and functional capacity.

Whenever possible, as determined by the information gained by a medical history, a physical exam, and an exercise stress test, the functional capacity of the individual with heart disease should be described according to the classification system of the New York Heart Association (NYHA). This system establishes four functional classes: Class IV—symptomatic at rest (no effort); Class III—symptomatic with minimal effort; Class II—symptomatic with moderate effort; Class I—asymptomatic at any effort level. This traditional functional classification is useful because it provides a common language and point of reference for all health professionals.

Treatment and Prognosis

The definite and ultimate treatment of coronary artery disease is the radical correction of the biopsychosocial failure that is at its root. Primary prevention (i.e., before any clinical event has taken place) of coronary heart disease should be a main mission of all health professionals and can be accomplished by the reduction or elimination of all of the risk factors for atherosclerosis.

An elevated serum cholesterol level is considered by some investigators to be the primary culprit in atherosclerosis. Some families have an autosomal dominant genetic condition called familial hypercholesterolemia. Patients who are homozygous for the gene have serum cholesterol levels as high as 1,000 mg/dl and have severe coronary and peripheral atherosclerosis in childhood and adolescence. Heterozygous individuals have a serum cholesterol level that ranges from 300 to 500 mg/dl. They also have premature and severe atherosclerosis. Homozygous individuals are only about one in a million and heterozygous only about 2 in a million of the U.S. population, however. Thus, the atherosclerosis epidemic is not the result of an unalterable genetic disorder but is the consequence of an atherogenic lifestyle that can be altered. It has been recently shown that chronic mental and emotional stress can elevate cholesterol. Numerous epidemiological and population studies, human trials of dietary intervention, and experimental animal investigations have shown the high causative correlation between an elevated serum cholesterol and atherosclerosis.

Cholesterol can be lowered below the recommended 200 mg/dl by weight loss and by reducing the consumption of animal fats that contain cholesterol and of saturated fats in general. It is now well documented that one of the lipoproteins that carry cholesterol in the blood, high-density lipoprotein (HDL), has an opposite and protective effect by scooping up circulating cholesterol and bringing it to the liver for degradation. HDL cholesterol can be raised by frequent exercise and by the judicious moderate daily drinking of alcoholic beverages. Hypertension can be lowered by weight loss, exercise, and a diet low in salt. When these natural measures are not successful, or while they are being undertaken, aggressive control of the elevated blood pressure with medication is indicated. Few are the individuals who cannot attain blood pressure control by a combination of interventions.

Most adult-onset diabetic patients have their metabolic disease because of obesity. Weight reduction significantly lowers serum glucose levels in these patients even to normal levels. It is still controversial whether obesity by itself is an independent risk factor. There can be no argument, however, that obesity has a causative relation with all of the atherosclerotic risk factors except for smoking. The smoking of cigarettes doubles the risk of coronary heart disease. Beyond being a causative factor for atherosclerosis, it may constitute an additional separate risk for myocardial infarction. The reduction of risk for infarction may be an astounding 50% within only 1 year after complete smoking cessation. Multiple studies have shown that exercise, through many mechanisms, results in reduced atherosclerosis and in a lower risk of clinical events if atherosclerosis is already present. Coronary heart disease, however, is usually first treated with medications. The medical therapy of stable angina pectoris is based on an understanding of its pathophysiologic basis: ischemia from an increased metabolic demand that cannot be met by a fixed supply.

Pharmaceutical intervention has as its goal the reduction or prevention of that ischemia through two main pharmacological means: an increased supply of blood to the heart muscle and a decreased demand of the heart muscle for that blood. These desired effects are accomplished by the three principal classes of cardiac pharmaceutical agents: nitrates, beta-receptor blockers, and calcium channel blockers. Nitrates are vasodilators. They exert their beneficial effects by dilating coronary arteries directly, thus increasing blood flow to the heart muscle. They also dilate peripheral veins, resulting in the peripheral pooling of blood, with a subsequent reduction in blood return to the heart, less stress on the heart wall, and finally a decreased need for oxygen. Beta-receptor blockers reduce oxygen demand by lowering the heart rate (or chronotropy) and are termed negative chronotropic agents. Calcium channel blockers combine the effects of the nitrates and the beta-blockers. Most of the calcium channel blocker agents available have both vasodilatory and chronotropic effects. Most patients with a stable angina pectoris syndrome can have their angina controlled and their functional impairment and disability eradicated with the use of one of these agents alone or with some combination or all three. Unless a contraindication exists, patients with coronary heart disease and also perhaps asymptomatic individuals with atherosclerosis risk factors should take low-dose prophylactic daily aspirin.

Patients with unstable angina pectoris require immediate hospitalization as they are at risk for an acute infarction. The treatment is based on its pathophysiologic basis: an unstable atherosclerotic plaque that creates a substrate for new thrombus and artery spasm which in turn may result in total vessel occlusion and heart muscle death. Treatment with intravenous heparin is directed at the inhibition of further thrombus formation. Treatment with intravenous nitrates aims to reduce and prevent arterial spasm.

Patients with an acute myocardial infarction should receive immediate intravenous thrombolytic therapy with either streptokinase or tissue plasminogen activator (TPA). The prompt breaking-up of the occluding thrombus results in a restoration of blood flow. If this is done within the first hour or two after the onset of symptoms there is considerable myocardial salvage. The earlier these agents are administered, the greater is the rescue of heart muscle and the patient's chance of survival. Non-medical therapy of coronary heart disease is percutaneous transluminal coronary angioplasty (PTCA) and coronary artery bypass grafting (CABG). About an equal number of these procedures are now performed in the United States yearly. Several randomized studies comparing the efficacy of each treatment are currently under way and preliminary reports indicate no clear superiority of one treatment modality over the other. In PTCA, a balloon-tipped catheter is introduced through a peripheral artery and then manipulated around the aortic arch and inserted into the coronary artery that has the occluding atheroma. The balloon inflation causes an increase of the overall vessel diameter and increased blood flow by the process of atheroma fracture and compression and by stretching of the vessel wall. The initial success rate is now greater than 90%, but re-stenosis occurs at a rate of about 25% within 1 year of the procedure. The recent development of stents, cylindrical rigid metal devices that are placed within a coronary artery at the site of an angioplasty, has decreased the frequency of post-PTCA re-stenosis.

In CABG, saphenous veins from the legs (or an internal mammary artery from inside the chest wall) are used as conduits to restore blood flow by bypassing the site of the atherosclerotic plaque. CABG is performed at present with an operative mortality rate approaching only 1%. More than 90% of operated patients achieve total or significant symptom relief. Progressive atherosclerotic occlusion of the vein grafts, through the same process that affected the native coronary arteries, is likely to occur within 10 years of surgery if the treated individuals do not change their lifestyles to reduce the risk factors for atherosclerosis.

Both procedures are indicated in patients with stable angina pectoris who cannot obtain symptom relief with medical therapy. Emergency PTCA should also be performed when medical treatment alone does not appear to arrest ongoing cardiac muscle damage in unstable angina or in acute myocardial infarction. Bypass surgery is indicated, regardless of symptoms, in patients who are found, by coronary angiography, to have significant disease of the main left coronary artery segment or to have severe triple-vessel disease, especially if they have impaired left ventricular function. Several studies have shown improved survival with surgical (compared to medical) therapy in these patient subgroups with more extensive coronary heart disease.

Newer alternative re-vascularization techniques include removal of the coronary atheroma by mechanical excision (coronary atherectomy) or by ablation using laser energy (laser angioplasty). Both procedures are considered experimental, but they hold great promise because both may supplant the major surgical procedure of coronary artery bypass surgery and solve the problem of re-stenosis in coronary angioplasty. Perhaps the most recent significant development in the management of coronary heart disease is the evidence that coronary atherosclerosis is reversible. It has now been convincingly shown by coronary angiography studies that coronary atherosclerosis can be reversed by lowering cholesterol with lipid-lowering agents or with changes in lifestyle.

The major determinants of prognosis in coronary heart disease are the extent and severity of the coronary atherosclerosis and of the ventricular dysfunction. Coronary artery disease can be best diagnosed and evaluated by exercise stress tests and by cardiac catheterization with coronary angiography. Echocardiography and nuclear ventriculography can assess the ventricular function. The lower the left ventricular ejection fraction (the percentage of blood in the left ventricle ejected with each heart beat, normal being 50% or higher), the worse the prognosis.

Even though the atherosclerotic epidemic still rages, there has been a significant decline in the age-adjusted mortality from all cardiovascular diseases over the past 20 years. The death rate from myocardial infarction alone declined by about 30% during the 1980s. This reduction in mortality is partly accounted for by the creation of hospital coronary care units, the development of sophisticated diagnostic tools, and the advances in medical and surgical therapies. Most of the reduction is the result of changes in lifestyle.

Psychological and Vocational Implications

There is an undisputed relationship between coronary heart disease and psychological disorders. Psychological disorders are definite contributors to atherosclerosis and the clinical syndromes of coronary artery disease. In turn, the diagnosis and treatment of coronary heart disease may create or worsen psychological disorders.

The mechanisms whereby psychological disorders cause or accelerate coronary atherosclerosis have not been well defined. Psychosocial stresses result in increased sympathetic nervous system activity, however, with a greater release of circulating catecholamines (epinephrine and norepinephrine). These, in turn, lead to elevated heart rates, elevated systemic blood pressures, and elevated cholesterol levels and also perhaps to enhanced platelet aggregation and thrombus formation. High catecholamine levels also lower the triggering threshold for ventricular arrhythmias.

Recent primate experiments appear to indicate that atherosclerotic vessels may respond with vasoconstriction when the experimental subjects are exposed to several psychosocial stresses. Moreover, far too many individuals in our society respond to mental or emotional stress by resorting to the immediate oral gratification of smoking or overeating. Poor dietary habits, with the wrong quality and quantity of foods, lead indirectly through obesity—and directly through elevated cholesterol, sugar, and salt intake—to a worse atherosclerosis risk profile.

More specifically, several studies have shown that emotional or mental stress precedes the clinical manifestations of coronary heart disease. There seems to be a positive correlation between an exacerbation of anxiety or depression just before the onset of the symptoms of stable angina and unstable angina, and prior to the occurrence of both fatal and nonfatal myocardial infarction and sudden electrical death. Psychiatric patients with previously diagnosed depression have been shown to have a much greater mortality from coronary heart disease than the general population. Social isolation, both of individuals and of large populations, seems to result in higher rates of sudden death.

Over the past 30 years perhaps the most studied relationship between the mind and the heart has been Type A behavior. Excessive drive, competitiveness, an exaggerated sense of time urgency, and free-floating hostility characterize this behavior. The earlier data seemed to support the thesis that such behavior was a significant independent risk factor for coronary heart disease. Then over the past decade, several major studies found no correlation. One investigation even suggested that Type A behavior may confer a survival advantage by reducing the death rate in survivors of myocardial infarction. Recently, a consensus seems to be developing that the subset of patients with Type A behavior who show cynical hostility and suppressed anger may be the only ones at risk for coronary disease. The conflicting findings may be a consequence of the differing methods (self-administered questionnaires, structure, interviews, videotaped observation of subjects) used in defining the behavior and evaluating the individuals who display it. The issue remains controversial.

Coronary heart disease leads to psychological distress and the development of psychiatric symptoms. Denial, a useful defense mechanism in some circumstances, may be injurious when it leads to self-destructive behavior—such as a delay in getting to the hospital after the first symptoms of a myocardial infarction. Denial is an acute adaptive and beneficial reaction during hospitalization, but when chronic it can be maladaptive and is detrimental because it may lead to noncompliance with prescribed medical therapy or risk factor modification. Anxiety, as both an appropriate response and as an inappropriate one when excessive, is seen during most diagnostic cardiac procedures from the most innocuous, such as echocardiography, to the most tedious and dangerous, such as electrophysiology testing.

An additional interface of psychological disorders and coronary heart disease occurs with the presentation of primary psychiatric disorders as cardiac disease when no cardiac disease exists. Such cardiac presentations are most commonly seen in patients who carry psychiatric diagnoses of hypochondriasis, chronic depression, and chronic anxiety. It is of interest that whereas in the United States anxiety disorders have a prevalence of about 10% in the population, a higher percentage of patients with anxiety disorders consult cardiologists. Specifically, patients with panic attacks are frequent visitors to emergency rooms and the offices of cardiologists. These patients can have many of the symptoms of an acute myocardial infarction: chest pain, palpitations, shortness of breath, dizziness, nausea, sweating, and a sense of impending doom. Many of them are treated erroneously, as if they had coronary heart disease. Indeed, as many as a third of all patients with chest pain syndromes referred for diagnostic coronary angiography who are found to have normal coronary arteries have a panic attack syndrome.

Coronary heart disease has significant vocational implications. Coronary heart disease causes more economic loss in the United States than any other disease or disorder. Millions of Americans are unemployed or underemployed because of the effects of coronary heart disease. The vocational counselor should consider, however, the magnitude of the problem in the context of the fact that the energy requirements of work have decreased in industrialized countries in this century. This is a result of the mechanization, automation, and computerization of labor. In 1950, 65% of all work was considered heavy labor; in 1990 only 5% was.

Therefore, through creative vocational counseling, if the economy and the job market allow, many now unemployed cardiac patients could rejoin the work force. The vocational counselor should take into account the individual's cardiac diagnosis; his or her functional capacity as determined by a careful history, personal observation, and the results of the exercise stress test; and an occupational history that incorporates physical, mental, emotional, and environmental job requirements. Whenever possible, the functional status should be expressed as an NYHA class.

Both the exercise tolerance on the stress test and the energy costs of work or other physical activities should be expressed in metabolic equivalents (METs). One MET is defined as the amount of oxygen consumed by an awake individual at rest. It is equivalent to 3.5 cc of oxygen per kilogram of body weight per minute. Stages of exercise and many vocational and recreational activities have been traditionally classified in terms of how many METs or multiples of the resting oxygen consumption are required by the activity. By the use of this method, results of the exercise stress test can be translated, though not precisely, to the level of exertion at work that the individual may safely perform.

Rates of return to work after a cardiac event or procedure have a range of 35% to 95%. Factors associated with a lower re-employment are severity of the cardiac condition; older age of the patient, social class, or educational level; coexisting psychological conditions; and family environment that is either not supportive or too protective. After a myocardial infarction men return to work at a rate of about 75%. Women have a lower rate of re-employment. Surprisingly the rate for patients after coronary bypass surgery is lower at about 60%. This is paradoxical because 100% of patients have reduced myocardial function after an infarction, and 90% of patients have improved myocardial blood flow after bypass surgery.

Formal rehabilitation programs with a multidisciplinary approach that incorporates supervised exercise, education, and nutritional and psychological counseling are increasingly proving to be beneficial in many aspects. They provide an excellent environment for the effective modification of atherosclerotic risk factors; they improve psychological status; and they increase rates of return to work. Moreover, several recent meta-analytic studies (in which data from similar randomized controlled studies are pooled and analyzed) indicate a secondary-prevention (the avoidance of a subsequent cardiac event) benefit of increased survival and decreased cardiovascular complications.

THE PERICARDIUM

THE PERICARDIUM IS the sac that contains the heart. It helps to fix the heart inside the thorax, protecting it from excessive movement. It prevents direct contact with other organs in the chest, reducing friction during constant cardiac motion. Perhaps it slows the spread of infection to the heart from other organs such as the lungs. Lack of a pericardium is quite compatible with life, however, and if removed, there are usually no clinical consequences.

Disease Description

The most common pericardial disease is pericarditis, or inflammation of the pericardium. This can be caused by infections with tuberculosis, bacteria, or viruses. Other causes are trauma, metabolic or autoimmune diseases, and adverse reactions to medications. Pericarditis can result in the accumulation of fluid within the two layers that make up the pericardium, termed pericardial effusion. When severe, it may result in cardiac tamponade—a choking of the heart that prevents its proper filling and emptying and may result in death. Tumors in the pericardium there either by adjacent spread or by metastasis from a distant site, can also cause pericardial effusion. Months after the acute episode of pericarditis, some patients, especially those with tuberculous pericarditis, may develop chrome constrictive pericarditis. As the inflamed pericardium heals, it scars, contracts, and constricts the heart, resulting in a condition similar to cardiac tamponade. The pericardium can be best visualized, and pericardial diseases diagnosed and evaluated, with echocardiography.

Function and Disability

Functional impairment and disability are usually not considerations in individuals with acute pericarditis because it is a short, limited process without sequelae. The most common symptom in the individual with acute pericarditis is chest pain, quite similar to that of angina pectoris. But it is usually the so-called pleuritic kind because, just as with inflammations of the pleura (the lining of the lungs), the pain comes about at rest, is of a sharp quality, and is worsened by motion, breathing, or coughing. Cardiac tamponade's main symptoms are similar to those of congestive heart failure. Chronic constrictive pericarditis presents with symptoms similar to tamponade, but its time course is more insidious. The patient may be ill for months, even years, and may appear emaciated, as if suffering from terminal cancer.

Functional impairment and disability in chronic constrictive pericarditis are similar to those of myocardial failure, with the notable exception that in chronic pericarditis the complete elimination of the functional impairment or disability may be possible by surgical excision of the constricting pericardium.

Treatment and Prognosis

The treatment of acute pericarditis is the direct treatment of the underlying disease causing the inflammation or infection. The threatening fluid of pericardial effusion or cardiac tamponade can be removed by inserting a small needle in the pericardial space. This procedure is called pericardiocentesis. A persistent or recurrent pericardial effusion of physiological import can be eradicated by the definitive curative procedure of surgical resection of the pericardium. This is also the treatment for chronic constrictive pericarditis. Great care must be taken that a patient with constrictive pericarditis not be medically managed as if ventricular failure was present. Such treatment may cause fluid depletion and dehydration and further decrease cardiac output, which will worsen symptoms and even lead to death.

Prognosis for patients with pericarditis is excellent; it depends on the nature of the condition causing the pericardial inflammation. Proper management of the acute condition, prompt recognition and drainage of pericardial fluid, and correct diagnosis and management of chronic constrictive pericarditis should result in a normal life span.

Psychological and Vocational Implications

The psychological and vocational implications of pericardial disease are not well studied or described. This is mainly because pericardial disorders are neither common nor chronic. The most usual psychological manifestation is the anxiety provoked by the pain of pericarditis because it is confused by the patients, their families, and even by health professionals, with the ischemic pain of angina or an acute myocardial infarction. This situation is particularly devastating because the majority of patients with viral or traumatic pericarditis are young people. Patients with chronic constrictive pericarditis often suffer from clinical chronic depression. Their vocational evaluation should include both physiological and psychological factors.

THE MYOCARDIUM

THE MYOCARDIUM IS the heart muscle itself. It is divided into the left ventricle and the right ventricle. The left ventricle receives oxygenated blood from the lungs via the left atrium, and then pumps that blood to the body via the aorta and its branches. The right ventricle receives deoxygenated blood from the body via the right atrium, and then delivers that blood to the lungs for re-oxygenation via the pulmonary artery.

Disease Description

Diseases of the myocardium are termed cardiomyopathy. There are three anatomical and physiological categories of cardiomyopathy: dilated (an enlarged heart with a thin or normal-thickness muscle wall), hypertrophy (a normal-size or only slightly enlarged heart with a thick muscle wall), and restrictive (a normal-size heart with a thick or normal muscle wall of increased rigidity). The cardiomyopathies are best diagnosed and evaluated with echocardiography.

In the United States dilated cardiomyopathies are usually caused by alcoholism, diabetes, and, principally, by coronary heart disease (ischemic cardiomyopathy). Another cause of dilated cardiomyopathy is inflammation of the myocardium, or myocarditis. This is most frequently caused by a viral infection and unfortunately occurs in young individuals. Some cardiomyopathies that were previously deemed idiopathic, or of unknown cause, are probably viral in origin.

Hypertrophic cardiomyopathies are most often the result of chronic untreated or improperly treated elevated blood pressure, or hypertension. These myopathies, secondary to pressure overloads, usually result in a symmetrical or concentric type of hypertrophy. A different type, asymmetric hypertrophy, which includes idiopathic hypertrophic subaortic stenosis (IHSS), has an unknown etiology, is often familial, and is associated with sudden death in young people.

Restrictive cardiomyopathies are the least common in the United States. They are caused by the infiltration or deposition of extraneous material in the heart muscle. In the case of patients with metabolic diseases or multiple blood transfusions, iron is an example of such extraneous material, as is amyloid in the case of those with chronic infections.

Function and Disability

The major determinant of impaired function and disability in myocardial disease is the degree of myocardial dysfunction. All of the cardiomyopathies, by definition, entail myocardial dysfunction. In dilated cardiomyopathies there is impaired ventricular contraction, or systole. In the hypertrophic and restrictive cardiomyopathies the initial dysfunction is in ventricular relaxation, or diastole. In their advanced stages, the latter two myopathies may also exhibit systolic dysfunction and cardiac dilation and may progressively begin to resemble, anatomically and physiologically, a dilated cardiomyopathy.

All of the cardiomyopathies may create a decreased cardiac blood output state that is insufficient to meet the metabolic needs of the peripheral tissues. This altered physiological state is called congestive heart failure. Congestive heart failure is usually the pathophysiologic endpoint of most cardiovascular diseases because eventually the myocardium is affected. Therefore, whether the initial disorder originated in the coronary arteries or in the cardiac valves or whether it was the result of a systemic condition such as diabetes or hypertension, it is myocardial failure that produces the symptoms that determine functional capacity and disability.

The decreased blood flow in congestive heart failure signals the kidneys to retain fluid. When the excess fluid accumulates in the lungs, it causes the most common symptom of heart failure: difficult breathing, or dyspnea. In the beginning stages of heart failure, when there is only mild impairment, dyspnea occurs only with significant exertion. As the condition becomes more severe and the ventricular function deteriorates, the dyspnea may occur with minimal effort and even at rest. When dyspnea occurs while the patient is lying down, it is termed orthopnea; when it suddenly wakens a patient, it is called paroxysmal nocturnal dyspnea. The excess fluid may also cause abdominal distension, or ascites. It may cause the liver to be enlarged, a condition called hepatomegaly. The fluid deposition in the legs, which usually begins about the ankle area, is termed edema. The symptoms of weakness, fatigue, and lethargy indicate even more severe heart failure and reflect a greatly decreased cardiac blood output.

Functional impairment and disability are best defined by placing a patient in an New York Heart Association class. This can be done by a careful interview, with special attention given to the patient's daily activities. Treadmill exercise stress testing can be useful in determining factional capacity in patients with cardiomyopathies and are of greatest help in those with dilated cardiomyopathies. They are not particularly useful in patients with restrictive cardiomyopathies because often their primary disease is the major contributor to their functional impairment and disability. Moreover, it must be specifically emphasized that patients with ideopathic hypertrophic sub-aortic stenosis (IHSS) should not (as a rule with occasional exceptions) undergo exercise stress testing. In the natural history of their disease, these individuals can have syncope and sudden death with exercise. To exercise them on purpose is a risk. This is particularly true if their ventricular obstruction to blood flow is physiologically significant.

For the assessment of functional capacity in the patient with a dilated cardiomyopathy, a gentler exercise is recommended. Before the test, it should be absolutely determined by interview and careful physical exam that the individual does not have active or decompensated congestive heart failure. Particularly useful and informative in these patients are exercise tests that use imaging of ventricular function such as nuclear ventriculograms or echocardiograms. The patient's ventricular function, including global ejection fraction and segmental wall motion, at rest and with exercise, can be easily, objectively, and safely determined with both techniques. Individuals whose ventricular function worsens with exercise are evidently more functionally limited and more likely to be disabled.

It is of great interest that a low left ventricular ejection fraction at rest, without question the best predictor of prognosis in any cardiovascular disorder, may not be predictive of functional capacity. Some patients with ejection fractions below 30% can have a normal exercise tolerance, whereas some patients with normal ejection fractions of greater than 50% can have a markedly reduced exercise tolerance. This seeming paradox is accounted for by the differing peripheral adaptation in different individuals. Those with higher exercise tolerance and greater functional capacity are more physically fit individuals because of their more efficient skeletal musculature and greater oxygen extraction capability.

Treatment and Prognosis

In the medical management of the patient with myocardial failure it is important to consider first the elimination of any conditions that might have helped to precipitate the failure. Such conditions may be internal stresses (e.g., anemia, fevers, infection, rhythm disturbances, and thyroid disorders) or they may be environmental stresses (e.g., high altitudes or excessive heat or cold). After such contributing factors are eradicated, therapy is aimed at creating the optimal hemodynamic milieu for myocardial function. This milieu can be best created by positively intervening in three components of myocardial mechanics and of congestive heart failure pathophysiology. This is accomplished by increasing inotropy, or myocardial contractility; by decreasing preload, or diastolic ventricular volume; and by decreasing afterload, or the stress or tension of the heart muscle wall during the ejection of blood. By improving one of the three, the two others are also improved.

Specific treatment includes nitrates to directly decrease preload, diuretics to eliminate excess fluid and indirectly reduce preload, digitalis to directly increase inotropy, and after-load reducing agents such as direct vasodilators or angiotensin converting enzyme (ACE) inhibitors. Most patients are also advised to restrict their salt intake because excessive dietary salt will cause fluid retention. There is no definite cure for myocardial failure other than complete cardiac transplantation. Patients referred for cardiac transplantation are those who prove refractory to the best possible combination of medical therapy and are in an NYHA Class IV functional status. Without transplantation, some of these individuals may have as high as a 90% 1-year mortality. This mortality is to be compared to the survival rates of transplantation, which are currently about 85% in 1 year and about 70% in 3 years.

The prognosis of patients with cardiomyopathies depends on the kind of cardiomyopathy and the degree of myocardial dysfunction and congestive heart failure present. Patients with a dilated cardiomyopathy have the worst average prognosis of all cardiomyopathies. Within that group, the individuals with the ischemic cardiomyopathies fare the worst. As a general rule, the worse the ventricular function, as assessed by resting left ventricular ejection fraction, the worse the prognosis and the greater the likelihood of death from end-stage congestive heart failure, cardiovascular collapse, and shock.

Psychological and Vocational Implications

The psychological and vocational implications of pericardial disease are not well studied or described. This is mainly because pericardial disorders are neither common nor chronic. The most usual psychological manifestation is the anxiety provoked by the pain of pericarditis because it is confused by the patients, their families, and even by health professionals, with the ischemic pain of angina or of an acute myocardial infarction. This situation is particularly devastating because the majority of patients with viral or traumatic pericarditis are young people. Patients with chronic constrictive pericarditis often suffer from clinical chronic depression. Their vocational evaluation should include both physiological and psychological factors.

THE ENDOCARDIUM

DISEASES OF THE HEART'S endocardium (its inner lining surface which is in contact with systemic blood) are mainly those of the four cardiac valves: the aortic, the mitral, the pulmonic, and the tricuspid. While rare diseases may primarily involve the endocardial lining and only secondarily the valves, these are quite uncommon in the United States

Disease Description

The principal etiologic factor of endocardial and valvular heart disease, in the developed as well as the developing countries of the world, has been rheumatic fever, a result of the body's immune response against a streptococcal infection. Rheumatic fever can result in both valvular insufficiency (or "leaky" valves) and valvular stenosis (or "tight" valves). With the introduction and widespread use of penicillin and other antibiotics to treat streptococcal infections, the incidence of rheumatic heart disease, and of valvular disease in general, has progressively and significantly decreased over the past half-century in economically developed nations. This decrease, at the same time that coronary atherosclerosis is on the increase, has limited endocardial and valvular disease to fewer than 10% of all cases of cardiovascular disease in these countries, while its prevalence remains high in underdeveloped areas of the world.

Mitral stenosis, with very few exceptions, is always secondary to rheumatic heart disease. About 70% of patients with mitral stenosis are women. Even though the left ventricle is usually normal in mitral stenosis, symptoms similar to those of congestive heart failure, such as dyspnea and orthopnea, begin in these patients when they are in their 40s or 50s. The elevated pressures in the left atrium and the pulmonary vasculature that must be generated to force the blood through the stenotic mitral valve cause these symptoms. Complications of mitral stenosis such as arrhythmias can lead to symptoms of palpitations. Mitral regurgitation is caused in 50% of cases by rheumatic fever. Pure rheumatic mitral regurgitation is more common in men than in women. Infective endocarditis, which preferentially attacks valves previously damaged by rheumatic disease, also leads to mitral regurgitation. Causative are also a variety of conditions that affect the supporting structures of the valve. There can be dilation or calcification of the mitral annulus, the ring-like orifice between the left atrium and ventricle that the valve occupies. Also there can be fibrosis of the papillary muscles, which through the netlike chordae tendinea attach the valve leaflets to the left ventricle. A unique disease entity of the mitral valve is the mitral valve prolapse syndrome. In this condition, the leaflets of the mitral valve prolapse into the left atrium during valve closure. Echocardiographic studies have suggested that the incidence of this condition may be about 5% in the female population.

Aortic stenosis may be caused by rheumatic fever, by degenerative calcification of the cusps, or by a congenital condition called bicuspid aortic valve. Bicuspid aortic valve is abnormal because it has two instead of three cusps. This abnormality, the most common congenital cardiac abnormality, occurs in about 2% of the population. In only a small portion of that group does this congenital condition result in clinical disease, however. As opposed to stenosis of the mitral valve, where mainly women are affected, about 80% of adult patients with isolated aortic stenosis are men.

Aortic regurgitation is mainly rheumatic in origin, especially when found in combination with mitral valve disease. Nearly 80% of patients with pure aortic regurgitation are men. Women are the majority of those who have concomitant mitral disease. A bicuspid aortic valve can also become insufficient. An increasing incidence of aortic regurgitation is caused by infective endocarditis. Diseases that result in the dilation of the aorta itself may also dilate the aortic valve annulus and lead to secondary aortic insufficiency. Disorders of the valves of the right side of the heart are far less common than those of the valves of the left side of the heart. Tricuspid stenosis is very uncommon and is usually secondary to rheumatic heart disease and found in association with disease of the other valves. Tricuspid insufficiency is more common than stenosis and results from either infective endocarditis in users of intravenous drugs or from right ventricular enlargement and accompanying tricuspid anular dilation. Of all valvular disorders, those of the pulmonic valve are the rarest. The most common pulmonic valve disorder is insufficiency secondary to pulmonary hypertension.

Function and Disability

The major determinant of impaired function and disability in endocardial disease is the severity of the valvular stenosis or insufficiency and the degree of secondary myocardial dysfunction.

Valvular insufficiency and valvular stenosis both interfere with normal cardiac blood flow. Valvular insufficiency leads to a volume overload and eventual dilation of the cardiac chambers. Aortic and pulmonic stenosis lead to a pressure overload and ventricular hypertrophy and atrial dilation. These overloads, if severe and if left untreated, will invariably lead to congestive heart failure. The time to onset of symptoms is related to the severity of the valvular lesion and also to the age and physical fitness of the individual patient.

Individuals with valvular disease may have the following symptoms: chest pain that has some of the features of angina pectoris, palpitations from both atrial and ventricular arrhythmias, and dyspnea most often when mitral regurgitation is present. In addition to the symptoms of congestive heart failure, patients with aortic stenosis can also have chest pain indistinguishable from angina pectoris and can also have sudden death as their only clinical presentation. Disease classification by NYHA criteria is similar to that of the patient with coronary heart disease or with a cardiomyopathy. If an appropriate functional history cannot be obtained, exercise stress testing is a good objective indicator of function in these patients. It should be noted, however, that exercise testing is relatively contraindicated in patients with mild to moderate mitral stenosis and aortic stenosis and absolutely contraindicated when the stenoses are severe. With exercise testing, those with stenotic valvular disease may develop acute pulmonary edema and those with aortic stenosis may also have syncope.

Treatment and Prognosis

Treatment is the surgical replacement of the diseased valve with either a porcine (pig) valve or a metal valve prosthesis. The use of porcine valves is rapidly falling into disfavor because it is becoming evident that they may become dysfunctional within 10 years after implantation. Replacement with a metal prosthesis results in the need for life-long anti-coagulation. Regurgitant valves can at times be surgically repaired, rather than replaced, in what essentially can be considered plastic surgery of the heart.

The treatment of patients with mitral valve prolapse is mainly reassurance that they have a good prognosis. Medical treatment with beta-blockers may be necessary to treat symptoms of palpitations from their benign yet symptomatic arrhythmias. A mitral valve prolapse patient with significant mitral regurgitation, like all other patients with valvular disease or with prosthetic valves, should have antibiotic prophylaxis before dental work or before surgery to prevent acquiring endocarditis from a potential bacteremia (the introduction of bacteria into the blood) that may happen with such procedures. The prognosis of patients with valvular disease is excellent as long as replacement, repair, or valvuloplasty is performed—before there is damage to the ventricles, the atriae, or the pulmonary vasculature. Once the chronic volume or pressure overloads have irreversibly damaged these structures, the surgical mortality is markedly increased, from about 1% in uncomplicated cases to greater than 15% in those with failing ventricles. These unfortunate individuals have a decreased life span even if the surgery is successful and the prosthetic valve has perfect function. Severely dysfunctional cardiac valves, if not repaired or replaced, usually will lead to death within 5 years.

Psychological and Vocational Implications

In many respects, the psychological and vocational implications of endocardial and valvular heart disease are the same as those of the dilated cardiomyopathies, especially when secondary ventricular dysfunction exists. Unique psychological situations in the valvular diseases arise because many of the patients with rheumatic valvular disease are young women of child-bearing age. Often, some patients who are childless must make a decision as to whether to become pregnant even though pregnancy may worsen their cardiac condition and lead to risk of death. At times, the stress-laden decision is not whether to become pregnant but whether to terminate an advanced wanted pregnancy. Psychological intervention and support is needed before, during, and particularly after the time of decision making. Patients with mitral valve prolapse present a difficult challenge to the psychologist. These individuals, with cardiac symptoms but with a good prognosis, are often disabled for psychological, not physiological, reasons. A team approach, with the cardiologist, psychologist, and other caregivers working together, is often more effective than an uncoordinated approach that often confuses the patient and results in further disabling distress.

Unique vocational implications exist with patients with valvular heart disease because this is the only group of cardiovascular diseases in which women constitute a majority. Patients with mitral valve prolapse and rheumatic mitral valve disease are often young women who have to care for a family and work outside the home in the context of their mitral disease. Surgical valve replacement often occurs in older women in their late 50s or early 60s who are near retirement age. Many do not return to work after the surgery. Many live alone because they have survived their husbands, who have already died from their own coronary heart disease. The rehabilitative and vocational challenges are great in this group of patients.

THE ELECTRICAL CONDUCTION SYSTEM

Disease Description
The cardiac conduction system, made of specialized fibers, has two functions. The main cardiac pacemaker, the sinus, or sinoatrial (SA) node, generates the rhythmic electrical impulse that is the basis of life. The other parts of the system include the atrioventricular (AV) node (the backup or auxiliary pacemaker), the bundle of His, the bundle branches, and the Purkinje fibers. They all ensure the sequential and uniform propagation of the electrical current so that the cardiac cycle of ventricular systole and diastole is an organized and effective activity.

Disease Description
Disorders of the electrical system can result in bradycardia (slow rates of less than 60 beats per minute), tachycardia (fast rates at greater than

100 beats per minute), or arrhythmias or dysrhythmias (irregular rhythms). Arrhythmias of a slow rate are brady-arrhythmias and those of a fast rate are tachy-arrhythmias. Dysrhythmias can be further classified as those with an abnormal current originating from the atriae or supraventricular arrhythmias, and those with an abnormal origin in the ventricles or ventricular arrhythmias. Supraventricular arrhythmias are paroxysmal atrial tachycardia (PAT), atrial flutter, atrial fibrillation, and multifocal atrial tachycardia (MAT). Although the atrial rates vary, the ventricular rate in these arrhythmias, even if untreated, is generally relatively slow, about 150 beats per minute, because the impulses are slowed or blocked at the level of the AV node and the His bundle. MAT occurs mostly in patients with pulmonary disease. PAT can occur in normal persons without heart disease and is most commonly precipitated by anxiety or by the ingestion of irritants such as alcohol and caffeine. Atrial flutter and fibrillation happen in patients with atriae that are enlarged either because of ventricular dysfunction or mitral or tricuspid valvular disease. An overly active thyroid gland, or hyperthyroidism, may cause atrial fibrillation.

Ventricular arrhythmias are evident in ventricular tachycardia and ventricular fibrillation. Ventricular tachycardia and fibrillation usually occur in patients with a dilated cardiomyopathy or a prior myocardial infarction. They are rare, but do occur, in people with normal ventricles.

A rare congenital anomaly of the conduction system occurs in the presence of an accessory pathway, an extra bundle with conduction properties akin to those of the conduction system. Such a bundle allows the electrical activity from the atriae to the ventricles to bypass the AV node and the bundle of His. Patients with these abnormalities, called pre-excitation syndromes, are usually young, are prone to episodes of PAT, and can have very fast ventricular rates with atrial fibrillation. There are two types of pre-excitation syndromes: Wolff-Parkinson-White (WPW) syndrome and Lown-Ganong-Levine (LGL) syndrome.

Cardiac electrical block is said to occur when either of the two cardiac pacemakers cannot generate a normal electrical impulse or when a normal impulse is not conducted correctly through the conduction system. Fibrosis of the conduction system, which is part of the aging process, is a cause of electrical blocks in the elderly. Most blocks, however, like most arrhythmias, are the result of coronary heart disease.

Function and Disability

The functional impairments and disabilities that result from the cardiac arrhythmias fall into two major categories. One is the physiologic disability from the ineffective ventricular contractions and decreased cardiac output that is secondary to a chronic arrhythmia that is too slow, too fast, or too disorganized. (Atrial fibrillation is the prototype and its symptoms place the functional considerations of this arrhythmia with those of congestive heart failure.) The other is the psychological disability secondary to an arrhythmia that is not chronic but acute. Such an arrhythmia is unpredictable. It arrives suddenly and without any warning. Ventricular tachycardia is the prototype. The individual may have no physiological functional limitation or disability with the activities of daily life yet may refrain from work because of fear of precipitating the arrhythmia with activity.

Patients with supraventricular arrhythmias have palpitation as their most common symptom. PAT and atrial flutter are acute and not chronic arrhythmias and therefore have no functional or disability implications when they are not present. Those with atrial flutter or fibrillation may develop syncope or symptoms of congestive heart failure, especially if they have the arrhythmias in the context of impaired ventricular function. Those with coexisting coronary artery disease may develop angina pectoris because the fast heart rates of the arrhythmia create metabolic demands that cannot be met by the compromised blood supply through the obstructed coronary arteries. Patients whose heart rate in atrial fibrillation is controlled at rest can still have exertional dyspnea, as in this condition the heart rate may rapidly increase with little exertion.

The chaotic atrial electrical activity of atrial fibrillation creates a combination of turbulence and stasis of blood in the atriae. This can lead to the complication of thrombus formation in the atriae. These thrombi can dislodge and be carried by the circulation to other parts of the body. Such a traveling thrombus, or embolus, may cause obstruction of blood flow to the eyes, leading to blindness, or to the kidneys, causing renal failure. When carried to the brain, it may result in cerebral infarction, or stroke.

If ventricular tachycardia is of a short duration (a few seconds), the patient may experience palpitation. If of a longer duration (a few minutes), syncope may occur. If sustained beyond a few minutes, degeneration to ventricular fibrillation is likely, and sudden death may ensue.

Individuals with the accessory pathway syndromes will experience palpitation when PAT is their acute arrhythmia. In them, atrial fibrillation, if of prolonged duration and of a very fast ventricular rate, may degenerate into ventricular fibrillation and lead to sudden cardiac death. The health professional should not be deceived into complacency because the patient looks young, healthy, and vigorous. Atrial fibrillation in a patient with a pre-excitation syndrome is dire. Severe bradycardia or high degrees of block, resulting in heart rates of less than 30 beats per minute, can cause fatigue and dizziness because of the decreased cardiac output and the resultant diminished cerebral perfusion. When the effective rate is even slower or when the bradycardia is sudden in onset, syncope may occur.

Treatment and Prognosis

The treatment of supraventricular arrhythmias involves their prevention, their quick termination, or the prompt and effective control of their fast rate. Avoiding stressful situations and the ingestion of alcohol or stimulants such as caffeine and antihistamines can prevent supraventricular arrhythmias. If the initiation of the arrhythmia is not preventable, then it may be terminated, or its fast rate controlled, by medications that slow electrical conduction through the AV node such as digitalis, beta-blockers, and calcium channel blockers. Individuals whose atrial fibrillation is chronic or recurrent (paroxysmal atrial fibrillation) need to take such medications for life to control their heart rates. Most of them will also require lifelong anticoagulation with warfarin (Coumadin) to prevent thrombus formation and embolization. If medication fails to abolish the arrhythmia or if the patient is severely ill because of angina pectoris, severe congestive heart failure, or shock, then prompt electrical cardioversion to normal sinus rhythm is indicated.

The treatment of sustained ventricular tachycardia and of ventricular fibrillation should be prompt electrical cardioversion to a normal rhythm. Only younger individuals with normal ventricular function can tolerate sustained ventricular tachycardia. Ventricular fibrillation is not compatible with life. Anti-arrhythmic agents to prevent these ventricular arrhythmias should be prescribed only by expert cardiologists who have evaluated the arrhythmia with invasive electrophysiological studies. It is no longer acceptable to treat such patients empirically, as these agents have been found to have a high pro-arrhythmic potential. In as high as 25% of the cases, they can precipitate the very arrhythmia they are supposed to prevent or even make it worse.

Patients with ventricular arrhythmias who do not respond to medical therapy may require surgical ablation of the myocardial focus from which the arrhythmia originates. Some, with recurrent episodes of ventricular fibrillation, may require the chronic implantation of an anti-arrhythmic device, similar to a pacemaker, called an implantable automatic defibrillator, to deliver an electrical shock whenever ventricular fibrillation occurs. The ultimate treatment of ventricular arrhythmias, however, lies in the prevention of coronary heart disease, which is present in about 80% of patients with malignant ventricular arrhythmias and sudden electrical death.

The treatment of patients with the pre-excitation syndromes is similar to that of those with supraventricular arrhythmias. However, great caution is needed when giving anti-arrhythmic agents to these patients because a paradoxical effect may result, that is, the arrhythmia may be made worse and faster rates may obtain if agents that would normally control the arrhythmia or slow down its rate are administered. In patients who arrhythmia is refractory to medical therapy or those who have the lethal trial fibrillation with a very rapid ventricular rate, ablation of the accessory pathway, possible nowadays by different techniques, is recommended.

Cardiac electrical blocks and symptomatic bradycardia are treated with the implantation of permanent pacemakers that substitute for the heart's own pacemakers and conduction system. In recent years, technology has led to the development of ever more sophisticated and smaller pacing devices that nearly duplicate the heart's electrophysiological mechanisms and allow for nearly normal ventricular hemodynamics.

The prognosis for patients with supraventricular arrhythmia under appropriate medical care is excellent. Their mortality depends on the physiological cause of the arrhythmia rather than on the arrhythmia itself. For example, those with normal hearts or with hyperthyroidism have a much better prognosis than do those whose arrhythmias are complications of structural heart disease, such as mitral stenosis or myocardial dysfunction.

The prognosis for the patient who is a survivor of sudden death and who has recurrent episodes of ventricular fibrillation or ventricular tachycardia is dismal. This is particularly the case for those with a dilated cardiomyopathy and a left ventricular ejection fraction of less than 20%. This poor prognosis has been ameliorated by the practice of medical therapy guided by electrophysiologic testing, by the newer surgical techniques, and by the use of the implantable defibrillators.

The prognosis in patients with pre-excitation syndrome is excellent because they usually have otherwise normal hearts. If the correct diagnosis is made and expert prompt treatment is rendered the few times it is needed, these individuals will have normal life spans. The prognosis of patients requiring pacemakers is excellent if the ventricular function is normal. If pacing was necessary because of severe coronary heart disease or from ventricular tachyarrhythmia with a normally functioning pacemaker in place.

Psychological and Vocational Implications

The psychological implications of cardiac arrhythmias are significant. Not only is the psychologist confronted with the psychological consequences of the arrhythmias, but perhaps more important, psychological disorders may trigger lethal arrhythmias.

As mentioned, a chronic depression or anxiety syndrome that may develop over time after repeated episodes of their sudden and unexpected tachyarrhythmia may disable patients with paroxysmal atrial fibrillation (PAT), recurrent ventricular tachycardia, and ventricular fibrillation. They may progressively and drastically curtail their range of activities as they associate the onset of their arrhythmias with particular events, places, or times. Phobias and a repertoire of superstitious behaviors may develop in many of these individuals. Intensive yet non-threatening psychological interventions are often necessary.

Particularly difficult is the control and prevention of the psychological precipitants of the arrhythmias. It is well documented that about 1% of all patients with malignant ventricular arrhythmias have no demonstrable structural heart disease, and the only causative factor for their arrhythmia is psychological. An even greater percentage of patients with known heart disease have their potentially lethal arrhythmias triggered by psychological factors. A few medical centers have laboratories and testing protocols that elicit and identify specific thoughts, ideas, or mental images that trigger the arrhythmias in a particular individual.

The judicious use of anti-arrhythmic agents, in combination with beta-blockers and directed and focused psychological intervention, has proved quite successful in preventing or reducing the frequency of arrhythmias in such patients. The vocational implications of cardiac arrhythmias are also significant. The vocational counselor must undertake a careful evaluation of the work situation, with special attention given to any environmental, emotional, or mental stress that may precipitate or aggravate the arrhythmia.

DISEASES OF THE VASCULAR SYSTEM

THE VASCULAR SYSTEM, also know as the peripheral vascular system, is responsible for the circulation of blood from the heart to the rest of the body and back again to the heart. Its components are the aorta, the arteries, the arterioles, the capillaries, and the veins. In this chapter, only diseases of the aorta will be considered. Disease of specific vessels and of the smaller vasculature are covered in other chapters of this book.

THE AORTA

THE AORTA, THE largest artery in the body, receives the blood from the heart and then, through its branches, delivers that blood to the rest of the body. Because of its large size and its unique function as the receiving conduit for blood directly from the left ventricle, the walls of the aorta experience greater tension and stress than do other blood vessels. Therein lies the anatomical and physiological substrate for its diseases.

Disease Description

Arteriosclerosis develops in the aorta just as it does in the coronary arteries. Such is the extent of the process that nearly all adults in the United States are believed to have some measure of aortic arteriosclerosis. Even children and adolescents have been shown to have aortic fatty streaks, the earliest lesion of aortic arteriosclerosis. The vast majority of patients with clinical aortic disease are hypertensive men who smoke cigarettes. There are three main diseases of the aorta: aneurysms, dissections, and obstructive disease. Diseases of the aorta and its branches are best evaluated by angiography. The new technique of trans-esophageal echocardiography (TEE) is particularly useful for the evaluation of diseases of the thoracic aorta.

An aortic aneurysm is an abnormal dilation of the aorta that is susceptible to acute rupture. Aneurysms can be found in the thoracic aorta (in both its ascending and descending segments) and also in the abdominal aorta. Ascending aortic aneurysms are the ones that are least likely to be caused by arteriosclerosis.

Before our age of antibiotics and organized prevention of sexually transmitted diseases, ascending aortic aneurysms were mainly caused by syphilis. At present the most common cause of ascending aneurysms is damage of the middle layer of the aortic wall, the media. This condition is termed cystic medial necrosis and is of unknown etiology. Aneurysms of the descending thoracic aorta and of the abdominal aorta are nearly all caused by arteriosclerosis. Many patients who have thoracic aneurysms also have abdominal aneurysms, and about 10% of those with abdominal aneurysms have more man one.

Aortic dissections can occur anywhere in the aorta. A dissection takes place when the innermost of the three layers of the wall of the aorta, the intima, breaks and allows blood to flow into the wall of the aorta itself. The pressure of the blood separates the layers of the aorta. Hypertension plays a significant role in aortic dissections regardless of their location. Surgeons categorize dissections into three types: Type I dissection involves the entire aorta, from its ascending portion, around the arch, and into the abdominal aorta. Type II dissection is limited to the ascending aorta. Type III dissection is limited to the descending aorta. Aortic obstructive disease, like coronary artery obstructive disease, impedes the adequate flow of blood. Obstruction in the aorta is most frequently noted in its terminal portion, usually at its bifurcation into the iliac and femoral arteries, the vessels that supply the lower extremities.

Function and Disability

Most patients with aortic aneurysms and dissections are free of functional impairments and disability because they are asymptomatic until the moment of the acute event. Aortic aneurysms are most often found on routine abdominal physical exam or by x-rays. Symptoms, when they do exist, may be only those of a lower back pain syndrome. Some patients may actually have been misdiagnosed as having lumbar vertebral disease.

Obstructive aortic disease does cause disability and chronic functional impairment. The most common symptom is claudication. This is pain of one or both legs, usually in the muscles of the calves, with walking. Patients may be able to walk only a few feet before disabling pain impedes further walking. They may also have pain of the thighs and buttocks with walking and at rest. They often have impotence. The functional capacity of patients with claudication and the degree of their vascular stenosis can be evaluated by Doppler ultrasound of the legs. This is performed before and after treadmill walking, using special test protocols different from those used for the evaluation of the impairment in coronary heart disease.

Treatment and Prognosis

The treatment of aortic aneurysms, of dissections, and of severe obstructive disease is always surgical. The acute rupture of an aortic aneurysm is nearly always a fatal event. When an abdominal aneurysm has a diameter of less that 6 cm, the probability of rupture is about 15% over a 10-year period, but if the aneurismal diameter is 6 cm or greater, there is a 50% probability of rupture in a shorter time span. The operative mortality of elective abdominal aneurysm resection is less than 10%. Resection of aneurysms of the ascending aorta or of the aortic arch carries a greater operative mortality. There is about a 20% mortality in the surgical treatment of aortic dissections.

The surgical treatment of obstructive disease of the main branches of the aorta to the lower extremities is aortic-femoral bypass grafting, using synthetic conduits to restore circulation to the legs. Excellent results are achieved with little mortality and morbidity, and claudication is abolished or decreased in about 90% of patients. As in coronary disease, an alternative treatment is percutaneous balloon angioplasty, most recently with the additional placement of vascular metal stents. This procedure is particularly feasible in the dilation of discrete lesions of the iliac arteries.

The prognosis of patients with any type of arteriosclerotic disease of the aorta and its branches can be best determined in the context of their coexisting coronary artery arteriosclerosis. It is the extent and severity of the coronary disease that is the major determinant of both the operative mortality and of the long-term survival of patients who undergo successful aortic or peripheral vascular surgery.

Psychological and Vocational Implications

There are usually no psychological implications in aortic disorders before the acute events of aortic aneurysm rupture and of aortic dissection because the patterns are usually asymptomatic up to that time. Most of these patients had denied the potential consequences of their smoking or of their uncontrolled hypertension. The acute event has perhaps no match in all of medicine as a truly terrifying experience. Most survivors of the event, and the subsequent surgery, experience a reversal of their present psychological mind-set, become acutely aware of their mortality, and may develop chronic depression and even excessive anxiety and an over-vigilant state. Such individuals can benefit from psychological intervention. A group of patients with a similar problem are those who are informed of the presence of an abdominal aortic aneurysm that is still too small to undergo surgical resection. They may spend months or even years in watchful waiting before surgery is finally indicated. Psychological implications in patients with obstructive aortic disease usually focus on their loss of self-esteem because of their inability to walk and work and principally because of impotence.

There are important vocational implications in aortic diseases. The patients who have had surgical repair of an aortic aneurysm or dissection have an even lower rate of return to work than do those who have had coronary bypass surgery. This may be due to the advanced age of these patients, most of whom are in their 60's and 70's. It may also be because the surgical procedure that was performed on them is perceived as, and is in fact, more complex than coronary bypass surgery. Patients with occlusive disease have specific vocational considerations because they are unable to perform most work activity that entails walking or prolonged standing. They may be employed in jobs that require the performance of work only with the arms, and only while sitting and with infrequent walking for short distances.

SUMMARY

THE CHALLENGE OF cardiovascular disorders will continue to grow as long as their prevention is not given emphasis and priority. If present trends continue the diagnostic and therapeutic advances of the past decades may reduce cardiovascular mortality without a reduction of the prevalence of cardiovascular disease and its attendant functional limitation and disability. The need of individuals with cardiovascular disease for medical, psychological, rehabilitative, and vocational services may be greater than ever.

RECOMMENDED READINGS

General

Braunwald, G., Zipes, D., Libby, P., & Bonow, R. (2004). *Braunwald's heart disease: A textbook of cardiovascular medicine* (7th ed.). Philadelphia: Elsevier and Saunders.

Braunwald, E. (1997). The Shattuck Lecture—Cardiovascular medicine at the turn of the millennium: Triumphs, concerns, and opportunities. *New England Journal of Medicine, 337,* 1360–1369.

Braunwald, E. (2004). Cardiology: The past, the present, and the future. *Journal of the American College of Cardiology, 42,* 2031–2041.

Kleinman, N., & Califf, R. (2000). Results from late-breaking clinical trials at the sessions of the American College of Cardiology in 2000. *Journal of the American College of Cardiology, 36,* 310–325.

Stafford, R., & Radley, D. (2003). The underutilization of cardiac medications of proven benefit (1990 to 2002). *Journal of the American College of Cardiology, 41,* 56–61.

Mosca, L., Appel, L., Benjamin, E., et al. (2004). Evidence-based guidelines from cardiovascular disease prevention in women. *Circulation, 109,* 672–693.

Mosca, L., Collins, P., Herrington, D., et al. (2001). Hormone replacement therapy and heart disease: A statement for healthcare professionals from the American Heart Association. *Circulation, 104,* 499–503.

The Coronary Arteries

Ross, R. (1999). Atherosclerosis—An inflammatory disease. *New England Journal of Medicine, 340,* 115–126.

Ridker, P. (2001). High sensitivity C-reactive protein—A potential adjunct for global risk assessment in the primary prevention of cardiovascular disease. *Circulation, 103,* 1813–1818.

Danesk, J., Wheeler, J., Gideon, M., Hirschfield, G., Shinich, E., Guday, E., et al. (2004). C-reactive protein and other markers of inflammation in the prediction of coronary disease. *New England Journal of Medicine, 350,* 1387–1397.

Deedwanna, P. (2004). Metabolic syndrome and vascular disease. Is nature or nurture leading the new epidemic of cardiovascular disease? *Circulation, 109,* 2–4.

James, S., Lindhal, B., & Siegkahn, A. (2003). Natriuretic peptide and other risk markers for the separate prediction of mortality in patients with unstable coronary artery disease. *Circulation, 108,* 278–283.

Gibbons, R., Abrams, J., Chaterjee, K., et al. (2003). American College of Cardiology and American Heart Association guidelines update for the management of the patient with angina: Summary article. *Circulation, 107,* 149–158.

Expert panel on detection, education, and treatment of high blood cholesterol in adults; Executive summary (2002). *Circulation, 6,* 3143–3421.

Jacobs, A. (2003). Primary angioplasty for acute myocardial infarction. *New England Journal of Medicine, 349,* 798–800.

Melo, L., Pachoi, A., Kong, D., et al. (2004). Myocardial gene therapy: Molecular and cell based therapies for protection, rescue, and repair of ischemic myocardium. *Circulation, 109,* 2386–2393.

Verma, S., Fedah, P., Weisel, R., et al. (2004). Off-pump coronary artery bypass surgery: Fundamentals for the clinical cardiologist. *Circulation, 109,* 1206–1211.

Gidron, Y., Gilutz, H., Berger, H., et al. (2002). Molecular and cellular interface between behavior and acute coronary syndromes. *Cardiovascular Research, 56,* 15–21.

Wulsin, L., & Singal, B. (2003). Do depressive symptoms increase the risk for the onset of coronary disease: A systematic quantitative review. *Psychosomatic Medicine, 5,* 201–210.

Wilson, P. (2004). Prediction of coronary heart disease events: The contribution of life style factors. *Cardiology Rounds, 8,* 2–12.

The Myocardium

Redfield, M. (2002). Heart failure—An epidemic of uncertain proportion. *New England Journal of Medicine, 347,* 1442–1444.

Levy, D., Kenchaiah, S., Larson, M., et al. (2002). Long term trends in the incidence and survival with heart failure. *New England Journal of Medicine, 347,* 1397–1402.

Young, J. (2004). Top trials in heart failure today. *Cardiology, 4,* 9–38.

Hunt, S., Baker, D., Chin, M., et al. (2001). The American College of Cardiology and American Heart Association guidelines for the evaluation of chronic heart failure in the adult: Executive summary. *Journal of the American College of Cardiology, 38*(7), 2101–2113.

Nohria, A., Lewis, E., & Stevenson, L. (2002). Medical management of advanced heart failure. *Journal of the American College of Cardiology, 39,* 83–89.

Abraham, W., Fisher, W., Smith, A., et al. (2002). Cardiac resynchronization in chronic heart failure. *New England Journal of Medicine, 346,* 1845–1853.

Frey, N., Katus, H., Olson, E., et al. (2004). Hypertrophy of the heart: A new therapeutic target. *Circulation, 109,* 1580–1589.

Shan, K., Constantine, G., Swananthan, M., et al. (2004). Role of cardiac magnetic resonance imaging in the assessment of myocardial viability. *Circulation, 109,* 1328–1334.

Kasper, E., Gertenblith, G., Hefter, G., et al. (2002). A randomized trial of the efficacy of multidisciplinary care in heart failure patients at high risk of hospital readmission. *Journal of the American College of Cardiology, 39,* 471–480.

The Endocardium

Cheitlin, M., et al. (2003). *American College of Cardiology and American Heart Association guidelines update for the clinical application of echocardiography.* Retrieved from http://www.acc.org/clinical/guidelines/echo

Rahimtoola, S. (2004). The year in valvular heart disease. *Journal of the American College of Cardiology, 43,* 491–504.

Sedrakyan, A., Vaccarino, V., & Paltiel, A. (2003). Age does not limit quality of life improvement in cardiac valve surgery. *Journal of the American College of Cardiology, 42,* 1208–1214.

The Electrical Conduction System

Wattinney, W., Mensah, G., & Croft, J. (2003). Increasing trends in hospitalization for atrial fibrillation in the United States (1985–1999). *Circulation, 108,* 711–716.

Fuster, V., Ryden, L., Asinger, R., et al. (2001). American College of Cardiology and American Heart Association guidelines for the management of patients with atrial fibrillation: Executive summary. *Journal of the American College of Cardiology, 38,* 1231–1266.

Gregoratis, G., Abrams, J., Epstein, A., et al. (2002). American College of Cardiology and American Heart Association guidelines update for implantation of cardiac pacemakers and anti-arrhythmic devices: Summary article. *Circulation, 106,* 2145–2161.

9

Chronic Pain Syndromes

ANDREW R. BLOCK, PhD, EDWIN F. KREMER, PhD,
AND ANN M. KREMER, PhD

O NE OF THE United States' most significant health problems is
chronic pain, pain of 6 months or longer duration. Approximately
30% of the U.S. population experiences a chronically painful condition (Bonica, 1990). Frymoyer and Durett (1997) estimate that over $125
billion is expended annually on hospital and medical treatment of chronic
pain. Approximately 50 million Americans are partially or totally disabled
by chronic pain with the disability lasting for weeks to many years.

Chronic pain is associated with a wide variety of medical conditions
and can affect every organ system in the body. The International
Association for the Study of Pain has developed a *Classification of Chronic
Pain* (Merskey & Bogduk, 1994). This classification system identifies over
600 pain syndromes: these include 66 syndromes involving the head and
neck, 35 the upper extremities, 154 the thoracic and cervical systems, 136
the lumbar, sacral, and coccygeal, spine, 85 the trunk, and 18 lower extremities. Thirty-six generalized syndromes are identified. These syndromes
affect more then three painful sites. Obviously, with such a plethora of
conditions, a single chapter can not approach comprehensive coverage.
By examining a few common syndromes, however, much can be learned
about the assessment and treatment of chronic pain in general.

INCIDENCE OF CHRONIC PAIN

LARGE-SCALE EPIDEMIOLOGICAL research details the prevalence of the various chronic pain syndromes (see Crombie, Croft, Linton, LeResche, & VonKorff, 1999). Two common syndromes are chronic back pain and headaches. Research by Luo, Pietrobon, Sun, Liu, and Hey (2003) used a national household survey of people 18 years and older in 1998. In that year, 25.9 million adults reported back pain. The average age was 48 years and there were slightly more females (55%) than males.

The greater incidence of females with low back pain has been found in other studies (Kopec, Sayre, & Esdaile, 2002; Smith, Elliot, Hannaford, Chambers, & Smith, 2004) but this is in no sense a universal finding (Frank, Kerr, & Brooker, 1996; Burdorf & Sorock, 1997).

Headaches are more prevalent than back pain. Migrainous headache 1-year prevalence rates range from 12.9% to 17.6% in women and from 3.4% to 6.1% in men (see Stewart, Shechter, & Rasmussen, 1994, for a review). Tension-type headaches are even more frequent, occurring each year in up to 92% of women (aged 25–34) and 49% of older men (aged 55–64). Migrainous headache has a clear heritability estimated at 38% for men and 48% for women (Svensson, Larsson, Waldenlind, & Pedersen, 2003).

Several other pain syndromes occur with lesser but still significant frequency. A review by Drangsholt and LeResche (1999) found prevalence of temporomandibular disorder ranging from 3.2–10% for males and from 4.9–14% for females. Abdominal pain has a 6-month prevalence rate of approximately 14% in 18–24-year-old men and 31% in women of that age group, decreasing to 7% among men and 12% among women aged 65 or older (VonKorff, Dworkin, LeResche, & Kruger, 1988). Finally, chronic widespread pain is also a condition which is quite common. This condition is defined as pain of greater than 3-months duration occurring in two centralized quadrants of the body. When widespread pain is accompanied by tender points in at least 11 of 18 specific physical sites, the syndrome is fibromyalgia. Fibromyalgia is typically accompanied by sleep disturbance, fatigue, depression, and hypersensitivity to a variety of stimuli in addition to blunt pressure to the tender points (Petzke, Clauw, Ambrose, Khine, & Gracely, 2003). In a review of the literature, Macfarlane (1999) found the prevalence of widespread pain to be 11–13% of various study populations with incidence greater in women than men and increasingly prevalent in both genders as a function of age. Fibromyalgia tends to be somewhat less prevalent but follows the same general pattern.

BIOPSYCHOSOCIAL MODEL OF CHRONIC PAIN

IT IS NOW widely accepted that chronic pain regardless of the specific syndrome is a biopsychosocial disorder (see Figure 9.1). The biopsychosocial model (Loesser, 1982) views nociception (the stimulation of pain receptors due to pathophysiology) as the cornerstone on which the pain experience and associated suffering is built. Pain perception, suffering, and pain behavior can grow well beyond the initial pathophysiology to engulf the patient's life. By virtue of chronicity, the patient's pain report and pain behavior can be influenced by a host of variables other then just nociception. Thus, it is not uncommon to see some patients report high levels of pain and display dramatic pain behavior but have only minimal tissue damage. In the same token, the opposite can also be the case. Understanding the individual patient then requires thorough evaluation, examining all dimensions of the biopsychosocial model.

Following the tenets of the biopsychosocial model, a thorough evaluation would entail a medical examination to precisely define the underlying pathophysiology or pain generator. Associated with the medical exam, there also must be a determination of other physical factors that have developed as a result of the chronic pain experience such as gait deviation, deconditioning, etc. A second component of the evaluation would assess the psychological impact of chronic pain and disability on the patient. Some of these psychological factors might involve mood changes such as depression, anxiety, or fear of the tortuous episodes of severe pain. Finally, evaluation of the social context in which the pain experience is occurring is necessary. For example, how does the patient's pain impact his or her role as a worker, parent, or partner? Moreover, how does the reaction of the employer, child, or partner influence the patient? Clearly, then, the psychosocial model implies that successful treatment of chronic pain not only involves ameliorating the pathophysiological condition underlying the pain, but also the psychosocial sequelae of the protracted suffering must be addressed.

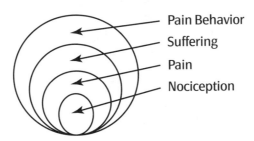

FIGURE 9.1   The biopsychosocial model of chronic pain (adapted from Loeser, 1982).

To illustrate both the physical basis of chronic pain and the utility of the biopsychosocial model, the current chapter will examine two archetypal syndromes—low-back pain and functional gastrointestinal pain. More comprehensive treatment of the depth and breath of chronic pain syndromes can be found in Block, Kremer, and Fernandez (1999).

LOW-BACK PAIN

ONE MODEL FOR understanding the pathological anatomy of low-back pain is termed the cascade of degeneration. The spinal column is composed of segments, each containing two adjoining bones, the vertebrae. The vertebrae are joined in the front by two bony joints, the facets. Together these joints form a three-pronged connection, much like a stool with three legs. On the back or posterior side of the vertebra, bony protrusions known as spinous processes provide the location for muscular attachments. The muscles can move the vertebral bodies in order to twist, turn, and bend. Pain usually arises in the spine beginning with the front of the disc, and later involving the facets. It is this progression beginning in the discs and proceeding to the facets that has come to be known as the degenerative cascade.

Some spinal pain does not fit this model. There are numerous other causes including cancer, visceral problems (e.g., pancreatitis), vertebral fractures, and some congenital conditions that can cause pain. Most spinal conditions, however, can be classified as derangements of one or more of the structures. Derangements in the front or anterior of the spine often begin as a prolapse or displacement of the internal gel-like substance. Known as disc herniation, this gel may directly compress peripheral nerves in the spinal column and cause back and lower extremity pain. Additionally, disc herniation often elicits an inflammatory response, producing more pain. Removal of the displaced gel through a procedure known as discectomy eliminates the compression of nerves and reduces the inflammatory response. In a discectomy procedure, only the 5–10% displaced portion will be removed, with the remaining stable portion left undisturbed. Laminectomy/discectomy represents the most common of surgical spinal treatments. Taylor, Deyo, Cherkin, and Kreuter (1994) report that of the approximately 280,000 spine surgeries performed in the United States during 1990, approximately 200,000 involved discectomy. Unfortunately, discectomy is not always successful and the inflammation may persist for reasons poorly understood, becoming a contributor to back pain syndromes.

Sometimes the degenerative cascade continues and the disc space diminishes in height, collapsing to rest on the two posterior facets. In turn, these facets can become painful because they are forced to carry a disproportionate load. If this occurs, the facets may enlarge in response to the increased mechanical stress and block the opening for nerves to exit the spinal column, leading to nerve root compression and pain. This process is known as stenosis. Its surgical treatment is more radical than a simple discectomy and involves removing part of the facet and part of the disc, in a procedure termed decompression. The goal is to free all compressed neural structures.

Finally, the degeneration may progress sufficiently that the normal alignment of the spine is disturbed. When the spine becomes misaligned in the forward or lateral plates, the condition is termed spondylolisthesis. If the spine is also twisted, the condition is scoliosis. As the vertebrae become misaligned, nerves in the spinal column are compressed or stretched. Surgery is preformed to prevent further slippage or misalignment of the vertebrae. This is accomplished by surgically constructing a bridge between the vertebrae, in a spinal fusion procedure. To accomplish the fusion, bone is typically scraped from the iliac crest of the pelvis and placed between the vertebral bodies. To correct alignment, hooks, screws, and/or rods are permanently implanted in the bony structure of the spine. As the fusion develops, a mass of bone eventually grows over the implants.

The term "failed spine syndrome" is applied to the patient who continues to experience disabling pain syndromes despite surgical treatment. Various factors can lead to failed spine syndrome, such as infection, vascular event, or damage to the neural structures during decompression. Additionally, on occasion, the spine fusion may fail to consolidate (much like concrete must set), causing pain. Inability to fully decompress the nerve is also a common cause of failure. Many patients develop failed spine syndrome as a result of inadequate postoperative rehabilitation. For many patients who fail to recover following surgery, it is the impact of psychosocial variables that militates against recovery.

Only about 1% of back pain sufferers requires surgery (Spitzer, 1987). Most patients with an episode of back pain recover with 2–3 days of bed rest and anti-inflammatory medication (Deyo, Diehl, & Rosenthan, 1986). A small proportion of patients, however, are responsible for a great deal of difficulty in managing low-back pain. Leavitt, Johnson, and Beyer (1971) found that 25% of patients with job-related injuries were responsible for 87% of total treatment costs. Similarly, Spitzer found that 7.4% of all industrial back claims were responsible for 86% of total costs. Many of these patients have no identifiable basis for pain (termed nonspecific low-back pain) or have pathophysiology that could not be expected to respond to surgery. Though there are non-operative treatment options for such patients, it is likely that some of these patients have significant psychosocial issues influencing both the perception of pain and its influence on the patient's behavior.

FUNCTIONAL GASTROINTESTINAL PAIN SYNDROME

A VERY DIFFERENT TYPE of chronic pain is seen in patients with functional gastrointestinal pain syndromes including irritable bowel syndrome (IBS), noncardiac chest pain (NCCP), and nonulcer dyspepsia (NUD). For most patients with these syndromes, pathophysiology is not evident (Crowell & Barofsky, 1999). These patients most frequently present to the physicians with complaints of nausea, vomiting, bloating, altered bowel patterns, and, most commonly, chronic intermittent pain. It is now generally accepted that such patients are hypersensitive to pain signals (hyperalgesia) arising from the gut. For example, Barish, Castell, and Richter (1986) utilized ballon distension of the esophagus in patients with NCCP and found that distention caused pain in 56% of patients, compared with 20% of normal controls (see also Deschner, Maher, Catlin, & Benjamin, 1990). Similarly, Coffin, Azpiroz, Guarner, and Malagelada (1994) found that patients with NUD demonstrated greater sensitivity to ballon distention of the stomach than did normals, and patients with IBS were more sensitive than normals to distention of the colon (Whitehead et al., 1990) and of the small bowel (Moriarity & Dawson, 1982).

The key to understanding the nociceptive process in gastrointestinal syndromes is an appreciation of the nature of pain receptors in the gut. Essentially, there are three types of receptors in the gut (see Crowell & Barofsky, 1999, for a more complete understanding). First, there are low-threshold intensity neurons which identify and send information about regulatory functioning and nonpainful stimulation of the gut to the brain. These fibers appear to provide important information from both the stomach and colon and show gradations in sensation and perception from mild distention, to fullness, to intense pain. Second, there are high-threshold intensity-coding neurons, also known as dedicated nociceptors, that are activated only when the intensity of stimulation in the low-threshold receptors exceeds a predefined level, indicating actual damage to an organ. Finally, a third type of neuron, the silent nociceptor, is generally quiet, providing neither regulatory nor nociceptive information. The silent nociceptor, however, can become activated through injury or inflammation and, once sensitized, can respond to even mild stimulation. Thus, the sensitized silent nociceptor can transmit pain signals in response to even normal regulatory activity in the gut and may provide the mechanism for persistent pain even in the absence of identifiable pathophysiology.

In an interesting assessment of the role of neural input from rectum/colon to the hyperalgesic pain experience in IBS patients, Verne, Robinson, Vase, and Price (2003) examined the effect of intrarectal lidocaine on response to rectal distention and thermal stimulation of the foot. Intrarectal lidocaine reduced reported rectal and cutaneous foot pain in all IBS patients but not in controls. These results indicate that visceral hyperalgesia and secondary cutaneous hyperalgesia in IBS reflect central sensitization mechanisms that are dynamically maintained by tonic impulse input from rectum/colon. Consistent with the secondary cutaneous hyperalgesia, many IBS patients exhibit extra-intestinal pain symptoms such as back pain, migrainous headache, dyspareunia, and muscle pain likely reflecting central hyperalgesia mechanisms (Mayer & Gebhart, 1994).

Generally, treatment of patients with functional gastrointestinal pain syndromes also follows a biopsychosocial model, which recognizes that "psychosocial factors such as depression and anxiety may influence visceral perception through brain-gut neurotransmitters and modulate descending pathways to increase or decrease pain perception" (Crowell & Barofsky, 1998). A "brain-gut" interaction was further demonstrated in an elegant study by Vase, Robinson, Verne, and Price (2003). Irritable bowel syndrome patients were given verbal suggestions for pain relief and then rated expected pain levels and desire for pain relief for both evoked visceral and cutaneous pain. Rectal lidocaine reverses visceral and cutaneous hyperalgesia. Adding a verbal suggestion for pain relief increased the magnitude of placebo analgesia to that of an active agent.

The specific types of biopsychosocial interventions used with patients depend on the severity of the patient's symptoms. In mild cases, patients may benefit from educational efforts, reassurance, and dietary or medication changes. For patients with moderate symptoms, pharmacotherapy, relaxation exercises, biofeedback, and psychotherapy are often utilized. Patients with intractable symptoms are treated through a combination of social support, realistic goal setting, changing expectations, teaching the patient to cope with pain as a long-term problem, and the elimination of unnecessary tests.

PSYCHOLOGICAL ASPECTS OF CHRONIC PAIN

THE TWO ARCHETYPAL syndromes of low-back pain and functional gastrointestinal pain exemplify the diversity of the pathophysiological processes underlying pain. As research on these and other pain syndromes makes clear, it is the psychosocial aspects of each individual's case that influence, in large part, both pain perception and functional ability. Also, there is now fairly strong literature demonstrating that, at least for some medical interventions, psychosocial variables are more potent indicators of treatment outcome than medical variables (e.g., spine surgery, see Block, Gatchel, Deardorff, & Guyer, 2003).

EMOTIONAL ASPECT

Depression

All chronic pain syndromes can be associated with significant emotional disturbance. The most frequent emotional difficulty is depression. An early study by Lindsay and Wyckoff (1981) found that 85% of their chronic pain study population achieved the diagnostic criteria for clinical depression. Other studies fail to find such a large percentage but still find a significantly greater percentage of chronic pain patients clinically depressed than non-pain patients (Dworkin & Gitlin, 1991; VonKorff & Simon, 1996; Fishbain, Cutler, Rosomoff, & Rosomoff, 1997). There are some studies, moreover, that find a percentage of patients had depression premorbid to their pain (Polatin, Kinney, Gatchel, Lillo, & Mayer, 1993). A compelling question, of course, is whether the depression is a consequence of the pain or whether it served as a risk factor for development of chronic pain. Indeed, research by Carroll, Cassidy, and Cote (2004) demonstrated "an independent and robust relationship between depressive symptoms and onset of an episode of pain." Obviously, this would be a very important medico-legal issue. In a review of the literature, Fishbain et al. (1997) found that for the preponderance of patients, depression was a product of the chronic pain experience; this is referred to as the *consequences hypothesis*. Recent work by Dersh, Gatchel, Polatin, and Mayer (2002) in a large study population (*N* = 1595) confirmed this finding.

This high incidence would be anticipated. Chronic pain typically involves some loss of role function (i.e., disability). Harris, Morley, and Barton (2003) found that pain patients who experienced greater losses of role function in measured domains of friendship, occupation, leisure, and family were more likely to be significantly depressed. Furthermore, Blackburn-Munro and Blackburn-Munro (2001) provide a compelling analysis of the relationship among chronic pain, chronic stress, and depression. This analysis involved changes in neuroendocrines and neurotransmitters that are set in motion by the chronic pain experience and result in the emergence of a biological depression. Treatment for depression in chronic pain typically involved both problem-solving psychotherapy for role and life changes and pharmacotherapeutics for neurotransmitter changes.

The pharmacology of depression has evolved dramatically over the past 15 years with greater than half of available antidepressants introduced during this time (Richelson, 2001). In a review of the literature, Salerno, Browning, and Jackson (2002) found that treatment with tricyclic antidepressant in chronic pain patients not only ameliorated symptoms of depression (e.g., dysphoria, weeping, anergia, sleep disturbance, change in appetite, etc.) but also resulted in a small but significant decrease in neuropathic pain. Because there is a fairly high probability of reoccurrence of depression once an episode has occurred (DSM IV), there is a strong argument for continued treatment beyond resolution of symptoms. Frank, Johnson, and Kupfer (1992) found that patients treated with imipramine for 3 years were four times more likely to remain depression-free than those treated with placebo after remission.

Anger

Another common emotional difficulty experienced by chronic pain patients is intense anger. Fernandez, Clark, and Ruddick-Davis (1999) report that 86% of outpatient chronic pain patients experience anger and that this anger is of greater intensity than that reported by age-matched pain-free individuals. This and subsequent research has found that the anger was directed primarily at the health care system and insurance companies. The target of the pain patient's anger is significant, for it may influence treatment outcome. DeGood and Klerman (1996) found that chronic pain patients who placed blame for the injury on the employer had poorer pain treatment outcomes, as well as higher levels of mood disturbance than those who did not make such attributions. Turk and Fernandez (1995) have suggested that patients who are angry blame others for their difficulties, and are rebellious toward authority figures may respond more poorly to treatment because they fail to form a therapeutic alliance with the health care team.

Pain Sensitivity

The most problematic emotional factor associated with chronic pain is pain sensitivity (also known as sensitization). It has long been felt that chronic, unremitting physical complaints, especially when associated with minimal identifiable physiological problems, are the result of psychological difficulties. Freud (Breuer & Freud, 1895) and neo-Freudians (Engle, 1959) consider that such protracted physical complaints arise from the conversion of unconscious psychological conflicts into physical symptomatology. Although there is little direct evidence to support such a contention (Gamsa, 1994), there is a converging body of evidence demonstrating that at least a large portion of chronic pain patients may be excessively sensitive to pain. First, research using the Minnesota Multiphasic Personality Inventory (MMPI) indicates that the most common personality profile for chronic pain patients involves elevations in the Hypochondriasis and Hysteria scales (Keller & Butcher, 1991) that assess disease conviction, sensitivity to physical symptoms, and denial of psychological problems (Graham, 1990). Patients with such MMPI profiles respond poorly to both conservative treatment (Kleinke & Spangler, 1988) and surgical intervention (see Block et al., 2003). Second, controlled research has documented excessive pain sensitivity in chronic pain patients. Schmidt (1987; Schmidt & Brand, 1986), for example, subjected chronic low-back pain patients to cold pressor tests (immersion of the forearm into ice water bath). Results showed that the patients both reported higher pain levels and tolerated the ice water for a shorter period of time than did a control, nonpatient group. In our own laboratory, we have found that MMPI Hysteria and Hyperchondriasis elevations are associated with false-positive reports of pain in patients undergoing discography, a presurgical diagnostic test for disc herniation (Block, Vanharanta, Ohnmeiss, & Guyer, 1996). If chronic pain patients display such pain sensitivity, it is not surprising that their pain conditions should be so protracted.

Behavioral Factors

Wilbert Fordyce (1976), in his pioneering text *Behavioral Methods in Chronic Pain and Illness*, conceptualized chronic pain from a behavioral perspective. From this perspective, the pain sensation itself is immeasurable and unobservable. Pain behavior, however, is measurable and observable and, therefore, should be subject to operant principles of reinforcement. That is, behaviors such as limping, grimacing, or groaning, if followed by positive consequence (e.g., desired attention, avoidance of the distasteful task, etc.), should increase in probability of occurrence. Similarly, chronic pain behavior resulting from injuries sustained in a motor vehicle accident could be sustained by the anticipation of financial gains from litigation. Work by Jolliffe and Nicholas (2004) supports this basic premise with subjects reporting greater levels of pain over trials, regardless of whether cuff pressure was stable or decreasing, if they were verbally reinforced to do so relative to subjects who were not so reinforced.

Spousal Reinforcement

The power to influence chronic pain behaviors rests perhaps most strongly with the patient's spouse or significant other. It is the spouse with whom the patient interacts most and the spouse who can provide the reinforcement for pain in addition to discouraging alternative well behaviors. Research in our laboratory has demonstrated that spousal reinforcement may strongly affect pain behaviors. In this study (Block, Kremer, & Gaylor, 1980), chronic pain patients were given a questionnaire assessing spousal reinforcement of pain behavior and were divided into high and low reinforcement groups. Patients with highly solicitous spouses reported higher pain levels in the presence of their spouse than in the presence of the ward clerk, whereas the opposite result obtained for patients with minimally solicitous spouses. This result demonstrated that the solicitous spouse could act as a discriminative stimulus for the patient to display an increase in pain behavior. More recent research found that pain patients show decreased walking time on a treadmill as well as greater pain reports in the presence of solicitous spouses compared to patients with nonsolicitous spouses (Lousberg, Schmidt, & Groenman, 1992). Kerns et al. (1991) demonstrated these same findings with functional tasks. Interestingly, solicitousness and perceived support appear to have a positive affect for the post-surgical patient, with these patients recovering more quickly (Mutran, Reitzes, Mossey, & Fernandez, 1995) and reporting greater pain relief (Schade, Semmer, Main, Hora, & Boos, 1999).

Vocational Factors

Aspects of the patient's employment situation may act in a number of ways, both to maintain pain behavior and as a disincentive to recovery. First, vocational attitude may influence the onset of pain. A prospective study of 3,000 aircraft workers by Bigos et al. (1991) found that workers who reported a high level of job dissatisfaction were 2.5 times more likely to incur a job-related back injury than were workers who enjoyed their work. Once back pain occurs, patients who blame the employer for the original injury have been shown to have a higher level of mood disturbance and poorer outcome of treatment for chronic pain than do patients who place blame on other individuals, on themselves, or on no one in particular (DeGood & Kierman, 1996). Finally, the occurrence of a job-related injury can be associated with some apparent disincentives for improvement. Patients injured on the job typically receive worker's compensation benefits, medical coverage for their injury, and partial replacement of lost wages if they are unable to work due to the injury. Patients receiving worker's compensation benefits often have a poorer outcome of treatment for pain (Glassman et al., 1998; Klekamp, McCarthy, & Spengler, 1998). Frymoyer and Cats-Baril (1987) contend that "compensability" is one of the strongest predictors of excessive disability among chronic pain patients. The bold truth, however, is that in many if not most worker's compensation cases, the factors militating against recovery are not as simple as mere financial disincentives. The injured worker faces the potential lack of accommodated work, nonsupportive attitude of coworkers, threatened job security, and an adversarial relationship with the employer and worker's compensation carrier (Pransky et al., 2002; Schultz et al., 2002; Schultz et al., 2004; VanDerWeide, Verbeek, Salle, & VanDijk, 1999). Thus, one must be very prudent in considering each case as to what the true incentives and disincentives are to recovery.

Fear Avoidance

Although the evaluation of fear has a long history (Vlaeyen & Linton, 2000), the fear-avoidance concept as it applies to pain and disability is relatively recent (Lethem, Slade, Troup, & Bentley, 1983). Simply put, this concept suggests that the patient's fear of pain results in avoidance of those activities which they feel would exacerbate their pain. The avoidant behavior is reinforced as pain increases are not experienced. Unfortunately, if the avoidant behavior involves refraining from exercise, the patient would become progressively deconditioned and experience greater levels of disability. Waddell, Newton, Henderson, Somerville, and Main (1993) developed a Fear-Avoidance Beliefs Questionnaire (FABQ) and were able to demonstrate that specific fear-avoidance beliefs about work were strongly related to work loss due to low-back pain. Crombez, Vlaeyen, Huets, and Lysens (1999) found that chronic low-back pain patients' pain-related fear measures reliably predicted self-reported disability as well as poor performance on a task involving lifting a 5.5 kg bag. Interestingly, pain-related fear was more predictive of physical performance than current pain intensity and experienced pain increase; pain-related fear is more disabling than pain itself.

Linton, Vlaeyen, deJong, and co-workers (Vlaeyen, deJong, Geilen, Heuts, & Van Breukelen, 2001; Linton, Overmeer, Janson, Vlaeyen, & deJong, 2002; Boersma, Linton, Overmeer, Jansson, Vlaeyen, & deJong, 2004) conceptualized fear-avoidance as a phobia. This follows the notion of kinesiphobia which Kori, Miller, and Todd (1990) defined as "an excessive, irrational and debilitating fear of physical movement and activity resulting from a feeling of vulnerability to painful injury or reinjury." Consistent with the extensive literature on behavioral treatment of phobias, these workers reasoned that graded exposure in vivo would be an effective treatment. Using the photograph series of daily activities (PHODA) (Kugler, Wijn, Geilen, DeJong, & Vlaeyen, 1999), patients developed a hierarchy of the 98 standardized cards from least to most fear provoking. Patients were asked to opine as to the outcome of performance of the task illustrated on a particular card. They were also asked to state a probability of the opined outcome. The patient was then asked to perform the task. After their performance, the patient was asked to rate the actual outcome and determine whether the fear was warranted. The goal was for patients to learn that specific activities were not dangerous and will not result in exacerbation of their pain. Over a number of studies, Linton, Vlaeyen and co-workers (see Boersma et al., 2004) were able to demonstrate decreases in rated fear and avoidance beliefs while function increased substantially. George, Fritz, Bialosky, and Donald (2003) followed the guidelines of Vlaeyen and Linton (2000) to develop a Fear-Avoidance-Based physical therapy intervention. Patients tested with this intervention showed significant decrease in disability at 1 and 6 months following treatment. They also showed significant change in fear-avoidance beliefs and fear-avoidance beliefs about physical activity.

Cognitive Factors

The behavioral model of chronic pain emphasizes the relationship between overt manifestations of pain (pain behaviors) and the response of others in the patient's environment to such behaviors. This model does not incorporate any aspects of the patient's thought process. An alternative approach, the cognitive-behavioral model, focuses on the influence of patient's *beliefs* about pain and *coping strategies* for dealing with pain. According to this model, such cognitive factors can serve to either minimize or magnify the impact of pain on behavior, mood, and recovery.

According to the cognitive-behavioral model, some patients hold *irrational* beliefs about pain. In considering pain, such patients may "catastrophize" (believe that a minor setback indicates the occurrence of a major injury), "personalize" (inappropriately believe that they are the cause of the injury or continued pain), or have "emotional reasoning" (believe that their feelings about the pain must be true). There is now considerable research (see Sullivan et al., 2001) demonstrating that catastrophizing accounts for significant amounts in the variance in pain ratings. This relationship holds across a variety of measures and diverse patient groups (e.g., those with low-back pain, dental procedures, burn dressing changes, and whiplash injuries). Further, catastrophizing is predictive of high levels of disability. Goubert, Crombez, and VanDamme (2004) found that catastrophic thinking and pain-related fear resulted in hypervigilance to pain resulting in greater pain severity. Sullivan, Adams, and Sullivan (2004) also found that catastrophizers tend to use pain behavior to communicate their pain dilemma. These researchers compared high and low catastrophizers in the presence of an observer or alone. Pain was induced with a cold pressor procedure. High catastrophizers displayed communicative pain behaviors (e.g., facial displays, vocalizations) for longer duration when an observer was present relative to high catastrophizers when alone. Moreover, with an observer present, high catastrophizers used fewer cognitive coping strategies than low catastrophizers.

Coping strategies are the second set of cognitive factors that have been the focus of a great deal of attention among researchers in chronic pain. Coping strategies refer to specific thoughts or behaviors that people use to manage their pain or emotional reactions to pain (Brown & Nicassio, 1987). The Coping Strategies Questionnaire (CSQ; Rosentiel & Keefe, 1983) is the most widely used questionnaire for assessing these strategies. The CSQ contains three basic dimensions (Lawson, Ressor, Keefe, & Turner, 1990): conscious cognitive coping (including ignoring the pain and coping self-statements), self-efficacy (including the ability to control and the ability to decrease pain), and pain avoidance (including diverting attention and hoping and praying). Research on the CSQ has found that higher self-efficacy is frequently associated with lower pain intensity and greater physical functioning (Jensen, Turner, Romano, & Karoly, 1991). Other strategies such as hoping and praying are maladaptive and lead to poor pain treatment outcome (Rosensteil & Keefe; Waddell et al., 1993).

McCracken, Vowles, and Eccleston (2004) have developed the Chronic Pain Acceptance Questionnaire (CPAQ) and have tested the notion that acceptance of one's pain condition leads to enhanced emotional and physical functioning in chronic pain patients beyond the influence of depression, pain intensity, and coping. In an earlier study, McCracken and Eccleston (2003) studied chronic pain patients waiting to begin interdisciplinary treatment. These researchers found that acceptance of chronic pain was a better predictor of pain, depression, disability, pain-related anxiety, and patient physical and vocational functioning than were measures of coping. In many senses, acceptance appears the opposite of catastrophizing and suggests that getting on with it might be more productive than swimming against the tide as it were. In any event, it is an exciting area for future study.

MULTIDISCIPLINARY PAIN TREATMENT

THE EARLIEST MODERN attempts to treat chronic pain patients were made by John Bonica (1985), who described his great frustration in attempting to treat chronic pain in the military during World War II. There was no coherent literature addressing the treatment of chronic pain, treatment efforts were piecemeal, and communication among the various treatment providers was sporadic. It was during this time that Bonica developed the concept of multidisciplinary treatment for chronic nonmalignant pain. All clinical specialties would be physically located in a single clinical setting, thereby optimizing communication among specialists and coordination of care.

It was not until 1961, however, that Bonica and Lowell White, a neurosurgeon, established the first multidisciplinary pain treatment program at the University of Washington in Seattle (Bonica, 1975). The following years, Wilbert Fordyce, PhD, joined the program. As already noted, Fordyce's (1976) text describing the application of behavioral principles to the treatment of chronic pain served as the philosophical underpinning of the program. Fordyce argued that the disease model in medicine, though perhaps appropriate for infectious disease, was not particularly helpful in providing guidance in the case of chronic pain. In the disease model, observed symptoms reflect some underlying pathology. Treatment, in turn, is directed at the underlying pathology. In contrast, it had already been well established that pain behavior is "subject to influence by a host of factors besides so-called underlying pathology" (Fodyce, p. 33). Further, there are instances, such as nonspecific low-back pain, where a pain generator can not be identified. Alternatively, a pain generator may be identified, but the pain complaint is far out of proportion (i.e., somatoform pain disorder). Finally, even in the presence of obvious, objectively confirmed pathophysiology, psychosocial factors may exert a significant influence on pain perception and response to treatment. For Fordyce, the salient relationship in chronic pain is between pain behavior and its consequences, rather than between pain behavior and some putative pain generator.

MULTIDISCIPLINARY BEHAVIORAL TREATMENT

FORDYCE (1976) APPLIED a richly developed literature in learning theory to patients with chronic pain syndrome. This syndrome can be defined as excessive pain behavior, overuse of pain medications, overutilization of the health delivery system, and a low level of activity. Treatment in an inpatient setting was designed to maximize control over stimuli and reinforcers; pain behaviors were no longer rewarded and well behaviors such as walking to a quota distance were rewarded. Spouses and families were educated to discontinue often unwitting reinforcement of pain behavior and disability. Medications were scheduled on a time basis rather than a take-as-needed basis, as the latter protocol creates a reinforcement contingency between pain complaint and medication. Problem medications, such as narcotic analgesics and minor tranquilizers, were placed in a "cocktail" to maintain stimulus constancy and gradually tapered over time. Careful and detailed record-keeping was required so that patients could track their progress and benefit from the motivational effects of the progress.

The 1970s and 1980s witnessed the development of numerous pain programs based on Fordyce's model. Flor, Fydrich, and Turk (1992) conducted a meta-analysis of a number of studies reporting outcomes of treatment in multidisciplinary pain treatment programs based at some level on Fordyce's model. The results of this analysis provide clear evidence as to the efficacy of the approach. More recent work (Okifuji, Turk, & Kalauokalani, 1999) provides further support for the efficacy of multidisciplinary behavioral treatment as well as a cogent analysis of the cost effectiveness of multidisciplinary pain treatment relative to surgery. Taking into account treatment costs, surgical and medical costs, disability payments, and return-to-work, the cost-effective index score for surgery was only 0.29 relative to an index of 0.83 for the multidisciplinary treatment. Importantly, Patrick, Altmaier, and Found (2004) reported that patients maintained their treatment gains in a 13-year follow-up. Work by Taimaela, Diederich, Hubsch, and Heinricy (2000) suggests that continued regular exercise habits are probably critical to maintaining programmatic gains over time.

COGNITIVE-BEHAVIORAL TREATMENT

PARALLELING THE APPLICATION of behavioral principles to the evaluation and treatment of chronic pain, cognitive learning theory was proving of greater neuristic value than traditional learning theory. Not surprisingly, the application of cognitive psychology to the clinical enterprise occurred in short order in the development of cognitive-behavioral theory. Turk, Meichenbaum, and Genest (1983) cogently synthesized these various influences in their work, *Pain and Behavioral Medicine: A Cognitive-Behavioral Perspective*. Behavior and behavioral change are seen as end products of cognitive events, affect, behavior, and consequences. Cognitions can be changed by reframing or reconceptualizing a problem for the patient, by teaching problem-solving skills, and by education. Behavior can be changed by altering consequences, working to quotas, modeling, and rehearsal. As patients successfully perform target behaviors, they become increasingly confident and develop feelings of self-efficacy and self-control (Bandura, 1977). Faced with a situation that once was overwhelming and impossible to manage, patients can acquire the skills and problem-solving ability to control the situation.

The case of John exemplifies the cognitive-behavioral approach to chronic pain. John is a 30-year-old engineer who is beginning a new job. Understandably, he is concerned about his performance and about making a good impression. John has a history of migrainous headaches, and these headaches are more frequent and more intense when he is under stress. John worries that he will have a headache, miss work, and make a poor first impression. He has had this problem in the past. He also knows that medication can not entirely rescue him from his dilemma as it dramatically reduces his performance.

In a cognitive-behavioral intervention, John first has to be educated to the fact that many migraine headache sufferers can learn to control their headaches. At present, if he begins to feel the early signs of headache, he worries that it will escalate and cause him to miss work. He knows there is nothing he can do to control the course of the headache. Worry and defeat are cognitions that can increase activity in the sympathetic nervous system and thereby promote headache. John can be taught relaxation exercises and imagery or be trained with biofeedback to acquire skills that can decrease activity in the sympathetic nervous system and abort headaches. Further, he can learn to be problem-or-solution focused. As John acquires headaches, he worries less about missing work. This reduces the stress and worry of a bad first impression, further decreasing the likelihood of headache. Kremer, Hudson, and Schreifer (1999) describe a cognitive-behavior headache treatment program using the aforementioned strategies. Results reported by Kremer and Kremer (1995) found decreases in pain, depression, and anxiety, greatly diminished medication use, increased feelings of control (self-efficacy), and decreased feelings of disability. Scharff and Marcus (1994) and Scharff, Marcus, and Turk (1996) found similar results.

Turk et al. (1983) noted the effectiveness of application of cognitive-behavioral therapy not only to pain treatment but also to risk factors such as essential hypertension, type-A coronary-prone behavior patterns, obesity, smoking, and alcoholism, as well as disease areas such as cancer and diabetes mellitus. McCracken and Turk (2002) note that there has been a number of reviews of the cognitive-behavioral literature over the years (Malone & Strube, 1988; Turner, 1996; Morley, Eccleston, & Williams, 1999). Generally, these reviews demonstrate that CBT and/or programs that have a CBT component result in significant improvement for chronic pain patients but not in all areas assessed. For example, Morley, Eccelston, and Williams found improvement in pain experience, positive coping strategies use, and pain behavior, but not in mood, negative coping and appraised responses, or social functioning. As McCracken and Turk correctly note there is a need for considerable research before we can have a clear understanding of exactly which patients will benefit from specific treatments and precisely what outcome to anticipate.

FUNCTIONAL RESTORATION MODEL

THE MOST RECENT development in the evolution of multidisciplinary treatment of chronic nonmalignant pain is the functional restoration model (Mayer & Gatchel, 1988). While incorporating many aspects of Fordyce's model and of cognitive-behavioral therapy, the functional restoration model specifically focuses on the use of sports medicine technology to assess physical capability and to design treatment protocols to enhance functional capability, the most common goal being return to work.

Mayer et al. (1987) described the functional restoration program at the Productive Rehabilitation Institute of Dallas for Ergonomics (PRIDE). Staffing comprises a directing physician, a physical therapist, an occupational therapist, a psychologist, and a nurse. As with the Fordycian model, evaluation and treatment in a single clinical setting is critical. Beyond this, functional restoration focuses on objective, quantifiable measures of both physical and psychosocial function that are relevant to the functional goal. Development of measures with such parameters allows a more or less precise definition of the patient's capability and a comparison of this capability to the rational standard of a normative database. The remaining consideration in measurement of performance is an "effort factor" so that suboptimal effort is not confused with the patient's true level of ability or disability.

Obviously, the focus of each discipline is somewhat different, although the overall functional goal is the same. The physical therapist is responsible for supervision of the patient's individualized physical therapy program, which is designed to treat the specific injuries and hence enhance functional capability. Occupational therapy focuses on functional tasks through work hardening and work simulation. In the program, the occupational therapist also addresses any financial, legal, or work-related barriers to successfully return to work. The psychologist addresses psychosocial and behavioral issues through a Multi-Modal Disability Management Program (MDMP). This program is individualized but can consist of group and family counseling, behavioral stress management training (including relaxation training and biofeedback), and cognitive-behavioral skills training. The nurse serves as an extension of the physician, checking and ordering medications and injections and making a preliminary evaluation of medical problems affecting a patient's ability to participate in the physical reconditioning program. Team members confer on a biweekly basis to ensure a high level of communication.

There are four phases in the treatment. The preprogram phase can be of a varying number of sessions; it addresses issues of compliance, motivation, and other barriers to functional recovery. The core program consists of 3 weeks of daily 10-hour sessions. The follow-up phase is 0–20 sessions over 0–6 weeks and consists of a variety of interventions to reinforce and maintain the pain management habits and functional skills acquired during the first two phases of the program. Finally, the outcome tracking phase can consist of periodic, repeated quantitive functional evaluations (QFEs), structured phone contact, and an annual interview.

Hazard (1993) reviewed outcome date for patients treated at the PRIDE program by Dr. Mayer and his team. He also reported outcome date of his own functional restoration program at the New England Back Center (NEBC). Using return to work as an index of success at 1 year post-treatment, the PRIDE program had 86% of their treated patients at work or in training, and the NEBC had 81% of their patients working. These outcomes were compared to various control groups where return-to-work rates varied between 20% and 45%. At 2-year follow-up, the PRIDE program found its success rate maintained with 85% of program graduates at work. Also, the PRIDE-treated patients had significantly fewer visits to health professionals than comparison patients at both 1- and 2-year follow-up.

More recent work is less impressive but still supports the efficacy of the functional restoration philosophy. A review article by Guzman, Esmail, Karjalainen, et al. (2001) reports that "there is strong evidence that intensive multidisciplinary biopsychosocial rehabilitation with functional restoration improves function when compared with inpatient or outpatient non-multidisciplinary rehabilitation" (p. 1511). There appears to be some argument for more intense programs (more than 100 hours of therapy) being more effective then less intense programs. Other research would support this contention (Jousset, Fanello, Bontoux, Dubus, Billabert, et al., 2004). One also has to be sensitive to outcome as a function of the accurate duplication of the PRIDE program in every aspect. Obviously, duplication would not only have to include treatment but also cultural considerations such as differences in the workers' compensation laws that vary from state to state and can constrain ability to return an injured worker to a productive life.

ISSUES FOR THE FUTURE

THE ISSUE OF support and sponsorship for multidisciplinary pain treatment outlined in the first edition of this text remains a most pressing and unresolved problem. Kulich and Lande (1997) noted that the advent of managed care has not provided a congenial environment for access to multidisciplinary pain treatment. As noted in this chapter, both the efficacy and cost-effectiveness of multidisciplinary pain treatment is well established. Unfortunately, as Gordon and Dahl (2004) note, there continues to be limited access to and reimbursement for adequate pain care. In an article by Fortner et al. (2003), the Zero Acceptance of Pain (ZAP) Quality Improvement Project is described. This project demonstrates that the technology to improve pain care is very much available. Harden (2002) expressed the concern that market forces might be propotent in determining pain management practices. Obviously, efforts have to continue to provide humane pain relief to anyone who suffers even if this provides only a slim profit margin.

Another area of pressing concern is behavior which increases risk for painful medical conditions. The specific concern can range from obvious life-style issues such as obesity and smoking to use of heavy backpacks by school children. Obesity has now reached epidemic proportions in the United States and, at this time, there is ample data to demonstrate that obese individuals are at risk for back pain, respond less well to treatment, and are at greater risk for co-morbid complicating medical conditions (Fanuele, Abdu, Hanscom, & Weinstein, 2002). Obviously, any initiative to reduce obesity will impact the incidence of back pain.

Akmal et al. (2004) have demonstrated the dose- and time-dependent changes in cellular integrity which explicitly define nicotine effect on disc degeneration. Effectively, nicotine dramatically accelerates age-related changes in intervertebral discs (Boos et al., 2002). Beyond this, nicotine use has far-reaching negative effects on health (Vogt, Hanscom, Lauerman, & Kang, 2002). Again, any initiative to reduce nicotine use will impact the incidence of pain conditions related to spine pathology.

The depth and breadth of need for cultural change is exemplified by the literature addressing back pain in children. The increased incidence of back pain in children has been recognized for some time (Balague, Troussier, & Salminen, 1999). Recent work finds that between 30% and 54% of students carry greater than 15% of their body weight with a backpack (Limon, Valinsky, & Ben-Shalom, 2004). This exceeded guidelines set for adults in industry! Moreover, Negrini and Carabalona (2002) have found that postural stresses resulting from students seating–teacher teaching orientation can result in pain problems. For example, one finding was that in 74% of classes, students sat with their side facing the teacher. As attending school is not discretionary, we have an obligation to our young to be thorough in application of ergonomic principles to the school setting.

REFERENCES

Akmal, M., Kesani, A., Anand, B., Abhinav, S., Wiseman, M., & Goodship, A. (2004). Effect of nicotine on spinal disc cells: A cellular mechanism for disc degeneration. *Spine, 29,* 568–575.

Balague, F., Troussier, B., & Salminen, J. J. (1999). Neurospecific low back pain in children and adolescents: Risk factors. *European Spine Journal, 8,* 429–438.

Bandura, A. (1977). Self-efficacy: Toward a unifying theory of behavior change. *Psychological Review, 84,* 191–215.

Barish, C. E., Castell, D. O., & Richter, J. E. (1986). Graded esophageal balloon distention: A new provocative test for noncardiac chest pain. *Digestive Diseases and Service, 31,* 1292–1298.

Bigos, S. J., Battie, M. C., Spengler, D. M., Fisher, L. D., Fordyce, W. E., Hansson, T., et al. (1991). A perspective study of work perceptions and psychosocial factors affecting the report of back injury. *Spine, 16,* 1–6.

Blackburn-Munro, G., & Blackburn-Munro, R. E. (2001). Chronic pain, chronic stress and depression: Coincidence or consequence? *Journal of Neuroendocrinology, 13,* 1009–1023.

Block, A. R., Gatchel, R. J., Deardorff, W. W., & Guyer, R. D. (2003). *The psychology of spine surgery.* Washington, DC: American Psychological Association.

Block, A., Kremer, E. E., & Fernandez, E. (1999). *Handbook of pain syndromes: Biopsychosocial perspectives.* Mahwah, NJ: Lawrence Erlbaum Associates.

Block, A. R., Kremer, E. F., & Gaylor, M. (1980). Behavioral treatment of chronic pain: The spouse as the discriminative cue for pain behavior. *Pain, 9*, 243–252.

Block, A., Vanharanta, H., Ohnmeiss, D., & Guyer, R. (1996). Discographic pain report: Influence of psychological factors. *Spine, 21*, 334–338.

Boersma, K., Linton, S., Overmeer, T., Jansson, M., Vlaeyen, J., & deJong, J. (2004). Lowering fear-avoidance and enhancing function through exposure *in vivo*: A multiple baseline study across six patients with back pain. *Pain, 108*, 8–16.

Bonica, J. J. (1975). Organization and function of a multi-disciplinary pain clinic. In M. Wersburg & B. Tersky (Eds.), *Pain: New perspectives in therapy and research*. New York: Plenum Press.

Bonica, J. (1985). History of pain concepts and pain therapy. *Seminars in Anesthesia, 3*, 189–208.

Bonica, J. J. (Ed.). (1990). *The management of pain* (2nd ed.). Philadelphia: Lea & Febiger.

Boos, N., Weisbach, S., Rohrbach, H., Weiler, C., Spratt, K., & Nerlich, A. (2002). Classification of age-related changes in lumbar intervertebral discs. *Spine, 27*, 2631–2644.

Breuer, J., & Freud, S. (1895). *Studies in hysteria*. New York: Basic Books.

Brown, G. K., & Nicassio, P. M. (1987). Development of a questionnaire for the assessment of active and passive coping pain strategies in chron pain patients. *Pain, 31*, 53–64.

Burdorf, A., & Sorock, G. (1997). Positive and negative evidence of risk factors for back disorders. *Scandinavian Journal of Work and Environmental Health, 23*, 243–256.

Carroll, L., Cassidy, J., & Cote, P. (2004). Depression as a risk factor for onset of an episode of troublesome neck and low back pain. *Pain, 107*, 134–139.

Coffin, B., Azpiroz, F., Guarner, F., & Malagelada, J. R. (1994). Selective gastric hypersensitivity and reflux hyperactivity in functional dyspepsia. *Gastroenterology, 107*, 1345–1351.

Crombez, G., Vlaeyen, J., Huets, P., & Lysens, R. (1999). Pain-related fear is more disabling than pain itself: Evidence on the role of pain-related fear in chronic back pain disability, *Pain, 80*, 329–339.

Crombie, I., Croft, P., Linton, S., LeResche, L., & VonKorff, M. (Eds.). (1999). *Epidemiology of pain: Task force on epidemiology*. Seattle, WA: IASP Press.

Crowell, M. D., & Barofsky, I. (1999). Functional gastrointestinal pain syndromes. In A. R. Block, E. F. Kremer, & E. Fernandez (Eds.), *Handbook of pain syndromes: Biopsychosocial perspectives*. Mahwah, NJ: Lawrence Erlbaum Associates.

DeGood, D. E., & Klerman, B. (1996). Perception of fault in patients with chronic pain. *Pain, 64*, 153–159.

Dersh, J., Gatchel, R. J., Polatin, P., & Mayer, T. (2002). Prevalence of psychiatric disorders in patients with chronic work-related musculoskeletal pain disability. *Journal of Occupational and Environmental Medicine, 44*, 459–468.

Deschner, W. K., Mahar, K., Catlan, E. L., & Benjamin, S. (1990). Intraesophageal ballon distention versus drug provocation in the evaluation of noncardiac chest pain. *American Journal of Gastroenterology, 85,* 938–943.

Deyo, R. A., Diehl, A., & Rosenthan, M. (1986). How many days of bedrest for acute low back pain? *New England Journal of Medicine, 315,* 1064–1070.

Drangshoff, M., & LeResche, L. (1999). Temporomandibular joint pain. In I. Crombie, P. Croft, S. Linton, L. LeResche, & M. VanKorff (Eds.), *Epidemiology of pain.* Seattle, WA: IASP Press.

Dworkin, R. H., & Gitlin, M. J. (1991). Clinical aspects of depression in chronic pain patients. *Clinical Journal of Pain, I,* 79–94.

Engle, G. (1959). "Psychogenic" pain and the pain-prone patient. *American Journal of Medicine, 26,* 899–918.

Fanuele, J. M., Abdu, W., Hanscom, B., & Weinstein, J. (2002). Association between obesity and functional status in patients with spine disease. *Spine, 27,* 306–312.

Fernandez, E., Clark, T., & Ruddick-Davis, D. (1999). A framework for conceptualization and assessment of affective disturbance in pain. In A. R. Block, E. F. Kremer, & E. Fernandez (Eds.), *Handbook of pain syndromes: Biopsychosocial perspectives.* Mahwah, NJ: Lawrence Erlbaum Associates.

Fishbain, D. A., Cutler, R., Rosomoff, H. L., & Rosomoff, R. S. (1997). Chronic pain associated depression: Antecedent or consequence of chronic pain: A review. *Clinical Journal of Pain, 13,* 116–137.

Floor, H., Fydrich, T., & Turk, D. D. (1992). Efficacy of multidisciplinary pain treatment centers: A meta-analytic review. *Pain, 49,* 221–230.

Fordyce, W. E. (1976). *Behavioral methods in chronic pain and illness.* St. Louis, MO: C. V. Mosby.

Fortner, B. V., Okon, T. A., Ashley, S., Kepler, G., Chavez, J., Taver, K., et al. (2003). The Zero Acceptance of Pain (ZAP) quality improvement project: Evaluation of pain severity, pain interference, global quality of life, and pain related costs. *Journal of Pain Symptom Management, 25,* 334–343.

Frank, E., Johnson, S., & Kupfer, D. (1992). Psychological treatment in the prevention of relapse. In S. Montgomery & F. Rovillon (Eds.), *Long term treatment of depression.* New York: Wiley.

Frymeyer, J. W., & Cats-Baril, W. L. (1987). An overview of the incidences and cost of low back pain. *Orthopedic Clinics of America, 22,* 263–271.

Frymeyer, J. W., & Durett, C. T. (1997). The economics of spinal disorders. In J. W. Frymoyer (Ed.), *The adult spine: Principles and practices* (2nd ed.). Philadelphia: Lippincott-Raven.

Gamsa, A. (1994). The role of psychological factors in chronic pain: A critical appraisal. *Pain, 57,* 17–29.

George, S. Z., Freutz, J. M., Bialosky, J. E., & Donald, D. (2003). The effect of a fear-avoidance-based physical therapy intervention for patients with acute low back pain: Results of a randomized clinical trial. *Spine, 28,* 2251–2560.

Glassman, S. D., Minkow, R. E., Dimar, J. R., Puno, R. M., Raque, G. H., & Johnson, J. R. (1998). Effect of prior lumbar discectomy on outcome of lumbar fusion: A prospective analysis using the SF-36 measure. *Journal of Spinal Disorders, 11*, 383–388.

Gordon, D., & Dahl, J. (2004). Quality improvement challenges in pain management. *Pain, 107*, 1–4.

Goubert, L., Crombez, G., & VanDamme, S. (2004). The role of neuroticism, pain catastrophizing and pain-related fear in vigilance of pain: A structural equations approach. *Pain, 107*, 234–241.

Graham, J. R. (1990). *The MMPI2: Assessing personality and psychopathology.* New York: Oxford University Press.

Guzman, J., Esmail, R., Karjalainen, K., Melmivaara, A., Irvin, E., & Bambardier, C. (2001). Multidisciplinary rehabilitation for chronic low back pain: A systematic review. *British Medical Journal, 322*, 1511–1516.

Harden, R. N. (2002). Pain management: Where is the evidence? *American Pain Society Bulletin, 12*, 5.

Harris, S., Morley, S., & Barton, S. B. (2003). Role loss and emotional adjustment in chronic pain. *Pain, 105*, 363–370.

Hazard, R. G. (1993). Functional restoration treatment outcomes. In T. J. Mayer, V. Mooney, & R. J. Gatchel (Eds.), *Contemporary conservative care of painful spinal disorders.* Philadelphia: Lea & Febiger.

Jensen, M. P., Turner, J. A., Romano, J. M., & Karoly, P. (1991). Coping with chronic pain: A critical review of the literature. *Pain, 47*, 249–283.

Jolliffe, C., & Nicholas, M. (2004). Verbally reinforcing pain reports: An experimental test of the operant model of chronic pain. *Pain, 107*, 167–175.

Jousset, N., Fanello, S., Bontoux, L., Dubus, V., Billabert, C., Vielle, B., et al. (2004). Effects of functional restoration *versus* 3 hours per week physical therapy: A randomized controlled study. *Spine, 29*, 487–494.

Keller, L., & Butcher, J. (1991). *Assessment of chronic pain patients with the MMPI-2* (MMPI-2 Monographs, Vol. 2). Minneapolis: University of Minnesota Press.

Kerns, R., Southwick, S., Giller, E., Haythornthwaite, J., Jacob, M., & Rosenberg, R. (1991). The relationship between reports of pain-related social interactions and expressions of pain and affective distress. *Behavioral Therapy, 22*, 101–111.

Kleinke, C. L., & Spangler, A. S. (1988). Predicting treatment outcome of chronic back pain patients in a multidisciplinary pain clinic: Methodological issues and treatment implication. *Pain, 33*, 41–48.

Klekamp, J., McCarty, E., & Spengler, D. (1998). Results of elective lumbar discectomy for patients involved in the workers' compensation system. *Journal of Spinal Disorders, 11*, 277–282.

Kopec, J. A., Sayre, E. C., & Esdaile, J. M. (2003). Predictors of back pain in a general population cohort. *Spine, 29*, 70–77.

Kori, S. H., Miller, R. P., & Todd, D. D. (1990). Kinisophobia: A new view of chronic pain behavior. *Pain Management, Jan./Feb.*, 35–43.

Kremer, E. F., Hudson, J., & Schreifer, T. (1999). Headache. In A. R. Block, E. F. Kremer, & E. Fernandez (Eds.), *Handbook of pain syndromes: Biopsychosocial perspectives*. Mahwah, NJ: Lawrence Erlbaum Associates.

Kremer, E. F., & Kremer, A. M. (1995). *Psychological factors influencing medical treatment outcome: Headache*. Paper presented at the Annual Scientific Meeting of the American Pain Society, Los Angeles, CA.

Kugler, K., Wijn, J., Geilen, M., DeJong, J., & Vlaeyen, J. (1999). *The Photograph Series of Daily Activities* (PHODA). Haartem, Netherlands.

Kulich, R., & Lande, S. D. (1997). Managed care: The past and future of pain treatment. *American Pain Society Bulletin, 7,* 1–5.

Lawson, K., Ressor, K., Keefe, F. J., & Turner, J. A. (1990). Dimensions of pain related cognitive coping: Cross validation of the factor structure of the Coping Strategies Questionnaire. *Pain, 43,* 195–204.

Leavitt, S. S., Johnson, T. L., & Beyer, R. D. (1971). The process of recovery patterns in industrial back injury: Costs and other quantitative measures of effort. *Industrial Medicine and Surgery, 40,* 7.

Lethem, J., Slade, P., Troup, J., & Bentley, G. (1983). Outline of a fear-avoidance model of exaggerated pain perceptions. *Behavior Research Therapy, 21,* 401–408.

Limon, S., Valinsky, L., & Ben-Shalom, Y. (2004). Risk factors for low back pain in the elementary school environment. *Spine, 29,* 697–702.

Lindsay, P., & Wyckoff, M. (1981). The depression pain and its response to anti-depressants. *Psychosomatics, 22,* 571–577.

Linton, S., Overmeer, T., Janson, M., Vlaeyen, J., & deJong, J. (2002). Graded *in vivo* exposure treatment for fear-avoidant pain patients with functional disability: A case study. *Cognitive Behavioral Therapy, 31,* 49–58.

Loeser, J. D. (1982). Concepts of pain. In M. Stanton-Hicks & R. Boas (Eds.), *Chronic low back pain*. New York: Raven Press.

Lousberg, R., Schmidt, A., & Groenman, N. (1992). The relationship between spouse solicitousness and pain behavior: Searching for more evidence. *Pain, 51,* 75–79.

Luo, X., Pietrobon, R., Sun, S., Liu, G., & Hey, L. (2003). Estimates and patterns of direct health care expenditures among individuals with back pain in the United States. *Spine, 29,* 79–86.

Macfarlane, G. (1999). Fibromyalgia and chronic widespread pain. In I. Crombie, P. Croft, S. Linton, L. LeResche, & M. VonKorff (Eds.), *Epidemiology of pain*. Seattle, WA: IASP Press.

Malone, M. D., & Strube, M. J. (1988). Meta-analysis of nonmedical treatment of chronic pain. *Pain, 34,* 231–244.

Mayer, T., & Gatchel, R. (1988). *Functional restoration for spinal disorders: The sports medicine approach*. Philadelphia: Lea and Febiger.

Mayer, T. G., Gatchel, R. J., Mayer, H., Kishino, N. D., Keeley, J., & Mooney, V. (1987). A prospective two year study of functional restoration in industrial low back injury. *Journal of the American Medical Association, 258,* 1763–1768.

Mayer, R. A., & Gebhart, G. F. (1994). Basic and clinical aspects of visceral hyper- algesia. *Gastroenterology, 107,* 271–293.

McCracken, L., & Eccleston, C. (2003). Coping or acceptance: What to do about chronic pain? *Pain, 105,* 197–204.

McCracken, L., & Turk, D. C. (2002). Behavioral and cognitive-behavioral treat- ment for chronic pain: Outcome, predictors of outcome, and treatment process. *Spine, 27,* 2564–2573.

McCracken, L., Vowles, K., & Eccleston, C. (2004). Acceptance of chronic pain: Component analysis and a revised assessment method. *Pain, 107,* 159–166.

Merskey, H., & Bogduk, G. (Eds.). (1994). *Classification of chronic pain: Descriptions of chronic pain syndromes and definition of pain terms* (2nd ed.). Seattle, WA: IASP Press.

Moriarity, K. J., & Dawson, A. M. (1982). Functional abdominal pain: Further evi- dence that the whole gut is affected. *British Medical Journal, 284,* 1670–1672.

Morley, S., Eccleston, C., & Williams, A. (1999). Systematic review and meta- analysis of randomized controlled trials of cognitive-behavior therapy and behavioral therapy for chronic pain in adults, excluding headaches. *Pain, 80,* 1.

Mutran, E., Reitzes, D., Mossey, J., & Fernandez, M. (1995). Social support, depres- sion and recovery of walking ability following hip fracture surgery. *Journal of Gerontology, 50B,* 5354–5361.

Negrini, S., & Carabalona, R. (2002). Backpacks on! School children's percep- tions of load, associations with back pain and factors determining this load. *Spine, 27,* 187–195.

Okifugi, A., Turk, D. C., & Kalauokalani, D. (1999). Clinical outcome and eco- nomic evaluation of multidisciplinary pain centers. In A. R. Block, E. F. Kremer, & E. Fernandez (Eds.), *Handbook of pain syndromes: Biopsychosocial perspectives.* Mahwah, NJ: Lawrence Erlbaum Associates.

Patrick, L. E., Attmaier, E. M., & Found, E. M. (2004). Long-term outcomes in multidisciplinary treatment of chronic low back pain: Results of a 13- year follow-up. *Spine, 29,* 850–855.

Petzke, F., Clauw, D., Ambrose, K., Khine, A., & Gracely, R. (2003). Increased pain sensitivity in fibromyalgia: Effects of stimulus type and mode of pres- entation. *Pain, 105,* 403–413.

Polatin, P. B., Kinney, R. K., Gatchel, R. J., Lillo, E., & Mayer, T. G. (1993). Psychiatric illness and chronic low back pain. *Spine, 18,* 66–71.

Pransky, G., Benjamin, K., Hill-Fotouhi, C., Fletcher, K. E., Himmelstein, J., & Katz, J. N. (2002). Work-related outcomes in occupational low back pain. *Spine, 27,* 864–870.

Richelson, E. (2001). Pharmacology of antidepressants. *Mayo Clinic Proceedings, 76,* 511–527.

Rosenstiel, A., & Keefe, F. (1983). The use of coping strategies in chronic low back pain patients: Relationship to patient characteristics and current adjustment. *Pain, 17,* 33–44.

Salerno, S., Browning, R., & Jackson, L. (2002). The effect of antidepressant treatment on chronic back pain. *Archives of Internal Medicine, 162,* 19–24.

Schade, V., Semmer, N., Main, C. J., Hora, J., & Boos, N. (1999). The impact of clinical, morphological, psychosocial and work-related factors on the outcome of lumbar diskectomy. *Pain, 80,* 239–249.

Scharff, L., & Marcus, D. (1994). Interdisciplinary outpatient group treatment of intractable headache. *Headache, 34,* 73–78.

Scharff, L., Marcus, D., & Turk, D. C. (1996). Maintenance of effects in the nonmedical treatment of headaches during pregnancy. *Headache, 36,* 285–290.

Schmidt, A. (1987). The behavioral management of pain: A criticism of a response. *Pain, 30,* 285–291.

Schmidt, A., & Brand, A. (1986). Persistence behavior of chronic low back pain patients in an acute pain situation. *Journal of Psychosomatic Research, 30,* 339–346.

Schultz, I. Z., Crook, J. M., Berkowitz, J., Meloche, G. R., Milner, R., Zuberbier, O. A., et al. (2002). Biopsychosocial multivariate predictive model of occupational low back disability. *Spine, 27,* 2720–2725.

Schultz, J. Z., Crook, J., Meloche, G. R., Berkowitz, J., Milner, R., Zuberier, O. A., et al. (2004). Psychosocial factors predictive of occupational low back disability: Towards development of a return-to-work model. *Pain, 107,* 77–85.

Smith, B. H., Elliott, A. M., Hannaford, P. C., Chambers, W. A., & Smith, W. C. (2004). Factors related to the onset and persistence of chronic back pain in the community. *Spine, 29,* 1032–1040.

Spitzer, W. O. (1987). Scientific approach to the assessment and management of activity-related spinal disorders. *Spine, 12*(Suppl.), 1.

Stewart, W. F., Shechter, A., & Rasmussen, B. K. (1994). Migraine prevalence: A review of population-based studies. *Neurology, 44*(Suppl. 4), 517–523.

Sullivan, M., Adams, H., & Sullivan, M. (2004). Communicative dimensions of pain catastrophizing: Social cueing effects on pain behavior and coping. *Pain, 107,* 220–226.

Sullivan, M., Thorn, B., Haythornthwaite, J., Keefe, F., Martin, M., Bradley, L., et al. (2001). Theoretical perspectives on the relation between catastrophizing and pain. *Clinical Journal of Pain, 17,* 52–64.

Svensson, D. A., Larsson, B., Waldenlind, E., & Pedersen, N. (2003). Shared rearing environment in migraine: Results from twins reared apart and twins reared together. *Headache, 43,* 235–244.

Taimela, S., Diederich, C., Hubsch, M., & Heinricy, M. (2000). The role of physical exercise and inactivity in pain recurrence and absenteeism from work after active outpatient rehabilitation for recurrent or chronic low back pain: A follow-up study. *Spine, 25,* 1809–1816.

Taylor, V. M., Deyo, R. A., Cherkin, D. C., & Kreutler, W. (1994). Low back pain hospitalization: Recent United States trends and regional variations. *Spine, 19*, 1207–1212.

Turk, D. C., & Fernandez, E. (1995). Personality assessment and the Minnesota Multiphasic Personality Inventory in chronic pain: Undeveloped and overexposed. *Pain Forum, 4*, 104–107.

Turk, D. C., Meichenbaum, D., & Genest, M. (1983). *Pain and behavioral medicine: A cognitive-behavioral perspective*. New York: Guilford Press.

Turner, J. A. (1996). Educational and behavioral interventions for back pain in primary care. *Spine, 21*, 2851–2859.

VanDerWeide, W. E., Verbeek, J. H., Salle, H. J., & VanDijk, F. J. (1999). Prognostic factors for chronic disability from acute low-back pain in occupational health care. *Scandinavian Journal of Work and Environmental Health, 25*, 50–56.

Vase, L., Robinson, M., Verne, G., & Price, D. (2003). The contributions of suggestion desire, and expectation to placebo effects in irritable bowel syndrome patients: An empirical investigation. *Pain, 105*, 17–25.

Verne, G. N., Robinson, M. E., Vase, L., & Price, D. D. (2003). Reversal of visceral and cutaneous hyperalgesia by local rectal anesthesia in irritable bowel syndrome (IBS) patients. *Pain, 105*, 223–230.

Vlaeyen, J., deJong, J., Geilen, M., Heuts, P., & Van Breukelen, G. (2001). Graded exposure *in vivo* in the treatment of pain related fear: A replicated single-case experimental design in four patients with chronic low back pain. *Behavioral Research and Therapy, 39*, 151–166.

Vlaeyen, J., & Linton, S. (2000). Fear-avoidance and its consequences in chronic musculoskeletal pain: A state of the art. *Pain, 85*, 317–332.

Vogt, M., Hanscom, B., Lauerman, W. C., & Kang, J. (2002). Influence of smoking on the health status of spinal patients. *Spine, 27*, 313–319.

VonKorff, M., & Simon, G. (1996). The relationship between pain and depression. *British Journal of Psychiatry, 30*(Suppl.), 101–108.

Waddell, G., Newton, M., Henderson, I., Somerville, D., & Main, C. J. (1993). A fear-avoidance beliefs questionnaire (FABQ) and the role of fear-avoidance beliefs in chronic low back pain and disability. *Pain, 52*, 157–168.

Whitehead, W., Holtkotter, B., Enck, P., Hoelzi, R., Holmes, K., Anthony, J., Shabsin, H., & Schuster, M. (1990). Tolerance for rectosigoid distention in irritable bowel syndrome. *Gastroenterology, 98*, 1187–1192.

10

Diabetes Mellitus

DAVID G. MARRERO, PhD, AND
JOHN C. GUARE, PhD

DIABETES IS A major health problem in the world today. Current estimates indicate that 18 million people in the United States have the disease (Centers for Disease Control and Prevention [CDC], 2004). Diabetes is considered the seventh leading cause of death, and the sixth leading cause of death by disease (National Institutes of Health [NIH], 1995, CDC). Individuals with diabetes are significantly more likely than their nondiabetic peers to develop macrovascular (large blood vessel) disease as well as the microvascular problems of retinopathy, neuropathy, and nephropathy. Such multiple morbidity problems can lead to various forms of functional limitation and disability. The combined direct and indirect costs attributable to diabetes care in 2003 were estimated at $132 billion (CDC).

Diabetes is most accurately viewed as a family of diseases characterized by the body's inability to effectively metabolize glucose. This inability is the result of defects in insulin secretion and/or insulin action. The result is chronic hyperglycemia (elevated blood glucose). The chronicity and degree of elevated glucose is associated with many of the long-term diabetes-related health problems (Eastman, 1995; Klein & Klein, 1995).

CLASSIFICATION OF DIABETIC CONDITIONS

DIABETES IS NOT a single, homogenous disease. Both the National Diabetes Data Group (NDDG, 1979) and the World Health Organization (WHO, 1980) have suggested that diabetes should be defined by five different classifications: (1) insulin-dependent diabetes mellitus, termed "type 1," which is characterized by beta-cell destruction typically mediated by the immune system with a resulting need for exogenous insulin, (2) non-insulin-dependent diabetes mellitus, termed "type 2," that is characterized by defects in insulin resistance and/or insulin secretion, (3) gestational diabetes mellitus (GDM) which occurs in women only during pregnancy, (4) malnutrition-related diabetes mellitus, and (5) "other types." Each is characterized by fasting hyperglycemia or elevated glucose concentrations in response to a glucose challenge. The 1979 NDDG classification also included the category of impaired glucose intolerance (IGT), defined by an elevated 2-hour glucose value in response to an oral glucose tolerance test (OGTT) that is above normal but below the value used to determine a diagnosis of diabetes (Expert Committee on the Diagnosis and Classification of Diabetes Mellitus [ECDCDM], 1997).

DIAGNOSTIC CRITERIA

THE DIAGNOSTIC CRITERIA for diabetes are based on glucose levels in the blood. The diagnosis of diabetes can be based on any of the following three glucose values (ECDCDM, 1997): (a) fasting plasma glucose (FPG) $\geq$ 126 mg/dl; (b) a random plasma glucose value $\geq$ 200 mg/dl plus the presence of classic symptoms, for example, polyuria, polydipsia; or (c) elevated plasma glucose in response to an OGTT performed according to WHO guidelines $\geq$ 200 mg/dl at the 2-hour time period. Confirmation on a subsequent day of any of these three criteria is strongly recommended. In clinical practice, however, diagnostic confirmation on a subsequent day is rare if the person presents with values significantly above the minimum values.

PREDIABETES

INCREASING EVIDENCE suggests that there are several factors whose presence significantly increases the risk for developing type 2 diabetes. These include age (older persons have increased risk), race/ethnicity (persons of color have greater risk), previous gestational diabetes (GDM), a family history of diabetes, body fat distribution (with central adiposity being associated with higher risk), obesity, physical inactivity, and elevated fasting glucose and/or impaired glucose tolerance (Edelstein, 1997). Recent data suggest that the presence of IGT results in a conversion to type 2 diabetes of approximately 11% per year (DPP Research Group, 2002). Additional research, however, has demonstrated that the onset of type 2 diabetes can be significantly delayed or even prevented in persons with IGT by use of selected medication or by intensive lifestyle modification that results in weight loss and increased physical activity (DPP Research Group; Pan et al., 1997; Tuomilehto, Lindström, Eriksson, et al., 2001).

As a result, a new diagnostic criterion for "prediabetes" has been introduced (Vendrame & Gottlieb, 2004) that indicates the person is at significantly increased risk for developing type 2 diabetes and should be considered for intervention. A diagnosis of prediabetes is established by a fasting blood glucose of greater than 110 mg/dl but less than 126 mg/dl or a 2-hour glucose following a 75 gram glucose challenge via an OGTT between 140 and 199 mg/dl (American Diabetes Association [ADA], 2003).

PREVALENCE AND INCIDENCE

IT IS CURRENTLY estimated that more than 18 million Americans, or approximately 6% of the U.S. population, have some form of diabetes, with greater than 90% having type 2 diabetes. These statistics are skewed with age: 13% of the population older than age 40 and 19% of the population older than age 65 have type 2 diabetes (CDC, 2004). Moreover, the incidence is increasing rapidly. The number of persons with diabetes (and the corresponding prevalence rate) has increased five-fold since 1958 (*Diabetes Overview*, 1996; Kenny, Aubert, & Geiss, 1995) reaching what the Centers for Disease Control term an "epidemic rate." The CDC now estimates that in 2004, every 24 hours there will be 3,600 new cases of type 2 diabetes, 580 deaths attributable to the disease, 225 amputations, 120 persons entering kidney failure and 55 new cases of blindness (CDC).

In the U.S., the lifetime risk for developing diabetes for individuals born in 2000 is 32.8% for males and 38.5% for females. Moreover, lifetime risk is higher among minority groups at birth and all ages. The lifetime risk at birth for Hispanic males is 45.4% compared to 26.7% for non-Hispanic whites. In females, the lifetime risk is 52.5% for Hispanics compared to 31.2% for non-Hispanic whites (Narayan, Boyle, Thompson, Sorenson, & Williamson, 2003).

This high-risk rate is largely due to a corresponding increase in associated risk factors such as obesity and sedentary lifestyle that have occurred over the past decade (Narayan, Imperatore, Benjamin, & Engelgau, 2002). There is a well-documented relationship between body mass index (BMI) and risk of developing type 2 diabetes. That risk increases at higher BMI levels (Knowler, Pettitt, Savage, & Bennett, 1981).

Type 1 diabetes is much less common than type 2, with approximately 120,000 individuals ≤ 19 years of age and 300,000–500,000 persons of all ages diagnosed with type 1 diabetes. Although studies vary in their estimates, it is generally accepted that 1.7 per 1,000 individuals have type 1, making this one of the most prevalent chronic diseases of childhood.

Incidence estimates in the United States suggest a rate of 30,000 new cases per year (LaPorte, Matsushima, & Chang, 1995).

Gestational diabetes mellitus occurs in approximately 4% of all U.S. pregnancies (Cousins, 1995). Testing for GDM between weeks 24–28 of gestation is therefore an important part of obstetric care for women who are at increased risk, for example, those with above normal body weight or a family history of diabetes (ECDCDM, 1997). Identification of GDM is important in order to reduce the associated fetal morbidities and mortality complications.

RISK FACTORS FOR THE DEVELOPMENT OF DIABETES

IN GENERAL, THE stress–diathesis model of illness applies to the development of both type 1 and type 2 diabetes—a genetic predisposition interacts with one or more environmental factors, conferring the expression of diabetes. Many factors thought to increase the risk of diabetes have been studied, including demographic, genetic, environmental/lifestyle, and physiologic. Risk factors are very different for type 1 and type 2, reflecting the differences in etiology between the two forms of the disease. Type 1 is viewed as an autoimmune disease caused by a pathogen that results in the destruction of beta cells responsible for the production of insulin. Type 2 is understood as a problem in insulin action (decreased insulin sensitivity) and/or insulin secretion (in a relative rather than absolute manner).

TYPE 1 RISK FACTORS

Gender, Age, Race/Ethnicity

Males and females have similar incidence rates, indicating that gender is not a risk factor for type 1 diabetes. The odds of developing type 1 is greatest at the age of puberty (age 10–14, depending on gender). This increased risk period is thought to be a result of hormonal changes or growth activity (Dorman, McCarthy, O'Leary, & Koehler, 1995). Whites are generally more susceptible to type 1, with the countries of Finland and Sweden having the highest prevalence of the disease (Dorman et al.). LaPorte et al. (1995) examined racial differences in type 1 incidence across several studies and found a significantly higher rate in Whites compared to either Blacks, Hispanics, or Asians.

Genetic

Only 20% of new cases of type 1 diabetes are linked to a family history of the disease. The risk of diabetes before age 30 for those with siblings, parents, or offspring with type 1 is 1%–15% compared to < 1% for those without a family history of the disease (Dorman et al., 1995). The concordance rate for identical twins is 25%–50% compared to 10% for a sibling of a person with diabetes (ADA, 1996). The identical-twin concordance rates (substantially less than 100%) reflect the importance of environmental factors.

Deoxyribose nucleic acid (DNA) research has implicated the human lymphocyte antigen (HLA) region of chromosome 6 in type 1 diabetes. Class II antigens include the DR locus antigens, and roughly 95% of individuals with type 1 have the DR3 and/or the DR4 antigen (Dorman et al., 1995). Persons with certain genetic factors have increased risk for developing type 1 diabetes.

Environmental/Lifestyle

There is a seasonal tendency toward greater type 1 diagnosis during winter months. Because flu strains are more common in winter, this lends evidence to a viral agent or other pathogen as a contributing factor. Coxsackie B viruses (B2, B3, B4, and B5) and cytomegalovirus have been implicated in type I onset, but their potential contribution is not well understood (Dorman et al., 1995).

Nutrition may play a part in the onset of type 1 diabetes, for example, consumption of cow's milk. The putative mechanism is a link between bovine serum albumin (BSA) antibodies and diabetes. (BSA may trigger an autoimmune response involving the beta cells of the pancreas.) Scott, Norris, and Kolb (1996) examined animal and human dietary evidence and suggest that there are at least three type 1 diabetogenic foods—wheat, soy, and cow's milk. More research is needed to better understand the potential contribution of nutritional factors in the onset of type 1 diabetes.

Physiologic

Compared to people without diabetes, individuals with type 1 are much more likely to exhibit islet cell cytoplasmic antibodies (ICAs), antibodies to insulin, and/or antibodies to the enzyme glutamic acid decarboxylase (GAD) (Dorman et al., 1995). It is not known if these antibodies are directly or indirectly involved in the pathophysiology of type 1.

TYPE 2 RISK FACTORS

Gender, Age, Race/Ethnicity

Although some studies suggest a greater prevalence of type 2 in women than men (ADA, 1996), such observations can be attributable to other risk factors rather than gender per se. When variables such as obesity and greater use of health care services are considered (both more common in women), the female: male ratio approaches 1 (Pareschi & Tomasi, 1989). Regarding age, the onset of type 2 has historically been rare before age 30. The rapid increase in obesity among children, however, has resulted in a rapidly increased observation of type 2 diabetes in children (Aye & Levitsky, 2003). After 30, age is directly and strongly related to the development of type 2 in most populations (Rewers & Hamman, 1995). Reaven and Reaven (1985) suggest much of the association can be attributed to age-related variables such as obesity and physical inactivity (discussed in the "Environmental/lifestyle" section that follows).

Prevalence rates of type 2 vary markedly depending on race and ethnic group. The highest rates are found in the American Pima Indians (50%), compared to the near zero prevalence rate in traditional societies such as the Mapuche Indians in Chile (Rewers & Hamman, 1995). U.S. data indicate African Americans and Hispanics have rates nearly twice that of non-Hispanic Whites (ADA, 1996).

Genetic

There is an 11% chance of developing type 2 diabetes by age 70 with no family history of the disease (ADA, 1996). This increases to 45% if both parents have type 2 diabetes. In reviewing studies assessing both monozygotic (MZ) and dizygotic (DZ) twin data, Rewers and Hamman (1995) noted at least a doubling of the concordance rate for MZ versus DZ twin pairs. The MZ concordance rates ranged from 34%–80% in these reports, with the mean rate substantially lower than 100%. Thus, environmental factors are important in the onset of type 2 diabetes.

Racial admixture data also reflect the (indirect) influence of genetic predisposition toward type 2. The percentage of Native American admixture across different groups (e.g., Pima Indians 100%, Barrio Mexican Indians 46%, mid-income Mexican Americans 27%) is strongly related to the prevalence rate of type 2 in each group (ADA, 1996). Potential group differences in environmental/lifestyle factors may also play a role in developing the disease.

More than 50 studies have investigated candidate genes for type 2 diabetes (Rewers & Hamman, 1995). Given the methodological challenges involved in this kind of research, how type 2 diabetes is inherited remains unclear. Overall, the data indicate polygenic influences rather than a single major locus influence.

Environmental/Lifestyle

The question of whether specific dietary components (e.g., high sugar, high fat, low fiber) are diabetogenic has generated much research. Interpretation of such studies is difficult because of methodological concerns. Perhaps the biggest concern is that few dietary components appear to promote diabetes independent of obesity. An exception is a prospective study by Marshall and Hamman (1988), who reported a sevenfold increased risk for a 40 g/day higher fat intake controlling for obesity and other factors. Overall, however, the available longitudinal (prospective) data do not support the hypothesis that dietary composition per se promotes the onset of type 2 diabetes (e.g., Bennett, Knowler, Baird, Butler, & Reid, 1984).

Physical inactivity may be a risk factor for type 2 diabetes. Research using a prospective epidemiological design has found that increased caloric expenditure is significantly related to a decreased risk of type 2 diabetes (Helmrich, Ragland, Leung, & Paffenbarger, 1991; Manson et al., 1992). Acute exercise enhances insulin sensitivity, but insulin sensitivity benefits diminish or disappear after only 3 days of inactivity (Schneider, Amorosa, Khachadurian, & Ruderman, 1984). Such evidence suggests adopting a lifestyle of physical activity (e.g., every 2–3 days) for both preventing and controlling type 2 diabetes.

As previously noted, obesity is a strong risk factor for type 2 diabetes. This is a very robust finding and has been observed in many populations worldwide. Prospective epidemiologic research demonstrates that the risk of developing type 2 diabetes is significantly related to being overweight and that increased risk occurs at even relatively low levels of obesity (Knowler et al., 1981). In addition, obesity is an independent predictor of type 2 onset when other assumed risk factors (e.g., age, blood glucose, family history of diabetes) are statistically controlled (Ohlson et al., 1988; Westlund & Nicolaysen, 1972). It is important to note, however, that most overweight individuals do not develop diabetes, and conversely, nonobese persons are diagnosed with type 2.

The distribution of a person's adipose (fat) tissue has been repeatedly shown to predict the presence of diabetes. A common index of body-fat distribution is the waist-to-hip ratio (WHR), obtained by dividing the circumference of the waist by the circumference of the hip. WHR is a significant predictor of type 2 diabetes (Vague, DeCastro, & Vague, 1986). Intra-abdominal fat assessed by computer tomography (CT) scans has also been shown to predict the onset of type 2 (Bergstrom et al., 1990).

Physiologic

Between 1%–11% of persons with impaired glucose tolerance develop type 2 each year (ADA, 1996; DPP Research Group, 2002). Thus, although the majority of patients with IGT either remain so or revert to normal glucose tolerance, elevated blood or plasma glucose is a risk factor for diabetes. Insulin levels have been studied, as impairment of insulin secretion/usage is considered a primary metabolic abnormality in these patients. Both reduced insulin secretion (Kadowaki et al., 1984) and hyperinsulinemia (Haffner & Stem, 1989) have been found to predict diabetes development.

THE PREVENTION OF DIABETES

B ECAUSE OF THE fact that several of the risk factors for diabetes are potentially modifiable, a number of trials have been conducted to determine if either type 1 or type 2 diabetes can be prevented or delayed. The results to date have been variable. The Diabetes Prevention Trial for type 1 investigated whether administration of insulin, either by injection or orally, would in effect "rest" the beta cell in persons with increased risk as defined by the presence of ICA antibodies (Morales, She, & Schatz, 2001; Schatz & Bingley, 2001; Sperling, 1997). Unfortunately, the results of these studies do not suggest that the prevention or even delay of type 1 diabetes is possible using these methods.

The case for the prevention of type 2 diabetes, however, is quite different. An increasing number of studies suggest that type 2 diabetes can be significantly delayed or possibly prevented by either the use of medications or lifestyle modification that results in weight loss in persons with IGT.

Three studies have demonstrated the ability of medications to delay or prevent the development of diabetes. The STOP-NIDDM trial compared Acarbose vs. placebo showing a 21% reduction in diabetes conversion in subjects receiving the active medication (Chiasson et al., 2003). The Traglitizone in Prevention of Diabetes (TRIPOD) study investigated the use of the first generation thiazolidinedione, an oral hypoglycemic agent, on the prevention of type 2 in women who were at increased risk by virtue of having had gestational diabetes mellitus (Buchanan et al., 2002). The results showed that using traglitizone resulted in a 44% reduction of risk, an effect that persisted over a 1-year period after the drug was stopped due to an unacceptable adverse event profile requiring that it be withdrawn from the marketplace.

The most rigorous randomized trial conducted to date that evaluated the effectiveness of a medication in preventing type 2 diabetes was the Diabetes Prevention Program (DPP) (DPP Research Group, 2002). The DPP compared in a randomized trial the effectiveness of metformin and lifestyle intervention on the reduction of diabetes in persons with IGT. The results of the study demonstrated a 31% reduction in diabetes risk when taking metformin and a 58% reduction associated with the lifestyle intervention. The lifestyle was relatively modest in its goals: a 7% loss of body weight from baseline entry into the study and a minimum of 150 minutes per week of physical activity equivalent to brisk walking.

The impressive reduction in diabetes risk resulting from lifestyle modification in the DPP has been corroborated by a study conducted in Finland that also observed a 58% reduction in diabetes risk when a similar lifestyle modification intervention as that used in the DPP was implemented (Tuomilehto et al., 2002).

FUNCTIONAL PRESENTATION OF DIABETES

TYPE 1: AT ONSET

THE ONSET OF symptoms for a person with type 1 diabetes is acute. The classic symptoms are polyuria (frequent urination), polydipsia (frequent drinking), polyphagia (frequent eating), and weight loss. Because the beta cells in the pancreas are no longer producing insulin, the body is unable to transfer glucose from the bloodstream into the organs, muscles, etc. Although there is plenty of fuel (glucose) available in the blood, it cannot reach the target tissues without insulin.

Unable to effectively use and store food intake, the individual is caught in a vicious cycle. The sensation of hunger promotes polyphagia. Because of polyphagia and lack of insulin, the high concentration of glucose circulates through the kidneys. At or above concentrations of 160–180 mg/dl (the renal threshold), the overload of glucose is excreted in the urine (glycosuria). The body's drive to eliminate excessive glucose promotes polyuria. In turn, the person experiences dehydration, which promotes polydipsia. Caloric loss via glycosuria can be substantial and promote weight loss. In addition, because circulating glucose cannot be used as energy, the body begins to break down fat stores (lipolysis) as an energy source, further promoting weight loss. Lipolysis causes an increase in the blood level of free fatty acids and ketone bodies. Depending on the severity of symptoms, a person may reach a state of diabetic ketoacidosis (DKA), which reflects a dangerously high level of acid in the bloodstream. Although DKA is preventable and treatable, coma and possibly death may result if diagnosis and treatment are delayed.

TYPE 2: AT ONSET

THE ONSET OF symptoms for a person with type 2 diabetes is much less acute and oftentimes not clinically evident for several years after onset of the disease. Because increasing age is associated with type 2 diabetes, many individuals perceive the slow onset of symptoms such as loss of energy, getting up at night to urinate, vision difficulties, and so on, as signs of aging. Individuals with type 2 rarely experience DKA because they do not suffer from absolute insulin deficiency. Given the insidious development of type 2, the discrepancy for some patients between meeting the diagnostic criteria for diabetes and actual diagnosis can be years. This explains in part the large number of undiagnosed cases in the United States.

THE COMPLICATIONS OF DIABETES

BOTH TYPE 1 and 2 diabetes are associated with a variety of acute and longer term complications. Individuals with poorly controlled type 1 diabetes are at risk for DKA, a very serious metabolic problem that can result in death but is generally preventable and correctable. Hospital discharge records note DKA on 3%–4% of all diabetes admissions (ADA, 1996). Hypoglycemic (i.e, low blood glucose also called "insulin reactions") episodes are fairly common in persons with type 1 diabetes, but may also occur in individuals with type 2 taking insulin or oral medication. Two acute though rather rare metabolic conditions associated with type 2 are hyperosmolar hyperglycemic nonketotic syndrome (HHNS) and lactic acidosis (LA). In addition, people with diabetes are at greater risk for various forms of infections.

There are a number of morbidities associated with diabetes that typically take years to develop. Patients with diabetes are very susceptible to microvascular disease, which can result in damage to the eye (retinopathy), kidney (nephropathy) and nerve functioning (neuropathy). Compared to nondiabetics, individuals with diabetes are 25 times more likely to become blind, 17 times more likely to develop renal disease, and 20 times more likely to develop gangrene (Davidson, 1986). It is believed that chronically elevated glucose levels (duration of diabetes interacting with degree of hyperglycemia) are primarily responsible for these problems (Diabetes Control and Complications Trial [DCCT] Research Group, 1993).

Retinopathy is a particularly common complication of diabetes. It is a leading cause of new cases of blindness in adults (12% of all new cases) (ADA, 1996). Klein and Klein (1995) reported 97% of insulin-taking and 80% of noninsulin-taking persons who have had diabetes for 15 or more years suffer some form of retinopathy. Bembaum and Albert (1996) note that many diabetes patients with proliferative retinopathy are not referred for vision-related rehabilitation services by their ophthalmologist or diabetes care provider. There is a strong need to improve referrals to such services.

Nephropathy and renal disease are common complications of diabetes affecting approximately 10%–21% of persons with the disease.

Progression of nephropathy can lead to end-stage renal disease (ESRD). Diabetes is the primary cause of ESRD and is responsible for approximately one third of all new cases annually. From 1982 to 1991, the percentage of ESRD cases attributable to diabetes increased from 23% to 36%. In a parallel fashion, the mortality rate for diabetes-related renal disease doubled between 1979 and 1990. ESRD is usually seen ≥ 25 years duration and requires dialysis or a kidney transplant for survival (ADA, 1996). Individuals with type 2 diabetes constitute the majority of new ESRD cases that are related to diabetes.

The general definition of neuropathy refers to nerve damage, and there are many forms of diabetic neuropathy. Approximately 60%–70% of individuals with type 1 and type 2 diabetes suffer from subclinical or clinical neuropathy (Eastman, 1995). The various neuropathic conditions can have pervasive effects throughout the body. The most common form is peripheral sensory neuropathy, affecting the hands, feet, and legs. Fifty-four percent of individuals with type 1 and 45% of those with type 2 have this form. Carpal tunnel syndrome affects one third of persons with diabetes. Impotence, delayed gastric emptying, and bladder and bowel dysfunction are examples of autonomic neuropathy. Increased risk of silent myocardial infarction and sudden death in patients with diabetes is caused in part by autonomic neuropathy (ADA, 1996).

Macrovascular Complications

Persons with type 2 diabetes are at increased risk for large blood vessel disease, the leading cause of mortality in this population. Individuals with diabetes are 2 to 12 times more likely to suffer from cardiovascular disease and 2 to 4 times more likely to die from heart disease compared to those without diabetes (ADA, 1996). Peripheral vascular disease (PVD) affects about 10% of all patients with diabetes, but the rate is much higher with a disease duration > 20 years. PVD interferes with blood and oxygen flow to the lower extremities. PVD in concert with peripheral sensory neuropathy can lead to foot ulcerations, gangrene, and amputation. Approximately half of all nontraumatic amputations in the United States occur in patients with diabetes (ADA; Palumbo & Melton, 1995). In addition, stroke is 2 to 4 times more common, making cerebrovascular disease another significant morbidity associated with diabetes.

Mortality

Portuese and Orchard's (1995) review indicates > 15% of persons diagnosed with type 1 in childhood will be dead by the age of 40, reflecting a mortality rate some 20 times that seen in the general population. Mortality in type 2 individuals is also elevated compared to the general U.S. population but to a lesser degree. When type 2 onset occurs in middle age, these persons are observed to lose about 5 to 10 years of life expectancy. The onset of type 2 in people ≥ 70 years of age has negligible effects on life expectancy (Geiss, Herman, & Smith, 1995).

ECONOMIC COSTS OF DIABETES

GIVEN THE EXTENSIVE morbidity and mortality problems related to diabetes, estimates of the direct and indirect costs attributable to the disease in 2003 totaled $135 billion (CDC, 2003). The following is based on the data collected by the Centers for Disease Control and Prevention. In descending order of attributable cost, direct medical expenditures ($92 billion) were due to (a) excess prevalence of general medical conditions (e.g., flu), (b) excess prevalence of chronic complications, and (c) acute glycemic care. Over 50% of all indirect costs were incurred by persons 65 years of age and older. Indirect costs ($43 billion) were caused by disability and premature mortality. The cost of lost productivity was $39.8 billion. The average per capita cost of caring for a person with and without diabetes was $13,243 and $2,560, respectively, more than a fivefold difference.

REDUCING/PREVENTING LONG-TERM COMPLICATIONS

UNTIL RECENTLY, IT was not known if improving glycemic control would prevent or delay the progression of long-term complications associated with either type 1 or 2 diabetes. This was the impetus for the Diabetes Control and Complications Trial (DCCT) (DCCT Research Group, 1993) and the United Kingdom Prospective Diabetes Study (UKPDS) (UKPDS Group, 1998).

The main purpose of the DCCT was to determine if intensive treatment of patients with type 1 diabetes would decrease the likelihood of the three main microvascular complications, particularly retinopathy. Two cohorts were recruited: those with and without retinopathy. Patients without retinopathy allowed for the assessment of prevention, whereas the other cohort allowed for the assessment of progression. Patients within each cohort were randomly assigned to either intensive therapy (IT) or conventional therapy (CT). The former condition was designed to achieve optimal glycemic control, and used intensive self-monitoring of blood glucose (SMBG), frequent treatment contact, and either multiple daily injections (MDI, defined as $\geq$ 3/day) or an insulin pump. The CT group was treated with one or two daily insulin injections with a lower frequency of SMBG and treatment contact.

Compared to the CT condition, IT demonstrated a 76% reduction in risk of developing retinopathy (primary-prevention cohort). The progression of retinopathy was slowed by 54% in the secondary-intervention cohort. Both cohorts combined showed that IT provided (a) a 39% mean reduction in the occurrence of microalbuminuria (nephropathy indication), and (b) a 60% mean reduction in clinical neuropathy. There were no significant differences between the two treatment conditions in neuropsychological functioning or quality of life. Risks associated with IT included a threefold increase in severe hypoglycemia and a greater likelihood of becoming overweight. In sum, IT was extremely successful in preventing/managing long-term complications. The associated risks may interfere with the adoption of such treatment in certain patients, however (e.g., persons with difficulty detecting hypoglycemia, young women who are more concerned about weight gain than glycemic control).

The UK Prospective Diabetes Study was a 20-year trial which recruited 5,102 patients with type 2 diabetes in 23 clinical centers based in England, Northern Ireland, and Scotland (UK Prospective Diabetes Study Group, 2000) who were studied over a 10-year period. The objective was to determine the relation between glucose levels over time and the risk of macrovascular or microvascular complications in patients with type 2 diabetes. The primary outcome was any end point or deaths related to diabetes and all cause mortality. Secondary measures included aggregate outcomes: myocardial infarction, stroke, amputation (including death from peripheral vascular disease), and microvascular disease (predominantly retinal photo-coagulation). The results showed that the incidence of clinical complications was significantly associated with glycemia. Each 1% reduction in updated mean HbA1c was associated with reductions in overall risk of 21% for complications, 21% for deaths related to diabetes, 14% for myocardial infarction, and 37% for microvascular complications. No threshold of risk was observed for any end point.

The UKPDS also studied the relationship of tight blood pressure control to macrovascular and microvascular complications. The study demonstrated that reductions in risk in the group assigned to tight control compared with that assigned to less tight control were 24% in diabetes related end points, 32% in deaths related to diabetes, 44% in strokes, and 37% in microvascular end points. There was also a non-significant reduction in all cause mortality. After 9 years of follow-up the group assigned to tight blood pressure control also had a 34% reduction in risk in the proportion of patients with deterioration of retinopathy by two steps and a 47% reduced risk AU: text missing here?

TREATMENT OF DIABETES

ALTHOUGH DIABETES IS a medical problem, effective management relies heavily on the patient to perform the appropriate self-care behaviors. Given the complexity and chronicity of diabetes self-management, coupled with the lack of an effective health care model for managing diabetes (Etzwiler, 1997), most patients with diabetes do not achieve proper glycemic control.

TREATMENT GOALS

TYPE 1 AND type 2 diabetes are characteristically different in terms of age at onset (and hence developmental challenges), level of obesity, lipid abnormalities, and other factors. Consequently, the focus of treatment is not identical for both forms of the disease.

The primary goals of treatment for type 1 diabetes are to (a) establish and maintain medical and psychological well-being; (b) avoid severe and frequent episodes of hypoglycemia, symptomatic hyperglycemia, and DKA; and (c) promote proper growth and development in children and adolescents (ADA, 1994a). A secondary goal is to provide the individual/family with the resources required to achieve optimal glycemic control in order to prevent/delay the diabetes-related micro- and macrovascular complications. The primary goals are viewed as very reasonable; the secondary goal requires much more effort and resources to achieve, though also providing greater benefits.

Primary treatment goals for patients with type 2 diabetes are to (a) promote normal metabolism (glucose and lipid), and (b) prevent or minimize micro- and macrovascular complications (ADA, 1994b). Because the majority of patients with type 2 diabetes are obese, normalizing lipid levels, blood pressure, and body weight are important for managing potential macrovascular complications.

TREATMENT COMPONENTS

THERE ARE FOUR basic components to the treatment of diabetes: medication (insulin, oral hypoglycemic agents), nutrition therapy, exercise, and self-monitoring of blood glucose (SMBG). Each component must be individualized for the patient. Medication, food intake, and exercise must be carefully balanced so the person maintains desirable glucose levels and avoids hypo- and hyperglycemia. SMBG is used as feedback to determine which aspects of the treatment regimen need adjustment.

Medication

For type 1 diabetes, all patients must take exogenous insulin to survive, as they have an absolute or near-absolute deficiency in endogenous insulin production. The optimal goal of insulin administration is to mimic normal insulin secretion. This requires multiple daily injections (MDI) ($\geq$ 3/day) or use of an insulin infusion pump. Many type 1 patients do not want such an intensive regimen and opt for a twice-daily regimen, mixing both short-term and long-term insulins in each injection. In general, a twice-daily regimen yields poorer glycemic control compared to an MDI or pump approach (ADA, 1994a). The diabetes health care team and the patient must work together to determine an insulin administration plan that is acceptable to both parties while achieving the best possible glycemic control.

Medication for patients with type 2 includes oral agents and insulin. Some type 2 patients are able to control their blood glucose with diet and exercise and do not need medication. This is a small minority, however. When diet alone is not successful, oral agents and possibly insulin are typically introduced in a stepped care approach.

Medical Nutrition Therapy

Regarding type 1 diabetes, current guidelines for macronutrient intake suggest calories be distributed as follows: protein 10%–20%; fat < 10% from saturated fat, $\geq$ 10% from polyunsaturated fat; this leaves the remaining 60%–70% to come from carbohydrate and monounsaturated fat (ADA, 1998b). These guidelines are much more flexible than those used in the past. Consequently, terms such as "medical nutrition therapy" (MNT) or "meal planning" are used to better convey the current approach of determining proper caloric intake according to a set of nutrition-related goals. The primary aim of MNT is to promote proper glucose metabolism. Additional MNT goals for type 1 include healthy lipid levels, distribution of calories and types of foods to promote normal growth and development in children and adolescents, and prevention/treatment of hypoglycemic episodes (ADA). All of these goals are developed with the individual while considering the person's health status, eating habits, cultural food preferences, and exercise habits.

MNT goals for persons with type 2 diabetes emphasize problems commonly seen in this population, for example, obesity, hypertension, and elevated lipid levels. Thus, in addition to normalizing glucose levels, primary goals for type 2 include modifying the quantity and quality of food intake to reduce weight, blood pressure, and blood lipids.

Exercise

Exercise is recommended for individuals with diabetes. The potential benefits may include (a) decreased risk of cardiovascular disease via reducing obesity, blood pressure, and elevated lipid levels, and by increasing HDL levels; (b) increased insulin sensitivity, which may enhance glycemic control and decrease dosage of antidiabetic medication; (c) improvements in mood and self-esteem; (d) enhancing quality of life and activities of daily living by improving muscle strength and joint flexibility; and (e) promoting weight reduction and maintenance of weight loss (ADA, 1994a, 1994b).

Potential risks associated with exercise for patients with diabetes are also numerous. These may include (a) cardiovascular effects such arrhythmias caused by ischemic heart disease, significant increases in blood pressure, and orthostatic hypotension following exercise; (b) microvascular problems such as retinal hemorrhage and increased proteinuria in patients with such preexisting problems; (c) metabolic decompensation such as promoting hyperglycemia caused by too little insulin when exercise is started, or hypoglycemia if too much insulin is present; and (d) musculoskeletal and related problems such as aggravating preexisting joint disease, and orthopedic injury and foot ulcers related to neuropathy (ADA, 1994a, 1994b). The benefit:risk ratio can be maximized by careful planning (with appropriate diabetes care providers) and tailoring physical activities to the person.

SMBG

Self-monitoring of blood glucose provides feedback regarding the effects of recent behavior (medication use, food intake, exercise) on blood glucose control. When used appropriately (i.e., accurate measurement and results properly used to modify regimen behavior), SMBG can be a powerful tool in optimizing glycemic control (DCCT Research Group, 1993). However, SMBG performance and/or use of the results to guide eating or insulin adjustments are used by a minority of type 1 patients seen in an outpatient clinic setting (Fekete, Guare, Marrero, & Orr, 1997). Thus, SMBG is best viewed as a self-management tool, and there is no reason to believe it will enhance glycemic control unless it is used properly.

PSYCHOLOGICAL AND VOCATIONAL IMPLICATIONS

THERE ARE A number of psychological/behavioral and vocational issues relevant to diabetes. This section addresses adherence, stress, depression, eating disorders, insulin manipulation for weight control, sexual dysfunction, and adjustment to disability. These topics are representative of the psychosocial concerns in the diabetes literature and should not be construed as exhaustive.

ADHERENCE

GIVEN THE MULTIPLE health behaviors involved in the self-management of diabetes, adherence should not be viewed as a unitary construct. Research has shown that an individual may adhere well to one behavior (e.g., SMBG) but not another (e.g., meal plan) (Johnson, 1994).

Consequently, attempts to measure diabetes adherence behavior should be domain specific. Partial or inconsistent adherence to one's diabetes treatment regimen is common (Kovacs, Goldston, Obrosky, & Iyengar, 1992). Patients often report the greatest difficulty in following the meal-plan component (Ary, Toobert, Wilson, & Glasgow, 1986). Recent research indicates that an average of 16% (range 0%–50%) of the foods patients report consuming in a typical week would promote hyperglycemia (Fekete et al., 1997). The least difficult aspect of the regimen involves taking medication. Though most patients take their medication, however, many do not wait the appropriate amount of time between insulin administration and eating (Johnson, 1994).

STRESS

PSYCHOLOGICAL STRESS HAS been thought to promote hyperglycemia and thus worsen glycemic control. Two mechanisms have been proposed to account for this hypothesis. Stress may indirectly affect blood glucose by interfering with one's behavior, for example, eating sweets and/or discontinuing exercise, which in turn promotes hyperglycemia. Another possibility is that glucose metabolism may be directly compromised by the neuroendocrine effects associated with stress, for example, increased catecholamine and/or cortisol levels.

Overall, the evidence that stress promotes metabolic decompensation in persons with diabetes is equivocal. The hypothesis that stress interferes with adherence to the type 1 regimen and consequently raises blood glucose has received mixed support (Hanson, Henggeler, & Burghen, 1987; Schafer, Glasgow, McCaul, & Dreher, 1983). Correlational studies have found that increased levels of stressful life events or daily hassles are significantly related to poorer glycemic control in persons with type 1 (Cox, Taylor, Nowacek, Holley-Wilcox, & Pohl, 1984) and type 2 diabetes (Aikens & Mayes, 1997). Conversely, lack of stress-induced hyperglycemia has been reported in laboratory research manipulating acute stressors in type 1 (Kemmer et al., 1986) and type 2 diabetes (Bruce, Chisholm, Storlien, Kraegen, & Smythe, 1992). Stabler, Morris, Litton,

258

DISABLING
CONDITIONS
and DISORDERS

Feinglos, and Surwit (1986) reported a greater blood glucose elevation in response to a competitive video task in Type-A-behavior vs. Type-B-behavior children with diabetes. Thus, the need to account for individual differences in response to stress is important.

DEPRESSION

INDIVIDUALS WITH DIABETES have to cope with the demands of managing an incurable disease, possibly putting them at risk for certain psychological problems. Depression has received the most attention in the area of diabetes. The finding that depression is more common in individuals with diabetes than in healthy persons is well established. Garvard, Lustman, and Clouse (1993) conducted a systematic review of the depression and diabetes prevalence literature (20 studies). They concluded that approximately 15%–20% of persons with type 1 or 2 diabetes experience major depression at some point during their lifetime, a rate several times that of the general population. It is unclear whether persons with diabetes are more likely to experience depression compared to persons with other chronic medical conditions, however. Thus, the question remains if the increased risk is the result of having a chronic disease or of having diabetes per se.

Griffith and Lustman (1997) note that the limited data addressing gender suggest depression in diabetes seems to follow the 2:1 female-to-male ratio seen in the general population. Given the recurring nature of depressive episodes and their significant impact on the person, diagnosing and treating depression in patients with diabetes should be an integral part of diabetes care. This is especially true for women.

EATING DISORDERS

THERE IS SUBSTANTIAL pressure on women in our society to be thin. Successful management of diabetes requires close attention to food intake. It has been hypothesized that young women with diabetes are at increased risk of eating disorders, especially bulimia nervosa. Initial research using self-report measures of eating-disordered behavior seems to support this hypothesis; however, two problems exist with self-report measures (Wing, Nowalk, Marcus, Koeske, & Finegold, 1986). One, although such measures are informative, they cannot be used to make a diagnosis of eating disorders. Two, persons with diabetes often endorse items that are appropriate for diabetes management, resulting in an artificially inflated score, for example, "I pay close attention to the food I eat."

Recent research using a structured-interview format and appropriate comparison subjects indicates that the prevalence of eating disorders is relatively low in women with diabetes and comparable to that of their nondiabetic peers (Peveler, Boller, Fairburn, & Dunger, 1992). Subclinical eating-disordered behavior is a substantial problem, however. For example, scores on the Bulimia test-revised (BULIT-R) were a significant and independent predictor of glycemic control in adolescents and young adult females with diabetes (Guare et al., 1997a).

INSULIN MANIPULATION FOR WEIGHT CONTROL

ADOLESCENT FEMALES WITH diabetes are significantly more dissatisfied with their weight/body shape than their male counterparts, and such attitude differences diverge even more as adolescence progresses (Guare & Orr, 1995). Individuals with type 1 diabetes can reduce/omit their insulin dose, which will promote loss of calories via glycosuria. Recent research indicates type 1 females aged 14–24 both decrease and skip their insulin dose specifically for weight-control purposes significantly more often than type 1 males (Guare et al., 1997b). Screening for weight dissatisfaction and possible insulin manipulation should be considered in type 1 females in this age category.

SEXUAL DYSFUNCTION

ERECTILE DYSFUNCTION OR impotence is reported by 50% of men with diabetes (Waxman, 1980). Both physiologic and psychologic factors may contribute to this problem. Women with type 2 (but not type 1) diabetes also report greater disturbance in sexual functioning compared to healthy women without diabetes in areas of sexual desire, orgasmic capacity, and lubrication (Schreiner-Engel, Schiavi, Vietorisz, & Smith, 1987). Research addressing sexual dysfunction in women with diabetes is relatively new and has produced mixed results. It is also not clear if diabetes has an organic contribution to sexual problems in women as it does in men. Future sexual-dysfunction research should stress the importance of assessing psychological and physiological factors and emphasize the study of women.

DISABILITY AND EMPLOYMENT

THE FOLLOWING IS based on a review of disability and diabetes by Songer (1995). Between 20%–50% of persons with diabetes report some form of disability, at rates substantially higher than in the general population. Activity limitations as well as restricted-activity days are reported 2 to 3 times more often by patients with diabetes. Increasing age and minority-group status are associated with greater impairment in activity and/or work. Reported activity limitations affect persons with type 2 (50.2%) more so than type 1 (42.3%), and are especially high for type 2 individuals taking insulin (63.5%). Long-term complications are a primary cause of disability.

Individuals with type 1 who are also disabled have higher rates of unemployment (49%) compared to nondisabled persons (12%). The same pattern holds true for absenteeism, 13.8 vs. 3.0 days per year. The average number of physician visits per year is double that for disabled persons with diabetes compared to those without disability. Activities of daily living (ADLs) are more likely to be limited by persons with diabetes (type 1: 8.8%; type 2: 4.9%) than without (2.3%).

SUMMARY AND FUTURE DIRECTIONS

DIABETES IS A serious medical disorder that places significant demands on the person and the health care system. This situation continues to worsen due to the increasing incidence and prevalence rates. The Centers for Disease Control and Prevention reported that 1 in 3 children born in 2000 will likely develop diabetes. The growing problem of obesity and physical inactivity in the United States must be addressed in order to curb these growing rates.

The good news is that behavioral and pharmacological interventions for persons with diabetes have been shown to significantly improve glycemic control, reduce the risk of diabetes-related morbidity, and improve quality of life. Recent clinical trials have also demonstrated that it is possible to prevent or significantly delay type 2 diabetes. Whether the health care system will support and patients choose an intensive lifestyle modification to prevent diabetes remains to be seen. Clearly, one of the most formidable challenges facing patients and the health care system is translating the results of clinical trials such as the DCCT and the DPP to the public health sector.

REFERENCES

Aikens, J. E., & Mayes, R. (1997). Elevated glycosylated albumin in NIDDM is a function of recent everyday environmental stress. *Diabetes Care, 20,* 1111–1113.

American Diabetes Association. (1994a). *Medical management of insulin dependent (type II) diabetes* (2nd ed.). New York: Author.

American Diabetes Association. (1994b). *Medical management of non-insulin dependent (type II) diabetes* (3rd ed.). New York: Author.

American Diabetes Association. (1996). *Diabetes vital statistics.* New York: Author.

American Diabetes Association. (1998a). Economic consequences of diabetes mellitus in the U.S. in 1997. *Diabetes Care, 21,* 296–309.

American Diabetes Association. (1998b). Nutritional recommendations and principles for people with diabetes mellitus. *Diabetes Care, 21*(Suppl. 1), S32–S35.

American Diabetes Association. (2003). Diabetes update. *Diabetes Care, 19* (Suppl. 1), 19–20, 24.

Ary, D. Y., Toobert, D., Wilson, W., & Glasgow, R. E. (1986). Patient perspective on factors related to non-adherence to diabetes regimen. *Diabetes Care, 9,* 168–172.

Aye, T., & Levitsky, L. L. (2003). Type 2 diabetes: An epidemic disease in childhood. *Current Opinion in Pediatrics, 15*(4), 411–415.

Bembaum, M., & Albert, S. G. (1996). Referring patients with diabetes and vision loss for rehabilitation: Who is responsible? *Diabetes Care, 19,* 175–177.

Bennett, P. H., Knowler, W. C., Baird, H. R., Butler, D. J., & Reid, J. M. (1984). Diet and development of noninsulin-dependent diabetes mellitus: An epidemiological perspective. In G. Pozza, P. Micossi, A. L. Catapano, & R. Pauletti (Eds.), *Diet, diabetes and atherosclerosis* (pp. 109–119). New York: Raven Press.

Bergstrom, R. W., Newell-Morris, L. L., Leonetti, D. L., Shuman, W. P., Wahl, W. P., & Fujimoto, W. Y. (1990). The association of elevated C-peptide level and increased intra-abdominal fat distribution with development of NIDDM in Japanese-American men. *Diabetes, 39,* 104–111.

Bruce, D. G., Chisholm, D. J., Storlien, L. H., Kraegen, E. W., & Smythe, G. A. (1992). The effects of sympathetic nervous system activation and psychological stress on glucose metabolism and blood pressure in subjects with type II non-insulin dependent diabetes mellitus. *Diabetologia, 35,* 835–843.

Buchanan, T. A., Xiang, A. H., Peters, R. K., Kjos, S. L., Marroquin, A., Goico, J., et al. (2002). Preservation of pancreatic beta-cell function and prevention of type 2 diabetes by pharmacological treatment of insulin resistance in high-risk Hispanic women. *Diabetes, 51*(9), 2796–2803.

Centers for Disease Control and Prevention. (2004). National diabetes fact sheet: General information and national estimates on diabetes in the United States, 2003 (rev. ed.). Atlanta, GA: U.S. Department of Health and Human Services, Centers for Disease Control and Prevention.

Chiasson, J. L., Josse, R. G., Gomis, R., Hanefeld, M., Karasik, A., & Laakso, M. STOP-NIDDM Trial Research Group. (2003). Acarbose treatment and the risk of cardiovascular disease and hypertension in patients with impaired glucose tolerance: The STOP-NIDDM trial. *Journal of the American Medical Association, 290*(4), 486–494.

Cousins, L. (1995). *Obstetric complications. Diabetes mellitus and pregnancy: Principles and practice* (2nd ed.). New York: Churchill Livingstone.

Cox, D. J., Taylor, A. G., Nowacek, G., Holley-Wilcox, P., & Pohl, S. (1984). The relationship between psychological stress and insulin-dependent diabetic blood glucose control: Preliminary investigations. *Health Psychology, 3*(1), 63–75.

Davidson, M. B. (1986). *Diabetes mellitus: Diagnosis and treatment.* New York: Wiley.

Devlin, J. T., Hirshman, M., Hurton, E. D., & Horton, E. S. (1987). Enhanced peripheral and splanchnic insulin sensitivity in NIDDM men after single bout of exercise. *Diabetes, 36,* 434–439.

Diabetes Control and Complications Trial Research Group. (1993). The effect of intensive treatment of diabetes on the development and progression of long term complications in insulin dependent diabetes mellitus. *New England Journal of Medicine, 329,* 977–986.

Diabetes Overview. October 1995 (updated 1996). NIDDK NIH publication no. 96-1468.

Dorman, J. S., McCarthy, B. J., O'Leary, L. A., & Koehler, A. (1995). Risk factors for insulin dependent diabetes. *Diabetes in America* (2nd ed.) [NIH publication no. 95-1468]. Bethesda, MD: U.S. Government Printing Office.

DPP Research Group. (2002). Reduction in the incidence of type 2 diabetes with lifestyle intervention or metformin. *New England Journal of Medicine, 346*(6), 393–403.

Eastman, R. C. (1995). Neuropathy in diabetes. *Diabetes in America* (2nd ed.) [NIH] publication no. 95-1468]. Bethesda, MD: U.S. Government Printing Office.

Edelstein, S. L. (1997). Predicators of progression from impaired glucose tolerance to NIDDM: An analyses of six prospective studies. *Diabetes, 46*(4), 701–710.

Etzwiler, D. D. (1997). Chronic care: A need in search of a system. *Diabetes Educator, 23,* 569–573.

Expert Committee on the Diagnosis and Classification of Diabetes Mellitus. (1997). Report of the expert committee on the diagnosis and classification of diabetes mellitus. *Diabetes Care, 20,* 1183–1197.

Fekete, D., Guare, G., Marrero, D., & Orr, D. (1997). Self-management of "off-diet" food intake by adolescents and young adults with insulin-dependent diabetes mellitus. *Diabetes, 46,* 265A.

Garvard, J. A., Lustman, P. J., & Clouse, R. E. (1993). Prevalence of depression in adults with diabetes: An epidemiological evaluation. *Diabetes Care, 16,* 1167–1178.

Geiss, L. S., Herman, W. H., & Smith, P. J. (1995). Mortality in non-insulin dependent diabetes. *Diabetes in America* (2nd ed.) [NIH publication no. 95-1468]. Bethesda, MD: U.S. Government Printing Office.

Griffith, L. S., & Lustman, P. J. (1997). Depression in women with diabetes. *Diabetes Spectrum, 10,* 216–223.

Guare, J. C., Marrero, D., Orr, D., Kakos-Kraft, S., Fineberg, N., & Friedenberg, G. (1997a). Predictors of diabetic control in male and female adolescents and young adults with IDDM. *Diabetes, 46,* 266A.

Guare, J. C., Marrero, D., Orr, D., Kakos-Kraft, S., Fineberg, N., & Friedenberg, G. (1997b). Bulimia symptomatology and insulin manipulation in males and females with IDDM. *Diabetes, 46,* 265A.

Guare, J. C., & Orr, D. P. (1995). Changes in weight-related attitudes over a 2-year period in male and female adolescents with IDDM. *Diabetes, 44,* 97A.

Haffner, S. M., & Stem, M. P. (1989). Hyperinsulinemia is associated with 8-year incidence of NIDDM in Mexican Americans. *Diabetes, 38*(Suppl. I), 92A.

Hanson, C. L., Henggeler, S. W., & Burghen, G. A. (1987). Model of associations between psychosocial variables and health-outcome measures of adolescents with IDDM. *Diabetes Care, 10,* 752–758.

Helmrich, S. P., Ragland, D. R., Leung, R. W., & Paffenbarger, R. S. (1991). Physical activity and reduced occurrence of non-insulin-dependent diabetes mellitus. *New England Journal of Medicine, 325,* 147–152.

Johnson, S. B. (1994). Methodological issues in diabetes research: Measuring adherence. *Diabetes Care, 15,* 1658–1667.

Kadowaki, T., Miyake, Y., Hayura, R., Akanuma, Y., Kajinuma, H., Kuznya, N., et al. (1984). Risk factors for worsening diabetes in subjects with impaired glucose tolerance. *Diabetologia, 26,* 44–49.

Kemmer, F. W., Bisping, R., Steingruber, H. J., Baar, H., Hardtmann, F., Schlaghecke, R., et al. (1986). Psychological stress and metabolic control in patients with type I diabetes. *New England Journal of Medicine, 314,* 1078–1084.

Kenny, S. J., Aubert, R. E., & Geiss, L. S. (1995). Prevalence and incidence of non-insulin-dependent diabetes. *Diabetes in America* (2nd ed.) [NIH publication no. 95-1468]. Bethesda, MD: U.S. Government Printing Office.

Klein, R., & Klein, B. E. K. (1995). Vision disorders in diabetes. *Diabetes in America* (2nd ed.) [NIB publication no. 95-1468]. Bethesda, MD: U.S. Government Printing Office.

Knowler, W. C., Pettitt, D. J., Savage, P. J., & Bennett, P. H. (1981). Diabetes incidence in Pima Indians: Contributions of obesity and parental diabetes. *American Journal of Epidemiology, 113,* 144–156.

Kovacs, M., Goldston, D., Obrosky, D. S., & Iyengar, S. (1992). Prevalence and predictors of pervasive non-compliance with the medical treatment among youths with insulin-dependent diabetes mellitus. *Journal of the American Academy of Child and Adolescent Psychiatry, 31,* 1112–1119.

LaPorte, R. E., Matsushima, M., & Chang, Y. (1995). *Diabetes in America* (2nd ed.) [NIB publication no. 95-1468]. Bethesda, MD: U.S. Government Printing Office.

Manson, J. E., Nathan, D. M., Krowleski, A. S., Stampfer, M. I., Coldlitz, G. A., Willett, W. C., et al. (1992). A prospective study of exercise and incidence of diabetes among U.S. male physicians. *Journal of the American Medical Association, 268,* 63–67.

Marshall, J. A., & Hamman, R. F. (1988). Low carbohydrate, high fat diet, and the incidence of non-insulin-dependent diabetes mellitus. *Diabetes, 37,* 115A.

Morales, A. E., She, J. X., & Schatz, D. A. (2001). Prediction and prevention of type 1 diabetes. *Current Diabetes Reports, 1*(1), 28–32.

Narayan, K. M., Boyle, B., Thompson, T., Sorenson, S., & Williamson, D. (2003). Lifetime risk for diabetes mellitus in the United States. *Journal of the American Medical Association, 290*(14).

Narayan, K. M., Imperatore, G., Benjamin, S. M., & Engelgau, M. M. (2002).

Targeting people with pre-diabetes. *British Medial Journal, 325*(7361), 403–404.

National Diabetes Data Group. (1979). Classification and diagnosis of diabetes mellitus and other categories of glucose intolerance. *Diabetes, 28,* 1039–1057.

National Institutes of Health. (1995). *Diabetes statistics* (NIH Publication no. 96-3926). Washington, DC: U.S. Government Printing Office.

Ohlson, L-O., Larsson, B., Bjorntorp, P., Eriksson, H., Svardsudd, K., Welin, L., et al. (1988). Risk factors for type II (non-insulin-dependent) diabetes mellitus. Thirteen and one-half years of follow-up of the participants in a study of Swedish men born in 1913. *Diabetalogia, 31,* 798–805.

Palumbo, P. J., & Melton, L. J. III. (1995). *Diabetes in America* (2nd ed.) [NIH publication no. 95-1468]. Bethesda, MD: U.S. Government Printing Office.

Pan, X. R., Li, G. W., Hu, Y. H., Wong, J. X., Yang, W. Y., An, Z. X., et al. (1997). Effects of diet and exercise in preventing NIDDM in people with impaired glucose tolerance: The Da Qing IGT and Diabetes Study. *Diabetes Care, 20,* 537–544.

Pareschi, P. L., & Tomasi, F. (1989). Epidemiology of diabetes mellitus. In M. Morsiani (Ed.), *Epidemiology and screening of diabetes* (pp. 77–113). Boca Raton, FL: CRC Press.

Peveler, R. C., Boller, I., Fairburn, C. G., & Dunger, D. (1992). Eating disorders in adolescents with IDDM. *Diabetes Care, 15,* 1356–1368.

Portuese, E., & Orchard, T. (1995). Mortality in insulin-dependent diabetes. *Diabetes in America* (2nd ed.) [NIH publication no. 95-1468]. Bethesda, MD: U.S. Government Printing Office.

Reaven, G. M., & Reaven, E. P. (1985). Age, glucose intolerance, and non-insulin dependent diabetes mellitus. *Journal of the American Geriatrics Society, 33,* 286–290.

Rewers, M., & Hamman, R. F. (1995). Risk factors for non-insulin-dependent diabetes. *Diabetes in America* (2nd ed.) [NIH publication no. 95-1468]. Bethesda, MD: U.S. Government Printing Office.

Schafer, L. C., Glasgow, R. E., McCaul, K. D., & Dreher, M. (1983). Adherence to IDDM regimens: Relationship to psychological variables and metabolic control. *Diabetes Care, 6,* 493–498.

Schatz, D. A., & Bingley, P. J. (2001). Update on major trials for the prevention of type 1 diabetes mellitus: The American Diabetes Prevention Trial (DPT-1) and the European Nicotinamide Diabetes Intervention Trial (ENDIT). *Journal of Pediatric Endocrinology & Metabolism, 14*(Suppl. 1), 619–622.

Schneider, S. N., Amorosa, L. F., Khachadurian, A. K., & Ruderman, N. B. (1984). Studies on the mechanism of improved glucose control during regular exercise in type II (non-insulin-dependent) diabetes. *Diabetologia, 26,* 355–360.

Schreiner-Engel, P., Schiavi, R. C., Vietorisz, D., & Smith, H. (1987). The differential impact of diabetes type on female sexuality. *Journal of Psychosomatic Research, 31,* 23–33.

Scott, F. W., Norris, J. M., & Kolb, H. (1996). Milk and type I diabetes: Examining the evidence and broadening the focus. *Diabetes Care, 19*, 379–383.

Songer, T. J. (1995). *Diabetes in America* (2nd ed.) [NIH publication no. 95-1468]. Bethesda, MD: U.S. Government Printing Office.

Sperling, M. A. (1997). Aspects of the etiology, prediction, and prevention of insulin-dependent diabetes mellitus in childhood. *Pediatric Clinics of North America, 44*(2), 269–284.

Stabler, B., Morris, M. A., Litton, J., Feinglos, M. N., & Surwit, R. S. (1986). Differential glycemic distress in type A and type B individuals with IDDM. *Diabetes Care, 9*, 550–552.

Tuomilehto, J., Lindström, J., Eriksson, J. G., Ville, T. T., Hamalainen, H., Ilanne-Parikka, P., et al. (2001). Prevention of type 2 diabetes mellitus by changes in lifestyle among subjects with impaired glucose tolerance. *New England Journal of Medicine, 344*, 1343–1350.

UK Prospective Diabetes Study Group. (1998). Intensive blood-glucose control with sulphonylureas or insulin compared with conventional treatment and risk of complications in patients with type 2 diabetes. *Lancet, 352*, 837–853.

UK Prospective Diabetes Study Group. (2000). *British Medical Journal, 321*, 405–412.

Vague, P., DeCastro, J. V., & Vague, J. (1986). The role of adipose tissue distribution in the pathogenesis of type II diabetes. In M. Serarano-Rios & P. J. Lefebvre (Eds.), *Diabetes 1985* (pp. 524–528). New York: Elsevier.

Vendrame, F., & Gottlieb, P. A. (2004). Prediabetes: Prediction and prevention trials. *Endocrinology & Metabolism Clinics of North America, 33*(1), 75–92.

Waxman, S. G. (1980). Pathophysiology of nerve condition: Relation to diabetic neuropathy. *Annals of Internal Medicine, 92*, 297–301.

Westlund, K., & Nicolaysen, R. (1972). Ten-year mortality and morbidity related to serum cholesterol. *Scandinavian Journal of Laboratory and Clinical Investigation, 30*(Suppl. 127), 3–24.

Williams, K. V., Kelley, D. E., Mullen, M. L., & Wing, R. R. (1998). The effect of short periods of caloric restriction on weight loss and glycemic control in type 2 diabetes. *Diabetes Care, 21*, 2–8.

Wing, R. R., Nowalk, M. P., Marcus, M. D., Koeske, R., & Finegold, S. (1986). Subclinical eating disorders and glycemic control in adolescents with type I diabetes. *Diabetes Care, 9*, 162–167.

World Health Organization. (1980). Report of the expert committee on diabetes [WHO Technical Report Series no. 646]. Geneva, Switzerland: Author.

11

Epilepsy

ROBERT T. FRASER, PhD, CRC, AND
JOHN W. MILLER, MD

EPILEPSY IS THE most common of the chronic neurological disorders. The term epilepsy derives from the Greek word for "to be seized." A seizure involves a disruption of the normal activity of the brain through neuronal instability. Neurons become unstable and fire in an abnormally rapid manner, and the excessive electrical discharging results in a seizure. A seizure may be confined to one area of the brain (a partial seizure) or may take place throughout the entire brain (a generalized seizure).

Seizures differ in their presentation, depending on the discharge focus within the brain. For some individuals, the focus of the electrical discharging can be in the motor cortex and simply involve some muscle twitching in a hand (simple partial seizure), whereas for others it involves most of the brain and results in a severe generalized tonic-clonic (formerly called grand mal) seizure. These seizures involve the whole body in convulsions and result in loss of consciousness.

Causes of epilepsy include traumatic brain injuary, birth trauma, anoxia, brain tumors, infectious diseases in the mother, parasitic infections (e.g., meningitis), vascular diseases affecting the brain's blood vessels, and high concentrations of alcohol or street drugs. The general incidence of epilepsy is between 1% and 4% varying with age groupings. In the Rochester studies (Hauser, Annegers, & Kurland, 1993), the cumulative risk for having epilepsy by age 80 was 4%, with the risk for having a single unprovoked seizure being 5%. Risk factors include alcohol abuse, hypertension, lower socioeconomic status, and depressive illness (Hauser, 1997). It should be underscored that epilepsy involves the occurrence of two or more seizures: the occurrence of one seizure is insufficient to make a diagnosis of epilepsy (Devinsky, 2002).

SEIZURE CLASSIFICATION

SEIZURES ARE GENERALLY classified by assessing clinical symptoms, supplemented by wake and/or sleep electroencephalograms (EEGs) and sometimes by more sophisticated procedures, such as 24-hour EEG-video monitoring. Seizures are generally categorized according to two types: generalized seizures, which affect both cerebral hemispheres, and partial seizures, which affect a specific part of the cerebral hemisphere. Partial seizures are further divided into simple partial seizures, in which consciousness is maintained, and complex partial seizures, which involve more than one symptom and in which consciousness is impaired. It is important to note that many partial seizures may secondarily evolve into generalized seizures. The classification proposed by the International League Against Epilepsy (ILAE) Commission on Classification and Terminology was published in 1981 and is provided in Table 11.1. This table provides the reader with a basic overview of the different types of seizure conditions in the generalized and partial categorizations. This classification schema is currently undergoing revision by the ILAE.

FUNCTIONAL PRESENTATION OF EPILEPSY

Generalized Seizures

Generalized seizures tend to involve both cerebral hemispheres and several areas of the brain (cerebral cortex, thalamus, brain stem structures, etc.) and are sub-categorized into a number of specific types. The individual loses consciousness with each type. The most common form of generalized seizure is the tonic-clonic convulsion that occurs in 10% or less of epilepsy cases (Penry, 1986). This type of seizure involves two stages: the tonic stage, in which the body becomes rigid for a period of seconds, and the clonic stage, in which the person experiences a series of convulsive and jerky movements. The entire seizure generally lasts about 1 to 3 minutes (Devinsky, 2002). It is this type of seizure that tends to be remembered by the general public.

Tonic–clonic seizures should be timed. If the actual seizure activity exceeds 5 to 10 minutes, patients may enter an emergency state called *status epilepticus*, in which they suffer a continuing, prolonged seizure or experience recurring seizures within a brief period. This is an emergency situation and requires immediate medical intervention. During the tonic-clonic seizure, it is best to discourage a crowd from gathering and to refrain from sticking anything into the person's mouth. It can be helpful to turn a person on one side and put a soft article of clothing under the head.

TABLE 11.1   An Abbreviated Classification of Epileptic Seizures

Generalized Seizures of Nonfocal Origin
　　Tonic–clonic
　　Tonic
　　Clonic
　　Absence
　　Atonic/akinetic
　　Myoclonic

Partial (Focal) Seizures
　　Simple partial seizures with elementary symptomatology (consciousness is not impaired)
　　　　a. With motor symptoms (including Jacksonism, versive, and postural)
　　　　b. With sensory symptoms (including visual, somatosensory, auditory, olfactory, gustatory, and vertiginous)
　　　　c. With autonomic symptoms
　　　　d. With psychic symptoms (including dysphasia, dysmnesic, hallucinatory, and affective changes)
　　　　e. Compound (i.e. mixed) forms

　　Complex partial seizures with complex symptomatology (consciousness is impaired)
　　　　a. Simple partial seizures followed by loss of consciousness
　　　　b. With impairment of consciousness at the outset
　　　　c. With automatisms

　　Partial seizures evolving to secondarily generalized seizures

Unclassified Seizures

The other commonly known type of generalized seizure is the simple absence seizure (traditionally known as petit mal seizure). It usually takes only a few seconds with a brief disruption of consciousness (less than 20 seconds) and autonomic symptoms such as pupil dilation and mild rhythmic movements of the eyelids. Although some simple absence seizures involve blank stares, most are accompanied by the eye blinking (Devinsky, 2002). Simple absence seizures are distinguished by the generalized spike-and-wave tracings on the EEG. Most patients with this type of epilepsy begin having such seizures before age 12. Although they involve less than 5% of epilepsy cases (Penry, 1986), it is important to intervene medically, because not only can seizures affect a child's learning and influence behavior, they can also change into generalized tonic-clonic. More severe generalized seizures can also occur as the child approaches adolescence.

A number of adults still believe that they have these "petit mal" seizures because they had them as children, and they appear more benign in presentation than other seizure types. Absence seizures are uncommon in adults. Often they simply do not know their precise seizure type, which may be complex-partial. On a vocational outreach grant at our center, between 25% and 30% of adults entering the study described their seizures as petit mal, which was generally not the case (Fraser & Clemmons, 1989). If patients do not know their seizure type, they may also be on an inappropriate medication.

Other types of seizures include tonic or clonic seizures, which are actually limited tonic-clonic seizures: atonic seizures, or brief drop attacks, which tend to affect children under 5 years of age; and generalized myoclonic jerks in adults, which arc brief shock-like contractions affecting the entire body or segmented to a part of the body.

Partial Seizures

Partial seizures, as described in Table 11.1, can be divided into three categories: simple partial seizures with elementary symptoms, complex partial seizures with diverse symptoms, and partial seizures evolving into secondarily generalized seizures. Simple partial seizures may be motor, sensory, or autonomic, or they may involve some combination of symptoms without impaired consciousness. Many individuals can function quite well with simple partial seizures that are only of a few seconds duration and do not impair consciousness (e.g., the person may pull over to the side of the road when driving).

Complex partial seizures or partial seizures with complex symptoms, however, present a significant problem. First, consciousness is impaired. These seizures are also known for having an associated aura, or warning, which can involve a strange odor, aphasia, dizziness, nausea, headache, unusual stomach sensations, or a deja vu experience. Common events include repetitive motor movements, fumbling with hands or clothing, lip smacking, and wandering. Complex-partial seizures without motor components are less common, but they can involve rapid emotional or sensory changes.

Approximately 60% of those with epilepsy have seizures classified in the partial seizure category (Pedley & Hauser, 1988). These patients are often not appropriately treated for their partial seizure but only for a later observed generalized (tonic-clonic) seizure into which the partial seizure has spread. Because of the impaired consciousness and strange characteristics of complex-partial seizures (clutching clothing, lip smacking, etc.), clients with complex-partial seizures are sometimes mistaken for psychiatric patients. This seizure type is often not appropriately identified in unsophisticated assessments. Accurate diagnosis is critical to appropriate medication treatment (e.g., from a clinical perspective an absence seizure and a complex-partial seizure may look the same— a brief period of unawareness and lack of response).

It should be noted that a subgroup of people initially diagnosed with chronic epilepsy are later determined to have "psychogenic" or "pseudo" seizures. These "nonepileptic seizures" truly mimic seizure activity. Kloster (1993) estimated this subgroup as between 10% and 20% of those initially diagnosed with syncope, hyperventilation, panic attacks, conversion disorders, dissociative events, and the like. More recent estimates have been 20% of those being assessed at epilepsy center inpatient units (Devinsky, 2002)—at the University of Washington Center this incidence is 28%. Diagnosis can sometimes be clarified by recording serum prolactin levels, which should be dramatically elevated 20–30 minutes post-seizure (Betts, 1997). About 5% of those with established seizures also have non-epileptic seizures (Betts). Martin et al. (1997) utilized a Minnesota Multiphasic Personality Inventory-2 (MMPI-2) stepwise discrimination function to successfully classify 81% of patients with and without epilepsy. Obviously, other clinical information must be considered.

TREATMENT AND PROGNOSIS

FOLLOWING AN INITIAL seizure, specifically a generalized tonic-clonic seizure, many individuals are briefly hospitalized or receive an initial outpatient evaluation. The physician may begin a medical treatment program or refer the individual to a general neurologist. If seizure control is not secured within 3 months, a neurological referral is recommended (National Association of Epilepsy Centers, 1990). Membership in the American Epilepsy Society (AES) is one indication of the physician's commitment to epilepsy treatment.

Neurological consultation includes physical examination, history-taking metabolic studies, and other evaluations, including routine EEG testing. Both awake and sleep EEGs provide the physician with a clearer definition of the nature of the abnormal neuronal discharging and have often confirmed a seizure diagnosis. When the diagnosis remains unclear in partial epilepsy, even when using two EEGs (approximately 25% of cases), other more specialized neuroradiological noninvasive techniques may be used to scan the brain and identify small focal lesions that may be the cause of partial seizures. Magnetic resonance imaging (MRI) is generally superior to computed tomography (CT), also known as CAT scan, because of its definitiveness and sensitivity in clarifying small lesions or cerebral cortex abnormalities, but in an acute situation, if MRI is not available or there are other technical difficulties, a CT scan may be used (International League Against Epilepsy, 1997). MRI, CT, single photon emission computed tomography (SPECT), or positive emission tomography (PET) clarify issues related to structural lesions. Multi-channel magnetoencephalography MEG) is a newer technique for measuring magnetic fields and appears to be more definitive in locating sources of epileptiform discharges.

It seizure control is not achieved by the general neurologist within 9 months, a referral to a tertiary- or fourth-level epilepsy center should be made (National Association of Epilepsy Centers, 1990). These centers have neurologists and allied health teams that specialize in epilepsy, and they address such areas as pharmacological problems; possible psychogenic or pseudoseizures; the potential for epilepsy surgery; the need for invasive, intracranial video/EEG recording; and the need for complementary psychological or psychiatric expertise. It is important to

TABLE 11.2   Epilepsy Types and Indicated Antiepileptic Drugs

---

Localization-related epilepsy (simple partial, complex partial, and secondarily generalized tonic–clonic seizures)

Primary drugs
  lamotrigine (Lamictal)
  carbamazepine (Tegretol, Carbatrol)
  oxcarbazepine (Trileptal)
  levetiracetam (Keppra)
  phenytoin (Dilantin)
  topirmate (Topamax)
  zonisamide (Zonegran)

Secondary drugs
  gabapentin (Neurontin)
  valproate (Depakote, Depakene)
  phenobarbital (Luminil)
  primidone (Mysoline)
  felbamate (Felbatol)
  tiagabine (Gabatril)
  methsuximide (Celontin)

Generalized epilepsies (myoclonic, absence generalized tonic clonic seizures)

Primary drugs
  valproate (Depakote, Depakene)
  lamotrigine (Lamictal)
  zonisamide (Zonegran)
  topiramate (Topamax)

Secondary drugs
  felbamate (Felbatol)
  clonazepam (Klonopin)
  acetazolamide (Diamox)
  ethosuximide (Zarontin)
  methsuximide (Celontin)

From Karceski, Morrel, & Carpenter (2001); Deray, Resnick, & Alvarez (2004).

acknowledge that antiepileptic medications are selectively effective for one or more different types of seizures (Wannamaker, Booker, Dreifuss, & Willmore, 1984). The neurologist matches the appropriate drug to the specific type. Table 11.2 presents an overview of the primary and secondary drugs that are most common for various seizure categories.

To achieve optimal daily life functioning for a patient (most effective treatment, fewer side effects), the normal course of treatment is the maximum tolerable dosage of one medication. A dosage should be established that maintains an appropriate concentration within the bloodstream throughout the day. Therapeutic ranges and toxicity levels have been established for the major recommended drugs. Table 11.3 shows pharmacological data on the major antiepileptic drugs.

Inappropriate or random taking of medications does not result in a steady state or maintenance of an appropriate level of the medication in the bloodstream. Excessive concentrations of medication (toxic ranges) can result in double vision, lethargy, impaired mental alertness/attention, coordination difficulties, weight gain, and other significant medical complications. Medication levels require periodic laboratory monitoring for assessing appropriate ranges. Even within appropriate ranges, drug side effects (such as facial hair on women or gum disease associated with phenytoin [Dilantin]) may require intervention.

Antiepileptic medications first came on the market in the United States in the 1970s, and the 1980s were a period of further research. In the 1990s we have a number of new compounds (viz., gabapentin, oxcarbazepine, felbamate, lamotrigine, tiagabine, topiramate, and yigabatrin), which were initially tested as "add on," or adjunctive drugs. All have shown effectiveness against complex partial and secondarily generalized seizures initially, but over time the majority have shown effec-

TABLE 11.3 Common Anticonvulsant Properties

Drug	Therapeutic range µg/ml	Half life (hrs)
carbamazepine	4–12	12–17
lamotrigine	4–20	11–61
levetiracetam	5–40	6–8
phenytoin	10–20	7–42
topiramate	4–10	19–23
valproate	50–130	9–12
zonisamide	15–40	60

From Deray et al. (2004). Half life may vary depending on age, hepatic or renal function, and interaction with other medications. Time to steady state is approximately 5 times the half life.

tiveness as monotherapeutic agents with generalized seizures. Although the potential side effects of medication need to be reviewed in each case, most of these medications (the "third generation" of anticonvulsants) tend to have minimal cognitive side effects, except for topirimate which tends to effect concentration. Brodie and Kwan (2002) indicate that 47% of patients respond to the first antiepileptic medication, 13% are seizure-free on the second, and only 1% respond to the third monotherapy choice. The best prognosis for seizure control is response to the first anticonvulsant. Only 3% were controlled with two simultaneous anticonvulsants and none with three.

In a staged approach to epilepsy management, Kwan and Brodie (2002, p. 86), emphasize the following:

1. tolerability and long-term safety are most important in choosing the first anti-epileptic.
2. if the first drug is poorly tolerated at low dosages or fails to improve seizure control, an alternative should be substituted.
3. if a well-tolerated drug does not completely abolish seizures, combination therapy may be tried.
4. work-up for epilepsy surgery should be considered after failure of two well treated regimens.

There are a number of considerations outside of epilepsy surgery, which is often not an option. The ketogenic diet for children is receiving more recent attention because new long-term studies indicate > 50% seizure reduction for 40%–50% of the children treated (Gaillard, Shields, Slafstrom, & Vining, 1997). The vagal nerve stimulator is implanted in the chest and stimulates the vagal nerve at an established cycle and at seizure onset. Approximately 50% of those using the stimulator achieve > 50% seizure reduction, 5%–8% are seizure free, and 30% have benefit but not less than half (Devinsky, 2002). Obviously, these individuals have very challenging seizure conditions. Much research, however, must be conducted in relation to these options, blended options, blended options and behavioral or cognitive-behavioral training approaches (e.g., relaxation).

A review of seizure relapse studies would suggest that patients treated with medication generally achieve a 65% to 80% seizure-free status (Hauser & Hesdorffer, 1990). Annegers (1988) indicates that 10 years after epilepsy diagnosis, 65% of patients seen are in seizure remission; at 20 years, 76%. Although the probability of achieving remission after 10 years exceeds 60%, the probability of achieving remission during the next 10 years for those patients not having seizure control at 5 years from diagnosis was only 33%. The most important prognostic indicator for the eventual control of seizures is the duration of seizure occurrences. Other factors include seizure cause, seizure type, and age of onset (Annegers).

For patients with medically intractable seizures, surgical intervention can be a consideration after 1–2 years. This will principally be a consideration for the 10% to 25% of patients with partial epilepsy, primarily partial complex epilepsy (Hauser & Hesdorffer, 1990). Surgery is occasionally a consideration for management of intractable seizure conditions without a focus, but this is infrequent. A series of diagnostic tests, including neuropsychological and continuous EEG/video monitoring are conducted, in addition to utilization of the previously mentioned neuroimaging techniques, so that medical staff and patients have a clear understanding of surgery's viability as specific to the situation. If surface EEG and neuroimaging techniques are unclear in relation to seizure focus, then depth electrodes, subdural grids, and direct intraoperative recording may he utilized (Hauser & Hesdorffer). In general, patients are chosen carefully for the operation and tend to have insignificant cognitive problems after surgery. Neuropsychological data, however, are reviewed very carefully, specifically in relation to memory and language functions. For some individuals, however, stopping the seizures is paramount.

There are two different approaches to the surgeries. As described by Schaul (1987), these include a standard temporal lobectomy and a Penfield technique, in which the surgical procedure is tailored to the individual patient's seizure focus. As identification of patients with surgically treatable epilepsy becomes easier with neuroimaging and other approaches, 80% of those undergoing surgery can become seizure-free through more cost-effective approaches (Engel, Wieser, & Spencer, 1997). To some degree, surgical outcome is not completely clear because of different means of establishing outcome across surgical centers. For example, warning auras (the beginning warning component of a seizure) may be counted at some centers and not at others. In Schaul's review, it is estimated that there may be up to 120,000 surgical candidates within the United States who could profit from this type of surgery. For those with successful, seizure-free outcomes, medications are generally tapered off over 2–5 years; obviously, this involves significant discussions among patient, significant others, and the allied health team.

NEUROPSYCHOLOGICAL ASSESSMENT

AT THE EPILEPSY Center of Michigan, over a 5-year period, Rodin, Shapiro, and Lennox (1977) found that only 23% of their medical referrals had epilepsy only; among the remainder, brain impairment was the largest presenting difficulty across other psychosocial adjustment issues. In establishing functional abilities, this can be an important area to assess. Approximately 40% of those applying to the University of Washington's Regional Epilepsy Center Vocational Services indicated on their program application form that they had had a head injury. Additional research has shown that if individuals have more than 75 life-time generalized tonic-clonic seizures or have an incidence of *status epilepticus* involving extended continuous seizure activity, their neu-ropsychological performance decreases (Dodrill, 1986).

It is reasonable to assume that those seeking vocational rehabilita-tion services would have diverse patterns of brain impairment that pres-ent more barriers to employment than would be common among a mainstream general or medical population. Rausch, Le, and Langfitt (1997) indicate that common cognitive concerns for individuals with epilepsy include attention, speed of mental processing, memory and learning, and cognitive flexibility. A neuropsychologist can be helpful in providing brain-related information relative to these deficits and also in identifying assets on which the vocational rehabilitation program can be established—assets often being most important. The neuropsy-chological evaluation moves beyond basic intellectual assessment to look at the more subtle aspects of problem solving, motor performance, sensory perceptual abilities, memory capacities, intentional capacities, language skills, visual/spatial abilities, and other self-regulating activity.

Commonly used neuropsychological batteries include the Halstead-Reitan Neuropsychological Battery (Reitan & Wolfson, 1985) and the Luria-Nebraska Neuropsychological Battery (Goldin, Hammeke, & Parisch, 1980). Dodrill (1978) has established a comprehensive battery of 16 discriminative measures more sensitive to brain impairment and epilepsy. This battery includes Halstead's Neuropsychological Battery for Adults, the Aphasia Screening Test, the Trail Making test, the Logical Memory and Visual Reproduction parts of the Wechsler Memory Scale, Form I, the Sensory-Perceptual Examination, the Stroop Test, and the Seashore Tonal Memory Test. Dodrill has also developed an abbreviated form of his battery that can be used as a screening instrument; although not allowing detailed neuropsychological analysis it is no less sensitive than the full battery in identifying brain impairment and providing a general indication of its overall extent. Neuropsychological testing is important both pre- and post-epilepsy surgery, particularly to assess surgical impact on memory and language functioning. The testing also can be helpful in clarifying epileptic foci.

It is important to emphasize that, among studies conducted at the University of Washington (Fraser, Clemmons, Dodrill, Trejo, & Freelove, 1986) with clients actively engaged in vocational rehabilitation services, it was aspects of brain impairment that discriminated between those who were able to go to work and maintain a job for 1 year and those who could not secure a job through our program (i.e., they tried to secure work through the program but were unsuccessful). Specifically, the impairments were visual/spatial problem solving and motor deficits. Most of these clients had job experience that was congruent with unskilled or semiskilled work, and the brain impairments were affecting their employability. These clients require longer training or coached work experience relative to accuracy and speed of functioning if they are to be able to secure and maintain a competitive job placement. They will also have to learn to use compensatory strategies to cope with their difficulties. For clients with a long history of generalized tonic-clonic seizures, neuropsychological test results can be very illuminating relative to rehabilitation planning.

PSYCHOSOCIAL ASSESSMENT

IN ASSESSING THE psychosocial functioning of clients with epilepsy, measures traditionally used in clinical environments certainly have their place and are useful in the assessment process. These assessment measures include MMPI-2, the Personality Assessment Inventory (PAI), the Millon Clinical Multiaxial Inventory (MCMI) III, computerized psychiatric diagnostic interviews (SC1D-II, DSR, etc.), and structured clinical interviews. For purposes of clinical interview, the reader might review the next section, on psychosocial adjustment, to identify risk factors to maladjustment that deserve attention in the interview. Depression, however, is the most common mood disorder and the single most important factor affecting quality of life in this population (Barry, 2004). Gillian (2004) in his review notes a suicide rate in excess of 11%. These are areas of concern worth examining.

It can be of particular benefit to use the Washington Psychosocial Seizure Inventory (WPSI) in assessing the psychosocial concerns of clients with epilepsy. This inventory, developed by Dodrill, Batzel, Queisser, and Temkin (1980), is helpful in identifying these concerns. It is an MMPI-like instrument in its development but has only 132 items, requiring 20 to 30 minutes for completion. Psychosocial concerns are identified across eight scales: family background, emotional, interpersonal, vocational, financial, adjustment to seizures, medicine and medical management, and overall psychosocial functioning. Other quality-of-life instruments have been developed more recently (e.g., Liverpool Quality of Life Battery, QOLIE-89 item, QOLIE-10 item), but these are more useful as outcome measures of medication changes or surgery outcome and are less helpful in guiding interventions.

PSYCHOLOGICAL AND VOCATIONAL IMPLICATIONS

INCIDENCE OF PSYCHOSOCIAL MALADJUSTMENT

IN DISCUSSING THE psychological and social adjustment issues of those with epilepsy, it is helpful to review findings using the WPSI. Trostle (1988) has found that most studies using the WPSI have identified 50% of the cases as having definite or severe problems on most of the WPSI scales. This author further indicates that maladjustment may approximate 50% to 60% of those sent for evaluation at a special epilepsy center, whereas overall psychosocial adjustment difficulties were identified for only 19% of a sample from Rochester, Minnesota (Trostle, Hauser, & Sharbrough, 1986). In general, it seems that referrals from private physicians have fewer adjustment difficulties than do clients referred from a medical center specializing in epilepsy treatment. The former may have less involved seizure conditions, lesser neuropsychological impairment, and simply may not be as much at risk psychosocially.

The WPSI is basically a screening instrument and can be helpful in initial planning. If there appear to be more significant psychiatric concerns, a referral for a structured psychiatric interview and the use of inventories normed on psychiatric populations (MMPI-2, MCMI III, etc.) can be more assistive.

FACTORS INFLUENCING PSYCHOSOCIAL ADJUSTMENT

THERE ARE A number of factors that have been established as relating to psychosocial adjustments for people with epilepsy. Hermann (1988) has synthesized the work of previous investigators in suggesting that four general forces affect adjustment among clients with epilepsy. These major influencing factors include biological, psychosocial, medication, and demographic factors. In Table 11.4, this multietiological model is presented with some additional factors identified by Fraser and Clemmons (1989). These factors cover most of those identified in the research literature as influencing the community adjustment of those with the disability. In the neurological category, items such as early age of onset, additional disabilities, associated neuropsychological impairment, type of seizure activity, and the like have been found to be important variables. Under the psychosocial category, a number of variables are identified, including perceived stigma and limitations, adjustment to seizures, vocational status, financial status, parental fears, limited socialization and recreation, divisive or dysfunctional parenting styles, and poor relationships with parents, siblings, and intrusive grandparents.

TABLE 11.4 Multietiological Predictor Variables

Neurological	Psychosocial	
Age at outset	Perceived stigma	Parental fears
Duration of Epilepsy	Perceived limitations	Divisive/dysfunctional parenting styles
Seizure type	Adjustment to seizures	
Neuropsychological impairment	Vocational adjustment	Limited recreation
Laterality of lesion	Financial status	Poor relationships with sibling, parents, grandparents
Presence/absence of multiple seizure types	Special education tracking	
Etiology	Locus of control Life event changes	Social support
Medications	Demographics	
Monotherapy vs. polytherapy	Age	
Presence of barbiturate medications	Gender	
Serum levels of medication	Education IQ	

Note. Reprinted with modifications with permission from the Epilepsy Foundation of America as found in Hermann (1988).

Other, more immediate issues, such as considerable life event changes, availability of social support, and perceived locus of control, seem to affect adjustment. Basic demographic issues such as age, gender, education, and intelligence also should be reviewed. Some older clients adapt well to the seizure condition because of positive prior life experiences and an integrated self-concept. For other individuals, despite their age, the onset of a seizure condition can be very unsettling. Young males tend to have more difficulties in adjusting than do females. It is of interest that the vocational interests and academic orientation of young males with more severe, early-onset seizures appear to be affected, compared to a norm group (Fraser, Trejo, Temkin, Clemmons, & Dodrill, 1985), but this is not true for young females. Special education tracking seems to relate to psychosocial maladjustment—this may be a masking variable for neuropsychological impairment (Goldin, Perry, Margolin,

Stotsky, & Foster, 1977). In the medication category, the number of medications an individual takes and the appropriateness of medication levels also can affect community adjustment.

As emphasized by Hermann (1988), this type of model simply increases the reader's awareness of the range of factors that can influence a client's mental health. When emotional difficulties occur, depression and anxiety appear to be among the most frequent. There also is a significant rate of sexual dysfunction, particularly among males, with a propensity toward those having complex-partial or temporal lobe seizures (Hermann).

Work at the University of Washington Regional Epilepsy Center has demonstrated that early vocational rehabilitation program dropouts can be discriminated from those who have successfully become employed on a number of specific items from the WPSI (Fraser, Trejo, Clemmons, & Freelove, 1987). These items identified increased depression and anxiety, financial difficulties, and lack of adjustment to one's seizure condition as being more prominent among program dropouts. New 12-hour interventions were tested at our center as precursors to vocational programming in order to stabilize dropouts (Fraser et al., 1990) but they were insufficient to render a difference. Other psychosocial adjustment concerns relate to epilepsy surgery—although a seizure free status is highly correlated with adjustment, some seizure free patients then experience a "burden of normality" (Fraser, in press). It would appear that careful psychological goal planning and intervention should occur before the surgical intervention.

VOCATIONAL IMPLICATIONS

IN EPILEPSY REHABILITATION it is very important to maintain an individualized approach to vocational evaluation and goal planning. Issues tend to arise around the seizure condition itself, associated disabilities, medication concerns, and seizure disclosure. Each of these salient issue categories is reviewed in the following section.

CLARIFICATION OF SEIZURE STATUS

IT IS VERY important that the counselor have a clear understanding of the client's seizure status. If a seizure status remains unclear, it is important that the client be referred to a major epilepsy center (to which one can be directed by the national Epilepsy Foundation, www.epilepsyfoundation.org) so that sophisticated testing and/or 24-hour EEG–video monitoring can be conducted. Some individuals will have nonepileptic seizures, which are emotionally rooted and require a different course of treatment. Recent advances in treatment of these seizures involve close interdisciplinary work and cognitive-behavioral individual and time-limited group intervention (Schöndienst, 2003). Some will have both real seizures, involving electrical discharges within the brain, and nonepileptic. This also deserves clarification because the nonepileptic seizures can be brought under control in many cases more quickly than the organically based seizure activity. In each case the counselor must understand the following:

1. The specific type of seizure the client currently has, with a clear description of what occurs during a seizure. Of particular importance is establishing whether there is a loss of consciousness.
2. What type of seizure control has the client achieved? If the seizures are not controlled, it is important to understand whether there is any pattern to their occurrence. Many individuals will have seizures only early in the morning, while sleeping, or when taking a break from the day's work activities. For some clients, certain precipitants seem to trigger the seizures. These can include fatigue, having flu or other illness, flickering lights or screens, certain levels of stress in the work environment (which certainly vary for each client), and other events or health-related issues.
3. Does the client have a specific warning or aura (actually the initial part of the seizure) before the occurrence of a full seizure? A warning can be a feeling of lightheadedness, an uneasy sick feeling, other strange sensations, or deja vu experiences. A consistent aura is very helpful in that it allows an individual to take safety precautions (e.g., sitting down, lying down, or otherwise removing oneself to a safe area before the seizure is in full progress).
4. What is involved in the recovery period? Some individuals can go directly back to work, others will require a brief nap, and some will have to take a sick day and spend the better part of the day recovering.
5. Has the client ever been otherwise injured as a result of a seizure? If not, this is very comforting for the employer.
6. Does the client have any other disabilities? In a recent study at our center (Fraser, Clemmons, Andrechak, Dodrill, & Temkin, 1991), 89% of the clients served had one or more additional disabilities. It is particularly important to note whether there has been an additional head injury that precipitated the seizures or whether a head injury came about as a result of seizure activity (e.g., due to a fall). The additional or associated disabilities will often require specific assessment (e.g., neuropsychological).
7. What type of medication is the client taking, is it appropriate, and is he or she complying with the recommended medication and dosages? Might the client with a clear focus and intractable seizures

be a surgical candidate? Is the medication evaluation recent? Might implanting of a vagal nerve stimulator be a desirable option?

If the psychologist can answer the above questions, he or she is in a better situation to serve the client more appropriately. For example, recently at our center, as the result of a misunderstanding on the part of a counselor about a seizure type (which he believed to be a minor partial type), an individual was placed in a loading dock position in which he fell during a seizure, breaking his nose and sustaining a significant number of facial contusions and lacerations. In fact, he had had relatively frequent generalized tonic-clonic seizures that resulted in loss of consciousness and falling. In consideration of the heavy physical work he had been assigned and the potential for falling from the dock, the job assignment was inappropriate. It is a good standing policy to confirm the seizure description with a family member or significant other. As discussed earlier, many clients do not understand their seizure type and may provide inaccurate information. Many of them have never even witnessed a seizure and do not understand what occurs. A recent report (Bryant-Comstock, Hogan, Shumaker, & Tennis, 1997) indicates that a client's own perception of seizure severity, using the Liverpool Seizure Severity Scale, may be a better discriminator of employability than other seizure variables (e.g., seizure frequency).

ADDITIONAL DISABILITIES

AS DISCUSSED EARLIER, a majority of clients with epilepsy coming for rehabilitation services will have an additional disability. This is most commonly some type of neuropsychological impairment that has to be clarified. In early work at our center, we would miss detailed information about head injuries and other brain-related difficulties, which would result in mismatching individuals in the job placement process. An example would be an individual who had significant memory deficits and was placed in a locksmith job-training program, requiring him to remember a large number of different key molds. Another individual, as a residue of epilepsy surgery, had a lower visual field cut that resulted in an accident while driving a bus. Clarification of some of these issues earlier would have redirected the placement effort or the effort would have begun with more compensatory strategies being utilized. As discussed previously, clients who drop out of our rehabilitation program tend to do so because of emotional difficulties, such as depression, anxiety, financial fears, and so on. Individuals who are placed through the program but lose jobs after they are hired tend to do so because of cognitive or neuropsychological deficits.

To clarify these issues, the neuropsychological or epilepsy battery

(Dodrill, 1978) that includes the Halstead-Reitan battery and other specialized measures is utilized to identify brain impairment issues. The WPSI is given to all clients in screening for emotional and psychosocial adjustment difficulties. Although neuropsychological issues and emotional concerns are more common, additional physical disabilities, mental retardation, cerebral palsy, and other medical concerns will be found in a subgroup of referrals. In review of some of these concerns, it becomes apparent that a number of clients will learn better in actual on-the-job training programs versus formal academic vocational/technical school training. Given specific cognitive deficits, it can be much easier to learn and retain the work tasks and requirements by training on the job site. This will be a counseling issue with clients who seek college training.

MEDICATION ISSUES

THE AREA OF medication management deserves significant attention. A number of clients are simply on the wrong medication when they come for vocational rehabilitation or are receiving too many medications, which results in poorly managed seizures and negative side effects. Common side effects can include double vision, blurred vision, balance difficulties, lethargy, behavioral changes, gingival growth, nausea, weight gain, and liver enzyme elevations. As discussed earlier, if a client is not achieving good seizure control and has not been evaluated at an epilepsy center or by a neurological group that specializes in epilepsy, it can be appropriate to make a referral for current medication evaluation. A number of clients referred to our center may still be receiving Dilantin and phenobarbital, prescribed by a general practitioner to manage their seizures, which is inappropriate. These instances occur more frequently in rural areas.

It is also very common that clients do not take their medication as prescribed and do not understand that it can take days (depending upon their medication) to achieve a steady state of the anticonvulsant within their bloodstream. Consequently, a number of them take medication infrequently or in larger doses that result in toxicity and other side effects. They must he cautioned that it is necessary to take their medication consistently. This situation can be improved by taking the medication at a specific time or by using a pill counter or a medication box that has an alarm to remind patients when to take the medications.

DISCLOSURE OF SEIZURE STATUS

DISCLOSURE OF A seizure condition is a very individual consideration. For most people, we recommend that seizures be clearly discussed if they could affect work performance, preferably at the end of the interview, after they have had the opportunity to discuss their work-related background and skills. Consequently, they generally do not mention epilepsy on the application, but they have the interviewer note it at the time of their actual meeting with the employer. There can be a number of different approaches to disclosing. Because they do not lose consciousness, only have a seizure while sleeping, or have some other mitigating circumstance, some do not really have to discuss the issue with an employer or co-worker. They may prefer to tell an employer or co-worker that they have a seizure condition after they have been on the job some time and have established credibility as a worker. Under the Americans with Disabilities Act, which was implemented in 1992, reasonable accommodation for many private-sector employers could involve minor modifications to the work site (layer of padding on a concrete floor or reassignment of work tasks [e.g., having a co-worker do some minimal driving that is required on the job if the client lacks a driver's license because of epilepsy]). Litigation under ADA is a slow moving process and persons with epilepsy (an intermittent disability, often stabilized) are not doing particularly well under ADA. It is better to try to negotiate an accommodation with the employer.

In general, most studies show that the attendance and performance records for people with epilepsy are equal to or better than those of the general working population (McLellan, 1987). Risch (1968) demonstrated that time lost as a result of seizures was approximately 1 hour for every 1,000 hours worked by individuals with active seizure conditions. A study by Sands (1961) indicated that over a 13-year period in the state of New York, there were more accidents in the workplace caused by sneezing or coughing on the job than accidents related to seizures. Hiring people with epilepsy does not increase industrial insurance. In addition, second injury funds in most states protect an employer from bearing responsibility for total disability if the client has a seizure on the job that results in inability to work again. Working around machinery is generally not a problem of any significant measure in today's society. Most machinery has plastic guards and other safety features. Even equipment such as farm tractors has been modified with toggle switches to kill the engine when an individual experiences seizure activity while driving. For some individuals with active seizure conditions, however, working around heights may not be a reasonable idea, and in some cases working around boiling or molten materials can also present certain concerns. In the latter case, however, flame-resistant or -retardant clothing materials may still enable an individual to perform the job. On issues of accommodation, the Job Accommodation Network (JAN) in West Virginia (www.jan.wvu.edu) or the university departments and their occupational therapeutic or assistive technologies can be contacted for accommodation or ideas specific to individual seizure-related concerns. The Epilepsy Foundation (EF) in Washington, DC, has a number of on-line website employment resources with some local EF affiliates having employment programs.

CONCLUSIONS

THIS CHAPTER HAS reviewed medical, psychosocial, and vocational implications of epilepsy as a disability. With greater understanding of third-generation anticonvulsants' benefits, people with epilepsy should be more employable. It is hoped that, by attention to a number of the concerns presented in this chapter, many human service professionals can be successful in working with the client having a seizure condition. In our experience, with good medical and psychosocial/vocational assessment and targeted intervention; the seizure condition itself and associated disabilities can be worked with and around, resulting in a successful job match and/or better general community adjustment.

REFERENCES

Anderson, V. E. (1988). Genetics of the epilepsies. In W. A. Hauser (Ed.), *Current trends in epilepsy: A self-study course for physicians (Unit 3)*. Landover, MD: Epilepsy Foundation of America.

Annegers, J. F. (1988). The natural history and prognosis of patients with seizures and epilepsy. In W. A. Hauser (Ed.), *Current trends in epilepsy: A self-study course for physicians (Unit 1)*. Landover, MD: Epilepsy Foundation of America.

Barry, J. J. (2004, December). *The link between mood disorders and epilepsy—Why is it important to diagnose and treat?* Paper presented at the Annual Meeting of the American Epilepsy Society, New Orleans, LA.

Betts, T. (1997). Psychiatric aspects of nonepileptic seizures. In J. Engel & T. A. Bedley (Eds.), *Epilepsy* (pp. 2101–2116). Philadelphia: Lippincott-Raven.

Brodie, M. J., & Kwan, P. (2002). Staged approach to epilepsy management. *Neurology, 58*(suppl. 5), 52–58.

Bryant-Comstock, I., Hogan, P., Shumaker, S., & Tennis, P. (1997). Relation of seizure severity to employment status and education [Abstract]. *Epilepsia, 38*(Suppl.), 135.

Deray, M., Resnick, T., & Alvarez, L. (2004). *Complete pocket reference for the treatment of epilepsy*. Miami, FL: CPR Educational Services, LLC.

Devinsky, O. (2002). *Epilepsy: Patient and family guide* (2nd ed.). Philadelphia: F. A. Davis.

Dodrill, C. B. (1978). A neuropsychological battery for epilepsy. *Epilepsia, 19,* 611–623.

Dodrill, C. B. (1986). Correlates of tonic-clonic seizures with intellectual, neuropsychological, emotional, and social functions in patients with epilepsy. *Epilepsia, 27,* 399–411.

Dodrill, C. B., Batzel, L. W., Queisser, H. R., & Temkin, N. R. (1980). An objective method for the assessment of psychological and social problems among epileptics. *Epilepsia, 21,* 123–135.

Engel, J., Wieser, H. G., & Spencer, D. (1997). Overview: Surgical therapy. In J. Engel & T. A. Bedley (Eds.), *Epilepsy* (pp. 1673–1676). Philadelphia: Lippincott-Raven.

Fraser, R. T. (in press). Psychosocial and vocational outcomes: A perspective on patient rehabilitation. In J. W. R. Miller & D. C. Silvergeld (Eds.), *Controversies in epilepsy surgery.* New York: Marcel Dekker.

Fraser, R. T., & Clemmons, D. C. (1989). Vocational and psychosocial interventions for youth with seizure disorders. In B. Hermann & N. I. Siedenberg (Eds.), *Childhood epilepsies: Neuropsychological, psychosocial, and intervention aspects* (pp. 201–220). Chichester, England: John Wiley & Sons.

Fraser, R. T., Clemmons, D. C., Andrechak, N., Dodrill, C. B., & Temkin, N. (1991, December). *Pre-vocational intervention in epilepsy rehabilitation: Outcome and pre/postintervention employability correlates.* Paper presented at the American Epilepsy Society meeting, Seattle, WA.

Fraser, R. T., Clemmons, D. C., Dodrill, C. B., Trejo, W., & Freelove, C. (1986). The difficult to employ in epilepsy rehabilitation: Predictors of response to an intensive intervention. *Eplepsia, 27,* 220–224.

Fraser, R. T., Clemmons, D. C., Prince, S., Dodrill, C., Nelson, H., & Lucas, L. (1990, November). *Preliminary report of an intensive intervention in epilepsy rehabilitation.* Paper presented at the American Epilepsy Society annual meeting, San Diego, CA.

Fraser, R. T., Trejo, W., Clemmons, D. C., & Freelove, C. (1987, November). *Psychosocial adjustment of early dropouts compared to competitive placements.* Paper presented at the annual meeting of the American Epilepsy Society, San Francisco.

Fraser, R. T., Trejo, W., Temkin, N. R., Clemmons, D. C., & Dodrill, C. B. (1985). Assessing the vocational interests of those with epilepsy. *Rehabilitation Psychology, 30,* 29–33.

Gaillard, W., Shields, W. D., Stafstrom, C., & Vining, E. P. G. (1997). Ketogenic diet: What is the evidence that it works clinically and how to study it mechanically [Abstract]. *Epilepsia, 38*(Suppl.), 2.

Gillian, F. G. (2004, December). *Understanding serious adverse outcomes of epilepsy.* Paper presented at the Annual Meeting of the American Epilepsy Society, New Orleans, LA.

Goldin, C. J., Hammeke, T. A., & Parisch, A. D. (1980). *The Luria-Nebraska Neuropsychological Battery: Manual.* Los Angeles: Western Psychological Services.

Goldin, C. J., Perry, S. L., Margolin, R. F., Stotsky, B. A., & Foster, J. C. (1967). *Rehabilitation of the young epileptic*. Lexington, MA: D. C. Heath.

Hauser, W. A. (1997). Incidence and prevalence. In J. Engel & T. A. Bedley (Eds.), *Epilepsy* (pp. 47–58). Philadelphia: Lippincott-Raven.

Hauser, W. A., Annegers, J. F., & Kurland, I. T. (1993). The incidence of epilepsy and unprovoked seizures in Rochester, Minnesota. 1935–1984. *Epilepsia, 34*, 453–468.

Hauser, W. A., & Hesdorffer, D. C. (1990). *Epilepsy: Frequency, causes, and consequences*. New York: Demos.

Hermann, B. P. (1988). Interrictal psychotherapy in patients with epilepsy. In W. A. Hauser (Ed.), *Current trends in epilepsy: A self-study course for physicians (Unit 1)*. Landover, MD: Epilepsy Foundation of America.

International League Against Epilepsy (Neuroimaging Commission). (1997). Recommendations for neuroimaging of patients with epilepsy. *Epilepsia, 38*(Suppl. 10), 1–2.

Karaceske, S., Morrel, M., & Carpenter, D. (2001). The expert concensus guideline series. *Epilepsy Behavior, 2*(Suppl.), A1–A50.

Kloster, R. (1993). Pseudo-epileptic versus epileptic seizures: A comparison. In L. Gram, S. Johannessen, P. Osterman, & M. Sillanpas (Eds.), *Pseudoepileptic seizures* (pp. 3–16). Petersfield, UK: Wrightson Biomedical.

Leppik, I. (1988). Drug treatment of epilepsy. In W. A. Hauser (Eds.), *Current trends in epilepsy: A self-study for physicians (Unit 3)*. Landover, MD: Epilepsy Foundation of America.

Marson, A. G., Kadir, Z. A., Hutton, J. L., & Chadwick, D. W. (1997). The new antiepileptic drugs: A systematic review of their efficacy and tolerability. *Epilepsia, 38*, 859–880.

Martin, R., Snyder, P., Gilliam, F., Roth, D., Fraught, E., & Kuzniecky, R. (1997). Classification accuracy of the MMPI-2 in the identification of patients with frontal lobe epilepsy and non-epileptic seizures [Abstract]. *Epilepsia, 38*(Suppl.), 159.

McLellan, D. L. (1987). Epilepsy and employment. *Journal of Social and Occupational Medicine, 3*, 94–99.

National Association of Epilepsy Centers. (1990). Recommended guidelines for diagnosis and treatment in specialized epilepsy centers. *Epilepsia, 32*(Suppl. 1), 1–12.

Pedley, T. A., & Hauser, W. A. (1988). Classification and differential diagnosis of seizures and of epilepsy. In W. A. Hauser (Ed.), *Current trends in epilepsy: A self-study course for physicians (Unit 1)*. Landover, MD: Epilepsy Foundation of America.

Penry, J. K. (Ed.). (1986). *Epilepsy: Diagnosis, management, and quality of life*. New York: Raven Press.

Porter, R. J., & Meldrum, R. J. (1997). Overview: Antiepileptic drugs. In J. Engel & T. A. Bedley (Eds.), *Epilepsy* (pp. 1381–1382). Philadelphia: Lippincott-Raven.

Rausch, R., Le, M. T., & Langfitt, J. L. (1997). Neuropsychological evaluation: Adults. In J. Engel & T. A. Bedley (Eds.), *Epilepsy*. Philadelphia: Lippincott-Raven.

Reitan, R. M., & Wolfson, D. (1985). *The Halstead-Reitan Test Battery: Theory and clinical interpretations*. Tucson, AZ: Neuropsychology Press.

Risch, F. (1968). We lost every game . . . but. *Rehabilitation Record, 9*, 16–18.

Rodin, E. A., Shapiro, H. L., & Lennox, K. (1977). Epilepsy and life performance. *Rehabilitation Literature, 38*, 34–38.

Sands, H. (1961). Report of a study undertaken for the committee on neurological disorders in industry. *Epilepsy News, 7*, 1.

Schaul, N. (1987). Epilepsy surgery. *New York Journal of Epilepsy, 5*, 14–15.

Schöndienst, M. (2001). Management of dissociative disorders in a comprehensive care setting. In M. Pfäfflin, R. T. Fraser, R. Thorbecke, V. Specht, & R. Wolfe (Eds.), *Comprehensive care for people with epilepsy* (pp. 67–76). London: John Libbey.

Trostle, J. A. (1988). Social aspects of epilepsy. In W. A. Hauser (Ed.), *Current trends in epilepsy: A self-study course for physicians (Unit 1)*. Landover, MD: Epilepsy Foundation of America.

Trostle, J. A., Hauser, W. A., & Sharbrough, F. (1986). Self-regulation of medical regimens among adults with epilepsy in Rochester. *Epilepsia, 27*, 640.

Wannamaker, B. B., Booker, H. E., Dreifuss, F. E., & Willmore, L. J. (1984). *The comprehensive clinical management of the epilepsies*. Landover, MD: Epilepsy Foundation of America.

Wilder, B. J. (1997). Vagal nerve stimulation. In J. Engel & T. A. Bedley (Eds.), *Epilepsy* (pp. 1353–1358). Philadelphia: Lippincott-Raven.

12

Speech, Language, Hearing, and Swallowing Disorders

PATRICIA KERMAN LERNER, MA, AND NANCY ENG, PhD

THE ABILITY TO share experiences, emotions, needs, and thoughts is a basic component of daily interactions between individuals and is a cornerstone to social structure. Indeed "the need for socialization is the core of human existence and the desire to communicate with others is the essence of that socialization" (Chapey, 2001, pp. 12–13). Therefore, impairment in the ability to communicate disrupts all aspects of the human experience: establishment and maintenance of relationships, participation in educational programs, pursuit and retention of employment, and the fulfillment of independence.

The ability to communicate is a complete and unique behavior that is influenced by interacting biological, psychological, and environmental factors. Communication requires adequate speech, language, and hearing, working in an integrated manner to produce an effective exchange of information. Unfortunately, many individuals have a disruption in their communication systems. It is conservatively estimated that over 38 million individuals in the United States have some form of communication impairment (Benson, 1990). Speech, language, and/or hearing disorders can impede economic self-sufficiency, academic performance, and employment opportunities.

In recent years, swallowing impairments often coexisting with a communication disorder have been identified, diagnosed, and remediated. The swallowing disorder often encompasses the same oral, pharyngeal, and laryngeal structures that are involved in the production of speech and language. Disorders of swallow function can be uncomfortable, embarrassing at times, and even life threatening. According to a major study in the *Journal of the American Medical Association* (Simmons, 1986), difficulty in swallowing affects more than 10 million Americans. Furthermore, approximately 1 in 17 persons suffers from swallowing difficulties at some point during his or her life span (Felt, 1999; Cook & Kahrilas, 1999).

Disorders of communication and swallowing can impose social isolation and personal suffering on an affected individual and may place enormous emotional and economic burdens on the individual's family and on society. Maximizing the ability of a person to communicate is integral to his or her education, vocational plans, and social interactions. Maintaining a person's ability to swallow foods and liquids is essential for his or her health, nutrition, and emotional well being.

Communication and swallowing deficits may be seen throughout the age spectrum. Discussion of all possible communication and swallowing disorders, including those that are congenital or acquired, functionally or organically based, is beyond the scope of this chapter. Therefore, only those impairments with a medical etiology that are frequently encountered by the rehabilitation specialist are reviewed. This chapter provides the reader with a description of the major communication and swallowing disabilities and their medical correlates, the treatment and prognosis for these disorders, and the subsequent psychological and vocational ramifications.

SPEECH AND LANGUAGE DISORDERS

APHASIA AND APRAXIA OF SPEECH

ESTIMATES OF 500,000–700,000 people sustain a cerebral vascular accident or stroke each year, and it is the third leading cause of death in the United States (Leary & Saver, 2003). Of this population, approximately two-thirds are believed to have the concomitant language deficit, aphasia. Aphasia is defined as an inability to express and/or comprehend language as a result of organic damage to the brain, usually in the left cerebral cortex. The person with aphasia demonstrates dysfunction in language content or meaning, language form or structure, and language usage or function, along with the underlying cognitive processes

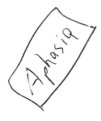

such as memory, reasoning, and recognition (Chapey, 1994). This dysfunction disrupts the individual's ability to listen and understand, read, speak, and write in varying degrees and is not attributable to confusion, hearing loss, or motor impairment.

Aphasia can also result from other neurological insults including, but not limited to, brain tumor, head trauma, subcortical infarcts, and infectious diseases. Infrequently, aphasia occurs following right hemispheric damage, especially in left-handed individuals, and as the result of focal subcortical lesions.

An elderly man who once delighted in reading now struggles to make sense of the morning headlines; the newsprint is clear, but the words appear to him like random squiggles on a page. A middle-aged woman speaks haltingly, groping for words that once flowed with ease. Thousands of alert, intelligent individuals find themselves suddenly plunged into a world of jumbled communication because damage to the brain has left them with aphasia. Aphasic symptoms are usually not restricted to deficits in one language modality. The aphasic individual has reduced abilities in all language areas, including oral expression, auditory comprehension, reading, writing, and even use and understanding of meaningful gestures. Generally, persons with aphasia have impairments of differing severity in both the receptive and expressive components of language.

Difficulty with verbal output and writing is commonly termed expressive aphasia; difficulty with comprehension of what is heard and/or read is often described as receptive aphasia. Central to a description and classification of aphasia is the ability to view verbal output as either fluent or nonfluent. Fluent forms of aphasia are marked by effortless speech with ease in articulation and the production of long strings of words in a variety of grammatical contexts. Words devoid of content, non-specific words–a pencil is called "a thing"—and circumlocutions frequently occur. Articulation skills are adequate. Normal speech rhythm and melody are usually preserved. Unfortunately, however, verbal output tends to be meaningless. At times, meaningless jargon is used.

In contrast, in the nonfluent aphasia, the flow of speech is impaired. The words uttered are usually limited in quantity, spoken slowly and with great effort, and frequently poorly articulated. The language may be telegraphic, containing only the information words (usually nouns) and excluding the grammatical words such as verb tenses and prepositions. These productions are frequently replete with word-finding difficulty (anomia) as evidenced by over-use of non-specific referring terms such as "that one," "those," "the whachamacallit," etc. The nonfluent aphasic knows what he wants to say but cannot find the words he needs; he has thoughts but cannot access or organize the language to express them (Kerman-Lerner, 1988).

*Global
Aphasia* (handwritten)

*Broca's
Aphasia
Wernicke's
Aphasia* (handwritten)

Apraxia (handwritten)

Occasionally, individuals show a severe impairment of communicative ability across all language modalities, resulting in little to no understanding or ability to communicate. This is termed global aphasia. These patients are unable to follow simple, one-level commands and are unable to produce any meaningful speech. Global aphasia usually results from extensive damage to the language areas of the left hemisphere or occasionally from a subcortical lesion.

One widely used descriptive system to classify aphasic speakers is the Boston classification schema (Goodglass, Kaplan, & Barresi, 2001) based on the speech output of the individual. Subtypes of aphasia in the Boston system include the more common Broca's aphasia (nonfluent aphasia), Wernicke's aphasia (fluent aphasia), and global aphasia, as well as the less common transcortical types.

Not all aphasias fit neatly into a single classification schema nor a specific aphasia syndrome. Variation of these syndromes occurs not only because lesions differ in location and extent but because the response to the same injury is not fixed among individuals. In addition, the symptoms and configuration of the aphasia may change as the time from onset increases and the severity decreases. Initially, the individual's language may have been diagnosed as a global aphasia yet may resolve toward a nonfluent aphasia with slow, labored, one- or two-word utterances during the acute stage. Following a period of therapeutic intervention, auditory comprehension and verbal expression may improve, approaching the cluster of symptoms seen in anomic aphasia.

A disorder that often coexists with aphasia is apraxia of speech. Apraxia was defined by Darley, Aronson, and Brown (1975) and by Duffy (1995) as a neurogenic speech disorder resulting from impairment in the capacity to program sensorimotor commands for positioning and movement of muscles for volitional production of speech. It can occur without significant weakness or neuromuscular slowness and in the absence of disturbances of conscious thought or language.

The person with apraxia can hear and comprehend a requested task and can perform a movement or series of movements reflexively. For example, he can pick up a glass of water and drink from it when he is thirsty. Yet, when given the command to "Show me what you do with a glass," this patient would have difficulty executing the series of movements needed. Similarly, when he attempts voluntary performance of a speech task such as repeating words, he cannot sequence and execute the movements. The speech pattern of a person with apraxia is usually slow and labored, with numerous vowel and consonant articulatory errors. In addition, patients with apraxia will demonstrate a qualitative difference in speech production when performing automatic tasks such as counting as compared to more volitional tasks such as word repetition (LaPointe, 1997). The speaker is often aware of his errors but is unable to modify or correct them.

Management Considerations

Language rehabilitation must be individualized to meet the communication needs of the client while being specific to the language deficits requiring remediation. The goal of aphasia treatment is to maximize the functional communication abilities of the person in daily living situations. Treatment tasks and goals depend on the nature and severity of the aphasia.

Remediation targets the achievement of a set of language skills and the generalization of these skills to the daily communication environment of the aphasic. Therapeutic approaches are derived from a theoretical framework based on a variety of linguistic models. These interventions may range from viewing language recovery in a holistic manner, to deficit specific approaches, or to a functional treatment regime which focuses on maximizing communication using any and all language modalities. Technology, such as the use of microcomputers with language-enhancing software, often furthers or supplements the treatment delivered (Duffy, 1995).

The prognosis for recovery from aphasia depends on many factors, including the age of the patient; the location, extent, and type of cerebral damage; the severity of language symptoms; and any additional associated impairments such as apraxia or dementia. The time post-onset of the brain damage also affects outcome predictions. Prognosis is generally more positive if therapy is initiated immediately after the brain injury. Behavioral factors, including motivation for recovery, error awareness, and ability to self-correct errors, all affect the ability of the individual to benefit from treatment. While a variety of different treatment approaches can be taken, the reader should be aware that although treatment may facilitate some improvement of language, total recovery from aphasia is rare (Holland & Reinmuth, 2002).

DYSARTHRIA

A MAJOR COMMUNICATION disorder that is often confused with aphasia is the motor speech impairment known as dysarthria. Dysarthria is manifested as a disruption in oral communication caused by a paralysis, weakness, abnormal tone, or incoordination of the muscles used in speech. It encompasses disorders of respiration, phonation, resonation, articulation, and prosody. Dysarthria does not refer to the symbolic language impairments that result from aphasia; rather, the person with dysarthria has retained the language symbols necessary for communication but speaks unclearly. Speech production may sound dis-

mastication

anarthria

dysarthria

Parkinsons

TBI

*6 major types
of dysarthria*

torted, unintelligible, or bizarre. In addition to the speech symptomatology, difficulty in mastication, swallowing, and controlling salivation are frequently observed.

The functional speech intelligibility of the client depends on the degree of neuromuscular disorder. Some individuals have only slightly distorted speech; they can communicate most needs verbally but may have to repeat an utterance or overarticulate for clarity. Others have an *over articulate* more marked impairment, with involved speech systems interacting inefficiently. Their speech sounds slow and labored, with imprecise consonant production and decreased control of vocal pitch and volume. In other situations, some persons have speech systems that are severely impaired; they can generate only minimally intelligible speech, even at the single word level. In its most severe form the individual cannot produce any intelligible words or even sounds, an impairment termed anarthria (Rosenbek & LaPointe, 1982).

Dysarthria results from a lesion or impairment of the central or peripheral nervous system, or both, including the cerebrum, cerebellum, brain stem, and cranial nerves. Some neurogenic disorders causing dysarthria are stable, whereas others are degenerative in nature. Speech characteristics will vary according to the site of neurological lesion and the severity of the physiological impairment.

The variation in neuromuscular disruption leads to differences in speech production. For example, in a person with Parkinson's Disease, intelligibility can be affected by imprecise articulation of sounds, low vocal volume, along with reduced rate and rhythm of speech. The person with traumatic brain injury, in contrast, will present with an "explosive speech pattern" characterized by sudden bursts of vocal volume, prolonged duration of words and phrases, and a generalized slurring of speech. A useful classification schema has been developed by Darley, Aronson, and Brown (1975), describing six major types of dysarthria associated with specific neuromuscular deficits and disordered speech subsystems, each having a unique cluster of deviant speech dimensions.

Management Considerations

The therapy program for persons with dysarthria focuses on increasing effective communication through improving speech intelligibility. For the mildly involved dysarthric speaker, whose speech is fairly intelligible in certain situations, treatment includes enhancing communication efficiency while maintaining clarity and speech naturalness. For those moderately involved dysarthric speakers who are able to communicate with speech but who are not completely intelligible, the primary goal of treatment is to maximize their speech intelligibility. Traditional behavioral methods have focused on improving the strength and coordination of the speech musculature. New technology, encompassing the use of microcomputers and instrumental biofeedback, has facilitated the modification of acoustic parameters in speech performance. In some instances, however, these methods produce only limited changes in function. Compensatory techniques to enhance speech intelligibility may also be employed, along with prosthetic devices to aid vocal intensity and/or resonance (e.g., palatal lift).

For the severely involved dysarthric speaker who has poor or nonfunctional speech intelligibility, little or no verbal, written, or gestural communication, as well as severe physical disabilities, treatment may include augmentative/alternative communication (AAC). The selection of an appropriate AAC system is dependent upon the communication needs as well as the physical and cognitive abilities of the person. Systems range from simple objects, letter or word boards (communication boards) where the user makes selections by pointing, to more complex computer-based systems that provide synthesized speech, printed output, and memory (Yorkston & Beukelman, 1988). The goals of treatment vary with the severity of the disability and, in some cases such as amyotrophic lateral sclerosis, with the progression of the disorder.

The prognosis for recovery from dysarthria depends on many factors, including whether the underlying neuropathology is stable or degenerative. With a stable neurological situation, functional gains may be realized; with a degenerative disorder, maintaining the current status and preparing for further decline is viewed as a favorable outcome. Other factors affecting prognosis include extent and type of neurological damage; additional impairments, such as aphasia or cognitive deficits; the ability of the individual to correct his errors; and the individual's motivation.

RIGHT HEMISPHERE DYSFUNCTION

INDIVIDUALS WITH RIGHT hemisphere dysfunction, in contrast to those with aphasia, demonstrate cognitive and higher-level language impairments as their primary communication disorder. Deficits include disturbances in attention, initiation of verbal utterances, left-neglect, visual memory, judgment, and the social use of language including understanding and use of humor and body language (Myers, 1997). Paucity in facial expression while speaking, poor eye contact, failure to use gesture, and a lack of vocal inflection all characterize their interaction style. Right hemisphere-impaired individuals are often labeled "difficult personalities." Problems with social interactions may develop. These patients may talk endlessly without noticing a change in conversational topic or may fail to recognize a listener's need for clarification (Stierwalt, Clark, & Robin, 2000). They often become isolated, with limited vocational options and family support.

Management Considerations

Higher-level language skills and improved cognition within a communicative context are the primary focus of therapeutic intervention for the person with right hemisphere impairment. Remediation of attention, recall, and initiation of conversation are three areas frequently addressed. Individuals often show a lack of awareness of communication style, resulting in a negative impact upon others. Therefore, activities that involve both clinician and peer feedback, role playing, and social interaction in group communication are valuable therapeutic tools.

TRAUMATIC BRAIN INJURY

TRAUMATIC BRAIN INJURY is the leading cause of death and disability for individuals under 40 years of age, with a mortality rate of approximately 56,000 deaths per year. For those who survive, 500,000 require hospitalization with an estimated cost of society of $25 billion each year (Kraus & McArthur, 1996; Adamovich, 1997). Such injuries may result from automobile accidents or penetrating wounds. The injury, whether a traumatic brain injury or a closed head insult, results in a wide range of disturbances. Unlike cerebrovascular accidents, damage to the cortex is often diffuse, affecting a variety of perceptual and linguistic behaviors. As a result, language is impaired as part of a complex constellation of memory and cognitive deficits instead of the isolated language impairment noted in aphasia.

Severity of the impairment depends on various factors including the length of comatose state (if applicable), extent of tissue damage, lack of oxygen to the brain, swelling of the brain, and the buildup of cerebrospinal fluid (Miller, 1984). Characteristics of the disorder often include impaired attention, perception, auditory comprehension, and recall. The individual may exhibit disorientation and confusion in verbal output, along with anomia (word-finding difficulty). Difficulty integrating, analyzing, and synthesizing information affect the person's abstract reasoning and problem-solving abilities. Subsequent to such impairments, almost all aspects of daily living and communication may be compromised. Functional disability ranges in severity from a comatose state, with little or no response to the environment, to mild brain injury or post-concussive syndrome, which results in subtle manifestation of deficits (Ylvisaker & Szekeres, 1986).

Management Considerations

Prognosis for recovery from traumatic brain injury depends on the nature and extent of cortical damage, the time post-onset of injury, the length of coma, and the nature of intact abilities. Significant restoration of function is frequently noted early in the process as a result of spontaneous recovery. Improvement in cognitive and linguistic function may be realized secondary to rehabilitation; in most cases some form of residual cognitive dysfunction will persist over the long term. For children, one can expect that at least 10% of such patients will experience residual memory deficits as compared to problems seen in 30% to 40% of adult patients (Klonoff & Paris, 1974). A 7-year follow-up study of 190 brain injury survivors conducted by Tennant, Macdermott, and Neary (1995) revealed that 7.4% had died post discharge, 17% had not achieved a good recovery, and 36% were failing to occupy their time in a meaningful way.

The majority of brain-injured victims are under the age of 30, with concomitant physical disabilities. As a result, treatment must be designed to address their current communication needs and to anticipate the cognitive demands of future educational and vocational endeavors. The direction of treatment is continually modified during the recovery process. Early intervention methods focus on remediation of deficit areas and instructional techniques aimed at restoration of skills. As recovery in function begins to plateau, efforts target implementation and training of compensatory strategies. The culmination of rehabilitation is directed toward carryover of skills and strategies into the everyday life of the client.

DEMENTIA

DEMENTIA IS VIEWED as a progressive diffuse pathology that results in chronic deterioration of intellect, memory, and communication function following neurological changes. The cluster of cognitive deficits most often associated with dementia include disorientation, impaired memory, emotional lability, and poor learning. Dementia not only affects the overall mental functioning of an individual but also the ability to use language to interact with caregivers and the environment. Davis (1993) describes three stages of dementia. In Stage I, patients are typically forgetful and demonstrate some vagueness in their language productions. In Stage II, short-term memory problems are more pronounced and auditory comprehension deficits become evident. By Stage III, patients are no longer able to store new information. Many become unresponsive to their surroundings and eventually become mute.

Dementia may result from a variety of progressive neuropathological conditions, including Alzheimer's disease, Pick's disease, Parkinson's disease, multi-infarct dementia, Huntington's chorea, acquired immune deficiency syndrome (AIDS), and multiple sclerosis. Deterioration of language function in dementia may be correlated with the progression of the disease (Bayles, Tomoeda, & Trosset, 1992).

Management Considerations

Treatment for dementia is directed toward compensation for lost skills, support of the remaining functional abilities, structure or control of the environment, and education of caregivers and families in effective communication techniques. Application of compensatory strategies in the environment facilitates enhancement of orientation, memory, and comprehension skills. Interactions are structured to be within the cognitive and linguistic abilities of the individual in order to reduce frustration and increase communication effectiveness. Within this context, nonverbal communication, such as touch, facial expression, eye contact, and gesture, can enhance communication effectiveness and foster interactions with patients who no longer respond to verbal stimuli (Hoffman, Platt, & Barry, 1988; Bayles, 1994).

VOICE DISORDERS

PHONATION, OR VOICE production, is a complex neuromotor activity that requires coordination of respiration, laryngeal function, and resonance. Disruption of any one of these processes can result in a disordered voice, termed dysphonia. Such conditions may result from pathological, neurological, traumatic, or behavioral conditions. This discussion is confined to those conditions that relate to a medical or neurological etiology.

Vocal fold pathologies disrupt the biomechanics of laryngeal function, thereby causing a phonatory disturbance. Vocal nodules, vocal polyps, contact ulcers, and laryngitis are the most prevalent benign conditions. Vocal fold pathologies are usually characterized by hoarse, breathy, strained, or harsh vocal quality and, at times, low vocal intensity. In addition, neurological or traumatic injury to the central nervous system or the larynx may result in vocal fold paralysis, resulting in a breathy voice quality, low intensity, or, in more severe cases, a total lack of phonation, which is termed aphonia. Laryngeal tumors of which approximately 80% are malignant, also may exist (English, 1976). Tumors are often suspected when there is a prolonged period of hoarse vocal quality combined with complaints of pain. Depending on the extent of surgical remediation for the tumor, the individual can be rendered dysphonic or even aphonic.

A common medical procedure that produces an aphonia is a tracheostomy. When the upper airway is compromised, an artificial airway, or tracheostomy, is surgically created below the cricoid cartilage of the larynx. Inhalation and exhalation take place below the larynx, precluding the passage of air through the vocal folds to produce voice. Individuals may undergo a tracheostomy for a variety of medical con-

copd   als

ditions, including chronic obstructive pulmonary disease, laryngeal trauma, or progressive neurological diseases such as amyotrophic lateral sclerosis or myasthenia gravis (Dikeman & Kazandjian, 2003).

Management Considerations

Management of voice disorders requires the coordinated efforts of a speech-language pathologist and various medical specialists including otolaryngologists. *otolarygologists* Treatment of noncancerous vocal fold pathologies often includes medical intervention (e.g., surgical resection) along with a period of vocal rest. When vocal abuse or misuse is identified as a cause of the pathology, voice therapy is recommended. The goal is the elimination of vocal abuse behaviors and the promotion of good vocal hygiene. Several techniques used may include breathing exercises, relaxation approaches, and digital manipulation/pressure.

In the case of vocal fold paralysis, remediation focuses on improving vocal fold approximation to produce voice. Spontaneous recovery is expected in many cases, usually within 6 months of onset (Tucker, 1980). In cases where recovery has not occurred, surgical interventions for paralysis include silastic tube implantation, thyroplasty, Teflon injections, or vocal cord repositioning to aid vocal cord closure (Colton & Casper, 1990). Voice therapy for this condition is usually employed to facilitate maximum gains. More recently, botox injections have been used experimentally to facilitate increased vocal fold function in specific phonatory disorders, such as spasmodic dysphonia.

Treatment for malignant vocal fold pathologies incorporates surgical resection, radiation and/or chemotherapy, and voice strengthening or restoration. A total laryngectomy, for example, requires the excision of the entire larynx, from the trachea to the base of the tongue. The laryngectomy renders the patient aphonic, and respiration takes place via a surgically created airway in the neck, the stoma. Restoration of *stoma* speech is usually accomplished by the use of an artificial larynx, esophageal speech, or a tracheoesophageal puncture (TEP).

For the tracheostomized individual with an intact larynx, voice restoration is the primary goal. Finger occlusion or capping of the tracheostomy tube is often adequate to redirect exhaled air through the vocal folds so that normal phonation is produced. Additionally, the use of prosthetic speaking valves or a two-way tracheostomy valve will facilitate the return of voice.

Prognosis for successful intervention depends on the etiology of the disorder, the severity of the dysphonia, and the regeneration of the vocal physiology. Of course, behavioral factors, including motivation and willingness to accept a modified but functional voice, are also important components. A summary of the functional presentation of the most common speech and language disorders is provided in Table 12.1.

TABLE 12.1   Summary of Functional Presentation

Disorder	Verbal expression	Writing	Auditory comprehension	Reading
Expressive aphasia	Impaired production of connected speech; may be able to produce greetings, yet has difficulty producing names and single words	Impaired production of single words or sentences; may be able to write name and numbers	Usually impaired, yet better than expressive language	Impairment is similar to that of auditory comprehension
Receptive aphasia	Verbal expression usually impaired due to comprehension deficits	May be impaired but often better than receptive language	Impairment in auditory comprehension, increasing with length and complexity; difficulties more pronounced with abstract or ambiguous language	Usually marked impairment, severity similar to that of auditory comprehension deficits
Global aphasia	Severely impaired expression; not able to produce single words or connected speech	Severely impaired writing; unable to write name, words, or numbers	Severely impaired auditory comprehension; difficulty with basic commands and questions	Severely impaired reading comprehension; unable to read single words
Right hemisphere syndrome	Basic language skills are intact; however, pragmatic language and initiation of verbal expression are often impaired	Intact	May present comprehension deficits due to cognitive impairment; difficulty understanding abstract language	Reading comprehension may be impaired
Head trauma	Expressive aphasia may be present with deficits in word retrieval, discourse cohesion and coherence, and pragmatic language	Difficulty with spelling, grammar, and paragraph formation may exist	Auditory attention and processing impairments often impact on comprehension; difficulty with abstract ideas, complex syntax, and humor	Same as receptive language; visual perceptual deficits may limit acuity and scanning of written material

300

Cognition	Motor speech	Voice	Swallowing
Intact	May present with apraxia or dysarthria of speech	Usually intact	Usually intact
Intact	May present with apraxia or dysarthria of speech	Usually intact	Usually intact
Cognitive impairment may coexist; unable to determine parameters due to severe language deficits	May present with apraxia or dysarthria of speech	Usually intact	Swallowing disorder may be present
Impairments in attention, initiation, memory, and abstract reasoning may be present; visual perceptual deficits often coexist	May have concomitant dysarthria ranging from mild to severe	Usually intact	Usually intact, although may be impaired especially when dysarthria coexists
Significant cognitive impairment affecting attention, memory, information processing, problem solving, organization, and abstract reasoning; difficulty with self-monitoring and awareness; may significantly impact on behavior	Apraxia or dysarthria of speech may coexist	Traumatic vocal fold damage or vocal cord paralysis may occur; aphonia due to tracheostomy may be present	Swallowing disorder may be present

(Continued)

301

TABLE 12.1 Summary of Functional Presentation *(Continued)*

Disorder	Verbal expression	Writing	Auditory comprehension	Reading
Dementia, Alzheimer's disease, Organic brain syndrome	Reduction in verbal output and syntactic complexity; word-finding difficulties evident; deficits increase in severity over time leading to scarce or no verbal output	Similar to verbal expression; writing difficulties increase over time to eventual loss of written expression	Comprehension deficits progressive in nature; initial difficulty understanding complex paragraphs progressing to difficulty understanding basic commands and questions	Same as receptive language; reading comprehension ability lessens over time
Parkinson's disease	Intact language skills; see Motor Speech	May be limited due to impairment of motor skills	Intact	May be limited by visual perceptual deficits
Other progressive neurological diseases	Intact language skills; see Motor Speech	Writing skills will progressively degenerate, with impairment of motor skills	Intact	Intact
Head and neck cancer	Intact language skills	Intact	Intact	Intact

From Lerner & Hauck (1999). Reprinted with permission.

302

Cognition	Motor speech	Voice	Swallowing
Progressive deficits in memory, orientation, problem solving, and learning new material; advances to global cognitive impairment over time	Intact	Intact	Swallowing physiology may be intact, yet oral feeding may be compromised by cognitive status
In later stages mild–moderate overall cognitive dysfunction may occur; cognition may also be reduced by side effects of medications	Speech becomes distorted with reduced articulatory precision, poor coordination with respiration and rushes of unintelligible speech	Progressive loss of vocal intensity and vocal inflection pattern	Swallowing impairment often results as disease progresses; diet modifications or nonoral feedings may be needed in later stages
Intact in amyotrophic lateral sclerosis; may have impairments in multiple sclerosis and Huntington's chorea, especially in later stages	Dysarthria progressing from mild to severe disability; speech will become unintelligible in late stages of disease and may evolve to anarthria	Volume and vocal quality may be reduced; strained erratic voicing pattern noted	Progressive degeneration of swallowing requiring diet modification; in later stages may require nonoral feeding
Intact	Resection of tongue, mandible, or other portions of the oral cavity may reduce intelligibility of speech depending on the extent of surgical excision	In cancer of the larynx, voicing may be moderately impaired (hemilaryngectomy), or absent (total laryngectomy); voice restoration may be possible via puncture or esophageal speech	Oral, pharyngeal, or laryngeal swallowing impairment may occur

303

Stuttering

Type & Frequency

non-speech behaviors

STUTTERING

STUTTERING REFERS TO the disruption of speech fluency. Fluent speech requires the uninterrupted rhythmic coordination of speech sounds, syllables, words, and phrases when one is talking. Interruption of this smooth flow can be perceived by listeners as stuttering or "stammering." The prevalence of this disorder is approximately 1% of the adult population: the incidence of this disorder is 5% (Guitar, 1998). The data suggests that many who may have stuttered at some time in their lives have recovered from the disorder. Stuttering therefore may best be described as a childhood disorder. The onset of stuttering can also occur in adulthood secondary to a discrete neurological, pharmacological, or psychological event. Stuttering tends to occur in males more than females, three of four stutterers being male, and it tends to run in families.

Though there is no known "cure" for stuttering, many patients report spontaneous recovery from the disorder. Yet for others, the disorder remains unresolved and it is maintained well into adulthood. While the impact of stuttering on one's communication, social, and emotional status cannot be ignored, there are many accomplished individuals who, despite their stuttering, have achieved success in their life's endeavors.

While all speakers will exhibit some disfluency in speech production, it is the *type* and *frequency* of disfluency along with associated (secondary) behaviors, if any, that determine whether a speaker is perceived as a "stutterer." Various aberrant speech behaviors that are considered stuttering may occur within the word while others occur in-between words. Within word disfluencies include part-word repetitions ("re-re-report"), sound prolongations ("w--eek"), and silent blocks where a sound is attempted but no phonation is heard. Between word disfluencies include whole-word repetitions ("he-he-he is home"); interjections ("he . . . um . . . um . . . um is sick"); and revisions ("I purch . . . bought a car"). Coupled with the frequency with which these behaviors occur, listeners make judgments about stuttering and fluency along with judgments about the severity of stuttering. Listeners' judgments may negatively impact on a speaker's fluency and emotional well-being.

Generally speaking, within-word disfluencies tend to draw more attention to the speaker, given the relatively disruptive nature of the behavior. That is, between-word disfluencies do not interrupt individual words so that these might be perceived as moments of word searching. In fact, interjections and revisions are not always judged to be "stuttering" by typical listeners (Wingate, 1959).

Associated or secondary non-speech behaviors refer to physical/visible behaviors that accompany disfluent speech. Examples of these include: finger-tapping, blinking, moving parts of the body, lip tension, and flaring of the nares. Initially, such behaviors were produced incidentally paired with the disfluent speech. Because the behaviors served as a distractor for the speaker, they seemed to decrease stuttering since they redirected the speaker's attention when speaking. Over time, the speaker draws an erroneous correlation between a behavior such as finger-tapping and fluency and the speaker begins to use finger-tapping to avoid stuttering. With overuse of such strategies, the novelty of the finger-tapping wears off but the stuttering persists. This results in the speaker incorporating finger-tapping as part of his stuttering behavior. For the person who stutters, there is a wide range of response to the interruption in the flow of speech. For some speakers, dysfluencies are not necessary troublesome; they do not rely on secondary behaviors or devices to escape or avoid stuttering. Yet for others, the dysfluencies may be so severe that speakers feel helpless and out of control. Embarrassment, fear, and shame are commonly reported by this group of speakers (Guitar, 1998). For this group, feelings and attitudes must be taken into consideration in the planning of treatment.

Management Considerations

Current literature divides therapy approaches for stuttering into two basic categories: stuttering modification therapy and fluency shaping therapy. The former focuses on teaching the client to modify his stuttering behaviors and to reduce the fear associated with speaking and stuttering. The client is taught to confront the stuttering, thereby reducing the avoidance of stuttering. The latter focuses on the establishment of a level of speech fluency followed by therapy activities with the primary gaol of integrating fluency into conversational speech (Guitar, 1998). The emphasis is on slow, easy flowing speech. More recently, fluency-enhancing devices have become available to those who stutter. These small units are worn in the ear canal (much like a hearing aid) and are based on the use of altered auditory feedback as means of reducing stuttering. Specifically, delayed auditory feedback (DAF) and frequency altered feedback (FAF) can be programmed into each unit to meet the particular needs of a client. Research has shown that these devices can markedly reduce and even eliminate stuttering within a brief period of time. Efficacy studies on these devices are currently being conducted so that the long-term benefits of this therapy can be assessed.

SWALLOWING DISORDERS

THE ABILITY TO swallow is a basic function essential to our health and well being, affording us both pleasure and nutrition. The act of swallowing encompasses the interaction of complex neurological and physiological systems. Even small alterations in the events, structures,

dysphasia

aspiration
mastication

or physiology involved in swallowing can have a profound influence on the process and significantly alter a person's quality of life.

Difficulty in swallowing, or dysphagia, affects people throughout the age spectrum with a wide range of medical etiologies. A person with dysphagia may have an unsafe swallow which causes food or saliva to enter his airway, termed aspiration. Or a person may have a weak and slow swallow resulting in difficulty taking in adequate food and liquids to insure proper nutrition. Mastication (chewing) may be impaired and some people may experience drooling. Other people may have difficulty propelling their foods through their pharynx and into the esophagus. These deficits create serious problems in sustaining a healthy and satisfying quality of life. Furthermore, profound changes in nutritional status may be seen. Consequences of dysphagia range from discomfort, e.g., throat pain, to coughing and choking or even life-threatening illness. Serious sequelae include silent aspiration, aspiration pneumonia, dehydration, and malnutrition.

Swallowing disorders are found in both the pediatric and adult population. Problems can arise from various causes, including neurological involvement; degenerative diseases; alteration of the anatomy and physiology following surgery, trauma or radiation therapy; cardiovascular and other systematic diseases; developmental disabilities; congenital defects; and failure to thrive.

Millions of individuals suffer from some type of swallowing disorder caused by a wide range of medical problems. Up to 50% of persons with head trauma (Lazarus & Logemann, 1987), 30% of patients who have suffered a cerebrovascular accident (CVA) (Groher & Bukatman, 1986; Veis & Logemann, 1985), 20% of patients with pneumonia, and 30% of patients with head and neck resections (Echelard, Thoppil, & Melvin, 1984) show a swallowing impairment. Research indicates that 12% to 15% of patients in acute care hospitals exhibit swallowing impairments (Groher & Bukatman). Thirty-five percent of patients in rehabilitation settings (Gordon, Hewer, & Wade, 1987) and up to 50% of individuals in nursing homes (Feinberg, Ekberg, Segall, & Tully, 1992; Jones & Donner, 1988) have difficulty with swallowing.

SWALLOWING STAGES

SWALLOWING IS A complex series of events involving the cerebral cortex, brain stem, six cranial nerves, and over 25 different facial and oral muscles, working together to initiate the swallowing process. Normal swallowing is a rapid, safe, and efficient process taking less than 2 seconds to move foods or liquids from the mouth, through the pharynx, and into the esophagus (Logemann, 1998). Swallowing occurs in three stages: oral (preparatory and oral transit), pharyngeal, and esophageal. The first stage is voluntary

3 stages of
Swallowing
Oral
Pharangeal
esophageal

and is controlled by cortical centers located in the brain. The next two stages are involuntary and are coordinated by brain-stem centers.

In the oral stage, food and liquids are mixed with saliva and, if solid, chewed to an appropriate size and consistency. Oral transit follows as the material is propelled toward the back of the mouth and then enters the pharynx. When material is in the pharynx (pharyngeal stage), several processes occur simultaneously to halt respiration, protect the airway, and transport the material being swallowed into the esophagus and stomach. Material must be efficiently transported in order to prevent delayed aspiration of foodstuffs into the airway and to assure adequate nutrition. The speed of the swallow encompassing both the oral and pharyngeal transit times is normally 2 seconds or less.

The final stage of swallowing, the esophageal stage, carries the swallowed material through the length of the esophagus, the gastro-esophageal junction, and into the stomach. The esophageal stage normally can take as much as 8–20 seconds. If the oral, pharyngeal, and esophageal stages of swallowing are not competent, it is unlikely that the patient will be able to obtain adequate nutrition by mouth to maintain good health.

Management Considerations

In recent years with technology-enhanced diagnostics and physiology-based treatment techniques, health care professionals have discovered that active intervention with the swallowing-impaired individual often aids in a person's return to normal feeding and swallowing (Groher, 1997). Treatment is designed to reestablish or increase oral intake, maintain adequate nutrition and hydration, improve the safety of the swallow, and eliminate aspiration. Therapy is usually directed at specific anatomical or physiological deficiencies detected from clinical and instrumental assessments. Intervention can include swallow rehabilitation and, if needed, specific medical/surgical techniques.

Remediation involves identifying problems and selecting correct swallowing techniques to address these problems. Through exercises and management strategies many individuals will eventually show improvement in swallowing function. Treatment can be divided into three types: 1) management of the impaired swallow by changing the type and consistencies of foods and liquids to aid intake and reduce risk of aspiration; 2) compensatory strategies to eliminate the symptoms of the swallowing problem while not necessarily changing the swallow physiology; and 3) specific therapy techniques, designed to change swallow physiology. Studies have shown that rehabilitation can be successful in returning over 80% of individuals with dysphagia to oral intake (Rademaker et al., 1993).

Compensatory strategies such as postural changes and diet restrictions alter the way food flows through the oral cavity and pharynx, permit-

Compensatory
Strategies

direct
strategies

ting a person to eat by mouth. The correct positioning of food in the mouth during eating and alternating solids and liquids to wash residue from the mouth or pharynx are examples of compensatory techniques. The advantage of compensatory strategies is that they can be put into effect quickly, enabling many people to immediately improve swallow function. In contrast there are a number of direct rehabilitation techniques designed to change the swallow physiology. They may include: (a) exercise programs to improve muscle strength, range of motion and muscle coordination; (b) enhancing sensory input to improve the awareness of food in the mouth or the speed at which the pharyngeal swallow is triggered; and (c) specific maneuvers, designed to change selected aspects of the pharyngeal swallow.

In many cases the individual is best managed when compensatory and direct treatment techniques are used simultaneously. That is, the patient is given a compensatory technique that enables him to eat by mouth while swallow treatment is initiated. The direct treatment will eventually improve oropharyngeal muscle function and enable the patient to eat without compensatory postures.

If swallowing therapy does not prove effective, there are limited prosthetic and surgical options which may be appropriate for select patients. To illustrate, a palatal lift elevates the soft palate to achieve separation between the oral and nasal cavity, thus preventing regurgitation of food through the nose. In the case of a vocal cord paralysis, injection of the vocal cord with Teflon or other substance to increase vocal cord closure may decrease the chance of aspiration. A cricopharyngeal myotomy is performed to allow greater opening into the upper cervical esophagus. A tracheostomy with a plastic tracheotomy tube and inflatable cuff may be the only option for some patients with intractable aspiration. Once in place, it provides a separate entrance for the airway and decreases the risk of aspiration. This procedure, however, deprives the patient of the ability to speak by diverting air from the vocal cords.

cricopharyngeal
myotomy

A multidisciplinary team approach enhances the diagnostic and treatment of a swallowing disability. Using the expertise of rehabilitation specialists and, when indicated, medical specialists such as a neurologist, gastroenterologist, pulmonologist, otolaryngologist, and radiologist affords the individual a comprehensive approach to a multifaceted disorder.

professionals
needed

HEARING DISORDERS

HEARING REQUIRES THE detection, transmission, analysis, and integration of sound into meaningful symbols. The act of hearing is an integral component of communication. Unfortunately more than 24 million Americans have some degree of hearing impairment (Benson

& Marano, 1995). This estimate includes over 2 million who have a profound hearing loss with little or no speech discrimination ability. These people are considered deaf. According to the National Institute on Deafness and Other Communication Disorders (1999), such numbers are expected to increase substantially in the next few decades due to the increase in longevity and consequent overall aging of the population. The U.S. Office of Technology Assessment has designated hearing impairment as the third most prevalent chronic condition among the older population in the United States (National Institute on Deafness and Other Communication Disorders, Better Hearing Institute, 1999).

Hearing impairments are classified on the basis of site of lesion in the auditory system. This provides information leading to appropriate diagnosis, prognosis, and aural rehabilitation for the hearing-impaired individual. Within this framework, there are three types of organic hearing loss: conductive, sensorineural, and mixed. The site of lesion indicated in a conductive hearing loss is in the outer or middle ear or both. A sensorineural hearing loss results from lesions to the cochlea and/or auditory nerve. The presence of sensorineural loss accompanied by conductive hearing loss in the same ear is referred to as a mixed hearing loss. In some cases, hearing loss is present with no organic pathology in the auditory system to validate this loss. The term functional hearing loss is applied in such cases.

CONDUCTIVE HEARING LOSS

PATHOLOGICAL CONDITIONS OF the outer and middle ear may produce a barrier to sound transmission, resulting in conductive hearing loss. In this instance sound energy is attenuated and not efficiently transferred to the inner ear. As a result, the individual perceives sound as muffled and of insufficient intensity. Speech sounds are not distorted; the individual is usually able to understand speech when it is increased in intensity.

Abnormalities of the outer ear tend to produce a hearing loss of varying degrees. Outer ear pathologies include malformations of the auricle or absence of the external auditory canal (meatus), which may be a hereditary condition, such as Treacher Collins syndrome, or the result of traumatic injury. Otitis externa (swimmer's ear) results in a conductive hearing loss caused by swelling of the skin lining in the external auditory canal. Tumors (both malignant and benign) and cerumen (ear wax) interfere with sound transmission when they completely obstruct the ear canal and eardrum.

As in the outer ear, any barrier or abnormality of the middle ear system often produces a conductive hearing loss. The most common condition arises from otitis media, an inflammation of the middle ear. In *[handwritten margin notes: tympanic membrane (ear drum), ostosclerosis, cochlear (sensory loss), auditory (neural loss), sensorineural (consonants), congenital, perinatal, presbycusis]*

chronic cases, fluid accumulation in the middle ear dampens the sound signal and can rupture the tympanic membrane (eardrum). Often, individuals with middle ear fluid report a "plugged up" sensation in the affected ear accompanied by a decrease in hearing sensitivity.

Structural abnormalities of the middle ear, such as fusion or absence of the ossicles, result in an inability to transmit sound from the middle to the inner ear. Otosclerosis is a progressive structural condition that results in the formation of spongy bone over the stapedial footplate, causing fixation of the ossicles. The disease can be unilateral or bilateral and may affect the anatomy of the inner ear. An individual with otosclerosis speaks in a very soft voice because he perceives his own voice as louder than normal (Sataloff, 1966). Damage to the ossicles also occurs as a result of trauma or perforation of the eardrum from tumors that invade the middle ear.

SENSORINEURAL HEARING LOSS

ABNORMALITIES OR DAMAGE to the cochlea (sensory loss) or to the auditory nerve (neural loss) result in sensorineural hearing loss. Determining whether the site of lesion is in the cochlea or auditory nerve will affect the individual's ability to benefit from amplification and indicate whether further exploration of the medical condition is required. A sensorineural loss, especially a high-frequency loss, will produce diminished clarity for specific sounds, making it difficult to distinguish consonants in connected speech. Consequently, word intelligibility may be significantly compromised, especially in noisy environments that mask consonant sounds. Word intelligibility becomes further compromised as the hearing deficit advances in severity. An individual with sensorineural loss frequently complains that he can hear but finds it difficult to understand speech even when the intensity of the speech is increased.

A sensorineural loss can result from a congenital condition or an acquired disorder. A congenital hearing loss results from either genetic factors (35%–50% of the cases) or prenatal or perinatal conditions (English, 1976). Prenatal conditions that result in hearing loss include rubella, RH incompatibility, anoxia, viruses, and the use of ototoxic drugs during the birth process. Genetic conditions that may result in hearing loss at birth or later in life (perinatal) include Waardenburg's syndrome, Crouzon's disease, and Pierre Robin syndrome.

An acquired hearing loss can be due to various conditions, including viruses, degenerative diseases, tumor, ototoxic drugs, or noise exposure. Common viruses which may produce a sensorineural hearing loss are measles, mumps, and meningitis. Degenerative changes to the auditory system associated with the aging process result in a progressive sensorineural hearing loss called presbycusis. Lesions of the auditory nerve (acoustic neuromas) are additional causes of acquired hearing loss. Lastly, prolonged and excessive use of well-known drugs such as aspirin, quinine, and antibiotics may produce temporary or permanent hearing loss (Martin, 1986).

Noise-induced sensorineural hearing loss usually results from excessive exposure to industrial or environmental noise. The severity is dependent upon the intensity and duration of the noise exposure. Hearing loss due to noise may be temporary, as with brief exposure to high levels of loud sound, or permanent if the exposure is repetitive over long periods (Martin, 1986). Noise exposure can worsen hearing loss in individuals taking toxic drugs.

One disease often seen clinically is Meniere's disease. Meniere's disease is characterized by fluctuating sensorineural hearing loss, accompanied by vertigo, vomiting, tinnitus, and fullness in the affected ear. The site of the lesion is cochlear; however, there is no definitive cause for this disease. In the course of Meniere's disease, either cochlear hearing loss or vestibular symptoms may be present but usually will not co-occur. Meniere's disease occurs at any age but is most prevalent in adults (Paparella, DaCosta, Fox, & Yoon, 1991).

[margin note: Meniere's disease]

FUNCTIONAL HEARING LOSS

OCCASIONALLY, IN DAILY practice, the professional evaluates a client whose hearing loss cannot be explained by organic pathology. The term functional hearing loss is frequently used to describe this behavior. A functional loss is also referred to as pseudohypoacusis, nonorganic hearing loss, psychogenic hearing loss, or hysterical deafness. The term malingering has been used and described in individuals who consciously falsify physical or psychological symptoms. The audiological evaluation may not be able to determine if a nonorganic hearing loss is the result of unconscious or conscious behavior. Financial gain, compensation, and psychological or emotional factors can contribute to this behavior. In fact, it is believed that some individuals with functional hearing loss have a nonorganic component superimposed on an organic loss (Katz, 2001).

[margin note: pseudohypoacusis]

CLASSIFICATION OF HEARING IMPAIRMENTS

CLASSIFYING HEARING IMPAIRMENTS by the degree and type of loss is a convenient method of interpreting audiological results and aids in determining the effect of the hearing handicap on communication. Although inferences can be made from interpreting the test results, the degree of impairment is affected by a variety of other factors, including the type, degree, and configuration of hearing loss, age of onset, cognitive status, educational background, and the individual's personality.

The following classification schema, with functional manifestations and a rating of hearing handicap, may be assistive to the professional's understanding of the hearing-impaired individual.

Mild Hearing Loss

The individual often has difficulty with faint speech, distant speech, or understanding conversational speech in background noise; slight hearing handicap.

Moderate Hearing Loss

The individual has difficulty understanding conversational speech, especially in noisy environments, if the distance between the speaker and listener is more than 3 feet; mild hearing handicap.

Moderately Severe Hearing Loss

The individual requires speech to be loud and may have difficulty understanding speech in most listening situations, unable to hear conversational speech; marked hearing handicap.

Severe Hearing Loss

The individual hears loud speech approximately 1 foot from the speaker and is aware of some environmental noises; speech sounds in conversation will not be heard; severe hearing handicap.

Profound

The individual's understanding of speech is poor; conversational speech is not audible, but some loud sounds may be heard; unable to rely on hearing as the only modality in communication situations; extreme hearing handicap.

MANAGEMENT CONSIDERATIONS

IT IS USEFUL to view management for the hearing-impaired population as either medical or surgical intervention, followed by appropriate aural rehabilitation as needed. One or all of these treatment modalities may be required to maximize the individual's functional communication capability. Medical intervention is indicated once a conductive or mixed hearing loss is identified. Hearing sensitivity is often improved or restored through treatment with antibiotics when a middle ear infection is present. Surgery is frequently the treatment of choice for structural or physiological etiologies. Outer ear pathologies are addressed through plastic surgery to create an ear canal or a more normal pinna. Surgical options for middle ear pathologies restore effective transmission of sound energy from the outer ear to the inner ear. The procedure implemented is dependent upon the location of the middle ear disruption and includes myringoplasty, tympanoplasty, stapedectomy, and insertion of myringotomy tubes (Miller, Groher, Yorkston, & Rees, 1988; Schein & Miller, 1990). Most sensorineural hearing losses are not amenable to medical or surgical intervention. A life-threatening tumor or disease associated with sensorineural hearing loss, however, can necessitate otologic surgery. Hearing preservation is not the primary concern in this situation.

Following the appropriate medical or surgical intervention, aural rehabilitation may be initiated. Aural rehabilitation includes amplification, speech reading, and auditory training. The aim of aural rehabilitation is to maximize the use of residual hearing in order for the hearing-impaired individual to function in social, educational, and vocational roles. A secondary purpose is to educate the individual to manage his or her hearing aid, to optimize communication strategies, and to prevent the possibility of further hearing impairment.

Amplification is central to a treatment program of aural rehabilitation. Amplification includes hearing aids that intensify the speech signal to a comfortable listening level for the hearing-disordered person. Hearing aids are frequency-specific, allowing for amplification of those frequencies in which hearing loss is present (Hartford, 1988). The most common styles of hearing aids are: Completely-in-the-Canal (CIC), In-the-Canal (ITC), In-the-Ear (ITE), and Behind-the-Ear (BTE) aids. The CIC, ITC, and ITE are custom-molded which provides acoustical benefits. Most recently, disposable aids have been introduced as a low-cost yet effective means of providing amplification (Preves & Dempesy, 2000).

In recent years, amplification has been improved with advances in hearing aid components. This has resulted in miniaturization of hearing aids with greater frequency specificity. In addition, technology has allowed for the development of programmable or digital hearing aids. These have the capacity to be programmed to acoustically accommodate different listening environments. In a noisy situation, for instance, the hearing aid wearer can adjust the aid to reduce low-frequency input in order to reduce background noise (Sammeth, 1990).

Cochlear implants, another breakthrough, are surgically implanted devices available for children and adults who present with severe to profound hearing losses. The cochlear implant is designed to amplify some of the speech spectrum information in an attempt to enhance lip reading ability (Boothroyd, Geers, & Moog, 1991; Staller, Dowell, Beiter, & Brimcombe, 1991). The components of a cochlear system include surgically implanted parts and an externally worn speech processor and headset (Zwolan, 2002). The internal components are surgically implanted into the mastoid area and the cochlea. Sounds are transformed into small electrical currents that stimulate auditory nerves found in the cochlea and produce hearing sensation.

In some situations, an individual can use both a traditional hearing aid and an assistive listening device. This device captures sound inches from the source and transmits it directly to the listener's ear without losing the sound intensity of the speech signal and without amplifying unwanted environmental sounds. For example, in a lecture hall, the lecturer wears a microphone inches from his or her mouth. The signal is transmitted through the air, by either infrared or FM waves, directly to the listener's hearing aid, a special FM unit, or a special infrared unit. Other assistive listening devices available include a closed caption decoder for television, flashing smoke detectors, flashing alarm clocks, and vibrator alarm beds.

For severely hearing-impaired or deaf individuals, sign language may be the primary method of communication. The most commonly used form of sign in the United States is American Sign Language (ASL). Sign language may be implemented as the sole means of communication, or used in conjunction with any combination of previously described management methods. An important piece of technology designed for this population is the telecommunication device for the deaf (TDD). The TDD allows direct interface with a phone line. The message is typed and either transmitted to a visual display screen or printed out at the receiver's TDD. Many phone companies provide toll-free numbers so that a hearing-impaired person using a TDD can communicate via telephone with a normal hearing person.

Finally, speech reading, traditionally called lip reading, consists of using visual cues for the recognition of speech sounds and incorporates the use of facial expressions, body movements, and gestures. Speech reading alone, however, is ineffective because only one-third of English speech sounds are visible. Auditory training, instructing the individual to maximize his residual hearing, in conjunction with speech reading, enables the person to use minimal auditory cues most effectively. The combination of speech reading, auditory training, and amplification offers the hearing-disordered individual enhanced comprehension of speech (Miller et al., 1988).

CULTURALLY AND LINGUISTICALLY DIVERSE CLIENTS

ADVANCES IN TECHNOLOGY are bringing people of the world closer together. United States immigration trends suggest that there continue to be significant increases in African Americans, Asians, and Hispanic groups. Government agencies, work settings, and schools are endeavoring toward breaking through cultural and linguistic barriers to improve relations among different cultural, linguistic, and ethnic groups. When working with people from culturally and linguistically diverse backgrounds, one must be aware of their belief systems, language differences, socioeconomic class, religion, gender, age, and sexual orientation. Such variables play a significant role in the provision and delivery of services to different groups of clients and provide clinicians with the opportunity to work with this unique population.

One of the major barriers in working with diverse groups is the clinician's limited understanding of how different cultures view disability. Medical, educational, and rehabilitation approaches for disabled individuals in this country place particular emphasis on individuality and equality, as profiled by the Americans with Disabilities Act. Individuals accessing such systems are drawn into a structure which is based on the beliefs and values of the majority, leaving little if any room for cultural differences. Unfortunately, without flexibility for negotiation, needy families and individuals may "opt out" of a system that is unfamiliar and foreign to them. Service delivery models incongruous with cultural beliefs are often why some individuals do not access readily available rehabilitative care. Being familiar with a client's belief system and the expectations of the service provider is of utmost importance.

An individual presenting with a disability is viewed differently across cultural groups. Some Chinese believe that, in a few cases, a child born with a disability is the result of the mother's behaviors during pregnancy. For example, a pregnant woman is warned against using sharp objects such as needles or scissors in bed for fear of bearing a child with a cleft palate. Similarly, looking at disabled individuals or animals will result in a child with a disability. Juarbe (1996) reported that in the Puerto Rican culture the mother may be blamed for not having taken proper care of herself during pregnancy. In other cultures, a handicapping condition is one that is "pre-determined" so that little can be done to reverse the situation. In fact, Central Americans view such a child as God's will (Boyle, 1996).

In cases of dysphagia where oral intake of food is prohibited for safety reasons, non-compliance might stem from the belief system of the family. The Chinese believe that food is the source of *chi* or "strength" and that strength is necessary for recovery from illness.

Awareness of cultural differences becomes evident during interviews and counseling sessions with clients. Clinicians should be prepared to spend time learning about a client's cultural and linguistic background and, at the same time, provide an opportunity for the client to become comfortable with the clinician. Avoiding technical language is useful in this respect. On occasion, despite the clinician's sensitivity, there are clients who simply feel "ill at ease" about revealing personal and confidential information about themselves to a stranger, especially to some-one of a different cultural or ethnic background. In such situations, maintaining a professional and consistent demeanor will help ease some of the concerns. Finally, one must be cautioned about *over*-emphasizing cultural or linguistic differences as being the explanation of a client's problems, thus running the risk of missing the real problem (Helman, 1994). Clinicians must consider the client's presenting symptoms in the context of culture and whether such behaviors are problematic within that context. Dialectal variation in a client's speech is an illustration of such a situation. Another would be the diagnosis of dyslexia. For Chinese readers, assessment of a reading problem cannot be based on knowledge about reading of alphabetic script such as English. Instead, attention must be given to specific features of writing that are likely to be affected following brain injury (Eng, 2002). Helman and others also challenge clinicians to determine whether presenting problems are the result of differences in communication or disorders in the communication process.

THE ROLE OF LANGUAGE IN PERSONS WITH COMMUNICATION DISORDERS

WORKING WITH BILINGUAL or non-English-speaking clients who present with a communication disorder requires extensive assessment in order to consider the impact of another language. Most of our knowledge about communication disorders, to date, has been based on speakers of English. In some situations, such knowledge and information can be generalized to linguistically diverse groups. However, the very notion of differences among languages triggers concern.

To illustrate, a client with dyslexia would present differently, depending on the writing system that he uses. Spanish, for example, has a highly consistent sound-to-letter-correspondence. This means that words can be easily decoded. By contrast, the Chinese writing system offers very few cues as to the pronunciation of written characters. This means that readers rely on skills such as visual memory and visual discrimination in the identification of printed words.

Because of the interplay among variables, such as age of second language learning, amount of exposure to different languages and code-switching, attitude towards different languages, and degree of literacy in each language, each factor must be considered in understanding a client's communication disorder. This begins by obtaining a bilingual assessment of the client's language abilities (Haynes & Pindozola, 2004). The American Speech-Language-Hearing Association (ASHA) has put forth position statements regarding the value of a comprehensive assessment of a client's language abilities. Assessment of communication and

ASHA

language skills must reflect language- and culture-specific features that separate one language and culture from another. Although there are not standardized tests available for every language, it is not appropriate to use an existing test translated into a different language. For example, English does not make a distinction between "feminine" and "masculine" nouns, unlike languages such as Spanish, French, and Italian. Merely translating an existing language evaluation from English into a different language would be fruitless and would not allow for a comprehensive assessment of the person's language skills.

Nonetheless, there are acceptable means of collecting information on the language behavior of non-English speakers. ASHA's most recent position paper (2004) regarding the knowledge and skills of clinicians working with such persons proposes that a clinician must be well versed in typical communication patterns and atypical manifestations in different cultural and linguistic populations.

PSYCHOLOGICAL AND VOCATIONAL IMPLICATIONS

A S HUMAN COMMUNICATION is central to an individual's feelings of well-being, a disruption in this ability has a significant impact on daily living. Most obvious is the limitation imposed on the ability of a person to express his wants and needs and to hear and understand the messages of others. When these difficulties are compounded by a swallowing disorder or even when difficulty with swallowing occurs in isolation, an individual's feelings of well-being and the ability to participate in all the vocational, social, and family events that take place around the ingestion of foods and liquids are disturbed. Individuals recount experiences of social isolation. Body image and physical vulnerability take on new importance since swallowing, a function so basic to living, is now fraught with difficulties.

The emotional reactions to a communication and/or swallowing disability depend upon a variety of factors, including its severity, its chronicity, and the extent of organic sequelae. Vocational expectations and pursuits may be jeopardized as a consequence of the disability. The personality style and coping patterns of the individual, as well as the acceptance and coping styles of significant others, will affect the psychological well-being of the client.

A severe communication disability frequently produces a strong emotional response from the impaired individual. For example, in receptive aphasia with auditory comprehension deficits, paranoia may develop around the individual's lack of verbal understanding. On the other hand, expressive aphasia may be accompanied by an agitated depression punctuated by explosive outbursts. Often, persons with severe cognitive impairments will have difficulty in making sense of their environment, as well as their disability and its impact on their lives. In addition, a severe dysarthric who is unable to produce even a single word yet has complete and accurate comprehension will experience a high degree of anxiety and anger. The swallowing-impaired individual may become withdrawn and depressed, refusing to attempt any nutrition by mouth when in the company of other people. At times, a catastrophic reaction to frustration and anger is seen with all of these disabilities.

Depending on the rate and extent of recovery, emotional reactions may lessen with improvement or become more intense and culminate in a depressive state should gains not meet the expectations and needs of the individual. Attainment of a productive vocational role is highly integrated into the individual's perception of recovery. Many become depressed and discouraged when the reality of a slow, painstaking, and typically incomplete recovery has to be faced, along with the awareness that complete restoration of function may never occur.

Significant issues of loss and mourning are noted in individuals with communication deficits and swallowing impairment secondary to chronic degenerative conditions and other neurological impairments. These reactions can be exacerbated by lack of productive employment. In some cases, the reactions of an individual to a stroke can be similar to that associated with bereavement or terminal illness, showing the stages of denial, anger, depression, and eventual acceptance.

In cases of head trauma, organically based psychological and behavioral deficits impact on one's ability to engage in interpersonal interaction and affect premorbid work and family roles. Posttraumatic psychosocial difficulties can represent a continuation or intensification of premorbid personality and behavioral patterns. Individuals who suffer head trauma report complaints of slowness, forgetfulness, excessive irritability, lability, fatigue, hypersensitivity, reduced frustration tolerance, anxiety, and depression (Ponsford, 1990). Such behavioral changes have been identified as elements commonly responsible for job loss in this population. The marked and persistent cognitive deficits following head injury limit the individual's return to premorbid employment and ability to develop new work roles. As a result, many head-injured clients are in a double-bind situation: they are faced with long-term and frequently permanent stressors without adequate personal coping resources (Myers, 1983; Moore, Stambrook & Peters, 1988).

The onset of a hearing loss forces an individual to make adjustments in interpersonal relationships, social activities, and vocational plans. Extra effort and an increase in visual awareness are required to follow a conversation. Anxiety results from a fear of misunderstanding what has been said. People with impaired hearing may also feel embarrassed by callous comments made by others. Hearing disability frequently becomes a factor affecting major life decisions concerning vocation, marriage, or retirement plans. Adults in the work force worry about the possibility of making costly errors, being unable to handle job demands, or meeting eligibility for career advancement. Employers may stereotype the hearing-impaired into work roles that are isolated and require minimal communication with others. Careful reevaluation of job tasks will frequently identify methods of modification that will compensate for the hearing loss (Schien, 1982).

The Americans with Disabilities Act (ADA) requires most employers to provide reasonable accommodations for the hearing-disabled person (e.g., devices such as the TDD, assistive listening devices, and amplifiers). Such adaptations, combined with consideration of the acoustic environment in the work setting, allow an individual to operate at his or her optimal potential.

The person who was born with or acquired a hearing loss prelingually may not feel the same sense of loss as would a postlingually deafened adult, nor experience the major life changes of an acquired disorder and the related denial and grieving period. On the other hand, an adult who loses all usable hearing will feel a great sense of loss and will go through the stages of grief mentioned earlier. The severely hard-of-hearing or deaf person may become isolated from colleagues at work and from neighbors. Most social contacts depend on quick, easy exchanges. When conversations have to be repeated or written out, frustration prevails.

The ability to return to work will affect overall adjustment to the disability. Not only is vocational satisfaction highly integrated with issues of self-esteem, it also has significant economic ramifications. Vocational outcomes are influenced by the nature and severity of the disability, the cognitive and communicative requirements of the job tasks, the work environment, and the individual's vocational expectations. Identification of appropriate vocational pursuits requires careful analysis of job tasks, the work setting, and the communication demands. Does the job require speech? Is auditory or reading comprehension an integral component? Is normal hearing required for safety or co-worker interaction? Is the individual required to put thoughts into written or verbal expression? Is a high level of memory or problem solving required? Following such a task analysis, the client's deficits and strengths are compared with the demands of the job. When there is a conflict between work requirements and the individual's abilities, methods of compensation for communication or cognitive deficits are explored. It is important to consider not only the feasibility of such compensation but also the ability of the environment to accept such adaptation. The work setting might be required to support additional equipment (e.g., augmentative systems or TDD) or methods (e.g., structured work lists or supervision), as well as provide social and emotional acceptance of such adaptations.

The personality characteristics that a communicatively or swallowing impaired individual brings to the disability will have a significant impact on the adjustment to the deficits and the subsequent life changes. Such life changes are highly integrated with the expectations of significant others and must be incorporated into the treatment process. Being able to modify expectations, develop new goals that incorporate the disability, alter family roles and vocational responsibilities, and apply socially acceptable defenses and behaviors are crucial components for a successful recovery from a speech, language, swallowing, or hearing disability.

REFERENCES

Adamovich, B. L. (1997). Traumatic brain injury. In L. LaPointe (Ed.), *Aphasia and related neurogenic language disorders* (2nd ed., pp. 226–237). New York: Thieme.

American Speech-Language-Hearing Association. (2004, April). Knowledge and skills needed by speech-language pathologists and audiologists to provide culturally and linguistically appropriate services. *ASHA, 24*(suppl.), 152–158.

Bayles, K. A. (1994). Management of neurogenic communication disorders associated with dementia. In R. Chapey (Ed.), *Language intervention strategies in adult aphasia* (2nd ed., pp. 540–543). Baltimore: Williams and Wilkins.

Bayles, K. A., Tomoeda, C. K., & Trosset, M. W. (1992). Relation of linguistic communication abilities of Alzheimer's patients to stage of disease. *Brain and Language, 42*, 454–472.

Benson, V., & Marano, M. (1995). Current estimates from the National Health Interview Survey, 1993. In *Vital and Health Statistics, Series 10*(190). National Center for Health Statistics.

Boothroyd, A., Geers, A. E., & Moog, J. S. (1991). Practical implications of cochlear implants in children. *Ear and Hearing, 12*(Suppl. 290), 815–895.

Boyle, J. S. (1996). Central Americans. In J. Lipson, S. Dibble, & P. Minarik (Eds.), *Culture and nursing care: A pocket guide* (pp. 222–238). San Francisco: UCSF Nursing Press.

Chapey, R., & Hallowell, B. (2001). Introduction to language intervention strategies in adult aphasia. In R. Chapey (Ed.), *Language intervention strategies in aphasia and related neurogenic communication disorders* (4th ed., pp. 12–13). Philadelphia: Lippincott, Williams and Wilkins.

Colton, R., H., & Casper, J. K. (1990). *Understanding voice problems: A physiological perspective for diagnosis and treatment.* Baltimore: Williams and Wilkins.

Cook, I., & Kahrilas, P. (1990). AGA technical review on management of oropharyngeal dysphagia. *Gastroenterology, 116*, 455–478.

Darley, F., Aronson, A. W., & Brown, J. R. (1975). *Motor speech disorders*. Philadelphia: W. B. Saunders.

Davis, G. A. (1993). *A survey of adult aphasia and related language disorders*. Englewood Cliffs, NJ: Prentice Hall.

Dikeman, K., & Kazandjian, M. (2003). *Communication and swallowing management of tracheostomized and ventilator-dependent adults* (2nd ed.). San Diego, CA: Singular Publishing Group.

Duffy, J. R. (1995). *Motor speech disorders: Substrates, differential diagnosis, and management*. St. Louis, MO: Mosby.

Echelard, P.D., Thoppil, E., & Melvin, J. (1984). *Rehabilitation of dysphagia*. Paper presented at the American Congress of Rehabilitation Medicine, Boston.

Eng, N. (2002). Acquired dyslexia in a biscript reader following traumatic brain injury: A second case. *Topics in Language Disorders, 22*(5), 5–19.

English, G. M. (1976). *Otolaryngology*. New York: Harper and Row.

Feinberg, M., Ekberg, O., Segall, L., & Tully, J. (1992). Deglutition in elderly patients with dementia: Findings of videofluorographic evaluation and impact on staging and management. *Radiology, 183*, 811–814.

Felt, P. (1999). The national dysphagia diet project: The science and practice. *Nutrition in Clinical Practice, 14*(Suppl.), 455–478.

Goodglass, H., Kaplan, E., & Barresi, B. (2001). *The assessment of aphasia and related disorders*. New York: Lippincott Williams and Wilkins.

Gordon, C., Hewer, R. L., & Wade, D. T. (1987). Dysphagia in acute stroke. *British Journal of Medicine, 295*, 411–414.

Groher, M., (1997). *Dysphagia: Diagnosis and management* (3rd ed.). Boston: Butterworth-Heinemann.

Groher, M. E., & Bukatman, R. (1986). The prevalence of swallowing disorders in two teaching hospitals. *Dysphagia, 1*, 3–6.

Guitar, B. (1998). *Stuttering: An integrated approach to its nature and treatment* (2nd ed.). New York: Lippincott, Williams and Wilkins.

Hartford, E. R. (1988). Hearing aid selection for adults. In M. Pollack (Ed.), *Amplification for the hearing impaired* (3rd ed., pp. 175–210). Orlando, FL: Statton.

Haynes, W. O., & Pindozola, R. H. (2004). *Diagnosis and evaluation in speech pathology* (6th ed.). Boston: Pearson Allyn and Bacon.

Helman, C. (1994). *Culture, health and illness* (3rd ed.). Oxford, England: Butterworth Heinemann.

Hoffman, S., Platt, C. A., & Barry, K. E. (1988). Comforting the confused: The importance of non-verbal communication in the care of people with Alzheimer's disease. *American Journal of Alzheimer's Care and Related Disorders and Research, 3*(1), 25–30.

Holland, A. L., & Reinmuth, O. M. (2002). Aphasia and related acquired language disorders. In G. H. Shames & N. B. Anderson (Eds.), *Human communication disorders: An introduction* (6th ed., pp. 510–544).

Jones, B., & Donner, M. (1988). Examination of the patient with dysphagia. *Radiology, 167*(2), 319–326.

Juarbe, T. (1996). Puerto Ricans. In J. Lipson, S. Dibble, & P. Minarik (Eds.), *Culture and nursing care: A pocket guide* (pp. 222–238). San Francisco: UCSF Nursing Press.

Katz, J. (2001). *Handbook of clinical audiology* (5th ed.). Philadelphia: Lippincott, Williams and Wilkins.

Kearns, K. P. (1997). Broca's aphasia. In L. LaPointe (Ed.), *Aphasia and related neurologic language disorders* (2nd ed., pp. 1–41). New York: Thieme.

Kerman-Lerner, P. (1988). Communication disorders. In J. Goodgold (Ed.), *Rehabilitation medicine* (pp. 681–714). St. Louis, MO: C. V. Mosby.

Klonoff, H., & Paris, R. (1974). Immediate, short-term and residual effects of acute head injury in children: Neuropsychological and neurological correlates. *Clinical neuropsychology: Current trends and applications.* Washington, DC: V. H. Winston.

Kraus, J. F., & McArthur, D. L. (1996). Epidemiologic aspects of brain injury. *Neurologic Clinics, 14*(2), 435–450.

LaPointe, L. (1997). *Aphasia and related neurogenic language disorders* (2nd ed.). New York: Thieme.

Lazarus, C., & Logemann, J. A. (1987). Swallowing disorders in closed head trauma patients. *Archives of Physical Medicine and Rehabilitation, 68*, 79–84.

Leary, M., & Saver, I. (2003). Annual incidence of first silent stroke in the United States. *Cerebrovascular Disease, 16*, 280–285.

Lerner, P., & Hauck, K. (1999). Speech, language, hearing, and swallowing disorders. In M. Eisenberg, R. Glueckauf, & H. Zaretsky (Eds.), *Medical aspects of disability* (2nd ed., pp. 245–272). New York: Springer Publishing Co.

Logemann, J. (1998). *Evaluation and treatment of swallowing disorders* (2nd ed.). Austin, TX: Pro-ed.

Martin, F. N. (1986). *Introduction to audiology* (3rd ed.). Englewood Cliffs, NJ: Prentice-Hall.

Miller, E. (1984). *Recovery and management of neuropsychological impairments.* New York: John Riley.

Miller, R. M., Groher, M., Yorkston, K. M., & Rees, T. S. (1988). Speech, language, swallowing and auditory rehabilitation in rehabilitation medicine. In J. A. DeLisa (Ed.), *Principles and practice* (pp. 118–134). Philadelphia: J. B. Lippincott.

Moore, A. D., Stambrook, M., & Peters, L. C. (1988). Coping strategies and adjustment after closed-head injury. A cluster analytical approach. *Brain Injury, 3*(2), 171–175.

Myers, P. S. (1983). Right hemisphere communication disorders. In W. H. Perkins (Ed.), *Current therapy in communication disorders* (pp. 213–229). New York: Thieme-Stratton.

Myers, P. S. (1997). Right hemisphere syndrome. In L. LaPointe (Ed.), *Aphasia and related neurologic language disorders* (2nd ed., pp. 201–225). New York: Thieme.

National Institute on Deafness and Other Communication Disorders, Better Hearing Institute. (1999). Bethesda, MD.

National Institute on Neurological Disorders and Stroke. (1990). *Aphasia: Hope through research* (pub. no. 90-391). Bethesda, MD.

Paparella, M., DaCosta, S., Fox, R., & Yoon, T. H. (1991). Meniere's disease and other labyrinthine diseases. In M. M. Paparella, D. A. Shumrick, J. C. Gluckman, & J. L. Meyerhoff (Eds.), *Otolaryngology* (3rd ed, pp. 291–321). New York: W. B. Saunders.

Ponsford, J. L. (1990). Psychological sequelae of closed-head injury: Time to redress the imbalance. *Brain Injury, 4*(2), 111–114.

Preves, D. A., & Dempesy, D. (2000). Speech recognition in noise results for a disposable hearing aid. *Hearing Review, 7,* 34, 36, 38.

Rademaker, A. W., Logemann, J. A., Pauloski, B. R., Bowman, J., Lazarus, C., Sisson, G., et al. (1993). Recovery of postoperative swallowing in patients undergoing partial laryngectomy. *Head and Neck, 15,* 325–334.

Rosenbek, J. C., & LaPointe, L. L. (1982). A physiological approach to the dysarthrias. *Journal of Speech and Hearing Disorders, 47*(3), 334.

Sammeth, C. A. (1990). Current availability of digital and hybrid hearing aids. *Seminars in Hearing, 11,* 91–100.

Sataloff, J. (1966). *Hearing loss.* Toronto, Ontario, Canada: J. B. Lippincott.

Schein, J. (1982). Group techniques applied to deaf and hearing impaired persons. In M. Seligman (Ed.), *Group psychotherapy and counseling with special populations* (pp. 143–161). Baltimore: University Park Press.

Schein, J., & Miller, M. (1990). Diagnosis and rehabilitation of auditory disorders. In F. J. Kottke & J. F. Lehmann (Eds.), *Krusen's handbook of physical medicine and rehabilitation* (3rd ed., pp. 935–966). Philadelphia: W. B. Saunders.

Simmons, K. (1986). Multidisciplinary approach aids successful swallowing. *Journal of the American Medical Association, 255,* 3209–3212.

Staller, S. I., Dowell, R. C., Beiter, A. L., & Brimcombe, I. A. (1991). Perceptual abilities of children with the Nucleus 22-Channel Cochlear Implant. *Ear and Hearing, 12*(4), 345–475.

Stierwalt, J. A. G., Clark, H. M., & Robin, D. A. (2000). Aphasia and related disorders. In J. B. Tomblin, H. L. Morris, & D. C. Spriestersbach (Eds.), *Diagnosis in speech-language pathology* (2nd ed., pp. 315–336).

Tennant, A., Macdermott, N., & Neary, D. (1995). The long-term outcome of head injury: implications for service planning. *Brain Injury, 9,* 595–605.

Tucker, H. M. (1980). Vocal cord paralysis—Etiology and management. *Laryngoscope, 90,* 585–590.

Veis, S. L., & Logemann, J. A. (1985). Swallowing disorders in persons with cerebrovascular accident. *Archives of Physical Medicine and Rehabilitation, 66,* 372–375.

Wingate, M. E. (1959). Calling attention to stuttering. *Journal of Speech and Hearing Research, 2,* 326–335.

Ylvisaker, M. S., & Szekeres, S. F. (1986). Management of the patient with closed head injury. In R. Chapey (Ed.), *Language intervention strategies in adult aphasia* (pp. 474–490).Baltimore: Williams & Wilkins.

Yorkston, K. M., Beukelman, D., & Bell, K. (1988). *Clinical management of dysarthria speakers*. San Diego, CA: College Hill.

Zwolan, T. A. (2001). Cochlea implants. In J. Katz (Ed.), *Handbook of clinical audiology* (5th ed., pp. 740–768). New York: Lippincott, Williams and Wilkins.

13

Hematological Disorders

BRUCE G. RAPHAEL, MD

N ORMAL BLOOD CELLS are produced in the bone marrow. A resting stem cell or progenitor cell will, under appropriate stimulus, divide and mature into the various blood cells. These include the red blood cells that carry oxygen to the tissues, the white blood cells that help fight infection, and the platelets, which are the blood-clotting cells. The white blood cells are further divided into a variety of cell types. The two most important white blood cell types are granulocytes, which fight bacterial infection, and lymphocytes, which make the antibodies, control the immune reactions, and help with viral infections. Cancers that develop because of abnormal proliferation of the white blood cells are called leukemia and lymphoma.

LYMPHOMA

DISEASE DESCRIPTION

LYMPHOMAS ARE A malignant proliferation of one of the white blood cell types, lymphocytes, which are divided into B lymphocytes and T lymphocytes. B lymphocytes are cells that go through a complicated maturation process in which only a portion of the genetic material that codes for antibody production is activated, so each B cell produces a single antibody against a specific foreign protein. T lymphocytes go through similar maturation, with activation of other portions of genetic

Lymphomas B and T

T - cells
helper cells
or suppressor

lymphoma - tumor

material. These cells then specialize in helping (helper cells) or suppressing (suppressor cells) the immune reaction. Once formed, these cells migrate to the lymph nodes, and when exposed to a foreign protein or an infectious agent, those lymphocytes programmed to make the specific antibody against the abnormal antigen will divide, enlarge, and multiply, producing large numbers of cells and antibodies to neutralize the invading organism. The T helper cells will aid this reaction. When the organism is cleared, T suppressor cells will inhibit the immune reaction, and the swollen lymph gland will shrink back to the quiescent state (Skarin, 1989).

When one of the maturing and dividing lymphocytes undergoes malignant change and divides uncontrollably, an accumulation of these cells occurs as a tumor, called a lymphoma. The cause of this malignant change is unknown, but certain viruses, the Epstein-Barr virus and T cell lymphotrophic virus, have been implicated in a small number of B and T cell lymphomas, respectively. Additionally, chromosomal breaks that occur during the division and maturation of each individual lymphocyte can lead to mutations of genes involved in proliferation and to uncontrolled growth (Williams, Butler, Erslev, & Lichtman, 1990). Three percent of all cancers in the United States result from lymphomas, with 70%–80% of B-cell origin and the rest derived from T cells (Skarin, 1989). There is a rising incidence of aggressive lymphoma in acquired immune deficiency syndrome (AIDS) patients and in patients on immunosuppressive drugs (i.e., post transplant state). The speculative cause of these lymphomas is excessive immune stimulation of B lymphocytes with chromosomal breaks and poor immune surveillance by the reduced T lymphocytes, which are destroyed by the AIDS virus (Raphael & Knowles, 1990).

PATHOLOGY

THE LYMPHOMAS ARE all classified by the appearance of malignant lymphocytes on biopsy of the tumor. As stated earlier, normal lymphocytes go through various stages of maturation. A lymphoma is an accumulation of malignant lymphocytes that are arrested at one stage of maturation. Clinical behavior of the tumor is often correlated with the level of maturation of abnormal lymphocytes. Hence, a recent classification of lymphomas is divided into three categories: (a) low, (b) intermediate, and (c) high grade (Rosenberg, 1982) (see Table 13.1). Low-grade lymphomas contain cells that are smaller, slower growing, and often asymptomatic. Intermediate-grade lymphomas have cells that are larger and faster growing. High-grade lymphomas are very fast growing, immature lymphocytes, which often present in extranodal as well as nodal tissues. Additionally, the tumor can present in a nodular (follicular) pat-

TABLE 13.1   Classifications of Lymphoma

Low grade
  Malignant lymphoma, small lymphocytic
  Malignant lymphoma, follicular, predominantly small cleaved cell
  Malignant lymphoma, follicular, mixed small and large cell

Intermediate grade
  Malignant lymphoma, follicular, predominantly large cell
  Malignant lymphoma, diffuse, mixed small and large cell
  Malignant lymphoma, diffuse large cell cleaved

High grade
  Diffuse large cell, immunoblastic
  Malignant lymphoma, lymphoblastic
  Malignant lymphoma, small noncleaved cell

tern or diffusely, replacing the architecture of the lymph node. Slower growth is associated with the former pattern, and more aggressive behavior is related to the latter (Rosenberg, 1982).

FUNCTIONAL PRESENTATION

PATIENTS PRESENT WITH swollen, growing lymph glands (nodal disease) or tumors in other organs (extranodal disease). Patients can be asymptomatic (A) or have one or more of the B symptoms, which include fever, drenching night sweats, loss of 10% of body weight, and pruritus. A staging evaluation is done to determine the extent of disease. This includes a proper physical examination to determine any lymph node group that is enlarged or any abnormal organ enlargement. Additionally, CT scans of chest, abdomen, and pelvis are done to determine internal organ and nodal involvement. A bone marrow biopsy is used to examine for bone marrow involvement by lymphoma. In the high-grade lymphomas, the central nervous system is more often involved, and spinal fluid analysis is required. Positive emission tomography (PET) scans have recently been added to the evaluation of lymphomas. Radioactive sugar is given intravenously, tumor cells use the sugar as fuel, and the cells accumulate radioactivity. The amount of activity can be followed during and after chemotherapy to determine completeness of response to therapy (Friedberg & Chengazi, 2003). The stage of disease is then determined by the number of lymph nodes involved and presence of disease in other organs (Table 13.2); once the type of lymphoma is known and patient stage and clinical presentation are determined, a decision on treatment can be made.

TABLE 13.2   Staging of Lymphoma

Stage	Characteristics
1	Involvement of a single lymph node region or single extra modal organ or site
2	Involvement limited to one side of the diaphragm with two or more lymph node regions
3	Involvement of lymph node regions on both sides of the diaphragm
4	Diffuse or disseminated involvement of one or more extralymphatic organs

TREATMENT AND PROGNOSIS

THE VAST MAJORITY of lymphomas present in multiple areas of the body, Stage 3 or 4, as the abnormal lymphocytes are free to travel to other areas of the body through the blood. Hence, localized treatment with surgery or radiation is rarely curative (Ruthoven, 1987; Skarin, 1989). Treatment is, therefore, primarily chemotherapy, in which chemicals are used to poison the growing malignant cells. Lymphomas are very sensitive to chemotherapy, but no drug is specific for only the tumor cell. This leads to the side effects of chemotherapy: normal-growing cells are affected as well as specific organs that are sensitive to the toxic effects of these agents. The disability that patients experience may in part be due to the presence of the tumor in a disease site, and alternatively may be related to the side effects of the chemotherapy. Prognosis is dependent on the grade and stage of the lymphoma. In general, the earlier the stage tumors (1 or 2) are more curable than more extensive disease as in later stage (3 or 4) lymphoma.

Additionally, other prognostic variables have been determined, including bulky disease of greater than 10-cm mass; performance status, which refers to degree of debilitation and symptoms; bone marrow and central nervous system involvement; and high level of lactic dehydrogenase, which is an enzyme correlated with rapid growth. Low-grade lymphomas can be controlled for many years, with average survival of 7 years, but are rarely curable (Skarin, 1989). The intermediate lymphomas now have a 50%–70% cure rate, depending on stage and prognostic factors, using combinations of multiple chemotherapy agents (Skarin; Williams et al., 1990). High-grade lymphomas are treated with intensive doses of chemotherapy, leading to a 30% cure rate but often to rapid death within a year for those who relapse (Skarin, 1989). In addition to chemotherapy and external irradiation to shrink disease, in the last 5 years biologic agents have been added to treatment regimens. These include manufactured antibodies directed at proteins on the cancer cell that attack the tumor cells directly, antibodies that are conjugated with a radioactive substance or toxin allowing preferential targeting of the tumor, and producing a vaccine from the tumor cells that stimulate an immune reaction by the patient against the cancer cell. It is hoped that these new agents when added to existing chemotherapeutic protocols can either cure or control the lymphoma growth (Berdeja, 2003).

For patients who do not respond to primary treatment, bone marrow transplantation is increasingly used. High-dose chemotherapy is used to kill the lymphoma that was resistant to conventional treatment. The bone marrow from the patient (autologous transplant) or from a tissue-matched relative (allogeneic transplant) is stored away before the procedure and given back to rescue the patient from the lethal effects on the bone marrow of high-dose chemotherapy. Other organs are damaged during the intensive therapy, infections are frequent, and immune suppressive drugs are sometimes needed. The result is a prolonged hospital stay with multiple complications and a lengthy recovery period requiring rehabilitation. Biological agents, such as antibodies that attack the tumor cells directly, as well as vaccine therapy that induces the body to make an immune reaction against the tumor cells, are now being tested as additional therapy to rid the body of residual tumor (Hsu et al., 1997).

LEUKEMIA

DISEASE DESCRIPTION

ACUTE LEUKEMIA IS characterized by an abnormal proliferation of immature white blood cells. As stated earlier, lymphoma represents an accumulation of lymphocytes arrested at one stage of maturation; leukemia is the accumulation of the earliest white blood cells, called blasts or progenitor cells. These cells normally divide and mature into the normal white cells that help fight infections, and they are continually renewed. Hence, the effect of lack of maturation is the presence of large numbers of these young cells in the bone marrow and lack of normal bone marrow cells. Patients then present with signs and symptoms of low red blood cell count (anemia), decreased white blood cells (granulocytopenia) with infection and fever, and a low platelet count (thrombocytopenia) with bleeding. Additionally, infiltration of various organs by these tumor cells can lead to enlargement of liver, spleen, and lymph nodes, as well as to gum hypertrophy and skin nodules.

The incidence of acute leukemia is 9 cases per 100,000 individuals, and the incidence rises with age (DeVita, Hellman, & Rosenberg, 1989). Unlike some other tumors, however, acute leukemia occurs in childhood and is the most common childhood malignancy. There are two main forms of acute leukemia: acute lymphoblastic leukemia (ALL) is a cancer of the earliest stages of lymphocyte maturation, and acute non-lymphoblastic leukemia (ANLL) usually is a malignancy of the progenitor of the granulocyte series called the myeloblast. ALL occurs more often in the young; ANLL is more common with adults. Cytogenetic studies show a variety of chromosomal breaks and mutations associated with different types of leukemia. The proteins encoded by these mutated genes cause dysregulation of division and maturation and hence accumulation of myeloblasts or lymphoblasts (Berman, 1997).

PATHOLOGY

PATIENTS' ROUTINE BLOOD tests show low blood counts (pancytopenia) and/or early white cell forms (blasts). Bone marrow analysis shows a hypercellular specimen with almost complete replacement by early white cell forms. Only a few remaining normally maturing blood cells can be found. The cells are analyzed by morphology, staining characteristics, biochemistry, and immunologic typing to differentiate between ANLL and ALL. Additionally, infiltration by leukemic cells may be detected in a variety of sites, such as gums, skin, lymph nodes, liver, and lungs.

FUNCTIONAL PRESENTATION

PATIENTS WITH LYMPHOMA present with tumor and related symptoms, but they generally have adequate normal blood cells and can tolerate chemotherapy as outpatients. Patients with acute leukemia usually present critically, with signs and symptoms of lack of normal blood elements. If they present late in the course of the disease, the white blood cell counts are high because the leukemic cells have multiplied and spilled into the blood, or there is organ dysfunction due to infiltration by the tumor cells. Hence, patients are admitted immediately and stabilized by correcting the anemia with red blood cell transfusions, treating any uncontrolled infection resulting from lack of mature white blood cells, stopping any bleeding with platelet transfusions, and starting chemotherapy to kill the leukemia cells. Although treatment for ANLL differs from treatment for ALL, the principle is the same. Induction therapy involves large doses of chemotherapy to poison the tumor cells (Gale & Foon, 1987; Hoelzer & Gale, 1987). However, these drugs are toxic to all blood cells, resulting in the death of the few remaining normal bone marrow cells and the development of aplasia in the bone marrow. Once chemotherapy stops and tumor cells die, the normal stem cells in the marrow that are resistant to chemotherapy divide, and their progeny cells mature and repopulate the marrow over the next 3 weeks. Until sufficient cells grow to produce the necessary mature, functioning peripheral blood cells, the patient is very sick and must receive antibiotics, fluids, and transfusions on a daily basis. Remissions occur in up to 80% of cases, but relapses are the rule, and additional consolidation chemotherapy is given after recovery to prevent recurrence (Gale & Foon; Hoelzer & Gale). The repetitive chemotherapy injury further slows recovery, adds days of admissions to the hospital, and results in more disability.

Furthermore, the chemotherapy drugs are toxic to other organs as well as bone marrow. Myopathy caused by steroids and neurotoxicity from the drug vincristine is common in the treatment of ALL. Heart damage from anthracycline chemotherapy drugs and fluid overload due to multiple intravenous fluids and transfusions are common to all patients. Finally, nausea, mouth sores, and gastric irritation are typical with this type of chemotherapy, making adequate nutritional intake difficult and further adding to the general level of debilitation. In cases of relapse, as well as in some experimental protocols for patients in remission, bone marrow transplantation is offered as a way of using very high doses of chemotherapy to rid the body of any remaining leukemia cells and to prevent any further relapses (Williams et al., 1990). The physical problems secondary to this intensive therapy are multiplied compared to conventional therapy. Hence, patients with leukemia face months of treatment and weeks of hospitalization with each treatment. The resulting physical, psychological, and financial toll is substantial.

PSYCHOLOGICAL AND VOCATIONAL IMPLICATIONS

A FURTHER DISCUSSION of the relationship of cancer and psychosocial adaptation will be found in another chapter in this book. However, several points that are unique to lymphoma and leukemia will be discussed here.

As stated earlier, lymphoma and leukemia affect a wider age range than do most cancers, and the psychosocial implications will vary with age. Younger adults ages 18 to 36 with leukemia and lymphoma were surveyed by Daiter et al. (Daiter, Larson, Weddington, & Ultmann, 1988). As might be expected, patients with less favorable prognoses experienced more stress but also significant personal growth and maturation. Additionally, family and friends who provided social support reported not only more stress when dealing with the sicker patient with poor prognosis but also sometimes expressed more prolonged anxiety after treatment was completed than did the patient. Psychological stress has been reported to be lower for leukemia than for breast cancer. Treatment with chemotherapy and radiation to young age patients with acute leukemia, particularly ALL, may add developmental disability to the list of long-term deficits. There is up to a 30% risk of school-related problems especially in those patients treated for central nervous system involvement (Mulhern, Friedman, & Stone, 1988). Adolescents require different types of support and negotiating treatment is more demanding (Penson et al., 2002).

Older patients have additional concerns about financial matters, how their spouses and children are coping and functioning, and interpersonal relationships at work. Depression, sleep disorder, and anxiety over personal appearance are common. Long-term survivors also have persistent problems; one study reported 73% of patients with Hodgkin's disease having at least one of five problems including decreased energy level, negative body image, depression, employment problems, and marital problems (Fobair et al., 1986). Additionally, the rising incidence of leukemia with age and secondary leukemia due to previous chemotherapy result in many difficult decisions concerning therapy and quality-of-life issues (Sekeres et al., 2004).

Finally, because bone marrow transplantation has become a common therapy for refractory lymphoma and leukemia, studies of the psychosocial morbidity of these procedures have been done. Jenkins, Linington, and Whittaker (1991) report a 40% prevalence of depression with impaired function, but most cases were temporary and resolved with resumption of normal activities and return to work. Wolcott, Wellisch, Fawzy, and Landsverk (1986) also reported that 15%–20% of bone marrow transplant recipients have a degree of psychological distress that would benefit from intervention. Somerfield et al. noted a list of most frequently endorsed fears of transplant patients, which included increased vulnerability to illness, uncertain future, reduced energy, and inability to have children (Somerfield, Curbow, Wingard, Baker, & Fogarty, 1996). Additionally, heightened concern over somatic symptoms leads to panic attacks that the cancer is returning. In particular, patients with continuing medical problems were more likely to need help. In addition to routine physical therapy, aerobic training has been tested in patients after high-dose chemotherapy and it reduced fatigue and enhanced physical performance (Dimeo et al., 1997).

In summary, patients with leukemia and lymphoma require intensive chemotherapy and, in some cases, repeated hospitalizations, which can lead to a host of psychological and vocational difficulties. Remarkably, most patients adapt well, but significant numbers may benefit from at least temporary counseling and rehabilitation services. Two recent studies show that recovery post bone marrow transplantation, both physical and emotional, is delayed with psychological symptoms persisting longer. Three to 5 years are required before most patients have fully recovered, and interventions such as physical, occupational, and psychological therapies are required to speed this process (Broers, Kaptein, Le Cessie, Fibbe, & Hengeveld, 2000; Skrjala et al., 2004).

DISORDERS OF HEMOSTASIS

HEMOSTASIS IS THE process by which blood clots in response to injury to the vessels. When a vessel is cut, it may constrict, reducing blood flow and bleeding. Platelets, the blood-clotting cells, then adhere to the open wound and clump together to form a plug. Coagulation factors are activated from an inactive proenzyme form, sequentially activating larger and larger numbers of other coagulation proteins until conversion of fibrinogen (Factor I) to fibrin occurs. Fibrin strands mesh with platelets, forming a stable clot that will not break down until the vessel repairs itself. Abnormal bleeding may occur when there is a defect in the number or function of the platelets or in any of the 13 coagulation factors. Hemophilia A and B are the most common congenital deficiencies of these plasma proteins, and we will discuss them in more detail as prototypes of a chronic bleeding disorder.

HEMOPHILIA

Disease Description

As stated previously, there are 13 coagulation factors. Factor XII is activated first, and then a series of factors are converted to their active form. This cascade of activation will be stopped or slowed if there is a deficiency of any one factor required to convert the next factor. Factor VIII is the most common congenital deficiency, accounting for 75% of hemophilias. It is a rare disease, however, with an incidence of 1 in 10,000 male births (Williams et al., 1990). A gene on the X chromosome encodes the protein; hence, males need inherit only one defective gene from the mother to be affected. Females, who have two X chromosomes, are rarely affected.

Hemophilia B, a deficiency of Factor IX, is also an X-linked recessive hemorrhagic disease. It occurs in 1 of 75,000 male births and clinically is indistinguishable from hemophilia A (Williams et al., 1990). The diagnosis of both of these disorders is made by functionally assaying the plasma for the level of either protein compared to normal plasma.

Functional Presentation

The genes controlling production of either Factor VIII or Factor IX may have one of many mutations. This can lead to no production, decreased production, or production of a defective protein. Hence, the patient can present with mild, moderate, or severe hemorrhagic disease, depending on the amount of active protein produced. Activity of the protein is measured in a timed clotting assay and compared to normal plasma. Mothers of hemophilia patients are obligate carriers and have 50% or greater activity. Mild hemophiliacs have 6%–25% activity, rarely bleed spontaneously, and usually are discovered after excessive bleeding secondary to trauma or surgery. Moderately affected individuals have 1%–5% levels of the active protein and have rare episodes of spontaneous bleeding but can hemorrhage with any trauma. Finally, patients with less than a 1% level have severe disease, with frequent spontaneous hemorrhage from early childhood (Williams et al., 1990). Patients can bleed anywhere, but bleeding into joints (hemarthrosis), soft tissue (such as muscle), urine (hematuria), and the brain are common. Chronic bleeding into joints or an acute bleed into the brain or spinal canal can lead to chronic disabilities, both functional and psychological.

Treatment and Prognosis

The general principle of treatment of hemophilia is, first, to avoid drugs that can interfere with clotting, particularly aspirin and other nonsteroidal anti-inflammatory agents that inhibit platelet function (Williams et al., 1990). Second, early recognition of bleeding episodes or potential trauma, and treatment with replacement Factor VIII or IX is imperative. Concentrates of these factors from normal plasma are commercially available. The number of units of coagulation protein infused depends on the initial level of the factor in the patient's plasma and the level of factor desired. Minor trauma or bleeding may require factor levels of only 20% of normal to stop bleeding, whereas major hemorrhage, especially intracranial, will require larger doses to raise levels of the factor to greater than 50% of normal (Kasper & Dietrich, 1985; Williams et al., 1990). If surgery is required, Factors VIII and IX must be raised before the operation. Because Factor VIII is degraded in the plasma, half the dose is gone in 8–12 hours; treatment is given every 12 hours for several days to allow healing and prevent late hemorrhage. Factor IX has a longer half-life, 18–24 hours, and reinfusion can take place less often.

Prognosis improved with the advent of factor concentrate treatment in the 1960s, with fewer severe bleeds, less crippling arthritis from hemarthrosis, and less intracranial bleeding. Complications of multiple transfusions, such as hepatitis and, more recently, AIDS, have greatly influenced the prognosis, however. Although new preparation techniques have eliminated the hepatitis and human immunodeficiency virus (HIV) from Factor VIII concentrates, many hemophiliacs, particularly those who are severely affected and who have had many transfusions, are infected by HIV and will ultimately die of AIDS. Additionally, because therapy has allowed normal growth and development, adult hemophiliacs are sexually active, and the risk of sexually transmitting the AIDS virus is problematic. New patients appear safe from transmission of these viruses because of the new concentrates, but it will be many years before the problem of transfusion-related viral infections in the older patients will disappear.

Psychological and Vocational Implications

The medical advancement of efficient factor replacement led to a great improvement in the psychosocial aspect of caring for hemophilia patients. A study from the Netherlands (Rosendall et al., 1990) showed that most patients consider their health and quality of life no different from that of the general population. Additionally, those who were employed had positions consistent with their education. In the older patient, however, joint damage correlated with increased disability and decrease in successful marriage and having children. Twenty-two percent of patients were unemployed and receiving some disability compensation. Vocational training should stress jobs that limit potentially hazardous situations. Patients who are on effective replacement therapy can compete equally for most jobs. It is clear that programs like home therapy slow the rate of progression of arthropathy, and most young hemophiliacs who are under appropriate medical care can and should be fully employed and leading normal lives.

However, the patients who were infected with the AIDS virus during therapy from 1980 to 1985 will require special psychological help and will experience greater disability. Social counseling for sexual partners is imperative. The impact of this tragic complication should be temporary as future patients are protected by the newer generation of coagulation factor replacement products.

SICKLE CELL DISEASE

Disease Description

Normal red blood cells have a biconcave shape with a pliable cell membrane and cytoplasm in the center filled with a protein called hemoglobin. This protein is a combination of two alpha-globin chains and two beta-globin chains (Hemoglobin A), forming a complex molecule that binds an iron containing heme molecule in the center, which allows the protein to bind oxygen. Hemoglobin is soluble in the cytoplasm, so the red cell shape can change and thereby squeeze through small vessels to deliver the oxygen to the tissues. Sickle cell disease occurs when the beta chain has one amino acid changed from a Glutamic acid to Valine in the sixth position of a 146-amino acid chain that makes up the beta globin protein molecule (Williams et al., 1990). This substitution of one amino acid for another results in another type of Hemoglobin S for sickle. Hemoglobin S has a conformation change producing stacking, forming a tubular insoluble structure, and causing the red cell to assume a nonpliable sickle shape. This process occurs only when the hemoglobin molecule has lost the oxygen molecule at the level of the tissue, and it can be reversed by reoxygenating the hemoglobin in the lungs as the blood returns to the left side of the heart. However, permanent membrane change occurs after several cycles of sickling and unsickling, resulting in an irreversibly sickled cell. The resultant cellular defect leads to the main manifestations of disease, which include (a) premature destruction of the cells, called hemolytic anemia; (b) vascular occlusion of vessels (due to plugging of vessels by sickle cells that cannot pass through the small capillaries) and subsequent tissue infarction; and (c) increased susceptibility to infection.

Sickle cell disease patients are homozygous for the abnormal gene controlling beta-chain production. Hence, both parents must be at least heterozygous for the abnormal gene. The frequency of one abnormal gene in the Black population of America is 1 in 12, and the incidence of sickle cell anemia is 1 in 650 in American Blacks (Williams et al., 1990). Milder forms of this disease can be seen with one sickle beta gene and either deletion of the other beta gene (thalassemia) or occurrence of a second type of sickle gene, called sickle C. The latter results from replacement of the Glutamic acid by lysine at the sixth position on the beta chain (Williams et al.).

FUNCTIONAL PRESENTATION

PATIENTS USUALLY PRESENT in the first decade of life with complications of the three main characteristics of sickle cell disorder. As stated earlier, anemia results from hemolysis secondary to irreversible shape change and the quick breakdown of blood cells, with large amounts of hemoglobin being released into the blood, converted into bilirubin, and secreted into the bile. Bile stones develop early, and the clinical picture is that of a patient with anemia, jaundice, and gallstone attacks. Also, the bone marrow expands, producing extra red blood cells to make up for the anemia, causing bone deformity. This hypercellular marrow is susceptible to vitamin deficiency and viral infection, leading to an abrupt decrease in production, a condition called aplastic crisis.

The second set of clinical symptoms results from the plugging of small blood vessels by the nonpliable sickle cells. Infarction of any organ or, particularly, bone results in a painful crisis. Additionally, strokes and cardiac and pulmonary infarction are major complications of the vascular occlusive disease. Leg ulcers develop for the same reason, heal poorly because of poor tissue perfusion, and can cause physical disability. Finally, the spleen, an organ that helps clear certain infectious agents from the blood, shrinks and is nonfunctional as a result of many infarctions in early childhood. The result is a susceptibility to infections, particularly pneumococcal pneumonia. Another infectious complication results from the combination of devitalized bone and a propensity for salmonella to lodge in the diseased gallbladder, leading to seeding of the bone and salmonella osteomyelitis.

TREATMENT AND PROGNOSIS

THERE IS NO specific treatment for sickle cell disease; hence, most therapy is supportive in treatment of the complications. Painful crises are treated with fluids, pain medication, and careful search for causes, such as an infection (Charache, 1974). Early recognition of infection, administration of prophylactic antibiotics, and vaccination may forestall or prevent other complications (Scott, 1985). If painful crisis persists or there is infarction of a major organ (brain, lung, or heart), exchange transfusion is performed to remove some of the sickle red cells. Normal red cells are transfused to lower the concentration of sickle hemoglobin to 50% (Charache). At this level no significant sludging, further thrombosis, or complications will occur. This effect is temporary, however, as the transfused red cells die and new cells with hemoglobin S are produced. Additionally, transfusion carries risks of infection, allergy, and sensitization to donor blood. Hence, this mode of treatment is used only for severe cases. Investigational approaches to therapy include inhibition of hemoglobin S polymerization, reduction of the intracellular hemoglobin concentration, and pharmacologic induction of gamma globin chain production leading to the production of Fetal Hemoglobin (HbF) as a substitute for hemoglobin S (Bunn, 1997). This has resulted in the use of hydroxyurea, an oral chemotherapeutic agent that can cause an increase in Hemoglobin F and reciprocal decrease in hemoglobin S. The decreased concentration of HbS then leads to reduced sickling and reduction in symptoms. The exposure to chemotherapy and potential complications has limited its use to patients with more frequent and severe attacks. In this group however efficacy and cost effectiveness has been established (Moore et al., 2000).

Bone marrow transplantation and possible gene therapy, in which the normal beta-globin gene is placed in the patient's stem cell, hold hope for the future, but may technical hurdles still remain. Prognosis has improved with good supportive care, and many patients survive into middle age. However, frequent admissions for painful crisis, the complication of sickle cell disease, narcotic use and abuse due to chronic pain, and absence from school and work lead to significant psychological and vocational problems.

PSYCHOLOGICAL AND VOCATIONAL IMPLICATIONS

SEVERAL AUTHORS HAVE documented the psychological impact on a patient with chronic painful disease (Barrett et al., 1988; Damlous, Kevess-Cohen, Charache, Georgopoulos, & Folstein, 1982). In one paper the findings suggested that a relationship between the chronicity and dependence on the medical care system was the best predictor of psychosocial functioning (Damlous et al.). Others have shown links between medical complications and psychopathology (Barrett et al.). The psychological impact can include drug addiction, hysterical conversion reaction, and malingering, as well as low self-esteem, dependency, and depression (Barrett et al.).

Adolescents with sickle cell disease must deal with defining their personal identity along with their chronic illness. Delays in sexual maturation and adolescent growth spurt contribute to poor self-image. Physical limitations, particularly in sports, also lead to low self-esteem. Fifteen percent of patients between the ages of 13 and 40 have been reported to be depressed (Kinney & Ware, 1996).

Physical limitations stemming from stroke in childhood, along with decreased IQ (Hariman, Griffith, Hartig, & Keehn, 1991) and medical complications, may contribute to both psychosocial and vocational limitations. The greatest dysfunction was found in areas of employment, finances, sleep habits, and performance of daily activities (Barrett et al., 1988). Hence, the implications of these findings suggest a strong need for vocational rehabilitation services, training in areas of communication and self-esteem (Barrett et al.), medical treatment, and psychological help for depression and drug dependence. The prevalence of this disease in the black population which is chronically underserved by the health care system and the difficulty of obtaining affordable insurance as well as maintaining a job with insurance benefits, has necessitated development of a national policy to pay for the costs and develop treatments for these patients (Nietert, Silverstein, & Abboud, 2002).

A national sickle cell disease program with 10 regional centers has been set up to provide the comprehensive care required, but many patients and families still have difficulty in obtaining the help they need (Scott, 1985). The centers provide cost-effective day treatment to handle the majority of patient complaints that are neither emergent nor life threatening. Additionally, the psychological, rehabilitation, and vocational services can be provided in a family setting for the patient (Koshy & Dorn, 1996).

REFERENCES

Barrett, D. H., Wisotzek, I. E., Abel, G. G., Rouleu, J. L., Platt, A. F., Pollard, W. G., et al. (1988). Assessment of psychosocial functioning of patients with sickle cell disease. *Southern Medical Journal, 81,* 745–750.

Berdeja, J. G. (2003). Immunotherapy of lymphoma: Update and review of the literature [Review]. *Current Opinion in Oncology, 15*(5), 363–370.

Berman, E. (1997). Recent advances in the treatment of acute leukemia. *Current Opinion in Hematology, 4,* 256–260.

Broers, S., Kaptein, A. A., Le Cessie, S., Fibbe, W., & Hengeveld, M. W. (2000). Psychological functioning and quality of life following bone marrow transplantation: A 3-year follow-up study. *Journal of Psychosomatic Research, 48*(1), 11–21.

Bunn, H. F. (1997). Pathogenesis and treatment of sickle cell disease. *New England Journal of Medicine, 337,* 762–769.

Charache, S. (1974). The treatment of sickle cell anemia. *Archives of Internal Medicine, 133,* 698–705.

Daiter, S., Larson, R. A., Weddington, W. W., & Ultmann, J. E. (1988). Psychosocial symptomatology, personal growth and development among young adult patients following the diagnosis of leukemia or lymphoma. *Journal of Clinical Oncology, 6,* 613–617.

Damlous, N. F., Kevess-Cohen, R., Charache, S., Georgopoulos, A., & Folstein, M. F. (1982). Social disability and psychiatric morbidity in sickle cell anemia and diabetes patients. *Psychosomatics, 23,* 925–931.

DeVita, V. T., Hellman, S., & Rosenberg, S. A. (Eds.). (1989). *Cancer, Principles and practice of oncology* (3rd ed.). Philadelphia: J. B. Lippincott.

Dimeo, F. C., Tilmann, M. H., Bertz, H., Kanz, L., Mertelsmann, R., & Kerl, J. (1997). Aerobic exercise in the rehabilitation of cancer patients after high dose chemotherapy and autologous peripheral stem cell transplantation. *Cancer, 79,* 1717–1722.

Fobair, P., Hoppe, R. T., Bloom, J., Cox, R., Varghese, A., & Spiegle, D. (1986). Problems in Hodgkin's disease survivors. *Journal of Clinical Oncology, 4,* 805–813.

Friedberg, J. W., & Chengazi, V. (2003). PET scans in the staging of lymphoma: Current status. *Oncologist, 8*(5), 438–447.

Gale, R. P., & Foon, K. A. (1987). Therapy of acute myologenous leukemia. *Seminars in Hematology, 24,* 40–54.

Hariman, L. M. P., Griffith, E. R., Hartig, A. L., & Keehn, M. T. (1991). Functional outcomes of children with sickle cell disease affected by stroke. *Archives of Physical Medicine and Rehabilitation, 12,* 498–502.

Hoelzer, D., & Gale, R. P. (1987). Acute lymphoblastic leukemia in adults: Recent progress, future directions. *Seminars in Hematology, 24,* 27–39.

Hsu, F. J., Caspor, C. B., Czerwinski, D., Kwak, L. W., Liles, T. M., Syrengelas, A., et al. (1997). Tumor-specific idiotype vaccines in the treatment of patients with B-cell lymphoma: Long term results of a clinical trial. *Blood, 89,* 3129–3135.

Jenkins, P. L., Linington, A., & Whittaker, I. A. (1991). A retrospective study of psychosocial morbidity in bone marrow transplant recipients. *Psychosomatics, 32,* 65–71.

Kasper, C. K., & Dietrich, S. L. (1985). Comprehensive management of hemophilia. *Clinics in Hematology, 14,* 489–512.

Kinney, T. R., & Ware, R. E. (1996). The adolescent with sickle cell anemia. *Hematology-Oncology Clinics of North America, 10,* 1255–1264.

Koshy, M., & Dorn, L. (1996). Continuing care for adult patients with sickle cell disease [Review]. *Hematology-Oncology Clinics of North America, 10,* 1265–1273.

Moore, R. D., Charache, S., Terrin, M. L., Barton, F. B., & Ballas, S. K. (2000). Cost-effectiveness of hydroxyurea in sickle cell. Investigators of the Multicenter Study of Hydroxyurea in Sickle Cell Anemia. *American Journal of Hematology, 64,* 26–31.

Mulhern, R. K., Friedman, A. G., & Stone, P. A. (1988). Acute lymphoblastic leukemia: Long-term psychological outcome [Review]. *Biomedicine & Pharmacotherapy, 42*(4), 243–246.

Nietert, P. J., Silverstein, M. D., & Abboud, M. R. (2002). Sickle cell anaemia: Epidemiology and cost of illness. [Erratum appears in *Pharmacoeconomics, 20*(12), 853]. [Review] [45 refs.]. *Pharmacoeconomics, 20*(6), 357–366.

Penson, R. T., Rauch, P. K., McAfee, S. L., Cashavelly, B. J., Clair-Hayes, K., Dahlin, C., et al. (2002). Between parent and child: Negotiating cancer treatment in adolescents. *Oncologist 7*(2), 154–162.

Raphael, B. G., & Knowles, D. M. (1990). Acquired immunodeficiency syndrome: Associated non-Hodgkin's lymphoma. *Seminars in Oncology, 17,* 361–366.

Rosenberg, S. A. (Chairman). (1982). National Cancer Institute sponsored study of classifications of non-Hodgkin's lymphomas: Summary and description of a working formulation for clinical usage. *Cancer, 49,* 2112–2135.

Rosendall, F. R., Smit, C., Varekamp, L., Brockervrunos, A. H., J. T., Van Dijck, J., Saurmeijer, T. P. B. M., et al. (1990). Modern hemophilia treatment: Medical improvements and quality of life. *Internal Medicine, 282,* 633–640.

Ruthoven, J. J. (1987). Current approaches to the treatment of advanced-stage non-Hodgkin's lymphoma. *Canadian Medical Association Journal, 136,* 29–36.

Scott, R. B. (1985). Advances in the treatment of sickle cell disease in children. *American Journal of Diseases of Children, 139,* 1219–1222.

Sekeres, M. A., Stone, R. M., Zahrieh, D., Neuberg, D., Morrison, V., De Angelo, D. J., et al. (2004). Decision-making and quality of life in older adults with acute myeloid leukemia or advanced myelodysplastic syndrome. *Leukemia, 18*(4), 809–816.

Skarin, A. T. (1989). Non-Hodgkin's lymphoma. *Archives of Internal Medicine, 34,* 209–242.

Skrjala, K. L., Langer, S. L., Abrams, J. R., Storer, B., Sanders, J. E., Flowers, M. E., et al. (2004). Recovery and long-term function after hematopoietic cell transplantation for leukemia or lymphoma. *Journal of the American Medical Association, 291*, 2335–2343.

Somerfield, M. R., Curbow, B., Wingard, J. R., Baker, F., & Fogarty, L. A. (1996). Coping with the physical and psychosocial sequelae of bone marrow transplantation among long-term survivors. *Journal of Behavioral Medicine, 19*(2), 163–184.

Williams, W. J., Butler, E., Erslev, A. J., & Lichtman, M. A. (Eds.). (1990). *Hematology* (4th ed.). New York: McGraw-Hill.

Wolcott, D. L., Wellisch, D. K., Fawzy, F. I., & Landsverk, J. (1986). Adaptation of adult bone marrow transplant recipient long term survivors. *Transplantation, 41*, 478–484.

14

Developmental Disabilities

RICHARD J. MORRIS, PhD, YVONNE P. MORRIS, PhD, AND PRISCILLA A. BADE WHITE, PhD

D EVELOPMENTAL DISABILITY CAN be traced to the work of Jean Itard, a French physician, and his attempts, beginning in 1799, to educate Victor, the Wild Boy of Aveyron (Itard, 1962). According to Humphrey (1962), Itard believed that Victor's condition could be cured. Itard felt that the reason for Victor's "apparent subnormality" was his lack of typical language experiences and social interactions that form an integral part of the development of a "normal civilized person." He placed Victor under his care for 5 years at the Paris institution where he worked. Although Victor improved over this period, he did not achieve Itard's initial expectations and predictions of becoming "normal."

Itard's work influenced the writings, research, and treatment practices of a number of early workers in the field of developmental disabilities, notably Edouard Seguin. Their writings, in turn, led directly to the building of residential schools and facilities for mentally retarded and other developmentally disabled persons in the United States. The first facility was established in Watertown, Massachusetts, in 1848 as part of the Perkins Institution for the Blind (MacMillan, 1982), and the second was built in Syracuse, New York, in 1851, as an independent facility for mentally retarded and other developmentally disabled persons. Although the primary residents of these facilities were children, adults and adolescents were placed in the same institutions. These persons were generally referred to as "feebleminded" or, more specifically, as either "idiots," "imbeciles," or "morons"—"moron" being applied to those people who were in the highest functioning category of feeblemindedness, followed by "imbeciles," who were in the middle range of functioning, and "idiots," who were in the lowest-functioning category (Kanner, 1948).

Seguin and others (e.g., Samuel Howe) intended these facilities to be established on an experimental basis as educational institutions rather than as custodial asylums. The hypothesis underlying this form of intervention was that after mentally retarded or other developmentally disabled people received training, education, or other forms of treatment to help them in their functioning in society, they would then be returned to their natural homes within the community. The hypothesis, however, was not supported by empirical data (Baumeister, 1970). In fact, few persons who entered these institutions ever returned to society, and by the beginning of the 20th century, the state educational schools became the state custodial institutions (Baumeister; Blatt, 1984; Brown et al., 1986; Kanner, 1964; Morris & Kratochwill, 1998; Wolfensberger, 1972). This custodial emphasis began to change in the late 1960s and early 1970s, with the introduction of behavior modification treatment (e.g., Ayllon & Azrin, 1968; Baer, Wolf, & Risley, 1968; Gardner, 1970; Lovaas & Bucher, 1974; Morris & McReynolds, 1986; Thompson & Grabowski, 1972), the deinstitutionalization and normalization movements (e.g., Blatt, 1968, 1984; Blatt & Kaplan, 1966; Nirje, 1969; Wolfensberger, 1969, 1972), and legal advocacy for individuals with mental retardation (e.g., Friedman, 1975; *Halderman v. Pennhurst*, 1977; *New York State Association for Retarded Children v. Rockefeller*, 1973; *Pennsylvania Association for Retarded Children v. Commonwealth of Pennsylvania*, 1971; *Wyatt v. Stickney*, 1971).

DESCRIPTION OF DISABILITY

DEVELOPMENTAL DISABILITY ENCOMPASSES a wide range of diagnostic conditions and behaviors (e.g., Blackman, 1983; Wright, 1987) and typically refers to those chronic or lifelong mental and/or physical conditions that develop prior to 18 years of age and require specific forms of agency services and intervention strategies that may occur over an extended duration (Ehlers, Prothero, & Langone, 1982; Scheerenberger, 1987). In addition, social adaptability and competence enter into the specific definition of one of these disabilities, mental retardation (American Association on Mental Retardation, 1992; Leland, 1991; Luckasson et al., 2002; Scheerenberger). The major forms of developmental disability are mental retardation, cerebral palsy, epilepsy and other types of seizure disorder, as well as pervasive developmental disorders, such as autism and Asperger's syndrome. Some of the common characteristics that are often found in persons with developmental disabilities are functional limitations in some or most of the following areas: self-care and self-help skills, receptive and/or expressive language, cognition and learning ability, mobility, self-direction, economic independence, and the ability to live on their own without assistance (see, for example, American Psychiatric Association, 1994; Cole & Gardner, 1993; Developmental Disabilities Act, 1984; Developmental Disabilities Assistance and Bill of Rights Act, 2000). In addition, these persons are often characterized as scoring in the subaverage range on individually administered standardized tests of intelligence. This chapter will focus on two broad types of developmental disability: mental retardation and pervasive developmental disorders.

FUNCTIONAL PRESENTATION

MENTAL RETARDATION

IN 1959, THE American Association of Mental Deficiency (AAMD)—now called the American Association on Mental Retardation (AMMR)—defined mental retardation in terms of a person's level of intellectual ability and level of adaptive behavior. This statement has been revised over the years; the current definition is as follows:

> Mental retardation is a disability characterized by significant limitations both in intellectual functioning and in adaptive behavior as expressed in conceptual, social, and practical adaptive skills. This disability originates before age 18. (Luckasson et al., 2002, p. 1)

This definition reflects the multidimensional underpinnings in approaching mental retardation as well as the expanding conceptualization of this condition. The dimensions included are intellectual abilities and adaptive behavior, with mental retardation being defined as state of intellectual and adaptive functioning that begins in childhood (Luckasson et al., 2002). Consistent with good testing practice, the evaluation of intellectual and adaptive functioning should be assessed in the context of environmental and personal factors, including culture, linguistic diversity, and sensory, motor, and behavioral factors.

Intelligence refers to overall mental ability including capacity to problem solve and learn. Limitations in "intellectual functioning" in mental retardation are generally assessed through the use of standardized individually administered IQ tests. Scores that are two or more standard deviations below the mean for the specific assessment instruments used, taking into consideration the assessment instrument's standard error of measurement (SEM), as well as the instrument's strengths and limitations, are viewed as falling into the mentally retarded range (Luckasson et al., 2002). As most IQ tests have a mean of 100, a standard deviation of 15, and an SEM of 5, the requisite IQ score for a diagnosis of mental retardation is generally 70 or lower. With the inclusion of the SEM criterion, the ceiling IQ score for mental retardation is raised to 75, with IQ being reported as a confidence band (e.g., 65–75) rather than a finite score (Luckasson et al.).

"Adaptive behavior" is defined by the AAMR (Luckasson et al., 2002) as the conceptual, social, and practical skills that people use in order to function in their everyday lives. Conceptual skills include communication skills, money and calculation skills, and self-direction. Social skills include interpersonal skills and the ability to understand and follow rules and laws. Practical skills include skills in personal and instrumental activities of daily living (e.g., eating, meal preparation, etc.), as well as occupational job-related skills (Luckasson et al.).

Tests of "adaptive behavior" usually assess these skills by observing the individual in situations where these skills are require, by interviewing those who know the individual well, or by a combination of these procedures. Adaptive behavior is typically assessed through the use of standardized tests of adaptive behavior that have been normed on the general population, including nondisabled and disabled individuals. "Adaptive functioning" limitations in mental retardation are generally conceptualized as scores on these standardized tests that are two or more standard deviations below the mean for adaptive behavior overall or for at least one of the three types of adaptive functioning: conceptual, social, or practical (Luckasson et al., 2002).

Mental retardation has traditionally been divided into levels of severity, with these levels linked to level of functioning or to IQ scores. In the early 1900s Goddard proposed a classification system for mental retardation based on the Binet-Simon concept of mental age. Individuals with mental deficiency with the lowest mental age level (less than 3 years of age) were identified as "idiots." "Imbiciles" had a mental age of 3 to 7 years of age, and "morons" had a mental age between 7 and 10 years of age (Mash & Wolfe, 1999). In 1959, Heber developed a classification system based on deficits in measured intelligence and adaptive behavior (personal-social and sensory-motor) (Heber, 1959). This system proved unworkable and in 1961 Heber revised the mental retardation classification manual (Brison, 1967). Heber (1959, 1961) linked his description of "retardation in measured intelligence" to the following IQ scores: "borderline" (IQ range of 70–84), "mild" (IQ range of 55–69), "moderate" (IQ range of 40–54), "severe" (IQ range of 25–39), and "profound" (IQ below 25).

In 1968, the American Psychiatric Association's (APA) *Diagnostic and Statistical Manual of Mental Disorders*, 2nd edition (DSM-II) (APA, 1968) linked IQ scores to levels of mental retardation, with "borderline men-

tal retardation" indicating IQ scores of 68 to 83, "mild mental retardation" indicating IQ scores of 52 to 67, "moderate mental retardation"
indicating IQ scores of 36 to 51, "severe mental retardation" indicating
IQ scores of 20 to 35, and "profound mental retardation" indicating an
IQ score under 20. Prior to 1973, the recommended IQ cut-off scores for
mental retardation were 84 or 85. With the publication of the AAMD's
Manual on Terminology and Classification in Mental Retardation (Grossman,
1973), the cut-off score was revised downward to approximately 70,
where it remains today.

In APA's *Diagnostic and Statistical Manual of Mental Disorders*, 4th edition (DSM-IV) (APA, 1994), a diagnosis of mental retardation is made when
a person has an IQ "about 70 or below . . . accompanied by significant
limitations in adaptive functioning in at least two [adaptive] skill areas"
(p. 39). In the DSM-IV, "mild mental retardation" encompasses an IQ range
of 50–55 to approximately 70, "moderate mental retardation" encompasses an IQ range of 35–40 to 50–55, "severe mental retardation" encompasses an IQ range of 20–25 to 35–40, and "profound mental retardation"
encompasses an IQ range below 20 or 25 (APA). Similar classification systems can be found in the World Health Organization's (WHO) *International
Classification of Diseases*: 10th revision (ICD-10) (WHO, 1992), and in educational classifications of mental disability (e.g., Individuals with
Disabilities Education Act (IDEA) (1991).

Beginning in 1992, the AAMR proposed a reconceptualization of the
levels of severity of mental retardation based on "intensities" of support a person required in order to function successfully in society. The
AAMR definitions of system levels of needed support are listed in Table
14.1 (AAMR, 1992; Luckasson et al., 2002).

The AAMR's "levels of intensities of supports" has not been as widely
accepted as the traditional system based on IQ scores (Conyers, Martin,
Martin, & Yu, 2002), and a number of concerns have been raised about
the differences between this system and state and federal statutes pertaining to mental retardation, which are usually comprised of wording
similar to the DSM-IV's severity levels and the AAMR's earlier conceptualization of mental retardation (see, for example, Gresham, MacMillan,
& Siperstein, 1995; Hodapp, 1995; MacMillan, Gresham, & Siperstein, 1993;
Matson, 1995). The AAMR (Luckasson et al., 2002) acknowledged these
concerns and added the caveat that clinicians may classify individuals
with mental retardation using support intensity, IQ range, adaptive
behavior limitations, etiology, mental health category, or other classification systems as necessary for the person with mental retardation to
meet statutory requirements to qualify for local, state, and federal services.

Estimates of the prevalence of mental retardation in the general population in the United States range between 1%–3% (Boyle et al., 1996;
Daily, Ardinger, & Holmes, 2000; Grossman, 1983; Lee et al., 2001;

TABLE 14.1 Definition and Examples of Intensities of Supports

Intermittent Supports. Supports on an "as needed basis." Characterized by episodic nature, person not always needing the support(s), or short-term supports needed during life-span transitions (e.g., job loss or acute medical crisis). Intermittent supports may be high or low intensity when provided.

Limited Supports. An intensity of supports characterized by consistency over time, time-limited but not of an intermittent nature; may require fewer staff members and cost less than more intense levels of support (e.g., time-limited employment training or transitional supports during the school-to-adult provided period).

Extensive Supports. This is characterized by regular involvement (e.g., daily) in at least some environments (such as work or home) and not time-limited (e.g., long-term support and long-term home living support).

Pervasive Supports. This is characterized by their constancy and high intensity, provided across environments, potentially life-sustaining in nature. Pervasive supports typically involve more staff members and intrusiveness than do extensive or time-limited supports.

Note: From American Association of Mental Retardation. (1992). *Mental retardation. Definition, classification, and systems of support* (9th ed.). Washington, DC. American Association of Mental Retardation. Copyright 1992 by the American Association of Mental Retardation. Reprinted with permission.

McLaren & Bryson, 1987). Prevalence rates for children in special education under the category "mental retardation" have dropped significantly over the past 25 years, to approximately 1% (U.S. Department of Education, 2000). This decline may reflect increased differentiation of these children from other children who have overlapping disabilities (e.g., autism), a reluctance to diagnose mild mental retardation, and an increased use of nondiagnostic multi-categorical classrooms. From a global perspective, in 1994 the World Health Organization (WHO) estimated a worldwide prevalence of mental retardation to be between 1% and 3% (WHO, 2001).

An appreciable amount of research has been devoted to determining the causes of mental retardation, as well as to developing techniques and strategies for its prevention and treatment (see, for example, AAMR, 1992; Aman & Singh, 1991; Berg, 1975; Cole & Gardner, 1993; Coulter, 1991; Curry et al., 1997; Daily et al., 2000; Gullone, King, & Cummins, 1996; Luckasson et al., 2002; Matson & Coe, 1992; Matson, Appelgate, Smirdo, & Stallings, 1998; Peterson & Martens, 1995; Williams, Kirkpatrick-Sanchez, & Crocker, 1994; Zigler & Hodapp, 1986). For example, over 1,000 recognized genetically-based syndromes associated with mental retardation are listed online in the *Online Mendelian Inheritance in Man* (OMIM, 2004) database. These genetically-based syndromes (e.g., Angelman Syndrome) as well as various non-genetically-based syndromic disorders (e.g., fetal alcohol syndrome) are associated with mental retardation. As a general rule, however, the more severe the mental retardation, the more likely the mental retardation can be attributable to an identifiable medical or physical condition or cause. The three major known causes of mental retardation are Down Syndrome, fetal alcohol syndrome, and fragile X syndrome. However, the etiology of 50% of all cases of mental retardation is presently unknown. For known cases, prenatal factors are implicated twice as often as perinatal or postnatal factors (McLaren & Bryson, 1987). Table 14.2 lists some of the physical conditions associated with mental retardation (Baraitser & Winter, 1996; Gorlin, Cohen, & Hennekam, 2001; Jones, 1997; Stevenson, Schwartz, & Schroer, 2000). For individuals whose mental retardation is not accounted for by known conditions, social deprivation and inadequate level of environmental stimulation are often considered to be primary etiological factors (Matson et al., 1998).

TABLE 14.2 Conditions or Events Which Are Often Associated with Mental Retardation

Period of development	Type of condition or event	Examples
Pre- and periconceptual	Brain malformation	Encephalocele Hydranencephaly Neural tube defects Agenesis of the corpus callosum
	Chromosomal abnormalities: trisomy	Down's Syndrome
	Chromosomal abnormalities: deletions	Prader Willi Syndrome Angelman Syndrome Wolf-Hirschoun Syndrome
	Chromosomal abnormalities: sex chromosome linked disorders	Fragile X Turner Syndrome Rett Syndrome Klenefelter Syndrome
	Chromosomal abnormalities: autosomal dominant conditions	Neurofibromatosis Tuberous sclerosis Williams Syndrome
	Chromosomal abnormalities: autosomal recessive conditions	Tay-Sachs Gaucher Nieman-Pick Lesch-Nyhan

(Continued)

TABLE 14.2 *(Continued)*

Period of development	Type of condition or event	Examples
Prenatal	Teratogens	Chemicals Radiation Maternal substance abuse (alcohol, drugs) Prescription medications (e.g., anticonvulsants, warfann)
	Infection	TORCH viruses: rubella, toxiplasmosis, cytome-galovirus, herpes simplex
	Fetal malnutrition	Mother with high blood pressure or kidney disease
Perinatal	Prematurity	Complications such as poor oxygenation of the brain and intracranial hemorrhage
	Metabolic abnormalities	Hypoglycemia Phenylketonuria
	Trauma	Misapplication of forceps
	Infection	Herpes simplex Encephalitis
Postnatal	Infection	Meningitis Encephalitis General inflammatory disease with high fever
	Trauma; Lack of oxygen	Automobile accidents Child abuse Near drowning Strangulation
	Severe nutritional deficiency	Kwashiorkor Iodine deficiency
	Environmental toxins	Lead Carbon monoxide Household products
	Environmental and social problems	Psychosocial deprivation Parental psychiatric disorders

Note. Adapted from: Blackman, J. A. (Ed.). (1983). *Medical aspects of developmental disabilities in children birth to three.* Iowa City: University of Iowa Press.

PERVASIVE DEVELOPMENTAL DISORDERS

PERVASIVE DEVELOPMENTAL DISORDERS (PDD) is an umbrella
term created by the APA (1980) to characterize a pattern of neurologically
based impairments in social interaction and communication, as well as
stereotyped patterns of behavior, activities, and/or interests. PDD is a
generic label (Szatmari, 2000) incorporating a wide range of impairments that a child is born with or born with the potential of developing (Frith, 1991). The DSM-IV (APA, 1994) includes five specific disorders
under the PDD umbrella: Autistic Disorder (or autism), Asperger's
Disorder (also referred to as Asperger's Syndrome), Rett's Disorder,
Childhood Disintegrative Disorder (CDD), and Pervasive Developmental
Disorder Not Otherwise Specified (PDDNOS). In this chapter we will
define all five types of Pervasive Developmental Disorders, but will focus
on Autism, Asperger's Disorder and Pervasive Developmental Disorder
Not Otherwise Specified. These three Pervasive Developmental Disorders
can be construed as existing on a continuum or spectrum, with problems in each of the three main symptom areas of social interaction,
communication, and behavior ranging from absent to severe (Attwood,
1998; Eisenmajer et al., 1996; Schopler, 1996). Collectively, these three disorders have been discussed in the literature as constituting the "Autism
Spectrum Disorders" (Fombonne, 2003a).

   Estimates of the prevalence of Autism Spectrum Disorders have varied widely, with the most recent literature suggesting that the range is
between 30 and 67 per 10,000 individuals (Bertrand et al., 2001; CDC,
2000; Chakrabarti & Fombonne, 2001; Fombonne, 2002; Fombonne,
2003b; Fombonne, Simmons, Ford, Meltzer, & Goodman, 2001; Yeargin-
Allsopp et al., 2003). Many of the more recent surveys also suggest an
increase in the prevalence of Autism Spectrum Disorders (e.g., Charman,
2002; Fombonne, 2003b; Fombonne et al., 2001; Mahoney et al., 2001;
Wing & Potter, 2002). For example, Fombonne (2003b) reported an estimated PDD prevalence rate of 30 per 10,000 children, but indicated
that this number is likely to be an underestimate of the true prevalence
of Autism Spectrum Disorder. He maintains that the prevalence figure
is more likely to be closer to 60 per 10,000 (approximately 425,000 children under 18 years of age in the United States), because (a) children
with milder or high-functioning types of Autism Spectrum Disorders
are often missed in surveys; (b) younger children are underrepresented
because assessment techniques used in the diagnosis of infants and pre-
school-aged children are less sensitive than techniques used for older
children; (c) older children are under-identified because the newer diagnostic criteria for Autism Spectrum Disorders were not in place when
they were diagnosed; and (d) with the increasing availability in the 1990s
of developmental disability services for children with Autism Spectrum

Disorders, as mandated by IDEA, schools and other educational services agencies have become more likely to identify and provide programs for children with Autism Spectrum Disorders.

However, assessing changes in the prevalence of Autism Syndrome Disorders over time is very difficult. Some of the reasons for this difficulty are the following: (a) surveys differ in their respective definitions of autism, (b) whether they are requesting information on each of the Autism Spectrum Disorders, and (c) the methods utilized to identify cases (e.g., some surveys rely on a single source or registry while other surveys rely on multiple methods for case identification). Another complicating factor is that the criteria for an Autism Spectrum Disorders diagnosis, including the criteria for a diagnosis of Autism, has changed over time—for example, Asperger's Disorder was first added to the DSM in 1994 (APA, 1994).

It is also possible that an increase in the prevalence of Autism Syndrome Disorders is due to an increase in the incidence of these disorders. Factors posited for such an increase include an increase in genetic sensitivity and exposure to environmental pathogens. It is difficult to assess the impact of these factors with prevalence studies as they are not experimental studies of hypothesized causes of Autism Spectrum Disorders. Comparative surveys investigating links between Autism and two proposed environmental factors, the triple vaccine for measles, mumps, and rubella, and vaccines containing Thimerosal (a mercury-based preservative) have failed to demonstrate such a relationship (e.g., Madsen et al., 2002; Hviid, Stellfeld, Wohlfahrt, & Melbye, 2003).

Autism

More than 50 years ago, Leo Kanner (1943) described a group of 11 children who displayed a similar pattern of specific symptoms that were significantly different from those of other childhood behavior disorders. Kanner called this form of childhood psychopathology "early infantile autism" and noted that among its characteristics were marked withdrawal; dislike of being held; unresponsiveness to people as well as to the environment; manipulation of objects in a rigid, stereotyped manner; lack of appropriate play; failure to acquire normal speech; echolalia and difficulties with pronoun use; anxious insistence on sameness in the environment; excellent rote memories; normal physical appearance; and good cognitive potential.

Currently, autism is characterized by the following: (a) qualitative impairment in reciprocal social interaction; (b) qualitative impairment in verbal and nonverbal communication, as well as in imaginative activity; (c) restricted and stereotyped patterns of behavior, interests, and activities; (d) delays or abnormal functioning in at least one of these areas, with onset prior to 3 years of age; and (e) the disturbance is not better accounted for by Rett's Disorder or Childhood Disintegrative

Disorder (pervasive developmental disorders in which there is a period of apparent normal functioning after birth, followed by the development of multiple specific deficits or marked regression in multiple areas of functioning) (APA, 1994).

Charlop-Christy, Schreibman, Pierce, and Kurtz (1998) have noted that the significant characteristics of autistic children include profound deficits in social behavior (including failure to develop relationships with people); problems in understanding the intentions, motivations, and beliefs of others or of themselves (i.e., an impaired "theory of mind"); ritualistic behavior and the insistence on sameness; abnormalities in response to the physical environment; self-stimulatory behavior; self-injurious behavior; limited intellectual functioning; problems in the development of speech and language (e.g., echolalia, pronominal reversal, failure to acquire functional speech) that affect the child's ability to learn, communicate, and develop relationships with others. Reportedly half of the individuals diagnosed with autism never develop meaningful speech (Tanguay, 2000).

It is estimated that 20 to 60 per 10,000 individuals are diagnosed with autism during their lifetime, with similar prevalence rates across socioeconomic and ethnic groups (Croen, Grether, Hoogstrate, & Selvin, 2002; Gillberg, 1999). Autism has consistently been found to be more prevalent in males than females, with a ratio of approximately 4:1 (Fombonne, 1999). Approximately 70% to 80% of individuals diagnosed with autism have IQ scores that fall within the mentally retarded range (APA 1994; Fombonne, 1999; Phelps & Grabowski, 1991; Ritvo & Freeman, 1978; Wing, 1991; Yeargin-Allsopp et al., 2003), with many of these individuals being dually diagnosed as having autism and mental retardation.

It is important to keep in mind that accurate assessment of intellectual functioning of individuals with autism may be difficult. Many individuals with autism have language impairments that depress performance levels on tests of abstract reasoning and symbolic logic. In addition, many individuals with autism demonstrate behaviors that are not consistent with and that interfere with test taking and, therefore, motivating individuals diagnosed with autism to comply with test directions and tasks may be difficult (L. K. Koegel, R. L. Koegel, & Smith, 1997; Schreibman & Charlop, 1987). Research regarding stability over time of IQ scores in children with autism is inconclusive, with some researchers (e.g., Rutter, 1978; Rutter & Bartak, 1973) reporting that IQ scores remain stable over time, while other researchers reporting that the I.Q. scores of individuals diagnosed with autism increase with age (Mayes & Calhoun, 2003).

Asperger's Syndrome
About the time Kanner (1943) was studying *early infantile autism* in the United States, Hans Asperger (1944/1991) in Austria identified a group

of young boys presenting with what he called *autistic psychopathy*. These children were described as having normal intelligence and language development, with autistic-like behaviors and deficiencies in social and communication skills. However, it was not until his research was translated from German to English in 1991 that it began to gain attention, with Wing (1991) describing children with Asperger's Disorder as tending to have "good grammatical speech from early in life, passive, odd, or subtly inappropriate social interaction and poor gross motor coordination on gait and posture" (Frith, 1991, p. 115).

Asperger's Disorder was not added to the DSM-IV until 1994 (APA, 1994). According to the DSM-IV, the clinical presentation of Asperger's Disorder includes (a) severe and sustained impairment in social interaction, (b) development of restricted, repetitive patterns of interest, behaviors, and activities, (c) the disturbances must cause clinically significant impairment in social, occupational, or other important areas of functioning, (d) no clinically significant delays or deviance in language acquisition, (e) no clinically significant delays in cognition during the first 3 years of life, and (f) the criteria are not met for another specific Pervasive Developmental Disability or for schizophrenia. The mean age for diagnosis of Asperger's Disorder is reported to be 8 years of age (Eisenmajer et al., 1996). It should be noted that the diagnostic criterion of no clinically significant delays in language development does not preclude the presence of unusual qualities in language skills. Speech and language peculiarities may be present and are most likely to involve difficulties in the areas of pragmatics and prosidy (Attwood, 1998; Safran, J. S., 2002).

Generally, individuals with Asperger's Disorder may move into the personal space of others failing to recognize body language and other nonverbal communicative gestures, and even verbal cues that he or she has failed to behave in a socially appropriate fashion (Safran, S. P., 2001; Safran, J. S., 2002). For example, the person with Asperger's Disorder may discuss pet topics at length despite cues from the listener that he or she is not interested (Safran, J. S., 2002). The person with Asperger's Disorder may not demonstrate every characteristic of this disorder. However, he or she will present with personal, motoric, and language characteristics of Asperger's Disorder and this feature will therefore separate these individuals from others with other Pervasive Developmental Disabilities.

Although individuals who have Asperger's tend to have a marginally late onset of speech, once it is acquired the person tends to have one-sided conversations and frequently uses questioning as a social tool (Attwood, 1998). Attwood explains that individuals with Asperger's Disorder are generally disinterested in games, sports, and play activities, are indifferent to peer pressure, and lack precision in expressing emotions. Issues regarding the differential diagnosis of Asperger's

Disorder, high functioning Autism, and nonverbal learning disabilities remain unresolved (see, for example, Rourke & Tsatsanis, 2000; Volkmar & Klin, 1998). At the present time there is no conclusive evidence regarding the etiology of Asperger's Disorder; it is thought to be a neurologically based syndrome.

Pervasive Developmental Disorder Not Otherwise Specified

Unlike Autism and Asperger's Syndrome, Pervasive Developmental Disorder Not Otherwise Specified (PDDNOS) does not have specific criteria for a diagnosis. According to the DSM-VI (APA, 1994), PDDNOS is considered an appropriate diagnosis "when there is a severe and pervasive impairment in the development of reciprocal social interaction, verbal and nonverbal communication skills, or the development of stereotyped behavior, interests, and activities, but the criteria are not met for a specific PDD" (pp. 77–78). A PDDNOS diagnosis is often used to diagnose individuals whose symptoms developed after 30 months of age and/or who present with atypical or fewer symptoms necessary for diagnosis (Tanguay, 2000). Children initially given a diagnosis of PDDNOS may develop additional diagnostic features as they mature, with many of these children receiving a subsequent diagnosis of autism (Tsai, 2000).

Rett's Disorder

Rett's Disorder was named for Austrian physician Adreas Rett, who in 1966 described two severely disabled young girls with stereotypical hand-wringing movements (Hagberg, Aicardi, Dias, & Ramos, 1983). It is a progressive neurodevelopmental disorder characterized by apparently normal prenatal and perinatal development for the first 6 to 18 months of life, followed by the development of clinical symptoms, including decreased head circumference growth and microcephaly, loss of muscle tone, and previously purposeful hand movements and characteristic hang-wringing stereotypical behaviors. Children with Rett's Disorder experience cognitive and functional regression (Mount, Hastings, Reilly, Cass, & Charman, 2003). Hagberg and his colleagues (Hagberg, 2002; Hagberg, Aicardi, Dias, & Ramos, 1983) have developed a detailed four-stage system of development of this disorder.

Rett's Disorder is caused by a genetic mutation of the MECP2 gene, which is located on the X chromosome (Amir et al., 1999). The protein encoded by this gene suppresses gene activation in neurons, and leads to developmental delays and neurological disorders. A genetic mutation in the MeCP2 gene can be identified in 80–85% of cases of Rett's Disorder, with unidentified aberrations in the MeCP2 gene region thought to be responsible for cases in which a genetic mutation is not apparent (Bienvenu et al., 2000).

[handwritten note at top: Was thought to only occur in girls but it does occur in boys as well]

[handwritten notes in left margin: Theodore Heller; 1908; after a period of 2 yrs normal development; rare / prevalence unknown]

Initially, it was thought that Rett's Disorder occurred exclusively in females. It is now known to occur at a much lower frequency in males. The true incidence and prevalence of Rett's Disorder is not known. It is thought to affect one in every 10,000 to 15,000 live female births. Although male fetuses can have Rett's Disorder, they are likely to be spontaneously aborted during pregnancy or to die shortly after birth. It is believed that Rett's Disorder males with an extra X chromosome may survive longer.

Childhood Disintegrative Disorder

Although the diagnostic category Childhood Disintegrative Disorder (CDD) was first added to the DSM in 1994 (APA, 1994), it has a long history and can be traced back to Theodore Heller's 1908 discussion of "Dementia Infantilis" (Hendry, 2000). Children with this disorder develop a condition similar to autism, with significant loss of skills in communication, social relationships, play, and adaptive behavior, after a period of at least 2 years of apparently normal development. According to the DSM-IV, the clinical presentation of CDD includes (a) significant loss, prior to age 10, of previously acquired skills in at least two of the following areas: expressive or receptive language, social skills or adaptive behavior, bowel or bladder control, play, or motor skills; and (b) abnormalities in functioning in at least two of the following areas: qualitative impairment in social interaction, qualitative impairment in communication, and restricted, repetitive, and stereotyped patterns of behavior.

CDD is a very rare disorder, and its prevalence is unknown. In his review of past epidemiological surveys of autism and other pervasive developmental disorders, Fombonne (2002) found four surveys that included CDD. Prevalence rates reported in those surveys ranged from 1.1 to 6.4 per 100,000 individuals. Fombonne calculated a pooled prevalence estimate for CDD, resulting in an estimated prevalence rate of 1.7 per 100,000 individuals.

TREATMENT AND PROGNOSIS

HISTORICALLY, TREATMENT PROGRAMS for individuals with developmental disabilities have been limited, with more severely impaired individuals typically living in institutional settings where they received custodial care. Educational programs may have been provided for higher functioning individuals within institutional settings, and community-based educational programs were likely to be found in private and church-related schools. Individuals functioning in the moderately and mildly mentally retarded range were likely to be educated in a segregated classroom setting (i.e., classrooms for the trainable and educable), and sheltered workshop activities, both within and outside the custodial institution, may have been available for older youths and adults. Psychotherapy and counseling services for individuals with developmental disabilities were not widely available (e.g., Cowen, 1963; Stacey & DeMartino, 1957).

Most contemporary approaches to the treatment of persons with developmental disabilities can be traced to the behavior modification treatment research of the early to mid-1960s (see, e.g., Ayllon & Azrin, 1968; Gardner, 1971; Matson & McCartney, 1981; Morris, 1976; Thompson & Grabowski, 1972; Ullmann & Krasner, 1965). Many contemporary behavioral treatment programs utilize an applied behavior analysis approach, and are based on the assumptions that the antecedents of a behavior, as well the consequences of a behavior, can be manipulated so that the likelihood that a behavior will be repeated is increased. Behavioral treatment programs have been widely used in helping individuals with developmental disabilities develop and strengthen their positive behavior skills, including adaptive behavior and coping skills, functional language skills, and social skills.

MENTAL RETARDATION

SO MUCH HAS been written about the relative effectiveness of behavior modification procedures with people who have mental retardation that few writers today would question its utility and the role that these procedures have played in assisting people to live more comfortable and humane lives, independent of their level of mental retardation (see, e.g., Alberto, Heflin, & Andrews, 2002; Brown et al., 1986; Carr, Turnbull, & Horner, 1999; Cole & Gardner, 1993; Matson et al., 1998; Matson & Schaughency, 1988; Wacker & Berg, 1988). Behavior modification procedures have been used successfully to develop and strengthen positive behaviors and to reduce and eliminate problem behaviors.

Reinforcement Procedures

Reinforcement is typically defined as an event that immediately follows a specific behavior that has been designated for change (called the target behavior) and that results in an increase in the frequency of occurrence of that behavior (e.g., Skinner, 1938, 1953). Because reinforcement is defined for our purposes in terms of its effects on the person, something that might be reinforcing to one person may not be reinforcing to another person. It is therefore very important when using reinforcement procedures to make sure that the clinician, teacher, or other care provider knows what is a reinforcer for the person with whom she or he is working.

There are typically five categories of *positive reinforcement*: social praise ("Very good," "That's right," "Fine," "You're terrific," etc.), nonverbal messages (smiling, tickling, hugging, kissing, etc.), edibles (small amounts of the person's favorite foods, snacks, or drinks), objects (pencil, paper, book, coupons, toys, cosmetics, etc.), and activities (playing catch, playing video games or other electronic games, going to the county fair, going to a shopping mall or park, etc.) (Morris, 1985). The positive reinforcers used by the clinician, teacher, or other care provider should be appropriate for the person's age, and if possible, the clinician or other behavior modifier should avoid the use of edibles or liquids.

Use of edibles and liquids is usually reserved for clients with severe to profound handicaps. The most commonly used method for distributing positive reinforcers is through the use of a conditioned reinforcer, called a token, within a token economy program (see, e.g., Ayllon & Azrin, 1968; Kazdin, 1994; Morris, 1985). A token is an object (such as a metal washer, poker chip, "credit card" receipt, or check mark on a personalized identity card) that can be earned by the client each time he or she engages in the target behavior and that has a quantitative relationship to the obtainment (i.e., "purchasing") of particular positive reinforcers such as those listed above.

Positive reinforcement can be applied on a continuous or intermittent basis but, whenever possible, should be applied on an intermittent basis. In addition, reinforcement can be applied when the client performs the target behavior or, in the case of *differential reinforcement of other behavior* (DRO) or *differential reinforcement of incompatible behavior* (DRI), when the client engages, respectively, in a behavior(s) other than the target behavior (DRO) or a behavior(s) that is incompatible with the target behavior (DRI). Another procedure, *shaping,* is used when the clinician or other behavior modifier wants to teach a complex target behavior to the client in successive steps, with each step gradually leading to an approximation of the desired behavior. For example, instead of attempting to teach a severely handicapped client a whole complex behavior pattern, the behavior modifier would break up the behavior into its component parts and teach each component in successive steps that lead eventually to the performance of the complex behavior pattern (Morris, 1985).

Each of these reinforcement procedures has been used successfully with persons with mental retardation to teach them a variety of target behaviors, such as self-help/self-care skills, social skills, reading, math, writing, job interview skills, job-finding skills, independent living skills, assertiveness, speech and sign language, and vocational/prevocational skills (see, e.g., Cole & Gardner, 1993; Matson et al., 1998; Matson & McCartney, 1981; Morris & McReynolds, 1986).

Behavior-Reduction Procedures

Behavior-reduction procedures involve the introduction of a dissatis-fying or unpleasant event immediately following a person's perform-ance of the target behavior that results in a decrease in the probability that the target behavior will occur again the next time that the same antecedent or situational stimuli are present (Skinner, 1938, 1953). The most commonly used behavior-reduction procedures are extinction, time-out from positive reinforcement, response cost, and overcorrec-tion (Morris, 1985). *Extinction* refers to the removal of the reinforcing consequences that normally follow a particular target behavior (Skinner, 1953). To use this procedure, the clinician, teacher, or other care provider must be able to (a) identify those consequences that are reinforcing or maintaining the client's undesirable behavior, (b) determine whether those consequences will follow the client's behavior each time the behav-ior is performed, (c) control the occurrence of those consequences, and (d) be consistent in the use of the procedure each time the target behav-ior is performed (Morris). If these conditions cannot be met, another behavior-reduction procedure should be used.

Time-out from positive reinforcement involves removing the person from an attractive and positively reinforcing situation (or withdrawing a pos-itive reinforcing activity) for a particular period of time immediately fol-lowing the client's performance of the undesirable target behavior. The type of time-out setting in which the client is placed is very important and should contain fewer positive aspects than the positive reinforcing area. Three types of time-out procedures have been applied with persons with mental retardation. "Contingent observation" involves having the client who performs the undesirable target behavior step away from the reinforcing setting (e.g., small group discussion, athletic event, group vocational activity) for a specified period and watch the other people in the setting perform appropriate behaviors and receive positive rein-forcement from the clinician or other behavior modifier. The client then rejoins the group after a specific time has elapsed. A second time-out method is called "exclusion time-out." In this method, the person is removed from the reinforcing setting for a specific time and placed in a situation that has a lower reinforcement value to the client each time he or she performs the undesirable target behavior. Typically, the client is not removed to another room or environment with this procedure; rather, he or she is placed in an isolated area in the same room with his or her back to the group activity. A third procedure is "seclusion time-out," in which the client is removed from the reinforcing situation for a specific period and placed in a supervised isolated area (e.g., vacant room, cubi-cle) that is separate from the reinforcing setting. The isolated area must be well ventilated, well lighted, and unlocked, and the person must be monitored on a regular basis (Kazdin, 1994; Morris, 1985).

*response
cost*

*Over
Correction*

Another behavior reduction procedure is *response cost*. This procedure is typically combined with a token-economy positive reinforcement method and involves placing a cost on a client's performance of a specific undesirable target behavior. Thus, this procedure consists of the removal or withdrawal of a particular quantity of reinforcers (tokens) from the person each time he or she performs the target behavior. *Overcorrection* is a procedure that includes both an educational and a response-suppression component (Foxx & Azrin, 1972). These components are "restitution" (the person corrects the environmental effects of the impact of his or her undesirable behavior to a vastly improved state) and "positive practice" (the person is required to intensely practice appropriate types of behavior in the environmental setting in which he or she performed the undesirable behavior).

These methods have been used effectively to decrease the frequency or eliminate the occurrence of a wide variety of target behaviors, including physical aggression, verbal aggression, disruptive behaviors, property destruction, stealing, noncompliance, head banging and other self-injurious behavior (SIB), and self-stimulation. However, they should be used only in conjunction with positive reinforcement procedures to teach alternative desirable target behaviors to clients (Kazdin, 1994; Morris, 1985).

Modeling/Imitation Learning Procedures

*Modeling
Bandura*

Imitation

Behavior change that results from the observation of another person has been typically referred to as *modeling* (Bandura, 1969; Bandura & Walters, 1963). The modeling procedure consists of an individual called the model (e.g., therapist, teacher, parent, aide) and a person called the observer (e.g., the client). The observer typically observes the model performing the desirable target behavior in a familiar setting, where the model experiences reinforcement for engaging in the behavior. Another approach to modeling follows Skinner's (1938, 1953) position, in which the clinician, teacher, or other care provider first demonstrates the target behavior and then reinforces the person for successfully imitating the target behavior of the therapist. Modeling or imitation learning often reduces the amount of time that a person needs to learn a particular behavior.

Although modeling and imitation learning have been found effective in teaching persons with mental retardation, there are certain preconditions that must be met for them to be helpful. First, the person should be able to attend to the various aspects of the modeling situation. Second, the person should be able to reproduce motorically the modeled behavior. Third, the person should be motivated to perform the target behavior that she or he has observed (Bandura, 1969; Rimm & Masters, 1979). If any of these factors is absent, the clinician should consider using another behavior modification procedure to teach the target behavior. Modeling has been used effectively to teach such behaviors as social skills, speech and related conversational skills, and recreational activities.

Self-Management Procedures

Self-management refers to a group of procedures in which the person becomes the primary agent directing and controlling his or her behavior to lead to preplanned and specific behavior changes and/or consequences (see, e.g., Goldfried & Merbaum, 1973; Kanfer, 1980; Karoly & Kanfer, 1982; Lloyd, Hallahan, Kauffman, & Keller, 1998; Matson et al., 1998). Self-management methods have the following as their common base: (a) the recognition of the contribution of cognitive processes to behavior change and (b) the view that individuals can regulate their own behavior. A third common base involves the presence of a clinician, teacher, or other care provider to motivate the person to begin the self-management plan and to teach him or her how, when, and where to use it (Kanfer).

The essence of a self-management approach involves the following general steps: (a) having the person with mental retardation discuss with the clinician or teacher the negative thinking styles that may be preventing the person from working effectively or that may lead him or her to become emotionally upset; (b) developing with the person specific self-statements, rules, or strategies that can be used to assist him or her in performing the appropriate target behavior, educational task, or work activity; and (c) providing the person with positive reinforcement and feedback for his or her use of the self-management procedure (e.g., Meichenbaum & Genest, 1980).

Self-management procedures represent a potentially effective approach for changing the behaviors of individuals with mental retardation (Ferretti, Cavalier, Murphy, & Murphy, 1993). The relative effectiveness of this approach, however, is tied not only to the level of structuring provided by the clinician but also to the receptiveness, interest, and motivational level of the client in implementing the procedure. Moreover, in some cases, if the level of cognitive functioning in the client is quite low, the procedures may be contraindicated—although there is research literature to suggest that they can also be used effectively with clients who have severe handicaps (e.g., Ferretti et al.; Rusch, McKee, Chadsey-Rusch, & Renzaglia, 1988; Shapiro, 1981, 1986). Self-management has been used effectively with teaching such behaviors as on-task activity, exercise skills, chores, and social skills.

PERVASIVE DEVELOPMENTAL DISORDERS

UNTIL THE MID-1960S it was commonly assumed that the basis for autism was a pathological parent-infant relationship (see, e.g., Bettelheim,

1950, 1967, 1974; Kanner, 1943, 1948). As a result, the most widely used therapeutic approach was psychoanalytically based treatment. Alternative theories regarding the etiology of autism and its treatment began to appear in the mid-1960s (Harris, 1988). An early alternative approach was associated with the organic theory of autism as proposed by Rimland (1964). After thoroughly reviewing the literature on autism, Rimland concluded that the disorder had a biological basis. His book stimulated a great deal of interest in the biological bases of autism, and treatment programs based on his assumption of a neurological or a biochemical dysfunction were developed (see, for example, Perry & Meiselas, 1988; Schopler, 1965; Schopler & Reichler, 1971).

More recent research on the biochemical basis of Autism Syndrome Disorders has focused on the role of the neurotransmitter serotonin, which is involved in the body's arousal system. Altered serotonergic function in individuals with autism has been reported by Freeman and Ritvo (1984), who note that 30% to 40% of autistic individuals maintain an elevated level of blood serotonin throughout their lifetime rather than demonstrating the expected decrease in serotonin level with maturation. Many studies have found similar increased levels of serotonin (Anderson, Horne, Chatterjee, & Cohen, 1990; Anderson et al., 2002; Cook et al., 1990; Minderaa et al., 1989), with this finding being considered one of the most robust and well-replicated in the neurobiology of autism (Buitelaar & Willemsen-Swinkels, 2000).

Some studies which have focused on pharmacological treatment to reduce blood serotonin levels (e.g., with fenfluramine) have reported improved eye contact, social awareness, attention, IQ scores, and sleep patterns in the children, as well as decreased hyperactivity and repetitive behavior (e.g., August, Raz, & Baird, 1985; Ritvo et al., 1984). However, other studies have failed to demonstrate behavioral or other improvements as a result of pharmacological treatment to decrease blood serotonin level (e.g., Duker et al., 1991; Ekman, Miranda-Linne, Gilberg, & Garle, 1989). Selective serotonin reuptake inhibitors (SSRIs), such as fluvoxamine and sertraline, have shown promising results with adults with autism who demonstrate rigid behaviors similar to those seen in patients with obsessive-compulsive disorder (Hellings, Kelley, Gabrielli, Kilgore, & Shah, 1996; McDougle et al., 1996). Response rates to SSRIs in children and adolescents diagnosed with Autism Syndrome Disorders have been low and these children and adolescents may be very sensitive to the stimulating side effects of SSRIs (Buitelaar & Willemsen-Swinkels, 2000). Little is known about the long-term effects of some of the medications for autism (Tanguay, 2000). In general, pharmacological treatment of children with Autism Syndrome Disorders has had limited success, with most drug treatments focusing on the reduction or alleviation of disruptive symptoms (Charlop-Christy et al., 1998; Tanguay, 2000).

In addition to studies on the biochemical basis of autism, other recent studies have focused on abnormal neuronal organization and brain development in individuals with autism (e.g., Waterhouse, Fein, & Mohdahl, 1996). Neuroimaging studies using MRIs and CT scans, as well as post-mortem examinations, have revealed a higher incidence of structural brain defects, particularly in the cerebellum, in individuals diagnosed with autism as compared to nondiagnosed individuals (e.g., Allen & Courchesne, 2003; Courchesne, 1989; Courchesne et al., 1994; Haas et al., 1996; Rapin & Katzman, 1998). The cerebellum is involved in the regulation of incoming sensation, and it has been suggested that decreased cerebellar volume in individuals with autism contributes to difficulties in coordinating and shifting attention (i.e., problems in "joint attention" and in shifting attention between people and between people and objects).

Dysfunction in the amygdala has also been suggested as an etiological source for the inability to interpret facial expressions and showing poor social judgment present in individuals with autism (Pickett, 2001). Recently, brain overgrowth has been associated with autism (Brambilla et al., 2003; Courchesne, Carper, & Akshoomoff, 2003). Based on a review of MRI studies of brain anatomy and development (Brambilla et al.), a larger total brain volume, as well as larger parieto-temporal lobe and cerebellar hemisphere volumes, were the most frequently replicated abnormalities found in individuals diagnosed with autism (Brambilla et al.).

Several studies have attempted to isolate the genetic underpinnings of pervasive developmental disorders. As noted earlier, the genetic basis of Rett's Syndrome was identified as mutation of the MeCP2 gene, which is located on the X chromosome (Amir et al., 1999). It is thought that most cases of autism are the result of a polygenic disorder with many genes contributing to the presentation of this disorder. Genetic markers for several behavioral conditions seen in autism have been identified. Chromosome 7 is hypothetically linked to communication dysfunction, chromosome 15 to ritualism and obsessive compulsive disorder, and chromosome 16 to social reciprocity deficits (Gillberg, 1999). Studies exploring the heritability of autism and Asperger's Disorder have found a high concordance rate in monozygotic but not dizygotic twins, suggesting that Autism Syndrome Disorders may be the result of an underlying autosomal recessive genetic disorder (e.g., Gillberg, 1999; Ritvo, Freeman, Mason-Brothers, Mo, & Ritvo, 1985; Ritvo, Spence et al., 1985). No genetically based treatment programs have been developed, but information on the heritability of pervasive developmental disorders may be of use in genetic counseling.

Most contemporary intervention programs for the treatment of pervasive developmental disorders are based on the use of *behavior modification procedures,* and the behavioral approach is reported to be the major treatment model that has been empirically demonstrated to be effective in treating children with autism (Charlop-Christy et al., 1998). Many contemporary behavior modification programs focus on a prescribed and structured teaching of objectively defined behaviors, skills, and facts. Focus is initially on student compliance with the teacher/adult, with rewards given for correct responses, with the behavioral program largely directed through oral language (Tanguay, 2000; Odom et al., 2003).

One of the earliest behavioral programs for the treatment of autism was proposed by Lovaas and his associates (e.g., Lovaas, 1977; Lovaas, Berberich, Perloff, & Schaeffer, 1966). They used behavior modification techniques to treat many of the behaviors associated with autism, including increasing the frequency of eye contact, developing functional speech and social skills, and reducing self-injurious and stereotypic behaviors. Lovaas and his associates used an approach called discrete trial training, in which every task given to the child consisted of a request to perform a specific action, followed by a response from the child, and a reaction from the therapist. Lovaas (1987) reported on the results of a treatment study in which preschool children with autism received intensive behavioral treatment (i.e., more than 40 hours per week of intensive one-to-one behavioral intervention), while similar children in a control group received less intensive treatment (i.e., 10 hours per week of behavioral treatment). Results indicated that 47% of the children in the intensive treatment group, compared to 2% of the children in the control group, achieved normal intellectual functioning and were placed in the regular first-grade education program.

A review of behavioral treatment programs for individuals with autism and related pervasive developmental disorders suggests that most studies have focused on the use of behavior modification procedures to reduce or eliminate behavior problems (e.g., tantrums, aggression, SIB, self-stimulation) and to develop and strengthen communication and social skills. Programs for treating behavior problems have typically used extinction, as well as such positive reinforcement techniques as DRO and DRI. In addition, many of the programs have included a functional analysis of the problem behavior prior to the start of treatment so that an appropriate replacement behavior, such as tapping the teacher to communicate with her rather than yelling, could be identified (e.g., Dunlap & Fox, 1999; Durand & Carr, 1991; Horner & Day, 1991; Keen, Sigafoos, & Woodyatt, 2001). One of the problems noted in initiating behavioral treatment programs for individuals who have been diagnosed with autism is that these individuals may not be motivated to learn the behaviors or skills to be taught (Charlop-Christy et al., 1998). In addition, it is often difficult to identify salient reinforcers—or any reinforcers other than food, liquids, and the avoidance of pain. Some researchers have utilized internal reinforcers (e.g., opportunities to engage in self-stimulatory behaviors) in teaching new skills (e.g., Charlop,

Kurtz, & Casey, 1990). The use of DRO and DRI is considered to be a well-established practice in the treatment of autism (Odom et al., 2003).

It has been estimated that approximately 50% of children with autism have very limited verbal skills or are nonverbal, and children with autism are diagnosed with receptive and expressive language deficits (Rimland, 1964). Behavioral programs for teaching language to these children have included both verbal language and sign language training (e.g., Carr, 1979; Carr, Kologinsky, & Leff-Simon, 1987; Fay & Schuler, 1980; Lovaas, 1977). Most such programs focus primarily on the development of functional language, using positive reinforcement and shaping procedures for imitating the clinician's vocalizations. Language enhancement programs, such as Natural Language Programming (NLP), also have been developed to teach nonverbal children with autism to talk (see, for example, R. L. Koegel, O'Dell, & Koegel, 1987). In NLP, language training through modeling and imitation takes place in a naturalistic setting, with the autistic children imitating the speech of the teacher/model as they play with high-interest toys or engage in high-interest activities. R. L. Koegel et al. have reported higher rates of imitated verbalization, as well as greater generalization of verbalizations to other settings, with the use of NLP than with the more traditional forms of functional language training.

Behavioral procedures are also used in teaching an augmentative communication program to nonverbal individuals. For example, the *Picture Exchange Communication System* (PECS) (Bondy & Frost, 1994) uses behavioral methods to teach functional communication skills. Nonverbal individuals are reinforced for exchanging a picture of something they want, such as an item (e.g., a glass of water) or an activity (e.g., swinging on a swing), for that item or activity. Programs that use visually-based communication systems and activity schedules have been found to promote language and decrease inappropriate behavior (Bondy & Frost, 1998, 2002; Charlop-Christy, Carpenter, Le, LeBlanc, & Kellet, 2002; Matson, Sevin, Box, Francis, & Sevin, 1993; Morrison, Sainto, BenChaaban, & Endo, 2002; Wood, Lasker, Siegel-Causey, Beukelman, & Ball, 1998). When compared to auditory presentation alone, visual strategies, such as picture icons, drawings, objects, and/or written word, provide a more concrete way of presenting information, support, and/or instruction (Hodgdon, 1996; MacDuff, Krantz, & McClannahan, 1993; Pierce & Schreibman, 1994). The use of visual strategies provides an effective procedure for developing language communication systems for individuals with autism and related pervasive developmental disorders (Odom et al., 2003).

Behavioral programs focusing on the development of social skills in individuals with Autism Syndrome Disorders also have utilized behavior approaches, such as modeling and imitation learning. For example, Strain and his associates (e.g., Odom, Hoyson, Jamieson, & Strain, 1985; Odom & Strain, 1984; Strain, Ken, & Ragland, 1979) integrated autistic and nonautistic peers in a naturalistic setting, with the socially competent children acting as peer models in initiating and carrying out social interactions. Laushey and Heflin (2000) created a class-wide buddy system wherein several students were assigned to support the social interaction of peers with autism. Other social skills studies have used adults to model social interactions, utilized verbal prompts to initiate social interaction patterns, and used self-management and self-reinforcement procedures for developing social interaction (e.g., R. L. Koegel & Frea, 1993; Krantz, MacDuff, & McClannahan, 1993).

Behavioral principles, including charting and reinforcement, have been incorporated into comprehensive curriculums for individuals with autism, such as the Treatment and Education of Autistic and related Communication-Handicapped Children (TEACCH) program developed at the University of North Carolina. This structured teaching program is heavily grounded in controlling the environment and providing routine. It utilizes visual strategies as part of the program (Schopler, Mesibov, & Hearsey, 1995).

Recently, treatment programs designed to teach social and interpersonal skills have been developed. These programs are based on the "theory of mind," and are designed to remediate deficits in the ability to understand or recognize feelings, points of view, or plans of others and to foster emotional development and the development of social skills. Two such programs are Carol Gray's "Social Stories" (e.g., Gray, 2000; Gray & Garand, 1993; Gray, White, & McAndrew, 2002) and Steven Gutstein's Relationship Development Intervention (RDI) program (Gutstein & Sheely, 2002a, 2002b). These programs, especially RDI, incorporate adult teacher and peer modeling. Controlled research documenting the efficacy of these programs is not currently available.

Other non-behavioral programs have been developed for use in teaching individuals with pervasive developmental disorders. These include social-pragmatic, child-centered, and incidental teaching methods that emphasize following the child's focus of attention and using what motivates him or her to build upon his or her current repertoire of social and communicative behaviors (see, for example, Greenspan, 1995; Lewy & Dawson, 1992; Rogers & Lewis, 1989). These procedures advocate the use of visual, verbal, and tactile cues, to motivate learning through shared experiences and naturally occurring events (Tanguay, 2000).

Other treatment procedures for individuals with pervasive developmental disabilities focus on addressing hyper- and hypo-reactivity to sensory stimulation, as well as problems with distortion of sensory input. As O'Neill and Jones (1997) have noted, there are many published firsthand accounts and published findings detailing the problems with multi-channel receptivity and processing of people with Autism Spectrum Disorders, especially autism (e.g., Grandin, 1986; Stehli, 1991;

Williams, 1992), and a wide variety of treatment programs aimed at improving the utilization of sensory information and alleviating problems associated with sensory input.

Perhaps the best-known and most widely utilized of these procedures is sensory integration therapy (Ayers, 1972, 1979), which focuses primarily on three senses, tactile (i.e., touch), vestibular (i.e., motion and balance), and proprioception (e.g., joints and ligaments). Although numerous anecdotal reports emphasize the beneficial effects of sensory integration therapy, empirical reviews of the efficacy of sensory integration procedures have not yet been able to document reliable treatment effects for any specific patient population (see, for example, Reilly, Nelson, & Bundy, 1983; Shaw, 2002). However, Miller (2003) has cogently argued that this lack of empirical documentation is the result of (a) the absence of controlled experimental studies of sensory integration treatments, (b) problems in developing measures to reliably and accurately assess the physiologic and behavioral manifestations of sensory processing impairments, and (c) difficulties in reaching conclusions based on studies that utilize different subject populations and different treatment protocols.

Specific treatment programs have also been developed to address problems in hypo- and hyper-sensitivity to auditory and visual stimuli as well as problems in sound discrimination and visual attention. Many auditory interventions, such as Berard's Auditory Integration Training (Berard, 1993) and the Tomatis method, focus on reducing oversensitivity to sound and involve repeated listening to a variety of different sound frequencies coordinated to the person's level of impairment. The most commonly used programs for the treatment of sensitivity to visual stimuli are vision training programs and the use of colored lenses (Irlen lenses) to minimize print distortions when reading. Formal vision training programs are usually directed by a developmental behavioral optometrist and involve visual-motor exercises. There have been a few studies supporting use of auditory intervention programs with individuals with Autism Syndrome Disorders (e.g., Bettison, 1996; Madell & Rose, 1994; Rimland & Edelson, 1994, 1995). There is no empirical research documenting the efficacy of vision training programs for individuals with Autism Syndrome Disorders or other pervasive developmental disabilities.

PSYCHOLOGICAL AND VOCATIONAL IMPLICATIONS

As a result of the deinstitutionalization and normalization movements that began in the late 1960s and early 1970s, as well as the research advances in behavior modification treatment, many individuals with developmental disabilities are living in group homes, semi-independent apartments/homes, or independent living residences rather than in institutional settings. Although this situation certainly reflects the advances that have taken place in the treatment of problems associated with developmental disabilities over the past 20–25 years, certain problems continue to plague the field (see, e.g., Brown et al., 1986; Cole & Gardner, 1993; Lovaas & Buch, 1992; Matson et al., 1998; Smith, Parker, Taubman, & Lovaas, 1992).

Two major issues remaining to be addressed involve the maximization of treatment gains through the generalization of behaviors that have been modified or successfully developed in persons with developmental disabilities in their natural environment (i.e., stimulus generalization) and the maintenance of treatment gains over time in the person's natural environment (temporal generalization). These issues have significant implications when assessing the long-term success of the psychological and vocational aspects of a person's treatment and habilitation process (see, e.g., Luce, Christian, Anderson, Troy, & Larsson, 1992; Matson & Coe, 1992; Matson et al., 1998; Perel, 1992; Wacker & Berg, 1988; Wetzel, 1992; Wetzel & Hoschouer, 1984). In addition, an overarching problem faced by all who work with individuals who have developmental disabilities concerns how we as a society and knowledgeable professionals can make the adult lives of persons with developmental disabilities more meaningful and fulfilling. The goal is for persons with developmental disabilities to lead meaningful and productive adult lives, including, if appropriate, gainful employment (Patton, 1988).

There is no cure for autism. Treatment and educational approaches reduce some of the challenges of the disability, including lessening disruptive behaviors and teaching self-help skills that allow for greater independence. Treatment is tailored to the child's behaviors and needs.

REFERENCES

Alberto, P., Heflin, L. J., & Andrews, D. (2002). Use of the timeout ribbon procedure during community-based instruction. *Behavior Modification, 26,* 297–312.

Allen, G., & Courchesne, E. (2003). Differential effects of developmental cerebellar abnormality on cognitive and motor functions in the cerebellum: An fMRI study of autism. *American Journal of Psychiatry, 160,* 262–274.

Aman, M. G., & Singh, N. N. (1991). Pharmacological intervention. In I. L. Matson & I. A. Mulick (Eds.), *Handbook of mental retardation* (2nd ed., pp. 347–372). New York: Pergamon Press.

American Association on Mental Retardation. (1992). *Mental retardation: Definition, classification, and systems of supports* (9th ed.). Washington, DC: Author.

American Association on Mental Retardation. (2002). *Mental retardation: Definition, classification, and systems of supports* (10th ed.). Washington, DC: Author.

American Psychiatric Association. (1968). *Diagnostic and statistical manual of mental disorders* (2nd ed.). Washington, DC: Author.

American Psychiatric Association. (1980). *Diagnostic and statistical manual of mental disorders* (3rd ed.). Washington, DC: Author.

American Psychiatric Association. (1994). *Diagnostic and statistical manual of mental disorders* (4th ed.). Washington, DC: Author.

American Psychological Association. (1994, August). *Resolution on facilitated communication by the Council of Representatives of the American Psychological Association.* Los Angeles: Author.

Amir, R. E., Ignatia, B., Van den Veyver, I. B., Wan, M., Tran, C. Q., Francke, U., et al. (1999). Rett syndrome is caused by mutations in X-linked MECP2 encoding mathyl-CpG-binding protein 2. *Nature Genetics, 23,* 185–188.

Anderson, G. M., Gutknecht, L., Cohen, D. J., Brailly-Tabard, S., Cohen, J. H. M., Ferrari, P., et al. (2002). Serotonin transporter and promoter variants in autism: Functional effects and relationship to platelet hyperserotonemia. *Molecular Psychiatry, 7,* 831–836.

Anderson, G. M., Horne, W. C., Chatterjee, D., & Cohen, D. J. (1990). The hyperserotonemia of autism. *Annals of the New York Academy of Science, 600,* 331–342.

Asperger, H. (1944). Die "autistichen psychopathen" in Kinder esatler. *Archive fur Psychiatrie und Nervenkrankheiten, 117,* 76–136. Translated by U. Frith (1991) (Ed.), *Autism and Asperger Syndrome* (pp. 37–92). New York: Cambridge University Press.

Attwood, T. (1998). *Asperger's syndrome: A guide for parents and professionals.* London: Jessica Kingsley Publisher.

August, G. J., Raz, N., & Baird, T. D. (1985). Brief report: Effects of fenfluramine on behavioral, cognitive, and affective disturbances in autistic children. *Journal of Autism and Developmental Disorders, 15,* 97–107.

Ayers, A. J. (1972). *Sensory integration and learning disorders.* Los Angeles: Western Psychological Associates.

Ayers, A. J. (1979). *Sensory integration and the child.* Los Angeles: Western Psychological Associates.

Ayllon, T., & Azrin, N. H. (1968). *The token economy: A motivational system for therapy and rehabilitation.* New York: Appleton-Century-Crofts.

Baer, D. M., Wolf, M., & Risley, T. R. (1968). Some current dimensions of applied behavior analysis. *Journal of Applied Behavior Analysis, 1,* 91–97.

Baraitser, M., & Winter, R. M. (1996). *Color atlas of congenital malformations.* London: Mosby-Wolfe.

Bandura, A., & Walters, R. H. (1963). *Social learning and personality development.* New York: Holt.

Bandura, A. (1969). *Principles of behavior modification.* New York: Holt.

Baumeister, A. A. (1970). The American residential institution: Its history and character. In A. A. Baumeister & E. Butterfield (Eds.), *Residential facilities for the mentally retarded* (pp. 1–28). Chicago: Aldine.

Berard, G. (1993). *Hearing equals behavior.* New Caanan, CT: Keats Publishing.

Berg, I. M. (1975). Aetiological aspects of mental subnormality: Pathological factors. In A. M. Clark & A. D. B. Clarke (Eds.), *Mental deficiency: The changing outlook* (pp. 81–117). New York: Free Press.

Bertrand, J., Mars, A., Boyle, C., Bove, F., Yeargin-Allsopp, M., & Decoufle, P. (2001). Prevalence of autism in a United States population: The Brick Township, New Jersey, investigation. *Pediatrics, 108,* 1155–1161.

Bettelheim, B. (1950). *Love is not enough.* Glencoe, IL: Free Press.

Bettelheim, B. (1967). *The empty fortress.* New York: Free Press.

Bettelheim, B. (1974). *A home for the heart.* New York: Knopf.

Bettison, S. (1996). The long-term effects of auditory training on children with autism. *Journal of Autism and Developmental Disorders, 26,* 361–374.

Bienvenu, T., Carrié, A., de Roux, N., Vinet, M., Jonveaux, P., Couvery, P. V., et al. (2000). MECP2 mutations account for most atypical forms of Rett syndrome. *Human Molecular Genetics, 9,* 1377–1384.

Blackman, J. A. (Ed.). (1983). *Medical aspects of developmental disabilities in children birth to three.* Iowa City: University of Iowa.

Blatt, B. (1968). The dark side of the mirror. *Mental Retardation, 6,* 42–44.

Blatt, B. (1984). Biography in autobiography. In B. Blatt & R. J. Morris (Eds.), *Perspectives in special education: Personal orientations* (pp. 263–307). Glenview, IL: Scott, Foresman.

Blatt, B., & Kaplan, F. (1966). *Christmas in purgatory: A photographic essay on mental retardation.* Boston: Allyn & Bacon.

Bondy, A., & Frost, L. (1994). The Delaware Autistic Program. In S. L. Harris & J. S. Handleman (Eds.), *Preschool education for children with autism* (pp. 37–54). Austin, TX: PRO-ED.

Bondy, A., & Frost, L. (1998). The Picture Exchange Communication System. *Topics in Language Disorders, 19,* 373–390.

Bondy, A., & Frost, L. (2002). *A picture's worth: PECS and other visual communication strategies in autism.* Bethesda, MD: Woodbine House.

Boyle, C. A., Yeargin-Allsopp, M., Doernberg, N. S., Holmgreen, P., Murphy, C. C., & Schendel, D. E. (1996). Prevalence of selected developmental disabilities in children 3–10 years of age: The Metropolitan Atlanta Developmental Disabilities Surveillance Program, 1991. *Morbidity and Mortality Weekly Report Surveillance Summaries, 45,* 1–14. Retrieved May 12, 2004 from www.cdc.gov/MMWR/preview/MMWRhtml/00040929.htm

Brambilla, P., Hardan, A., Ucelli di Nemi, S., Perez, J., Soares, J. C., & Barale, F. (2003). Brain anatomy and development in autism: Review of structural MRI studies. *Brain Research Bulletin, 61*(6), 557–569.

Brison, D. W. (1967). Definition, diagnosis, and classification. In A. A. Baumeister (Ed.), *Mental retardation* (pp. 1–19). Chicago: Aldine.

Brown, L., Shiraga, B., Ford, J. R., Nisbet, J., VanDeventer, P., Sweet, M., et al. (1986). Teaching severely handicapped students to perform meaningful work in nonsheltered vocational environments. In R. J. Morris & B. Blatt (Eds.), *Special education: Research and trends* (pp. 131–189). New York: Pergamon Press.

Buitelaar, J. K., & Willemsen-Swinkels, S. H. N. (2000). Medication treatment in subjects with autistic spectrum disorders. *European Child & Adolescent Psychiatry, 9*, 85–97.

Carr, E. G. (1979). Teaching autistic children to use sign language: Some research issues. *Journal of Autism and Developmental Disorders, 9*, 345–359.

Carr, E. G., Kologinsky, E., & Leff-Simon, S. (1987). Acquisition of sign language by autistic children: 3. Generalized descriptive phases. *Journal of Autism and Developmental Disorders, 17*, 217–229.

Carr, E. G., Turnbull, A. P., & Horner, R. H. (1999). *Positive behavior support in people with developmental disabilities: A research synthesis.* Washington, DC: American Association on Mental Retardation.

Center for Disease Control and Prevention. (2000). *Prevalence of autism in Brick Township, New Jersey. 1998: Community report.* Retrieved May 20, 2004 from http://www.cdc.gov/ncbddd/pub/BrickReport.pdf

Chakrabarti, S., & Fombonne, E. (2001). Pervasive developmental disorders in preschool children. *Journal of the American Medical Association, 285*, 3093–3099.

Charlop, M. H., Kurtz, P. F., & Casey, F. G. (1990). Using aberrant behaviors as reinforcers for autistic children. *Journal of Applied Behavior Analysis, 22*, 275–285.

Charlop-Christy, M. H., Carpenter, M., Le, L., LeBlanc, L. A., & Kellet, K. (2002). Using the picture exchange communication system (PECS) with children with autism: Assessment of PECS acquisition, speech, social-communicative behavior, and problem behavior. *Journal of Applied Behavior Analysis, 35*, 213–231.

Charlop-Christy, M. H., Schreibman, L., Pierce, K., & Kurtz, P. (1998). Childhood autism. In R. J. Morris & T. R. Kratochwill (Eds.), *The practice of child therapy* (3rd ed., pp. 271–302). Needham Heights, MA: Allyn & Bacon.

Charman, T. (2002). The prevalence of autism spectrum disorders: Recent evidence and future challenges. *European Child and Adolescent Psychiatry, 11*, 249–256.

Cole, C. L., & Gardner, W. I. (1993). Psychotherapy with developmentally delayed children. In T. R. Kratochwill & R. J. Morris (Eds.), *Handbook of psychotherapy with children and adolescents* (pp. 426–471). Boston: Allyn & Bacon.

Conyers, C., Martin, T. L., Martin, G. L., & Yu, D. (2002). The 1983 AAMR Manual, the 1992 Manual, or the Developmental Disabilities Act: Which do researchers use? *Education and Training in Mental Retardation and Developmental Disabilities, 37*, 310–316.

Cook, E. H. J., Leventhal, B. L., Heller, W., Metz, J., Wainwright, M., & Freedman,

D. X. (1990). Autistic children and their first-degree relatives: Relationships between serotonin and norepinephrine levels and intelligence. *Journal of Neuropsychiatry and Clinical Neuroscience, 2,* 268–274.

Coulter, D. L. (1991). Theoretical basis of the definition. In R. Luckasson (Ed.), *Classification in mental retardation: Draft—1991.* Washington, DC: American Association on Mental Retardation.

Courchesne, E. (1989). Neuroanatomical systems involved in infantile autism: The implications of cerebellar abnormalities. In G. Dawson (Ed.), *Autism: New perspectives on diagnosis, nature, and treatment* (pp. 119–143). New York: Guilford Press.

Courchesne, E., Carper, R., & Akshoomoff, N. (2003). Evidence of brain over-growth in the first year of life in autism. *Journal of the American Medical Association, 290,* 337–345.

Courchesne, E., Saitho, O., Yeung-Courchesne, R., Press, G. A., Lincoln, A. J., Haas, R. H., et al. (1994). Abnormality of cerebellar vermian lobules VI and VII in patients with infantile autism: Identification of hypoplastic and hyperplastic subgroups by MR imaging. *American Journal of Roentgenology, 162,* 123–130.

Cowen, E. (1963). Psychotherapy and play techniques with the exceptional child and youth. In W. M. Cruickshank (Ed.), *Psychology of exceptional children and youth* (2nd ed., pp. 526–592). Englewood Cliffs, NJ: Prentice-Hall.

Croen, L. A., Grether, J. K., Hoogstrate, J., & Selvin, S. (2002). The changing prevalence of autism in California. *Journal of Autism and Developmental Disorders, 32,* 207–215.

Curry, C. J., Stevenson, R. E., Aughton, D., Carey, J. C., Cassidy, S., et al. (1997). Evaluation of mental retardation: Recommendations of a consensus conference. *American Journal of Medical Genetics, 72,* 168–477.

Daily, D. K., Ardinger, H. H., & Holmes, G. E. (2000). Identification and evaluation of mental retardation. *American Family Physician, 61,* 1059–1065.

Developmental Disabilities Act. (1984). Washington, DC: U.S. Government Printing Office.

Developmental Disabilities Assistance and Bill of Rights Act, Pub. L. No. 106-402). (2000). Washington, DC: U.S. Government Printing Office.

Duker, P. C., Welles, K., Seys, D., Rensen, H., Vis, A., & van der Berg, G. (1991). Brief report: Effects of fenfluramine on communicative, stereotypic and inappropriate behaviors of autistic-type mentally handicapped individuals. *Journal of Autism and Developmental Disorders, 21,* 355–363.

Dunlap, G., & Fox, L. (1999). A demonstration of behavioral support for young children with autism. *Journal of Positive Behavior Interventions, 1,* 77–87.

Durand, V. M., & Carr, E. G. (1991). Functional communication training to reduce challenging behavior: Maintenance and application in new settings. *Journal of Applied Behavior Analysis, 25,* 251–264.

Ehlers, W. H., Prothero, J. C., & Langone, J. (1982). *Mental retardation and other developmental disabilities* (3rd ed.). Columbus, OH: Merrill.

Eisenmajer, R., Prier, M., Leekham, S., Wing, L., Gould, J., Welham, M., & Ong, B. (1996). Comparison of clinical symptoms in autism and Asperger's disorder. *Journal of the Academy of Child & Adolescent Psychiatry, 35,* 1523–1531.

Ekman, G., Miranda-Linne, F., Gillberg, C., & Garle, M. (1989). Fenfluramine treatment of 20 children with autism. *Journal of Autism and Developmental Disabilities, 19,* 511–532.

Fay, W. H., & Schuler, A. L. (1980). *Emerging language in autistic children.* Baltimore: University Park Press.

Fereitti, R. P., Cavalier, A. R., Murphy, M. J., & Murphy, R. (1993). The self-management of skills by persons with mental retardation. *Research in Developmental Disabilities, 14,* 189–206.

Fombonne, E. (1999). The epidemiology of autism: A review. *Psychological Medicine, 29,* 769–786.

Fombonne, E. (2002). Prevalence of childhood disintegrative disorder. *Autism, 6,* 149–157.

Fombonne, E. (2003a). Editorial. *Journal of the American Medical Association, 289,* 49.

Fombonne, E. (2003b). Epidemiological surveys of autism and other pervasive developmental disorders: An update. *Journal of Autism and Developmental Disorders, 33,* 365–382.

Fombonne, E., Simmons, H., Ford, T., Meltzer, H., & Goodman, R. (2001). Prevalence of pervasive developmental disorders in the British nationwide survey of child mental health. *Journal of the American Academy of Child and Adolescent Psychiatry, 40,* 820–827.

Foxx, R. M., & Azrin, N. H. (1972). Restitution: A method of eliminating aggressive-disruptive behavior of retarded and brain-damaged patients. *Behaviour, Research, & Therapy, 13,* 15–28.

Freeman, B. J., & Ritvo, E. R. (1984). The syndrome of autism: Establishing the diagnosis and principles of management. *Pediatric Analysis, 13,* 284–305.

Friedman, P. (1975). *The rights of the mentally retarded.* New York: Avon.

Frith, U. (1991). Asperger and his syndrome. In U. Frith (Ed.), *Autism and Asperger Syndrome* (pp. 1–36). New York: Cambridge University Press.

Gardner, W. I. (1970). *Behavior modification in mental retardation.* Chicago: Aldine.

Gardner, W. I. (1971). *Behavior modification in mental retardation.* Chicago: Aldine.

Gillberg, C. (1999). Neurodevelopmental processes and psychological functioning in autism. *Development and Psychopathology, 11,* 567–587.

Gillberg, C., & Wing, L. (1999). Autism: Not an extremely rare disorder. *Acta Psychiatrica Scandinavia, 99,* 399–406.

Goldfried, M. R., & Merbaum, M. A. (1973). A perspective on self-control. In M. R. Goldfried & M. Merbaum (Eds.), *Behavior change through self-control* (pp. 127–143). New York: Holt.

Gorlin, R. J., Cohen, M. M., & Hennekam, R. C. M. (2001). *Syndromes of the head and neck* (4th ed.). Oxford, England: Oxford University Press.

Grandin, T. (1986). *Emergence: Labeled autistic.* Novato, CA: Academic Therapy Publications.

Gray, C. A. (2000). *The new social stories book: Illustrated edition.* Arlington, TX: Future Horizons.

Gray, C. A., & Garand, J. D. (1993). Social stories: Improving responses of students with autism with accurate social information. *Journal of Autism and Developmental Disabilities, 23,* 593–617.

Gray, C. A., White, A. L., & McAndrew, S. (Eds.). (2002). *My social stories book.* London: Jessica Kingsley.

Greenspan, S. C. (1995). *The challenging child. Understanding, raising and enjoying the five "different" types of children.* New York: Addison-Wesley.

Gresham, F. M., MacMillan, D. L., & Siperstein, G. N. (1995). Critical analysis of the 1992 AAMR definition: Implications for school psychology. *School Psychology Review, 10,* 1–19.

Grossman, H. J. (Ed.). (1973). *Manual on terminology and classification in mental retardation.* Washington, DC: American Association on Mental Deficiency.

Grossman, H. J. (Ed.). (1983). *Classification in mental retardation.* Washington, DC: American Association on Mental Deficiency.

Gullone, E., King, N. J., & Cummins, R. A. (1996). Fears of youth with mental retardation: Psychometric evaluation of the Fear Survey Schedule for Children-II (FSSC-II). *Research in Developmental Disabilities, 17,* 269–284.

Gutstein, S. E., & Sheely, R. K. (2002a). *Relationship development intervention with children, adolescents and adults: Social and emotional development activities for Asperger Syndrome, Autism, PDD and NLD.* London: Jessica Kingsley.

Gutstein, S. E., & Sheely, R. K. (2002b). *Relationship development intervention with young children: Social and emotional development activities for Asperger Syndrome, autism, PDD, and NLD.* London: Jessica Kingsley.

Haas, R. H., Townsend, J., Courchesne, E., Lincoln, A. J., Schreibman, L., & Yeung-Courchesne, R. (1996). Neurologic abnormalities in infantile autism. *Journal of Child Neurology, 11,* 84–92.

Hagberg, B. (2002). Clinical manifestations and stages of Rett syndrome. *Mental Retardation and Developmental Disabilities Research Review, 8,* 61–65.

Hagberg, B., Aicardi, J., Dias, K., & Ramos, O. (1983). A progressive syndrome of autism, dementia, ataxia, and loss of purposeful hand use in girls. Rett's syndrome: Report of 35 cases. *Annals of Neurology, 14,* 471–479.

Halderman v. Pennhurst, 446 F. Supp. 1295 (1977).

Harris, S. L. (1988). Autism and schizophrenia: Psychological therapies. In J. L. Matson (Ed.), *Handbook of treatment approaches in childhood psychopathology* (pp. 289–300). New York: Plenum.

Heber, R. F. (1959). A manual on terminology and classification in mental retardation. *American Journal on Mental Deficiency, 64* (Monograph Suppl.).

Heber, R. F. (1961). Modications in the manual on terminology and classification in mental retardation. *American Journal on Mental Deficiency, 65,* 499–500b.

Hellings, J. A., Kelley, L. A., Gabrielli, W. F., Kilgore, E., & Shah, P. (1996). Sertraline response in adults with mental retardation and autistic disorder. *Journal of Clinical Psychiatry, 57,* 333–336.

Hendry, C. N. (2000). Childhood disintegrative disorder: Should it be considered a distinct diagnosis? *Clinical Psychology Review, 2,* 77–90.

Hodapp, R. M. (1995). Definitions in mental retardation: Effects on research, practice, and perceptions. *School Psychology Review, 10,* 24–28.

Hodgdon, L. A. (1996). *Visual strategies for improving communication.* Troy, MI: Qirk Roberts.

Horner, R. H., & Day, H. M. (1991). The effects of response efficiency on functionally equivalent competing behaviors. *Journal of Applied Behavior Analysis, 24,* 719–732.

Humphrey, G. (1962). Introduction. In J. M. C. Itard (Ed.), *The wild boy of Aveyron* (G. Humphrey & H. Humphrey, Trans.). New York: Appleton-Century-Crofts.

Hviid, A., Stellfeld, M., Wohlfahrt, J., & Melbye, M. (2003). Association between thimerosal-containing vaccine and autism. *Journal of the American Medical Association, 290,* 1763–1766.

Individuals with Disabilities Education Act. Amendments of 1991, Pub. L. No. 102-119, 20. (1991). USS 1400 *et seq. Federal Register, 137,* 1991.

Itard, J. M. C. (1962). *The wild boy of Aveyron* (G. Humphrey & H. Humphrey, Trans.). New York: Appleton-Century-Crofts.

Jones, K. L. (1997). *Smith's recognizable patterns of human malformations* (5th ed.). Philadelphia: W. B. Saunders.

Kanfer, F. H. (1980). Self-management methods. In F. H. Kanfer & A. P. Goldstein (Eds.), *Helping people change* (2nd ed., pp. 334–389). New York: Pergamon Press.

Kanner, L. (1943). Autistic disturbances of affective contact. *Nervous Child, 2,* 217–250.

Kanner, L. (1948). *Child psychiatry.* Springfield, IL: Charles C Thomas.

Kanner, L. (1964). *A history of the care and study of the mentally retarded.* Springfield, IL: Charles C Thomas.

Karoly, P., & Kanfer, F. H. (Eds.). (1982). *Self-management and behavior change: From theory to practice.* New York: Pergamon Press.

Kazdin, A. E. (1994). *Behavior modification in applied settings* (5th ed.). Homewood, IL: Dorsey.

Keen, D., Sigafoos, J., & Woodyatt, G. (2001). Replacing prelinguistic behaviors with functional communication. *Journal of Autism and Developmental Disabilities, 22,* 407–423.

Koegel, L. K., Koegel, R. L., & Smith, A. (1997). Variables related to differences in standardized tests outcomes for children with autism. *Journal of Autism and Developmental Disorders, 27,* 233–243.

Koegel, R. L., & Frea, W. D. (1993). Treatment of social behavior in autism through the modification of pivotal skills. *Journal of Applied Behavior Analysis, 26,* 369–377.

Koegel, R. L., O'Dell, M. C., & Koegel, L. K. (1987). A natural language teaching package for nonverbal autistic children. *Journal of Autism and Developmental Disorders, 17,* 187–200.

Krantz, P. J., MacDuff, M. T., & McClannahan, L. E. (1993). Teaching children with autism to initiate to peers: Effects of a script fading procedure. *Journal of Applied Behavior Analysis, 26,* 121–132.

Laushey, K. M., & Heflin, L. J. (2000). Enhancing the social skills of kindergarten children with autism through the training of multiple peers as tutors. *Journal of Autism and Developmental Disabilities, 30,* 183–193.

Lee, J. K., Larson, S. A., Lakin, K. C., Anderson, L., Lee, N. K., & Anderson, D. (2001). Prevalence of mental retardation and developmental disabilities: Estimates from the 1994/1995 national health interview survey disability supplements. *American Journal on Mental Retardation, 106,* 231–252.

Leland, H. (1991). Adaptive behavior scales. In J. L. Matson & J. A. Mulick (Eds.), *Handbook of mental retardation* (pp. 234–251). New York: Pergamon Press.

Lewy, A., & Dawson, G. (1992). Social stimulation and joint attention deficits in young autistic children. *Journal of Abnormal Child Psychology, 20,* 555–566.

Lloyd, K. W., Hallahan, D. P., Kauffman, J. M., & Keller, C. E. (1998). Academic problems. In R. J. Morris & T. R. Kratochwill (Eds.), *The practice of child therapy* (3rd ed., pp. 167–198). Needham Heights, MA: Allyn & Bacon.

Lorimer, P. A., Simpson, R. L., Myles, B. S., & Ganz, J. B. (2002). The use of social stories as a preventative behavioral intervention in a home setting with a child with autism. *Journal of Positive Behavior Interventions, 4,* 53–60.

Lovaas, O. I. (1977). *The autistic child.* New York: Irvington Publishers.

Lovaas, O. I. (1987). Behavioral treatment and normal education and intellectual functioning in young autistic children. *Journal of Consulting and Clinical Psychology, 55,* 3–9.

Lovaas, O. I., Berberich, J. P., Perloff, B. F., & Schaeffer, B. (1966). Acquisition of imitative speech by schizophrenic children. *Science, 151,* 705–707.

Lovaas, O. I., & Buch, G. (1992). Editor's introduction. *Research in Developmental Disabilities, 13,* 1–8.

Lovaas, O. I., & Bucher, B. D. (Eds.). (1974). *Perspectives in behavior modification with deviant children.* Englewood Cliffs, NJ: Prentice-Hall.

Luce, S. C., Christian, W. P., Anderson, S. R., Troy, P. J., & Larsson, E. V. (1992). Development of a continuum of services for children and adults with autism and other severe behavior disorders. *Research in Developmental Disabilities, 13,* 9–25.

Luckasson, R., Borthwick-Duffy, S., Buntinx, W. H. E., Coulter, D. L., Craig, E. M., Reeve, A., et al. (2002). *Mental retardation: Definition, classification, and systems of supports* (10th ed.). Washington, DC: American Association on Mental Retardation.

MacDuff, G. S., Krantz, P. J., & McClannahan, L. E. (1993). Teaching children with autism to use photographic activity sheets: Maintenance and generalization of complex response chains. *Journal of Applied Behavior Analysis, 26,* 89–97.

MacMillan, D. L. (1982). *Mental retardation in school and society.* Boston: Little, Brown.

MacMillan, D. L., Gresham, F. M., & Siperstein, G. N. (1993). Conceptual and psychometric concerns about the 1992 AAMR definition of mental retardation. *American Journal on Mental Retardation, 98,* 325–335.

Madell, J. R., & Rose, D. E. (1994, March). Auditory integration training. *American Journal of Audiology,* pp. 14–18.

Madsen, K. M., Hviid, A., Vestergaard, M., Schendel, D., Wohlfahrt, J., Thorsen, P., et al. (2002). A population-based study of measles, mumps, and rubella vaccination in autism. *New England Journal of Medicine, 347,* 1477–1482.

Mahoney, W., Szatmari, O., MacLean, J. E., Bryson, S. E., Bartolucci, G., Walter, S. D., et al. (2001). Reliability and accuracy of differentiating pervasive developmental disorder subtypes. *Journal of the American Academy of Child and Adolescent Psychiatry, 40,* 820–827.

Mash, E. J., & Wolfe, D. A. (1999). *Abnormal child psychology.* New York: Wiley.

Matson, J. L. (1995). Comments on Gresham, MacMillan, and Siperstein's paper "Critical Analysis of the 1992 AAMR Definition: Implications for School Psychology." *School Psychology Review, 10,* 20–23.

Matson, J. L., Appelgate, H., Smirdo, B., & Stallings, S. (1998). Mentally retarded children. In R. J. Morris & T. R. Kratochwill (Eds.), *The practice of child therapy* (3rd ed., pp. 303–324). Needharn Heights, MA: Allyn & Bacon.

Matson, J. L., & Coe, D. A. (1992). Applied behavior analysis: Its impact on the treatment of mentally retarded emotionally disturbed people. *Research in Developmental Disabilities, 13,* 171–187.

Matson, J. L., & McCartney, J. R. (Eds.). (1981). *Handbook of behavior modification with the mental retarded.* New York: Plenum.

Matson, J. L., & Schaughency, E. A. (1988). Mild and moderate mental retardation. In J. C. Witt, S. N. Elliott, & F. M. Gresham (Eds.), *Handbook of behavior therapy in education* (pp. 631–652). New York: Plenum.

Matson, J. L., Sevin, J. A., Box, M. L., Francis, K. L., & Sevin, B. M. (1993). An evaluation of two methods for increasing self-initiated verbalizations in autistic children. *Journal of Applied Behavior Analysis, 26,* 389–398.

Mayes, S. D., & Calhoun, S. L. (2003). Ability profiles in children with autism. *Autism: The International Journal of Research & Practice, 7,* 65–81.

McDougle, C. J., Naylor, S. T., Cohen, D. J., Volkmar, F. R., Heninger, G. R., & Price, L. H. (1996). A double blind, placebo-controlled study of fluvoxamine in adults with autistic disorder. *Archives of General Psychiatry, 53,* 1001–1008.

McLaren, J., & Bryson, S. E. (1987). Review of recent epidemiological studies of mental retardation: Prevalence, associated disorders and etiology. *American Journal on Mental Retardation, 92,* 243–254.

Meichenbaum, D., & Genest, M. (1980). Cognitive behavior modification: An integration of cognitive and behavioral methods. In F. H. Kanfer & A. P. Goldstein (Eds.), *Helping people change* (2nd ed., pp. 390–422). New York: Pergamon Press.

Miller, L. J. (2003, February). Empirical evidence related to therapies for sensory processing impairments. *National Association of School Psychologists Communique, 31*(5).

Minderaa, R. B., Anderson, G. M., Volkmar, F. R., Harcherick, D., Akkerhuis, G. W., & Cohen, D. J. (1989). Whole blood serotonin and tryptophan in autism: Temporal stability and the effects of medication. *Journal of Autism and Developmental Disorders, 19*, 129–136.

Morris, R. J. (1976). *Behavior modification with children: A systematic guide.* Cambridge, MA: Winthrop Publishers.

Morris, R. J. (1985). *Behavior modification with exceptional children: Principles and practices.* Glenview, IL: Scott-Foresman.

Morris, R. J., & Kratochwill, T. R. (1998). Historical context of child therapy. In R. J. Morris & T. R. Kratochwill (Eds.), *The practice of child therapy* (3rd ed., pp. 1–4). Needham Heights, MA: Allyn & Bacon.

Morris, R. J., & McReynolds, R. A. (1986). Behavior modification with special needs children: A review. In R. J. Morris & B. Blatt (Eds.), *Special education: Research and trends* (pp. 66–130). New York: Pergamon Press.

Morrison, R. S., Sainato, D. M., BenChaaban, D., & Endo, S. (2002). Increasing play skills of children with autism using activity schedules and correspondence training. *Journal of Early Intervention, 25*, 58–72.

Mount, R. H., Hastings, R. P., Reilly, S., Cass, H., & Charman, T. (2003). Toward a behavioral phenotype for Rett syndrome. *American Journal on Mental Retardation, 108*, 1–12.

New York State Association for Retarded Children v. Rockefeller, 357 F. Supp. 752, (1973).

Nirje, B. (1969). The normalization principle and its human management implications. In R. B. Kugel & W. Wolfensberger (Eds.), *Changing patterns in residential services for the mentally retarded* (pp. 179–195). Washington, DC: President's Commission on Mental Retardation.

Odom, S. L., Brown, W. H., Frey, T., Karasu, N., Smith-Canter, L. L., & Strain, P. S. (2003). Evidence-based practices for young children with autism: Contributions for single-subject design research. *Focus on Autism and Other Developmental Disabilities, 18*, 166–175.

Odom, S. L., Hoyson, M., Jamieson, B., & Strain, P. S. (1985). Increasing handicapped preschoolers' peer social interactions: Cross-setting and component analysis. *Journal of Applied Behavior Analysis, 18*, 3–16.

Odom, S. L., & Strain, P. S. (1984). Classroom based social skills instruction for severely handicapped preschool children. *Topics in Early Childhood Special Education, 4*, 97–116.

O'Neill, M., & Jones, R. S. (1997). Sensory-perceptual abnormalities in autism: A case for more research? *Journal of Autism and Developmental Disorders, 27*, 283–293.

Online Mendelian Inheritance in Man (OMIM). (2004). Trademarked by Johns Hopkins University. Retrieved May 12, 2004 from http://www.ncbi.nlm.nih.gov/entrez/query.fcgi?db=OMIM

Patton, P. (1988). Preparation for adulthood. In E. E. Lynch & R. B. Lewis (Eds.), *Exceptional children and adults* (pp. 588–618). Glenview, IL: Scott, Foresman.

Pennsylvania Association for Retarded Children v. Commonwealth of Pennsylvania, 334 F. Supp. 1257 (1971).

Perel, I. (1992). Deinstitutionalization at a large facility: A focus on treatment. *Research in Developmental Disabilities, 13,* 81–86.

Perry, R., & Meiselas, K. (1988). Autism and schizophrenia: Pharmacotherapies. In J. L. Matson (Ed.), *Handbook of treatment approaches in childhood psychopathology* (pp. 301–325). New York: Plenum.

Peterson, F. M., & Martens, B. K. (1995). A comparison of behavioral interventions reported in treatment studies and programs for adults with developmental disabilities. *Research in Developmental Disabilities, 16,* 27–42.

Phelps, L., & Grabowski, J. (1991). Autism: Etiology, differential diagnosis, and behavioral assessment. *Journal of Psychopathology & Behavioral Assessment, 13,* 107–125.

Pickett, J. (2001). Current investigation in autism brain tissue research. *Journal of Autism and Developmental Disorders, 10,* 91–103.

Pierce, K. C., & Schreibman, L. (1994). Teaching daily living skills to children with autism in unsupervised settings through pictorial self-management. *Journal of Applied Behavior Analysis, 27,* 471–481.

Rapin, I., & Katzman, R. (1998). Neurobiology of autism. *Annals of Neurology, 43,* 7–14.

Reilly, C., Nelson, D. L., & Bundy, A. C. (1983). Sensorimotor versus fine motor activities in eliciting vocalizations in autistic children. *Occupational Therapy Journal of Research, 3,* 199–211.

Rimland, B. (1964). *Infantile autism.* New York: Appleton-Century-Crofts.

Rimland, B., & Edelson, S. M. (1994). The effects of auditory integration training in autism. *American Journal of Speech-Language Pathology, 5,* 16–24.

Rimland, B., & Edelson, S. M. (1995). Auditory integration training: A pilot study. *Journal of Autism and Developmental Disorders, 25,* 61–70.

Rimm, D. C., & Masters, J. C. (1979). *Behavior therapy: Techniques and empirical findings.* New York: Academic Press.

Ritvo, E. R., & Freeman, B. J. (1978). National Society for Autistic Children definition of the syndrome of autism. *Journal of Autism and Childhood Schizophrenia, 8,* 162–167.

Ritvo, E. R., Freeman, B. J., Mason-Brothers, A., Mo, A., & Ritvo, A. (1985). Concordance for one syndrome autism in 40 pairs of affected twins. *American Journal of Psychiatry, 142,* 64–77.

Ritvo, E. R., Freeman, B. J., Yuwieler, A., Geiler, E., Yokota, A., Schroth, P., et al. (1984). Study of fenfluramine in outpatients with the syndrome of autism. *Journal of Pediatrics, 105,* 823–828.

Ritvo, E. R., Spence, M. A., Freeman, B. J., Mason-Brothers, A., Mo, A., & Marzarita, M. L. (1985). Evidence of autosomal recessive inheritance in 46 families of multiple incidences of autism. *American Journal of Psychiatry, 142,* 187–182.

Rogers, S., & Lewis, H. (1989). An effective day treatment model for young children with pervasive developmental disorders. *Journal of the American Academy of Child and Adolescent Psychiatry, 28,* 207–217.

Rourke, B. P., & Tsatsanis, K. D. (2000). Nonverbal learning disabilities and Asperger Syndrome. In A. Klin, F. Volkmar, & S. Sparrow (Eds.), *Asperger Syndrome* (pp. 231–253). New York: The Guilford Press.

Rusch, F. R., McKee, M., Chadsey-Rausch, J., & Renzaglia, A. (1988). Teaching a student with severe handicaps to self-instruct: A brief report. *Education and Training of the Mentally Retarded, 23,* 51–58.

Rutter, M. (1978). Diagnosis and definition of childhood autism. *Journal of Autism and Childhood Schizophrenia, 8,* 139–161.

Rutter, M., & Bartak, L. (1973). Special education treatment of autistic children: A comparative study. 11. Follow-up of findings and implications for services. *Journal of Child Psychology and Psychiatry, 14,* 241–270.

Safran, J. S. (2002). Supporting students with Asperger's syndrome in general education. *Teaching Exceptional Children, 34,* 60–66.

Safran, S. P. (2001). Asperger's syndrome: The emerging challenge to special education. *Exceptional Children, 67,* 151–160.

Scheerenberger, R. C. (1987). *A history of mental retardation.* Baltimore: Brookes Publishing.

Schopler, E. (1965). Early infantile autism and receptor processes. *Archives of General Psychiatry, 13,* 327–335.

Schopler, E. (1996). Are autism and Asperger's syndrome different labels or different disabilities? *Journal of Autism & Developmental Disabilities, 26,* 109–110.

Schopler, E., Mesibov, G. B., & Hearsey, K. (1995). Structured teaching in the TEACCH system. In E. Schopler & G. B. Mesibov (Eds.), *Learning and cognition in autism* (pp. 243–268). New York: Plenum.

Schopler, E., & Reichler, R. J. (1971). Psychobiological referents for the treatment of autism. In D. W. Churchill, G. P. Alpern, & M. K. DeMyer (Eds.), *Infantile autism* (pp. 327–335). Springfield, IL: Charles C Thomas.

Schreibman, L., & Charlop, M. H. (1987). Autism. In V. B. Van Hasselt & M. Hersen (Eds.), *Psychological evaluation of the developmentally and physically disabled* (pp. 155–177). New York: Plenum Press.

Shapiro, E. (1981). Self-control procedures with the mentally retarded. In M. Hersen, R. M. Eisler, & P. M. Miller (Eds.), *Progress in behavior modification* (vol. 12, pp. 265–297). New York: Academic Press.

Shapiro, E. S. (1986). Behavior modification: Self-control and cognitive procedures. In R. P. Banett (Ed.), *Severe behavior disorders in the mentally retarded* (pp. 259–276). New York: Plenum.

Shaw, S. R. (2002, October). A school psychologist investigates sensory integration therapies: Promise, possibility, and the art of placebo. *National Association of School Psychologists Communique, 31*(2), 5–6.

Skinner, B. F. (1938). *The behavior of organisms.* New York: Appleton-Century-Crofts.

Skinner, B. F. (1953). *Science and human behavior*. New York: Macmillan.

Smith, T., Parker, T., Taubman, M., & Lovaas, O. I. (1992). Transfer of staff retraining from workshops to group homes: A failure to generalize across settings. *Research in Developmental Disabilities, 13,* 57–71.

Stacey, C. L., & DeMartino, M. F. (Eds.). (1957). *Counseling and psychotherapy with the mentally retarded*. Glencoe, IL: Free Press.

Stehli, A. (1991). *The sound of a miracle: A child's triumph over autism*. New York: Doubleday.

Stevenson, R. E., Schwartz, C. E., & Schroer, R. J. (2000). *X-linked mental retardation*. New York: Oxford University Press.

Strain, P. S., Ken, M. M., & Ragland, E. U. (1979). Effects of peer-mediated social initiations and prompting/reinforcement procedures on the social behavior of autistic children. *Journal of Autism and Developmental Disorders, 9,* 41–54.

Szatmari, P. (2000). Children with autism spectrum disorder: Medicine today and in the new millenium. *Focus on Autism & Other Developmental Disabilities, 15,* 138–146. Retrieved 9/6/2003 from http://search.epnet.com/direct.asp?an=3584132&db=aph

Tanguay, P. M. (2000). Pervasive developmental disorders: A ten year review. *Journal of the American Academy of Child and Adolescent Psychiatry, 39,* 1079–1095.

Thompson, T., & Grabowski, J. (Eds.). (1972). *Behavior modification of the mentally retarded*. New York: Oxford University Press.

Tsai, L. (2000). Children with autism spectrum disorder: Medicine today and in the new millenium. *Focus on Autism & Other Developmental Disabilities, 15,* 138–147.

Ullmann, L., & Krasner, L. (Eds.). (1965). *Case studies in behavior modification*. New York: Holt.

U.S. Department of Education. (2000). *Twenty-second annual report to congress on the implementation of the Individuals with Disabilities Act*. Washington, DC: U.S. Government Printing Office.

Volkmar, F. R., & Klin, A. (1998). Asperger Syndrome and nonverbal learning disabilities. In E. Schopler & G. B. Mesibov (Eds.), *Asperger Syndrome or High Functioning Autism? Current issues in autism* (pp. 107–121). New York: Plenum Press.

Wacker, D. P., & Berg, W. K. (1988). Behavioral habilitation of students with severe handicaps. In J. C. Witt, S. N. Elliott, & F. M. Gresham (Eds.), *Handbook of behavior therapy in education* (pp. 719–737). New York: Plenum.

Waterhouse, L., Fein, D., & Mohdahl, C. (1996). Neurofunctional mechanisms in autism. *Psychological Review, 103,* 457–489.

Wetzel, R. J. (1992). Behavior analysis of residential program development. *Research in Developmental Disabilities, 13,* 73–80.

Wetzel, R. J., & Hoschouer, R. (1984). *Residential teaching communities*. Glenview, IL: Scott, Foresman.

Williams, D. (1992). *Nobody, nowhere: The extraordinary life of an autistic.* New York; Times Books.

Williams, D. E., Kirkpatrick-Sanchez, S., & Crocker, W. T. (1994). A long-term follow-up of treatment for severe self-injury. *Research in Developmental Disabilities, 15,* 487–501.

Wing, L. (1991). The relationship between Asperger's Syndrome and Kanner's autism. In V. Frith (Ed.), *Autism and Asperger Syndrome* (pp. 93–121). New York: Cambridge University Press.

Wing, L., & Potter, D. (2002). The epidemiology of autistic spectrum disorders: Is the prevalence rising? *Mental Retardation and Developmental Disabilities Research Review, 8,* 131–151.

Wolfensberger, W. (1969). The origin and nature of our institutional models. In R. B. Kugel & W. Wolfensberger (Eds.), *Changing patterns in residential services for the mentally retarded* (pp. 59–171). Washington, DC: President's Commission on Mental Retardation.

Wolfensberger, W. (1972). *The principle of normalization in human services.* Washington, DC: National Institute on Mental Retardation.

Wood, L., Lasker, J., Siegel-Causey, E., Beukelman, D., & Ball, L. (1998). An input framework for augmentative and alternative communication. *Augmentative and Alternative Communication, 14,* 261–267.

World Health Organization. (1992). *Manual of the international classification of diseases, injuries, and causes of death* (Vol. 1). Geneva, Switzerland: Author.

World Health Organization. (2001). *Fact sheet: The world health report 2001. Mental and neurological disorders.* Retrieved May 12, 2004 www.WHO.int/whr/2001/media_centre/en/whr01_fact_sheet1_en.pdf

Wright, E. B. (1987). Developmental disabilities. In C. R. Reynolds & L. Mann (Eds.), *Encyclopedia of special education* (vol. 1, pp. 486–488). New York: Wiley Interscience.

Wyatt v. Stickney, 325 F. Supp. 781 (1971).

Yeargin-Allsopp, M., Rice, C., Karapurkar, T., Doernberg, N., Boyle, C., & Murphy, C. (2003). Prevalence of autism in a US metropolitan area. *Journal of the American Medical Association, 289,* 49–55.

Zigler, E., & Hodapp, R. M. (1986). *Understanding mental retardation.* New York: Cambridge University Press.

15

Neuromuscular Disorders

Ludmilla Bronfin, MD

THIS CHAPTER WILL familiarize a general medical reader with the most common conditions involving the peripheral nervous system. Neuromuscular disorders include motor neuron diseases, nerve root and peripheral nerve disorders, neuromuscular junction disorders, and diseases of the muscle itself.

The peripheral nervous system (PNS) is made up of cranial nerves, spinal roots, plexuses, peripheral nerves, and autonomic ganglia. The initial segment of the motor peripheral neuron originates in the spinal cord. The motor cell body occupies the ventral gray matter. For the sensory system, the spinal ganglion or sensory cell body of the posterior nerve root lies in the intervertebral foramina. Autonomic ganglia are the sensory cell bodies of the peripheral autonomic nerve.

The PNS supplies efferent motor impulses to muscles and conveys sensory stimuli from skin and deep structures back to the spinal cord.

The motor spinal nerves arise from the spinal cord and are formed by the union of the dorsal and ventral nerve roots. The anterior and posterior nerve roots unite to form the mixed spinal nerve. The spinal nerve divides into an anterior ramus and posterior ramus. The posterior rami innervate the paraspinal muscles. The ventral rami supply the limbs and the front of the body. In the cervical and lumbosacral regions the ventral rami intermingle and form plexuses from which major peripheral nerves emerge.

Peripheral motor, sensory, and autonomic nerve cells are very long. The cell body is responsible for the synthesis of macromolecules. These macromolecules are transported along the length of the nerve by axonal flow. The rapid anterograde transport system is microtubule based and transports at a rate of 400 mm/day. The slow antegrade system for cytoskeletal elements transports at a rate of 0.5 to 3 mm/day. A retrograde transport system returns recycled vesicles from the periphery to the cell body at a rapid rate of 2 to 300 mm/day.

The well-being of the peripheral nerve depends on the integrity and well being of the Schwann cells which line up along its length, each one forming a protective internode of myelin. Anatomically, the metabolic conditions of the nerve are maintained by several structures including perineurium, endothelial capillaries, and physical barriers at the proximal and distal ends of the nerve. Endoneurial fluid pressure is maintained at a small positive pressure. This may rise dramatically in certain neuropathies producing endoneural edema.

MOTOR NEURON DISEASES

AMYOTROPHIC LATERAL SCLEROSIS (ALS)

AMYOTROPHIC LATERAL SCLEROSIS (ALS) is a progressive degenerative disorder that involves both the lower motor neurons (LMN) in the spinal cord and brainstem and upper motor neurons (UMN) in the motor cortex. The coexistence of both LMN and UMN findings is the distinctive picture of ALS. ALS is the most common motor neuron disease in adults.

Epidemiology

The incidence of ALS peaks between ages 55 and 75. Sporadic ALS has an annual incidence of about 1–2 per 100,000 population and is more common in men (Brooks, 1998). Familial ALS represents 5% to 10% of all ALS cases. Familial ALS is associated with a point mutation on the superoxide dismutase-1 (SOD1) gene in 25% of the cases. Familial ALS is usually autosomal dominant, with a mean age of onset of 47, 10 years earlier than sporadic ALS. In familial ALS, the ratio of men to women is 1:1.

Affected motor system components include:

* Upper motor neurons in the cortex (corticospinal and corticobulbar tracts) and brainstem (tectospinal, rubrospinal)
* vestibulospinal and reticulospinal that directly communicate with lower motor neurons
* The limbic motor neuron system
* The cerebellum and basal ganglia, which communicate with UMNs

* LMNs, which include motor nuclei in the brainstem and the anterior horn cells in the spinal cord
* Neuromuscular junctions
* Muscle fibers
* Proprioceptive input, which monitors the accuracy of the intended movement.

Only UMNs, LMNs and the limbic motor control system are affected clinically in ALS.

Clinical Features

Weakness is the most common presenting symptom in 60% of the patients with ALS. Other symptoms include muscle cramps, weight loss, fasciculations, respiratory distress, or difficulty swallowing. The signs of ALS are divided into UMN and LMN or are due to a combination of UMN and LMN degeneration.

Lower motor neuron features include atrophy, flaccid weakness, hyporeflexia. Weakness is more prominent when it is due to LMN degeneration rather than to UMN degeneration. Whereas early upper motor neuron degeneration may produce some stiffness and loss of dexterity, focal spread of LMN degeneration leads to initial prominent monoplegia. The degeneration often spreads to involve anterior horn cell on both sides, causing bilateral arm or leg weakness, before later involving the bulbar LMNs and causing bulbar palsy. Atrophy is associated with LMN weakness and is a prominent feature of ALS. The weakness is painless.

Muscles cramps are another common feature of ALS. The mechanism for muscle cramps is not entirely clear but may relate to axonal hyperexcitability. Muscle cramps commonly occur in calves, and less commonly in thighs, abdomen, jaw, and neck.

Fasciculations are one of the most well-known features of ALS. Fasciculations are caused by a spontaneous discharge of the entire motor unit. The mechanism is probably similar to that of muscle cramps. Fasciculations are not painful and are often noticed by a clinician as a rapid and irregular twitching movement of the skin. Fasciculations may be enhanced by tapping lightly with a finger over the muscle. It is important to note that fasciculations are common in people without neuromuscular disorders (benign fasciculations) and are rarely the initial presenting sign of ALS.

As stated previously, LMN degeneration results in greater clinical weakness than UMN degeneration. This pattern is true for bulbar palsy. Bulbar palsy is a result of LMN degeneration in the medulla (brainstem). Bulbar palsy is associated with atrophy and fasciculations of the tongue, absent jaw and gag reflexes, dysarthria, and dysphasia. Often patients have a mixture of bulbar (LMN) and pseudobulbar (UMN) palsy. The dysarthria has a nasal quality. Eventually speech may be completely lost. Patients with bulbar palsy are unable to move their tongue or open or close their mouth (due to weakness of the muscles of mastication innervated by cranial nerve V). Weakness of cranial nerves V, IX,X, XII produces dysphasia. In ALS, difficulty swallowing is usually more prominent with liquids.

ALS patients often report increased time necessary to complete a meal. As the disease progresses, the ability to cough diminishes which may lead to aspiration. Drooling is a common sign of bulbar palsy. Weight loss is also a common feature because of muscular atrophy.

Symptoms of respiratory insufficiency usually occur later in the disease, although respiratory failure may be a presenting symptom of ALS and is associated with poor prognosis. Early symptoms of respiratory insufficiency in ALS patients include difficulty lying flat in a bed, morning headaches, and exertional dyspnea. Following a patient's forced vital capacity (FVC) is important for monitoring the progression of respiratory failure.

Upper motor neuron degeneration produces muscle weakness, spasticity and pathologic reflexes. Muscle weakness results in difficulty with skilful movements and dexterity. This is usually described by a patient as "clumsiness" or "stiffness" of the extremities. As UMNs degenerate, the fusimotor neurons are no longer inhibited and they fire more frequently, resulting in increased LMN firing and spasticity. This mechanism is also responsible for increased muscle stretch reflexes and clonus. In addition, the loss of brainstem UMN inhibition results in spasticity that is most prominent in upper extremity flexors and lower extremity extensors.

Pathologic reflexes are reflexes present in normal infants that are lost as the central nervous system (CNS) matures. In a degenerative process such as ALS, when UMN are lost, these reflexes can reappear. The Babinsky sign (extensor plantar response) and Hoffmann sign (thumb flexion in response to a quick release after forceful flexion of the third finger) should be interpreted carefully.

Pseudobulbar palsy implies a UMN lesion above the bulb or medulla and represents degeneration of the bilateral corticospinal tracts which control cranial nerves. Symptoms include difficulty with mastication, articulation, and deglutition. Aspiration may be a life-threatening event in a patient with ALS mainly because of aspiration pneumonia and laryngospasm. Another related feature of ALS is difficulty controlling emotions, which results in spontaneous laughter or crying that is out of proportion to the emotional stimuli. Pseudobulbar palsy is often associated with brisk jaw jerk and gag reflexes.

Prognosis

Most patients die between 2 and 4 years after the onset of the symptoms. But a significant proportion of ALS patients (20%) live beyond 5 years after onset. Better prognosis is associated with younger age of onset, spinal onset, UMN or LMN involvement, absent respiratory impairment, fewer fasciculations, a long interval from onset to the diagnosis, milder muscle involvement, normal amplitude muscle potentials on nerve conduction, and psychological well-being (Mitsumoto, 1997). Low serum chloride levels are associated with poor prognosis. Certain types of SOD1 mutations are associated with short or long survival. Accurately predicting prognosis for an individual patient is impossible.

Specific Treatment

In 1995, riluzole (Rilutek) became the first drug approved by the FDA for treating ALS. This drug is reported to prolong survival and may slow the disease progression in patients with ALS (AAN Quality Standards Subcommittee, 1997). It is the only approved drug but its effects are minimal and the drug is expensive.

Riluzole may be more beneficial either in the first 12 months of the drug treatment or when given in the early stages of the disease. Therefore riluzole should be prescribed as soon as the diagnosis is established. The standard dosage of riluzole is 50 mg twice a day. A transient elevation of serum transaminase and rarely leucopenia have been reported. Thus, complete blood counts and liver function tests must be performed every month for the first 3 months and every 3 months thereafter. Generally, riluzole is an easily tolerated medication in terms of side effects.

Current drugs under investigation for possible usefulness in ALS include neurontin and myotrophin (Miller, 1997).

Symptomatic Treatment and Physical Rehabilitation

The majority of symptoms in patients with ALS are directly caused by degenerating motor neurons and include muscle paralysis, atrophy, cramps, fasciculations, and loss of key motor functions. Other symptoms are caused by the disease process and include joint pains secondary to contracture, depression, anxiety, and insomnia. Symptomatic treatment is very important for patients with ALS because, as mentioned above, specific pharmacotherapy in ALS is limited. The goal is to maintain a patient's independence. Rehabilitation involves active and passive exercise, the extent of it depending on the patient's muscle strength and tolerance.

Arm and hand function are essential for activities of daily living. Several orthoses (wrist extensor supports, mobile arm supports, thumb splints) are effective for patients with hand and arm weakness. For head extension weakness a soft cervical collar is effective support.

The ankle-foot orthosis is the most frequently used brace in patients with ALS. In the early stages of ALS, a cane is often helpful for gait difficulties. When the disease progresses, a walker may be required. When independent walking is impossible, a wheelchair becomes an important device. Whether to use a regular manual wheelchair or a motorized wheelchair depends on the individual needs of the patient.

Successful rehabilitation also includes evaluating the patient's home. Home equipment can preserve patient independence and safety. The education of patients and caregivers is an important aspect of rehabilitation. Successful rehabilitation promotes psychological well-being as well. ALS patients who are mentally fit have better survival.

Rehabilitation for patients with ALS requires a comprehensive approach. It is best achieved by a multidisciplinary team consisting of physical and occupational therapists, physiatrist, orthotists, nurses, speech pathologists, dietitians, social workers, pulmonologists, and neurologists (Sufit, 1997).

A major principle in ALS care is that patients must be followed up closely in order to detect impending problems in nutrition or respiration. Altering food consistency, a high-calorie food supplement, and percutaneous endoscopic gastrotomy (PEG) placement are essential steps in prevention of aspiration while maintaining nutritional status.

Home care is necessary when the patient's condition severely deteriorates. Hospice provides comfort care to patients and their families (Borasia, 1997).

Ethical Issues

Palliative care is primarily directed toward improving the quality of life for dying patients. Treatment to relieve pain and use of opioids is recommended to relieve significant discomfort.

POLIOMYELITIS

THIS DISEASE IS caused by a neurotropic enterovirus. The virus affects anterior horn cells and eventually destroys them. Poliomyelitis is a monophasic disease that leaves patient with severe disability due to LMN involvement.

Epidemics of poliomyelitis were commonplace worldwide until the introduction of the Salk vaccine between 1953 and 1956. Only a few cases of acute poliomyelitis have been seen in developed countries over the past 40 years. Because most of the patients in North America who had poliomyelitis acquired it before the mid-1950s, the youngest of these patients are now at least 40 years of age. Some of these patients have had new neuromuscular symptoms develop attributed to the postpolio syndrome. It can be very difficult, if not impossible, to diagnose any superimposed neuromuscular disorder such as ALS, radiculopathies, and myopathies, because of the severe, widespread motor unit action potential changes that result from poliomyelitis.

Spinal Muscular Atrophy

Werdnig-Hoffmann disease or spinal muscle atrophy type 1 (SMA-1), is a genetically determined anterior horn cell disorder that affects children younger than the age of 2 years. Wohlfart-Kugelberg-Welander disease or SMA-3 is the autosomal-recessive disorder that usually affects adolescents and young adults.

Segmental Motor Neuron Disease

This sporadic disorder was reported initially in 1959 (Donofrio, 1994). It is also called juvenile muscular atrophy of unilateral upper extremity, benign monomelic amyotrophy, juvenile amyotrophy, or segmental motor neuron disease. These terms reflect the hallmark characteristics—juvenile onset, localized muscle weakness and atrophy, and the nonprogressive nature of this disorder. The majority of patients are young males who describe an insidious onset of unilateral hand and distal forearm muscle atrophy and weakness that usually progresses over a 1- to 4-year period and is followed either by further slow progression or complete arrest.

PERIPHERAL NERVE DISEASE

Peripheral nerve injury or disease usually leads to the rapid onset of muscle atrophy unless there is a transient conduction block due to pressure. Hyporeflexia or areflexia occurs early in neuropathy and persists indefinitely, even after the return of motor power. This hyporeflexia must be differentiated from the markedly slowed reflexes of myxedema and the areflexia of muscles involved by a myopathy.

All modalities of sensation are impaired in peripheral neuropathies. Dissociation of sensory loss—where only one component is involved—are rare. Several patterns of dissociated sensory loss are worth highlighting.

In subacute combined degeneration (Vitamin B12 deficiency related) and in spinocerebellar degenerations such as Friedreich's ataxia, large-diameter primary sensory neurons degenerate early. Such patients lose touch-pressure, vibration, and joint-position sense but retain pain, light touch, and temperature sensation.

In contrast, in a variety of small-fiber neuropathies, the opposite is true. In amyloidosis, Fabry's disease, Tangier's disease, autonomic and diabetic neuropathy, and hereditary sensory neuropathy type I, pain sensation and thermal discrimination may be lost before touch-pressure, vibration, and joint-position sense.

Peripheral vasomotor and trophic changes include the objective sensation of warmth or coolness, redness, pallor or cyanosis (bluish discoloration), hyperhidrosis (increased sweating) or hypohidrosis (decreased sweating), edema (swelling), atrophy of the skin and subcutaneous tissues, hyperkeratosis, pigmentation or depigmentation, irregular growth of hair and nails, and ulcers (Dyck, 1993).

Dependent edema of the feet and ankles requires leg elevation or support hose for control.

MONONEUROPATHY

PATIENTS WITH DIFFERENT mononeuropathies present with corresponding types of pathophysiology. For example, sudden-onset mononeuropathies, regardless of the nerve affected, location, etiology, or severity, almost always are manifested pathophysiologically as conduction failure secondary to conduction block caused by demyelination. Rarely, such lesions produce conduction slowing. In contrast, chronic slowly progressive mononeuropathies are most often manifested as conduction failure due to axon loss. There are a few exceptions in which focal demyelination occurs. The most common exception is Carpal Tunnel Syndrome, in which focal demyelinating slowing is the characteristic presentation. In a third category of chronic lesion mononeuropathies, which include radiation plexopathies, multifocal motor neuropathy, and tourniquet paralysis, demyelinating conduction block occurs.

Mononeuropathy is a common result of injury. Because of the dramatic events associated with fracture, nerve injuries are often overlooked. The nerve is usually injured by the sharp edge of a bone. However, soft tissue may crush or stretch the nerve itself. Hemorrhage or exudate into a restricted space, particularly near a joint, may compress the nerve.

In fractures of the head of the humerus, the radial and ulnar nerves are involved most frequently. Intercostal neuropathy most commonly results from rib fractures. Fractures of the pelvis in the region of the sacroiliac joint may involve the sacral plexus. Hip fracture or dislocation causes sciatic nerve injury. Fractures of the femur or pelvis cause femoral nerve injury.

Trauma in athletes can be categorized by the types of sports involved (Sicuranza, 1992). Injuries to the brachial plexus commonly occur in motorcycle accidents, football, hockey, golf, acrobatics, and diving. The long thoracic nerve may be injured in wrestling, swimming, and tennis. The ulnar nerve is injured in bicycling, rowing, boxing, wrestling, football, and hockey. The radial nerve is injured in boxing, football, and hockey. The suprascapular nerve is injured in acrobatics, volleyball, baseball pitching, and bowling. In the lower extremities, the lumbosacral plexus may be injured in diving, football, or acrobatics. The sciatic nerve is usually hurt in golf or volleyball. Runners may experience peroneal nerve entrapment involving the nerve that travels under the fibrous edge of the peroneus longus muscle. Male bicycle riders may experience numbness of the penis and scrotum because of the pressure of a hard saddle on the pudendal nerve.

A variety of occupations may be associated with peripheral nerve involvement. For example, craftsmen, such as jewelers, engravers, and machinists who hold their tools tightly and exert hard pressure on the palm, suffer injury of the deep palmar branch of the ulnar nerve (progressive muscular atrophy of gold polishers). An occupational neuropathy generally disables the worker. Even when the work is stopped, the prognosis is not always good (Lederman, 1993).

Palsy may develop during sleep, especially after large doses of narcotics, sedatives, or alcohol. Developmental anomalies, an impaired nutritional state, and the surface on which the patient sleeps play a role. The nerves affected most often are the radial and the peroneal. Radial paralysis may result from sleeping with an arm hanging over the back of a chair ("Saturday night palsy"), with the head of another lying on the arm ("bridegroom's paralysis"), or with the patient's head resting on his arm. If the patient is in the habit of sleeping prone with arms raised above the head, the median, axillary, musculocutaneous, and long thoracic nerves may become involved owing to stretching or to compression by the head of the humerus. In the lower extremity, the bones of the opposite knee may compress the common peroneal nerve if the patient has slept while seated with knees crossed.

Postoperative neuropathy is the result of compression, section, traction, or ischemia (Dawson, 1983).

Early diagnosis is essential because medical measures can reduce the severity of deficit. Care in securing the arms and in providing protective pads has decreased the incidence of injury to the ulnar and radial nerves from a hard surfaces during anesthesia. A 15% incidence of ulnar neuropathy in patients undergoing coronary bypass surgery has been noted. Fortunately, physical therapy and time usually suffice to bring about recovery in many patients.

Birth trauma can cause brachial plexus injury. The upper arm is involved most frequently, and the lower arm less frequently. Erb's palsy or upper trunk plexopathy occurs in vertex presentations when the head is pulled laterally to free the shoulders from the pelvis. Paralysis of the lower arm (Klumpke's paralysis) usually occurs from overextension of the arm in cases of face or breech presentation or from traction made in the axilla in vertex presentation (Dodds, 2000).

Entrapment neuropathies occur when peripheral nerves are injured by mechanical pressure or ischemia at the points where they pass through rigid anatomic canals, beneath tight ligamentous or fascial bands; or where they enter, exit, or pass through muscle. Entrapment nerve trauma occurs more often when inflammation or degeneration is present in adjacent joints and tendons, as may happen in rheumatoid arthritis, myxedema, or acromegaly or when the nerves lie in shallow grooves, allowing them to be easily compressed or traumatized repeatedly. The presence of an underlying peripheral neuropathy often renders nerves more susceptible to compressive injury (Atroshi, Gummesson, Johnsson, et al., 1999). The deleterious effects of repetitive motion, vibration, and occupational factors has been mentioned above.

MONONEUROPATHY MULTIPLEX

IN MONONEUROPATHY MULTIPLEX, single peripheral nerves become involved sequentially. Typically, the patient has weakness and paresthesia and dysesthetic pain develops in the distribution of a peripheral nerve. Later, symptoms occur in the distribution of an additional nerve. A key feature is that the neurologic deficits are asymmetric. Mononeuropathy multiplex develops in diseases that produce a necrotizing angiitis (polyarteritis nodosa, rheumatoid arthritis, Wegener's granulomatosis, Churg-Strauss syndrome) but may be seen in diabetes mellitus, an inflammatory-demyelinating disorder, or a more benign vasculopathy.

When mononeuropathy multiplex develops in a patient with rheumatoid arthritis or a systemic disease involving collagen vascular tissue, a necrotizing angiopathy should be suspected. The sedimentation rate is usually elevated, above 50 mm/hr, and there is a raised titer to nuclear antibodies.

Patients with an inherited tendency to pressure palsy report weakness or sensory loss in the distribution of a mixed nerve after relatively mild compression to the nerve or sometimes even without compression. On physical examination, there is evidence of more widespread neuropathic involvement from previous injuries.

Multiple cutaneous nerve involvement, as occurs in leprosy, is generally distinguishable from the causes of multiple mononeuropathy listed above. In lepromatous leprosy, the discrete loss of pain and sensitivity to temperature over a region of skin coincides with a depigmented area.

BRACHIAL PLEXUS NEUROPATHY

THE ANNUAL INCIDENCE of brachial plexus neuropathy is of 1.64/100,000. The disorder is more common in men, and more common between the 3rd and 7th decades.

Brachial plexopathy begins suddenly with pain. The pain is located in the region of the shoulder, but may radiate down the lateral arm. The pain is severe and constant and may be described as sharp, stabbing, or aching, aggravated by coughing, sneezing and in rare instances by neck motion. It is accompanied by rapid development of muscle weakness and wasting.

Weakness affects shoulder girdle muscles predominantly, including the deltoid, supraspinatus, infraspinatus, serratus anterior, biceps, and triceps. Complete unilateral limb paralysis has been reported. Plexus involvement in bilateral cases is usually not symmetric. Sensory loss is much less prominent than are pain and muscle weakness. Muscle stretch reflexes may be diminished in weak muscles.

The cerebrospinal fluid (CSF) is normal except for a mild increase in the protein level. MRI scans of the brain and spinal cord are usually normal. MRI scans of the brachial plexus performed to exclude a mass lesion are also usually normal.

The etiology of this condition is unknown, though an allergic or autoimmune mechanism has been suspected. The prognosis is good. There is improvement in muscle strength within the first months after symptom onset with 90% recovery within 3 years. A few patients are left with minimal neurologic deficits. Recurrences are rare.

There is no evidence that steroids alter the course of this disease, although in some patients, steroids may result in relief of pain. Analgesics are needed for pain relief in any case. Early rehabilitation is important in order to prevent the development of shoulder joint periarthritis and to improve muscle strength.

POLYNEUROPATHY

SUSPECTING PERIPHERAL NEUROPATHY, the physician should ask the following questions:

What is the course?
Which populations of neurons or nerve fibers are affected?
What level of the neuron—is the proximal or the distal part affected?
What is the nature of fiber degeneration—axonal degeneration, segmental demyelination, or both?
With what other systemic symptoms or diseases is the neuropathy associated? (Differential diagnosis depends on a reliable history.)
With what other biochemical derangement is the neuropathy associated?

The medical, social, and occupational history and the clinical course are helpful in determining the type of neuropathy. Medications taken, possible exposure to industrial poisons, drugs that might have been taken for pleasure, or the infections to which the patient was exposed, are all possible causes.

An acute or subacute onset of a neuropathic process is typical of the inflammatory immune mediated neuropathies, various toxins and poisons, or certain metabolic conditions such as acute intermittent porphyria.

The clinical course determines whether the process is monophasic, recurrent, stepwise progressive, or slowly progressive. A recurrent course is seen particularly in chronic inflammatory polyradiculoneuropathy, in intermittent poisoning, or in a metabolic disorder such as acute intermittent porphyria. A slowly progressive course is typical of many inherited motor and sensory neuropathies.

It is necessary to know which population of motor neurons is affected in order to properly diagnose a motor peripheral polyneuropathy. Polyneuropathy presents with lower motor neuron degeneration, the same as is seen in progressive spinal muscular atrophy and amyotrophic lateral sclerosis. But polyneuropathy is associated with proximal and distal muscle weakness. Patients often have muscle weakness, cramps, and atrophy.

In inflammatory motor polyradiculoneuropathy, as is seen in Guillain-Barré syndrome, muscle weakness also may be proximal and distal, and tends to be symmetric. In this situation, the elevated protein in spinal fluid examination is helpful in determining the diagnosis.

Symptoms of paresthesia, hyperalgesia, tightness, aching, and burning are indicative of sensory neuropathy. These symptoms represent excessive neural activity related to the damaged fibers or regenerated sprouts.

Many mixed neuropathies also begin with these same sensory symptoms, even though motor and autonomic symptoms are also present. Diabetes mellitus, uremia, B_{12} deficiency, and hypothyroidism are common examples of mixed metabolic neuropathies.

Many toxic and medication-related neuropathies can begin with sensory symptomatology and then progress to include motor symptoms. In arsenic and thallium related neuropathies, gastrointestinal upset is often followed by a painful, burning, distal neuropathy with weakness. In thallium neuropathy, these symptoms are also associated with hair loss. Amyloidosis often presents with sensory symptoms.

Carcinomatous sensory neuropathy may begin with symptoms from loss of both large- and small-fiber function. Patients become unsteady and, in addition, have hyperalgesia, tight bandlike constrictions around toes and ankles, and hyperpathia.

Slowly progressive disorders may develop over many years. These inherited neuropathies are divided into two groups. The first group (spinocerebellar) involves mainly large fibers and produces ataxia. The second group includes predominantly small fibers. Patients may have mutilation of the fingers and toes, stress fractures, and a sequence of medical maladies including dry skin, repeated cellulitis, or chronic plantar ulcers.

Autonomic dysfunction in peripheral neuropathy can be varied and disabling. Dysautonomia is a major feature in the Riley-Day syndrome, a recessively inherited disorder in Jewish children. Acquired autonomic neuropathies are present in inflammatory-immune mediated neuropathy, α-lipoprotein deficiency (Tangier's disease), and in diabetes mellitus. Symptoms include dysfunction of tear production, temperature deregulation, dysphagia, and crampy abdominal pain. Lack of heart rate and blood pressure regulation is often found in patients with diabetes.

The most troublesome symptom of dysautonomia is postural hypotension. The patient's blood pressure falls on standing. Impotence may develop in the male. This symptom is commonly reported in various types of amyloidosis and in diabetes mellitus (Bastron, 1981).

Methods of Investigation

Nerve conduction and electromyography (EMG) should be done in all patients suspected of having a peripheral neuropathy (Dumitru, 1995). Spinal fluid is helpful in documenting protein elevation, malignant cells, or an elevation of gamma globulin. Biopsy of nerve tissue may help to determine an underlying process. Laboratory evaluation is helpful in the differential diagnosis of peripheral neuropathy and should include fasting and postprandial blood sugar, serum protein electrophoresis, 24-hour urine protein electrophoresis, serum lipids, and tissue estimation of specific heavy metals, medications, or toxins. DNA studies may prove necessary to diagnose inherited neuropathy (Dyck, 1993).

DISEASES OF THE NEUROMUSCULAR JUNCTION

MYASTHENIA GRAVIS

MYASTHENIA GRAVIS (MG) is the most common disorder of neuromuscular transmission. It is an acquired autoimmune disease characterized by the presence of antibodies toward acetylcholine receptors (AChR). Clinically, it is manifested by fluctuating and fatiguable weakness. The weakness may be limited to a few muscles, such as the extraocular muscles, or it may be generalized. The weakness is often worse with activity and improved by rest. The weakness is also made worse by drugs that inhibit acetylcholinesterase.

Pathogenesis

The reduction and blockade of AChR on the postsynaptic membrane of the neuromuscular junction by AChR antibodies play a major role in the pathogenesis of myasthenia gravis. The precipitating factors remain unknown. The implicating of the antibodies in the neuromuscular abnormalities is based on several lines of evidence including the presence of modulating or blocking antibodies in 85–90% of patients, and the beneficial effects of plasmapheresis in improving clinical symptoms.

The thymus gland appears to play a central role in the evolution of the disease as well as in its treatment. Thymic hyperplasia has been reported to occur in 65% of myasthenic patients and thymoma in up to 15%. There is a beneficial effect of thymectomy, especially in younger patients (Gutman, 1972).

Epidemiology

Myasthenia gravis is a fairly common disorder with an incidence of 2–6 per million population and a prevalence of 40 per million population. Although the incidence has not changed significantly, the prevalence has increased over the last 45 years, most likely due to longer life spans and improved therapies. There is no racial predominance.

Almost all cases occur sporadically, and familial clusters are rare. Patients are classified on the basis of age and the presence or absence of thymoma. In those without thymoma, there is a predominance among women under the age of 40 years (75%) and an increased association with HLA-A1, B8, and DRw3 antigens. Men predominate over the age of 40 years (60%), and there is an increased association with HLA-A3, B7, and DRw2 antigens.

Clinical Presentation and Diagnosis

The initial symptoms and signs of myasthenia gravis involve the extraocular muscles (ptosis, diplopia, blurred vision), leg weakness, generalized fatigue, dysphagia, slurred or nasal speech, difficulty chewing, and weakness of the face, neck, and arms.

When the extremities are affected, the proximal muscles are usually more severely involved than the distal ones. The fluctuating eyelid ptosis and extraocular muscle weakness does not occur in other illnesses. Ptosis involves one or both eyelids. Extraocular muscle weakness involves any combination of gaze abnormality. Facial weakness gives the patient an expressionless look. In severe cases, the patient may have to support his or her jaw manually because of the weakness of the jaw muscles. Nasal or slurred speech results from the weakness of the tongue and soft palate. Enfeebling of the muscles responsible for coughing and swallowing leads to dysphonia and choking on food and secretions.

Keeping the airway patent sometimes proves difficult, and fatigue of respiratory muscles leads to dyspnea at rest or with exertion.

Weakness can be provoked by exertion, exposure to heat or hot weather, infections, or emotional upset. Pregnancy causes a variable response, but the postpartum period is more likely to be associated with worsening symptoms.

Myasthenic crisis is most commonly provoked by a respiratory infection or a major surgical procedure. A poor vital capacity as a result of respiratory weakness and an inability to keep the airway patent are predictors of the crisis.

The disorder is limited to weakness of the skeletal muscles. It does not involve cardiac or smooth muscle, nor is there an alteration of cognitive skills, coordination, sensation, or tendon reflexes.

Prognosis

The prognosis for myasthenia gravis has improved dramatically over the past 50 years with the mortality rate dropping to 7%, and 90% of patients being either in remission, improved, or unchanged. The improvement in prognosis is a result of advances in respiratory care including the availability of positive pressure ventilators, sophisticated intensive care equipment, and the evolution of new therapeutic modalities.

New therapeutic modalities include early thymectomy, immunosuppressive drug therapy, and short-term immunotherapies (plasmapheresis, intravenous immunoglobulins).

Diagnosis

The distribution and fluctuating nature of the weakness, especially when it involves muscles innervated by cranial nerves, is characteristic of MG. The dramatic improvement following the intravenous injection of the rapidly acting acetylcholinesterase inhibitor edrophonium (Tensilon test) further demonstrates MG. Repetitive nerve stimulation studies confirm the diagnosis. Nerve conduction studies and EMG assist in ruling out other possibilities. Single fiber EMG is very sensitive to abnormalities of the neuromuscular junction. The presence of serum AChR antibodies is highly specific for myasthenia gravis.

The use of chest x-ray and chest CT scans are important in the evaluation and identification of those patients with thymoma. Assessment of antinuclear antibodies, rheumatoid factor, thyroid function studies, and vitamin B_{12} levels assist in the identification of associated autoimmune disorders.

Differential Diagnosis

The differential diagnosis includes the progressive external ophthalmoplegias, oculopharyngeal dystrophy, amyotrophic lateral sclerosis, progressive bulbar palsy, motor axonopathies, Lambert-Eaton syndrome

(Castaigne et al., 1977), botulism, congenital myasthenic syndromes, intracranial mass lesions compressing cranial nerves, and the intranuclear ophthalmoplegia of multiple sclerosis. Neurasthenia may be confused with myasthenia gravis if the distinction between decreased energy and actual muscle weakness (MG) is not made. Clinical features and laboratory studies help a discerning clinician to differentiate among these disorders.

Treatment

Anticholinesterase medications are given as the initial therapy. Pyridostigmine (Mestinon) is the most commonly used. These medications inhibit the action of acetylcholinesterase, allowing acetylcholine to remain longer at the neuromuscular junction. This increases the ability to generate a muscle action potential.

The usual starting dose of pyridostigmine is 30–60 mg every 4 hours. Some patients develop side effects that include abdominal cramps and diarrhea. These are usually treated with atropine 0.4 mg 3 times daily.

Thymectomy is now widely used early in the course of myasthenia gravis. In a large series of patients without thymoma, 96% improved. The maximum response occurred 1–4 years after the surgical procedure. Currently, thymectomy is recommended for almost all patients under the age of 50–55 years, except for those with only ocular involvement.

Prednisone therapy is a mainstay in the treatment of myasthenia gravis in those patients over the age of 50, and may be useful in those younger patients in whom anticholinesterase medication and/or thymectomy have not been sufficiently effective. It is being used more frequently in patients who have only ocular myasthenia gravis. Alternate-day therapy with 60–100 mg of prednisone is an effective and popular form of treatment with fewer potential side effects. Improvement usually occurs over several months, and is followed by a gradual taper of the medicine. Long-term use is often modified with other immunosuppressant agents including azathioprine, cyclophosphamide, or cyclosporine. Azathioprine (2–3 mg/kg) may be initiated at the same time as the prednisone, and has few side effects at this low dose. It may not be effective for several weeks. Leukopenia is uncommon at this dosage. The risk of neoplasm is a relatively small one.

Plasmapheresis is a relatively safe, but expensive, treatment modality and is usually reserved for the treatment of serious exacerbations of myasthenia crisis or for preparing a patient for a surgical procedure including thymectomy (Dau, 1982). The improvement produced by a course of plasmapheresis may range from mild, lasting for a few days, to marked, persisting for 3–6 weeks. Complications include hypotension, bleeding, sepsis, and embolism. It is not known whether there is a synergistic effect with plasmapheresis and immunosuppressive drugs.

Impending myasthenic crisis requires immediate treatment. Respiratory failure requires endotracheal intubation, careful bronchopulmonary care, and mechanical ventilation in an intensive care unit. Vital capacity is the most commonly followed parameter. Myasthenic crisis is usually self-limited, and spontaneous recovery is expected within a few days or weeks. The effectiveness of plasmapheresis in shortening crisis is not well established, but may be tried. In this setting, medications that adversely affect neuromuscular transmission should be used with caution. These include aminoglycoside antibiotics, procainamide, quinidine, b-adrenergic blocking agents, and lithium. Magnesium should be avoided.

MUSCLE DISEASE

MUSCLE WEAKNESS IS the most common sign of muscle disease. Patients with muscle disease often do not initially report muscle weakness. Clinicians should look for clues that suggest reduction in physical activities. Clinicians assess muscle function by observing the patient's ability to perform simple directed motor tasks.

Muscle disease classification includes muscular dystrophies, congenital myopathies, membrane myopathies, and metabolic myopathies.

MUSCULAR DYSTROPHIES

THE MUSCULAR DYSTROPHIES are hereditary myopathies characterized by progressive muscle degeneration. These include dystrophin deficient muscular dystrophies, congenital muscular dystrophies, limb girdle muscular dystrophies, fascioscapular muscular dystrophies, oculopharengeal muscular dystrophies, distal muscular dystrophies, Emery Dreifuss muscular dystrophies.

Dystrophin-Deficient Dystrophies
Duchenne muscular dystrophy and Becker muscular dystrophy (BMD) are the types of dystrophin-deficient dystrophies.

Duchenne Muscular Dystrophy
DMD, or pseudohypertrophic muscular dystrophy, was described in the mid-1800s. The incidence of DMD is about 30 per 100,000 live male births (Bonilla, 1988).

Etiology and Pathogenesis. DMD is transmitted by X-linked recessive inheritance. Women are carriers, since the likelihood of two transmitted genes is very low and would uniformly lead to death in utero. The extremely large size of the DMD gene may account for the high rate of spontaneous mutations.

The magnitude of dystrophin deficiency correlates with clinical severity. Dystrophin is an important cytoskeletal protein localized to the inner surface of the sarcolemma and it accounts for 2% of total sarcolemmal protein.

Clinical Features. Marked elevation of serum creatine kinase (CK) is common in the neonatal period. The disease does not become clinically apparent until age 2–4 years. Initial manifestations include a delay in walking, frequent falls, difficulty climbing stairs and getting up from the floor, and toe-walking due to heel cord contractures. Patients look muscular due to the pseudohypertrophic enlargement of the calves.

Between the ages of 8 and 12 years, there is a steady and progressive decline in functional motor capability. By age 10 years, most patients are dependent upon long-leg braces for ambulation. By 12 years of age, most patients become wheelchair bound. Following wheelchair confinement, there is an acceleration in the development of contractures and kyphoscoliosis. Increasing thoracic muscle weakness produces severe respiratory insufficiency that typically leads to death from a respiratory infection at about 20 years of age.

Dystrophin also has been identified in cardiac and smooth muscle, and in brain. There is a high frequency of cardiac involvement in DMD. The electrocardiogram is abnormal in up to 90% of patients.

Women who are carriers of the DMD gene may display partial manifestations of the disease and present with progressive, usually mild, limb-girdle weakness.

Diagnosis. Demonstration of the near-absence of dystrophin in muscle from biopsy specimens has become the gold standard to diagnose DMD. DNA analysis can also be used for the prenatal detection of DMD-affected fetuses.

A clinical diagnosis of DMD can be made in boys between the ages of 3 and 5 years who present with markedly elevated serum CK levels. By late adolescence, when skeletal muscle destruction is nearly complete, serum CK may decrease to near-normal levels. Electromyography (EMG) demonstrates a myopathic pattern.

Treatment. No specific treatment for DMD exists. Many drugs have been tried without convincing benefit. Prednisone and deflazacor have limited beneficial effects.

At present, the management of DMD patients utilizes a multidisciplinary approach involving physical therapy, bracing, and surgery.

Becker Muscular Dystrophy

Becker muscular dystrophy (BMD) was recognized as a benign form of X-linked dystrophy in the 1950s. BMD occurs one tenth as often as Duchenne's. Both BMD and DMD result from defects in the same dystrophin gene. The clinical course is not as severe with BMD, but the pattern of muscular involvement is similar. Pseudohypertrophy of the calves can be quite dramatic.

Onset of weakness typically occurs between the ages of 5 and 15 years, later than in DMD. The mean age of wheelchair confinement in BMD is in the fourth decade, and these patients tend to live twice as long as Duchenne's patients.

Cardiac involvement in BMD may lead to cardiomyopathy (Saito, 1996). Serum CK levels are markedly elevated. EMG demonstrates myopathic features but with less evidence of necrosis than in DMD. As with DMD, there is no known effective treatment, and management consists largely of symptomatic approaches.

Congenital Muscular Dystrophy

Congenital muscular dystrophy (CMD) is a heterogeneous group of disorders that become manifest at birth. Affected infants present with flaccidity, weakness, and/or restriction of joint function. The diagnosis is made by the demonstration of myopathic features on muscle biopsy and exclusion of other types of myopathies of the newborn.

CMD is currently classified by the presence or absence of associated clinical central nervous system involvement. Those without clinical CNS involvement are then distinguished by the presence or deficiency of merosin. Merosin is an extracellular matrix protein that is essential for the normal linkage between the muscle cytoskeleton and the extracellular matrix.

Even in mild CMD cases, symptoms may be present at birth. Weakness is greater proximally than distally and often involves the facial muscles. In severe cases, death may occur secondary to respiratory failure.

Serum CK is typically increased, but not to the levels observed in young DMD patients. EMG shows myopathic features. Treatment is symptomatic, including aggressive physical therapy to prevent contracture formation.

Limb Girdle Muscular Dystrophy

Limb girdle muscular dystrophy (LGMD) is a clinically and genetically diverse group of disorders involving proximal weakness and lacking the symptoms of the other distrophies (Shields, 1994). An autosomal dominant variety of LGMD with later onset (2nd to 4th decade) has been mapped to chromosome 5. The serum CPK, EMG, and muscle biopsy findings vary from mild to severe. There is no disease-specific treatment. Treatment modalities include: physical therapy, appropriate equipment, occupational canceling, support groups, and psychological interventions.

Facioscapulohumeral Muscular Dystrophy

Of the myopathies with a restricted distribution of involvement, facioscapulohumeral muscular dystrophy (FSHMD) is the most common. The genetic defect in FSHMD is transmitted in an autosomal dominant pattern and has been mapped to chromosome 4.

In familial cases, the age of onset appears to be earlier in successive generations (anticipation). The pathogenesis of FSHMD and the reasons for the restricted muscle involvement are unknown.

The weakness in FSH initially occurs in the face. Shoulder girdle weakness often develops next and is dominated by periscapular and pectoral weakness. Inability to fix the scapulae results in scapular winging. The patients have difficulty bringing their arms to the level of their face and raising them above their head. Characteristically, the deltoid muscles retain their bulk and strength. Humeral involvement, with wasting and weakness of the biceps and triceps, may produce a characteristic "Popeye" appearance due to the relative prominence of the forearm.

Serum CK levels are elevated in most patients, but may be within normal limits. The EMG typically demonstrates nonspecific myopathic features in the involved muscles.

Life expectancy, in general, is not adversely affected. There is no specific treatment for FSHMD. Physical therapy and bracing are employed symptomatically.

Oculopharyngeal Muscular Dystrophy

Oculopharyngeal muscular dystrophy (OPMD) is an autosomal dominant disorder. The genetic abnormality in OPMD has been located to chromosome 14. Originally associated with individuals of French-Canadian extraction, OPMD has now been found in different nationalities. The disease manifests late in life, during the 4th–6th decade.

Initial symptoms are upper eyelid weakness (ptosis), and difficulty swallowing (dysphagia). As the disease progresses, weakness of other extraocular and proximal skeletal muscles increases. Dysphagia is the most serious manifestation. Double vision is uncommon. Cardiac muscle is not involved.

Serum CK is generally normal, but may be mildly increased. EMG studies may show mild myopathic features.

Patients are at risk for malnutrition and aspiration. Treatment of OPMD consists of symptomatic measures such as glasses with eyelid crutches, blepharoplasty, cricopharyngeal myotomy, and surgical placement of feeding tubes.

Distal Muscular Dystrophy

Distal myopathies are exceptions to the general rule that myopathies affect mainly proximal muscles. Serum CK is generally normal, or only mildly increased. EMG demonstrates myopathic features that are more prominent in distal muscles.

While no specific treatment is available, patients may benefit from the use of ankle-foot orthoses.

Emery-Dreifuss Muscular Dystrophy

Emery-Dreifuss muscular dystrophy (EDMD) is an X-linked disorder that also involves only males.

Clinically, affected men develop progressive muscle weakness in the arms and legs in a humeroperoneal distribution during childhood. This disease is associated with prominent early contractures of the elbows, neck, and achilles tendons. EDMD also causes varying degrees of proximal girdle weakness.

Cardiac involvement can present with atrial rhythm disturbances, conduction defects, and occasionally complete heart block with sudden death. The skeletal muscle weakness is not life-threatening, but cardiac involvement may necessitate the insertion of a pacemaker.

The serum CK may be several times normal. EMG may show both neurogenic and myopathic features. The EDMD phenotype appears to be genetically heterogeneous.

No specific treatment is available. Physical therapy is used in an attempt to minimize contracture formation. Cardiac pacemaker placement may be required in patients with severe cardiac involvement.

Congenital Myopathies

The congenital myopathies often present in early infancy as the "floppy infant" syndrome. Luckily, many of these infants have a relatively benign course with the weakness and hypotonia remaining static or even improving. However, some infants have a progressive course leading to early death from respiratory complications.

In childhood onset of symptoms, muscular weakness and hypotonia are often accompanied by skeletal anomalies such as a high-arched palate, pectus excavatum, kyphoscoliosis, and dislocated hips.

Occasionally, these disorders start later in childhood or adult life. When diagnosed in adults, the congenital myopathies are usually asymptomatic or only mildly progressive.

Electromyography generally shows nonspecific myopathic features, and the serum muscle enzymes are only mildly elevated or normal. The individual disorders are delineated on the basis of characteristic morphologic features. Congenital myopathies include Central Core Disease, Multicore Disease, Nemaline Myopathy, Centronuclear Myopathy, Congenital Fiber Type Disproportion, Reducing Body Myopathy, Fingerprint Body Myopathy, Myopathies with Tubular Aggregates, Type 1 Myofiber Predominance.

MEMBRANE MYOPATHIES

THE MEMBRANE MYOPATHIES are muscle disorders that exert their pathophysiologic effect by altering the bioelectrical function of the muscle membrane, resulting in episodic weakness (in periodic paralyses), or repetitive discharge (in myotonia).

Hypokalemic Periodic Paralysis

In terms of treatment, potassium aborts acute attacks of hypokalemic periodic paralysis but is ineffective when administered chronically for prophylaxis. Because swallowing is rarely affected, potassium can be administered orally in the treatment of the acute attacks. In a patient with vomiting or an ileus, intravenous potassium may be cautiously given by slow infusion. Acetazolamide is often very effective in treating hypokalemic periodic paralysis. Significant improvement in muscle strength has also been noted with this treatment.

Dichlorophenamide, another carbonic anhydrase inhibitor, is also effective in improving the interictal strength. The mechanism for acetazolamide's beneficial effect in hypokalemic periodic paralysis remains incompletely understood. The protective effect may be due to acidosis. Metabolic acidoses modulates the influx of potassium into intracellular compartments. Nephrolithiasis is a potential complication of chronic acetazolamide use.

Spironolactone and triamterene may also be beneficial in hypokalemic periodic paralysis. However, concomitant administration of potassium during an acute attack may produce hyperkalemia. Acute attacks of weakness in Hyperkalimic periodic paralysis are often so brief that treatment is unnecessary. The prompt ingestion of carbohydrates at the onset of weakness will often abort attacks.Many patients learn to eat snacks or drink beverages at times when the attacks characteristically occur. Severe attacks have been treated successfully with intravenous glucose. Glucose and other measures known to alleviate attacks presumably ac by lowering serum potassium. Accordingly, epinephrine, calcium gluconate, salbutamol, insulin, metaproterenol, and glucagon have all proved effective. The chronic administration of the sodium potassium ion exchange resin, kayexalate, has not proved beneficial.

Hyperkalimic Periodic Paralysis

Paradoxically, acetazolamide is effective prophylaxis in many patients, although occasional nonresponders have been reported. The mechanism for this drug's beneficial effect may be acidosis. Thiazide diuretics are often preferable and appear to be as effective, although occasional nonresponders have been reported. The diuretics likely produce their beneficial effect by their kaliuretic action. Treatment of normokalimic periodic paralysis is essentially the same as hyperkalimic periodic paralysis.

Thyrotoxic Periodic Paralysis

Effective treatment requires treatment of the thyrotoxicosis. Attacks of paralysis cease when patients are euthyroid by medical or radioactive suppression or by surgical ablation of the thyroid. However, the underlying metabolic defect remains. Patients rendered eu-thyroid will experience recurrent attacks if given excessive thyroid supplementation. The treatment of acute attacks of thyrotoxic periodic paralysis with potassium is the same as in hypokalemic periodic paralysis. Acetazolamide, which is effective in the prophylaxis of attacks of hypokalemic periodic paralysis, appears to make induction of weakness easier, and the resultant weakness more severe in thyrotoxic periodic paralysis.

The principal myotonic disorders are myotonic dystrophy, myotonia congenita, and paramyotonia. No specific treatment is available for myotonic dystrophy. Therapy remains entirely symptomatic. Myotonia congenita was the first myotonic disorder to be described by Thomsen, 1876. A number of drugs, including quinine, phenytoin, procainamide, tocainide, mexiletine, nifedipine, and acetazolamide, have been used to treat myotonias with the exception of dystrophy. Tocainide is effective treatment for the cold-induced myotonia and weakness in paramyotonia congenita and paralysis periodica paramyotonica. Mexiletine, however, is as effective and has less potential toxicity. The optimal treatment of periodic paralysis in paramyotonia is not well defined. Chlorothiazide, a kaliuretic agent, has prevented attacks of weakness and alleviated myotonia in patients with paralysis periodica paramyotonica. On the other hand, chlorothiazide either caused weakness or had no effect in patients with paramyotonia congenita. Spironolactone, a potassium-sparing agent, decreased the frequency of attacks and severity of weakness in paramyotonia congenita, but had no effect on paralysis periodica paramyotonica. Potassium-sparing drugs may be beneficial in the prophylaxis of periodic paralysis in paramyotonia congenita, and kaliuretic drugs may be beneficial in the prophylaxis of periodic paralysis in paralysis periodica paramyotonica.

INFLAMMATORY MYOPATHIES

THE INFLAMMATORY MYOPATHIES are a heterogeneous group of diseases (Dalakas, 1991). These include the idiopathic inflammatory myopathies, and a smaller group caused by identifiable bacterial, mycotic, and viral pathogens. The idiopathic inflammatory myopathies are generally considered to be immunologically mediated. This interpretation is supported by the increased prevalence of certain human leukocyte antigen (HLA) groups among patients with these inflammatory myopathies, plus the relatively frequent association with other immunologically mediated disorders, and the favorable response in many patients to immunosuppressive therapy. Microscopically, the association is supported by the results of immunohistochemical and immunocytochemical studies that have been performed on muscle biopsy specimens. The treatment of both polymyositis and dermatomyositis is similar. High-dose daily steroids are a common initial therapeutic strategy in both disorders. Once weakness has begun to resolve, usually after several weeks, a gradual switch to alternate-day steroids is often started to limit steroid toxicity. Patients failing to respond to steroid therapy may benefit from the addition of other immunosuppressant therapy such as azathioprine, methotrexate, and cyclophosphamide. Azathioprine is often begun initially along with steroids for a "steroid-sparing" effect. High-dose intravenous immune globulin also has been utilized in the treatment of refractory myositis.

Polymyositis

Polymyositis can occur at any age, but it is most common in adults. Women are affected more often than men. The disease begins insidiously, and progresses gradually over a period of weeks to months. There may be spontaneous remissions and relapses.

Proximal weakness is the major clinical manifestation. Affected muscles are often tender, painful, and swollen. Sometimes these symptoms are severe and rapidly progressive. Dysphagia is common and results from involvement of pharyngeal and esophageal muscles. Cardiac involvement may lead to congestive heart failure. Respiratory dysfunction is found in about 10% of patients.

Serum CK is generally elevated when the disease is active but may decline during remission. Myoglobinuria occurs. The erythrocyte sedimentation rate is often elevated, but does not correlate with disease activity. Electromyography demonstrates a mixture of fibrillations and brief, small amplitude, polyphasic potentials (myopatic pattern). Muscle biopsy shows a variable number of necrotic myofibers.

Dermatomyositis

Skin lesions are found in one third of patients with idiopathic inflammatory myopathy. Skin lesions are the main clinical features that distinguish dermatomyositis from polymyositis. Most common are a heliotrope discoloration of the eyelids; an erythematous rash over the face, neck, and chest.

The distribution of muscle weakness, laboratory findings, and electromyographic abnormalities is similar to that encountered in patients with polymyositis.

Dermatomyositis is more common in children than adults. Malignant neoplasms, especially carcinomas of the lung, breast, and gastrointestinal tract, may occur with adult cases of dermatomyositis.

Muscle biopsy specimens show a distinctive pattern of myofiber atrophy described as perifascicular.

Treatment. The treatment of polymyositis and dermatomyositis is similar. High-dose daily steroids is an initial therapy in both disorders. A gradual switch to alternate-day steroids is often preferred to limit steroid toxicity. Addition of other immunosuppressant therapy such as azathioprine, methotrexate, and cyclophosphamide may be necessary in resistant cases. High-dose intravenous immune globulin has also been used in the treatment of refractory dermatomyositis (Griggs, 1995).

METABOLIC MYOPATHIES

THE METABOLIC MYOPATHIES are a heterogeneous group of disorders affecting all aspects of muscle metabolism. These include carbohydrate myopathies, lipid myopathies, mitochondrial myopathies, endocrine myopathies, and myalgic syndromes. The endocrine myopathies often have a treatable cause.

Endocrine Myopathy

Muscle dysfunction is identified in a wide variety of endocrine disorders. Myopathy occurs frequently in hyperthyroidism. Muscle weakness, cramps, pain, and stiffness are common complaints, though objective muscle weakness is uncommon. The serum CK is generally not elevated. Nonspecific myopathic features are commonly found on EMG and in muscle biopsy specimens. These symptoms resolve with successful treatment of the condition.

Patients with hyperparathyroidism may have mild generalized muscle weakness. Clinically, hyperparathyroid myopathy includes proximal weakness and wasting, occasional bulbar weakness, and preserved or even brisk reflexes. Serum CK is usually normal.

Muscle weakness, fatigue, and cramping are also frequent symptoms in patients with Addison's disease. Occasionally, the associated weakness is severe and it may be episodic. Treatment requires glucocorticoid and mineralocorticoid replacement and correction of the associated electrolyte abnormalities.

Patients with hyperaldosteronism may present with attacks of periodic paralysis and associated hypokalemia. Muscle weakness is a symptom in over 70% of these patients, but will cease if the underlying cause is corrected.

Muscle weakness occurs frequently in Cushing's syndrome and in patients exposed to glucocorticoids. The muscle weakness of steroid myopathy is typically insidious in onset and affects primarily proximal muscles. Unfortunately, the muscle damage from steroids is not reversible. Serum CK is usually normal. EMG may show minor myopathic changes.

REFERENCES

American Academy of Neurology. Quality Standards Subcommittee. (1997). Practice advisory on the treatment of amyotrophic lateral sclerosis with riluzole: Report of the quality. *Neurology, 49,* 657–659.

Atroshi, I., Gummesson, C., Johnsson, R., et al. (1999). Prevalence of carpal tunnel syndrome in a general population. *JAMA, 282,* 153.

Bastron, J. A., & Thomas, J. E. (1981). Diabetic polyradiculopathy: Clinical and electromyographic findings in 105 patients. *Mayo Clinic Proceedings, 56,* 725.

Bonilla, E., Samitt, C. E., Miranda, A. F., et al. (1988). Duchenne muscular dystrophy: Deficiency of dystrophin at the muscle cell surface. *Cell 54,* 447–452.

Borasia, G. D., & Voltz, R. (1997). Palliative care in amyotrophic lateral sclerosis. *Journal of Neurology, 244*(Suppl. 4), S11–S17.

Brooks, B. R. (1998). Clinical epidemiology of ALS. In J. E. Riggs (Ed.), *Neurology clinics* (Vol. 14, pp. 399–420). Philadelphia: W. B. Saunders.

Castaigne, P., Rondot, M., Fardeau, M., et al. (1977). Lambert-Eaton myasthenic syndrome: Clinical electrophysiological, histologic and ultrastructural studies. *Reviews in Neurology* (Paris), *133,* 513.

Dalakas, M. C. (1991). Polymyositis, dermatomyositis, and inclusion-body myositis. *New England Journal of Medicine, 325,* 1487–1498.

Dau, P. C. (1982). Plasmapheresis in myasthenia gravis. *Progress in Clinical Biological Research, 8,* 265–285.

Dawson, D. M., & Krarup, C. (1989). Perioperative nerve lesions. *Archives of Neurology, 46,* 1355.

Dodds, S. D., & Wolfe, S. W. (2000). Perinatal brachial plexus palsy. *Current Opinions in Pediatrics, 12,* 40.

Donofrio, P. D. (1994). Monomelic amyotrophy. *Muscle Nerve 17,* 1129–1134.

Dumitru, D. (1995). *Electrodiagnostic medicine.* Philadelphia: Hanley & Belfus.

Dyck, P. J., Giannini, C., & Lais, A. (1993). Pathologic alterations of nerves. In P. J. Dyck, P. K. Thomas, J. W. Griffin, et al., *Peripheral neuropathy* (3rd ed., p. 514). Philadelphia: W. B. Saunders.

Griggs, R. C., Mendell, J. R., & Miller, R. G. (1995). *Evaluation and treatment of myopathies*. Philadelphia: F. A. Davis.

Gutmann, L., Crosby, T. W., Takamori, M., et al. (1972). The Eaton-Lambert syndrome and autoimmune disorders. *American Journal of Medicine, 53,* 354.

Lederman, R. J. (1993). Entrapment neuropathies in instrumental musicians. *Medical Problems of Performing Artists, 8,* 35.

Miller, R. G., & Sufit, R. (1997). New approaches to the treatment of ALS. *Neurology, 48*(Suppl. 4), S28–S32.

Mitsumoto, H. (1997). Diagnosis and progression of ALS. *Neurology, 48*(Suppl. 4), S2–S8.

Mitsumoto, H., Chad, D., & Pioro, E. P. (1997). Amyotrophic lateral sclerosis. In *Contemporary neurology series, vol 49*. Philadelphia: F. A. Davis.

Sabin, T. D., & Jacobson, R. R. (1993). Leprosy. In P. J. Dyck, P. K. Thomas, J. W. Griffin, et al., *Peripheral neuropathy* (3rd ed., p. 1354). Philadelphia: W. B. Saunders.

Saito, M., Kawai, H., Akaike, M., et al. (1996). Cardiac dysfunction with Becker muscular dystrophy. *American Heart Journal, 132,* 642–647.

Shields, R. W. (1994). Limb girdle syndromes. In A. G. Engel & C. Franzini-Armstrong (Eds.), *Myology, basic and clinical* (2nd ed., pp. 1258–1274). New York: McGraw-Hill.

Sicuranza, M. J., & McCue, F. C. III. (1992). Compressive neuropathies in the upper extremity of athletes. *Hand Clinic, 8,* 263.

Sufit, R. (1997). Symptomatic treatment of ALS. *Neurology, 48*(Suppl. 4), S15–22.

16

Orthopedic Impairments

EDWIN F. RICHTER III, MD, AND
ROBERT DEPORTO, DO

O RTHOPEDIC IMPAIRMENTS ARE almost inevitable developments for most individuals. Routine activities of daily living stress
the musculoskeletal system. Degenerative changes accumulate
in joints over time. Environmental and lifestyle factors may influence
this process. In the geriatric population, osteoporotic weakening of
bones becomes increasingly evident. These forces may affect even the
healthiest members of the adult population.

Acute traumatic events can suddenly create an orthopedic problem.
Premorbid characteristics play major roles in shaping responses to such
developments. Psychological factors influence response to the acute
trauma, the medical treatment, and the rehabilitation process. Other
medical illnesses may limit treatment options or interfere with recovery.

Economic forces may act on patients, families, health care providers,
employers, and other institutions. Social support systems are challenged
when orthopedic impairments lead to disability.

FUNCTIONAL PRESENTATION OF
ORTHOPEDIC IMPAIRMENTS

M ANY ORTHOPEDIC IMPAIRMENTS develop gradually and often
cause only limited disability in early stages. Osteoarthritis is a
degenerative change seen in joints, commonly associated with frequent

and vigorous activity. Bearing the weight of the human body is a substantial stress over time. Even thin individuals load their body weight on and off their lower extremities each time they take a normal step. Running, carrying extra weight, exposure to hard surfaces, choice of footwear, and variations in anatomy may increase the stresses across the joints. Long-term use of crutches by active persons with gait disorders may lead to similar effects on the shoulders. The affected joints may initially be painful intermittently. Over time the severity, frequency, and duration of painful episodes typically escalate, sometimes leading to persistent pain even when the joint is at rest.

Rheumatoid arthritis is an autoimmune disease in which the immune system attacks joints. More than 2 million Americans have rheumatoid arthritis, with peak onset ages between 20–45 years. Women are almost 3 times more likely to develop this condition (American College of Rheumatology, 2003). Pain, stiffness, and swelling of joints are common symptoms. Traditionally joint deformity has been a much greater concern in this condition than osteoarthritis, with use of splints and adaptive equipment to preserve joint function. Use of disease-modifying medications has substantially improved pharmacologic management of this condition.

Many systemic diseases affect joints. Systemic Lupus Erythematosus is an example of another autoimmune disorder that attacks joints and other organ systems, including kidneys, lungs, heart, and central nervous system. Survival after 4 years was 50% in 1954 but has exceeded 90% with current treatments. Prevalence of this disease is 40–50 per 100,000, with over 85% female, and a greater prevalence among blacks (American College of Rheumatology, 2004). Treatment with corticosteroids or other immunosuppressive medications may control the disease, but exposes patients to increased risk of infection.

Concurrent loss of range of motion may occur in osteoarthritis and other joint pain syndromes. This may limit functional use of the joint. This depends on which joint is involved and the number of degrees lost in a particular plane of motion, as well as the specific tasks that the person needs to do (Triffit, 1998). Loss of mobility at a given joint may be due to contracture of the soft tissues around the joint, fusion of bony structures, or mechanical blockage (such as by a loose piece of cartilage blocking the swinging of the knee joint's hinge mechanism). Pain may also prompt a functional restriction of movement, which may take place without conscious effort. "Guarding" may also reflect apprehension or quests for secondary gain.

Other joints may be able to compensate for loss of normal motion at a site of pathology. This strategy is not without risk. Normal body mechanics can be altered to such a degree that other structures may be harmed. A more subtle but quite serious problem occurs when the energy efficiency of an important activity is impaired. Normal gait involves strategic movements at several joints to lower metabolic costs (Winter, 1983). Interference with this process may stress cardiovascular and pulmonary systems. Speed and endurance would be jeopardized.

Low back pain deserves special attention when considering orthopedic impairments. The overall incidence of back pain is high. At least one debilitating episode affects 80% of Americans by age 55 years (Frymoyer, 1988). It is the leading cause of activity limitation in patients under age 45 years, and the second most common cause for visits to physicians (Andersson, 1999). Fortunately, most episodes resolve with conservative management. For many individuals, back pain can be considered a recurrent problem with exacerbations and remissions (Deyo & Weinstein, 2001). The cost of this condition, however, remains quite high. The direct expense has been estimated to be from $20 to $50 billion in the United States (Nachemson, 1992). This has raised concerns among health care providers, insurers, employers, and government agencies.

Many potential risk factors for back pain have been reviewed. Increasing age has some association with increasing likelihood of episodes. There is interest in anthropometric factors (Battie, Bigos, & Fisher, 1990), but the predictive value of height and weight is limited. Abdominal and lumbar muscle strength has been studied (Gardner-Morse & Stokes, 1998), but biomechanical models do not always correspond well with clinical realities.

Much attention has been paid to risk factors related to the workplace. Direct trauma, overexertion, or repetitive stresses can cause injuries, while postural factors may be more relevant to those with sedentary occupations (Bendix & Biering-Sorensen, 1983). Attributing an individual worker's pain to a specific ergonomic problem is often a challenge. Psychosocial factors have been implicated. Occupational factors, including an injured employee's prior attitudes toward his work, must be considered (Battie, Bigos, & Fisher, 1989).

Problems in the clinical evaluation of back pain complicate the situation. Gross assessment of lumbar movement may be hindered by hip joint factors (such as tight hamstring muscles) or voluntary guarding. Physical examination maneuvers such as straight leg raising (Lasegue's test) to look for nerve root involvement rely on the patient's verbal response, as well as the examiner's assessment of facial expression and body language. Subtle abnormalities on neurological testing of sensory and motor function or reflex activity are difficult to quantify.

Differences of opinion between practitioners are common when evaluating and treating back pain. The Agency for Health Care Policy and Research (AHCPR) has promoted practice guidelines (Bigos, Bowyer, & Braen, 1994), but on surveys of practicing physicians from eight specialties that commonly treat such patients there was little consensus on selection of diagnostic tests (Cherkin, Deyo, Wheeler, & Ciol, 1994). Patients do not limit themselves to seeking care from allopathic physicians, introducing further potential controversies. One third of patients in a study conducted in North Carolina reported seeking care initially from a chiropractor (Carey et al., 1996).

Different anatomical structures may be involved in low back pain. Acute muscle strains may be accompanied by significant spasm and local tenderness. Most cases respond well to oral analgesics and possibly muscle relaxants, which may work primarily as central sedatives (Robinson & Brown, 1991), brief periods of rest, and limited physical therapy interventions.

Degenerative changes may affect the spine as well. Osteophytes (bone spurs) may compress critical structures, such as nerve roots. Many of these spurs, however, may look impressive on an x-ray without causing any clinical problem. Facet joint arthritis has been implicated as a source of pain, which may radiate down the lower extremities. An injection with local anesthetic may temporarily relieve such pain, helping to make this diagnosis (Gamburd, 1991). Some physicians treat this condition with radio frequency ablation of the local nerve supply.

An acute disk herniation may cause compression of the spinal cord or nerve roots. The size and location of the protruding disk material are essential factors. The size of the spinal canal is also important, as this determines how much extra room is available to accommodate any invading structure. Computerized tomography (CT) and magnetic resonance imaging (MRI) have represented major advances over plain radiographs and traditional myelograms (x-rays done after injection of dye) (Herzog, 1991). Abnormal findings on imaging studies of asymptomatic individuals remind us that such tests do not obviate the need for clinical judgment (Frymoyer & Haldeman, 1991). Electrodiagnostic testing yields physiologic rather than anatomic data, but can be painful. It can also be difficult to distinguish between new and chronic abnormalities.

Many competing theories have been advanced in the debate over treatment of herniated disks and other lumbar pathologies. At least a brief period of rest may be beneficial, but prolonged bedrest has risks that may outweigh its benefits. Trunk muscle weakness may follow such inactivity. As little as 2 days bedrest may be appropriate (Deyo, Diehl, & Rosenthal, 1986). Similar concerns have been raised about prolonged use of corsets. The efficacy of traction has been challenged, as considerable forces are required to provide distraction of the lumbar spine before any reduction of pressure within a disk could be achieved. Suspending as little as ten pounds from the apparatus is at best only a means of enforcing bedrest.

Therapeutic exercises are also the subject of different schools of thought. Some clinicians advocate strengthening flexor muscles or extensors, while others recommend both approaches. Hyperextended postures are utilized in some methods, such as the McKenzie technique, while body mechanics are stressed in the "back school" approach (Sinaki & Mokri, 1996). Programs aimed at dynamic lumbar muscular stabilization have been reported to be quite successful (Saal & Saal, 1991). That approach seeks a "neutral" position of the lumbar spine to minimize pain. Analysis of this controversy is beyond the scope of this chapter, but it is safe to assume that some patients are perplexed by the conflicting advice they receive. Systematic reviews of literature have shown some evidence for effectiveness of back school approaches, but not necessarily for cost-effectiveness (Van Tulder, Esmail, Bombardier, & Koes, 2004).

Another area of conflict is the role and timing of surgery. Patients with progressive neurologic disfunction, especially involving bowel or bladder control, require acute attention. Some physicians will try high-dose steroid treatment even in such scenarios before moving to surgical options, but great caution is required. Patients with less dramatic deficits are more likely to receive longer courses of conservative management before having invasive procedures.

Communication with patients involves selection of medical terms. Use of terms like "herniated," "ruptured," or "bulging" disks may be interpreted in various ways. Assuming that a patient understands the clinical significance of such words is inappropriate.

Acute back pain may result from osteoporotic vertebral body compression fractures. This situation initially warrants short periods of rest, analgesics, and efforts to prevent constipation. Spinal supports may help to maintain posture and reduce uneven distribution of forces on the vertebral body (Sinaki, 1995). During ambulation, some patients experience less pain when using a rolling walker to place more weight on their upper extremities, reducing the forces across the fracture site. New minimally invasive procedures to inject bone cement (vertebroplasty) or inflatable bone tamps (kyphoplasty) into fractured vertebra may offer faster pain relief and correction of deformity (Philips, 2003).

Reducing risk of osteoporotic fractures has become increasingly effective with use of biphosphonate medications (Licata, 1997). These drugs inhibit bone resorption, but may cause gastrointestinal irritation when taken orally.

Fracture management must consider the location and severity of the injury. Fortunately at least some fractures are relatively stable and can be treated symptomatically. Uncomplicated fractures of ribs or distal phalanges of the toes are often in this category. Other fractures are moderately unstable. Manipulation of the bone fragments may yield adequate positioning. (When done without surgery this is a closed reduction.) Maintaining alignment may require controlling the joint above and below the site (Zuckerman & Newport, 1988). Traditional plaster casting techniques have been augmented by use of fiberglass material.

The use of special braces for fracture care allows faster mobilization in some cases. This approach invokes the importance of mechanical forces across the fracture site. Control of surrounding soft tissues allows a limited degree of movement at the fracture, which facilitates the healing process (Kumar, 1995). Weight bearing causes small local electric fields, which may enhance new bone formation. Braces may also be used to limit weight bearing by shifting weight to appropriate structures. The ischial bone of the pelvis and the patellar tendon below the kneecap are capable of supporting weight through braces in selected cases. Orthotic designs utilizing plastic and metal components can be strong but light. They are often more comfortable than a cast and can be removed for inspection and hygiene. Noncompliant patients do find them easier to remove.

Some fractures will be quite unstable without operative intervention (Zuckerman & Newport, 1988). Open reduction and internal fixation (ORIF) allow direct access to the site. Various types of hardware have been developed. Various screws, nails, and pins can be used to directly secure fragments of bone. They are also used to anchor metallic plates, which span a fracture site, to healthy areas of bone. Rods may also be placed inside a long bone to span a fracture site.

An alternative method of using external fixation was pioneered by Ilizarov in the Soviet Union. This approach came into worldwide use during the 1980s (Bianchi, 1997). Pins can be placed above and below a fracture site and attached to a strong external apparatus. The sites where the pins puncture the skin must be carefully cleaned and monitored. The appearance of the device may be disconcerting to some patients but it can facilitate early mobilization.

There are several acute medical issues potentially associated with fractures (Duong, 1995). Infection may delay healing or even lead to amputation or death. Bleeding may be dramatic or gradual. Pressure from a collection of blood (hematoma) or watery fluid (edema) may compress nerves or blood vessels or may hinder wound healing. Inflammatory responses may be dramatic. These factors may all subsequently decrease adjacent joint mobility, even if the joints were not directly injured. Contractures are of great concern in this setting. A patient may be disabled long after a fracture heals if nearby joints never regain adequate range of motion.

Chronic pain may follow orthopedic injury via a number of mechanisms. Direct nerve injury or indirect compression may lead to chronic burning pain or hypersensitivity in the sensory territory of that nerve. Reflex sympathetic dystrophy is a more complicated syndrome involving pain and vasomotor instability. Skin changes, soft tissue atrophy, and osteoporotic changes may be seen (Subbarao & Blair, 1995). There are many controversies surrounding this subject, but early mobilization is suggested as a preventive measure.

Hip fractures are particularly associated with problematic complications. These fractures typically affect geriatric patients. Osteoporosis and increased risk of falling are the main risk factors. Bone mineral density below the fracture threshold level puts patients at risk from relatively low impact falls from seated or standing positions (Goh, Bose, & Das, 1996). Mortality rates have been measured at 20% at 1 year and 33% at 2 years after injury (Emerson & Andersson, 1988). The mortality rate has been linked with poorly controlled systemic disease, cognitive disorders, and surgery before medical stabilization (Lyons, 1997).

Deep vein thrombosis (DVT) is a special concern after hip fracture. Decreased mobility and perhaps slowing of venous return past the site of injury are implicated in the increased risk of blood clot formation. Estimates of incidence are as high as 70% (Cifu, 1995), although clinically significant cases are clearly somewhat less common. The main concern is that thrombotic material may break loose, reaching the vascular supply to the lungs. This can cause a potentially fatal pulmonary embolus. Patients with atrial septal defects have a hole between the upper chambers of the heart, which could allow an embolic stroke to occur.

Pharmacologic prophylaxis is the primary method of prevention (Agnelli & Sonaglia, 1997). Oral anticoagulation with warfarin is effective, but requires frequent blood tests and increases risk of bleeding. Subcutaneous injection of low molecular weight heparin has also been used effectively. It does not require monitoring with blood tests. This medication also increases bleeding complications (Greaves, 1997). Injections are not always feasible in home settings after discharge. Some patients are prophylaxed with aspirin, despite a lack of compelling evidence in medical literature. Patients who are at very high risk of clot formation can have a filter placed in the vena cava to block access to vital organs.

Hip fracture patients who avoid major medical complications must confront problems with mobility and self-care performance. The amount of weight they can bear on the affected extremity is determined by the orthopedic surgeon. The type of fracture and the hardware used to repair it influence this decision. Quality of bone at the fracture site is also important. Complete avoidance of weight bearing is very difficult or impossible for some elderly patients. Even toe touching for balance requires that almost all body weight be supported through the arms to advance the uninvolved leg. A walker is required in this situation, unless the patient has adequate coordination to utilize bilateral crutches. Climbing stairs is very difficult unless at least partial weight bearing is allowed.

Compliance with precautions is important. Excessive weight bearing increases risk of failure of the repair. Refusing to use adequate assistive devices also increases risk of another fall and further injury.

Mobility and self-care skills may never recover after hip fracture. In one study 1 year after hip fracture 40% of patients could not walk independently, 60% had difficulty with one or more activity of daily living, and 27% had entered nursing homes for the first time (Cooper, 1997). Premorbid dementia and postoperative confusional states decrease the likelihood of recovering walking ability (Lyons, 1997).

Rehabilitation efforts should begin as soon as possible. Reimbursement policies discourage lengthy stays in acute care hospitals. Patients who are not ready to go home directly and who can benefit from an active program typically have gone to acute rehabilitation services. Patients with limited endurance can receive less vigorous regimens at subacute programs, typically at skilled nursing facilities. Further restrictions on reimbursement for traditional inpatient rehabilitation programs may shift greater numbers of orthopedic patients to subacute care or day programs. Providers will likely seek outcome data to justify support for their form of care.

Patients who undergo elective hip replacement face some of the same challenges as hip fracture patients. (Some hip fracture patients receive joint replacement hardware if the injury is near the head of the femur and extensive degenerative changes are present.) The majority of the patients facing hip arthroplasty demonstrate very advanced joint disease. Osteoarthritis and rheumatoid arthritis are typical etiologies. Many patients are elderly and have some other chronic conditions, although very frail or medically unstable patients should be discouraged from having this procedure. Arthritic involvement of the upper extremities may hinder use of walkers or canes. Prior limitation of activity due to pain may have decreased exercise tolerance. Abnormal gait patterns may have developed.

Total hip replacement has become a popular procedure. Approximately 120,000 were performed annually in the early 1990s (Harris & Sledge, 1990; Poss, 1993) and interest has remained strong. Restoring ability to ambulate without pain is the usual goal.

Deep venous thrombosis is a potential major complication (Brandes, Stulberg, & Chang, 1994). Pneumatic compression boots can be used postoperatively. Elastic compression stockings are commonly used subsequently. The medications commonly used to prevent clots are the same as those used after hip fracture.

Anticoagulation does increase the risk of major bleeding at the operative site. Bleeding into the thigh may cause significant pain and swelling. This may cause nerve compression, possibly leading to muscle weakness. Major blood loss may require treatment with transfusions. Some patients will donate their own blood preoperatively in anticipation of postoperative anemia.

Heterotopic ossification may occur after any hip surgery, but is most likely to be seen after arthroplasty. Calcification within muscle tissue can lead to a serious loss of range of motion. Severe cases may require surgical resection, followed by prophylactic radiation therapy (Lo & Healy, 2001) or medication, such as indomethacin or etidronate, to prevent recurrence. These medications may have gastrointestinal side effects.

The implanted hardware includes a ball-and-socket joint that mimics the function of the original joint. Preventing dislocation of the prosthetic joint is critical. Standard instructions after a posterolateral approach include avoiding hip flexion past 90° and hip adduction or internal rotation past neutral. Triangular pillows can be placed between the legs to encourage compliance. High chairs and raised toilet seats reduce the need to flex the hips while sitting. Long handled shoehorns, sock pullers, and reachers are useful devices that facilitate safe dressing. Patients may require substantial reinforcement to use them correctly. Eventually the healing of soft tissues around the hip reduces the risk of dislocation. Patients who dislocate may need to be brought back to the operating room. Subsequent care may include a brace that holds the hip in abduction and limits flexion. Patients tend to find such devices uncomfortable.

Weight-bearing limitations depend on several factors. Use of cement to help bind the femoral component to the bone immediately may increase the amount of weight bearing that the surgeon allows. Weight bearing as tolerated may be ordered, with a walker being used for a standard period of time before advancing to less restrictive devices as the patient's comfort level permits. This faster mobilization may be offset by earlier loosening of the bond between hardware and bone in later years. Noncemented prostheses may have better long-term fitting of hardware to bone. Initial restrictions on bearing weight are usually more conservative, although substantial variations are noted, depending on the individual orthopedist's protocol. If the greater trochanter of the femur was cut as part of the surgical approach, which may be done for a revision, then active hip exercises may be restricted further (Brandes et al., 1994).

The durability of the replacement may depend on the activity level of the patient. Vigorous sports or active manual labor may hasten failure of the interface between hardware components and bone. Traditional concerns about variable levels of activity in patient populations have been supported by current research. Joint replacement patients less than 60 years old walked 30% more on average than those over 60 years old (Schmalzried et al., 1998). The plastic lining of the acetabular cup may wear. The metal elements are very unlikely to break, since they are stronger than the surrounding bone.

Total knee replacements are also commonly performed at many centers. Postoperative swelling and pain may respond well to cold modalities. Wounds are monitored closely for signs of infection. Initial ambulation orders may specify partial weight bearing. Adaptive equipment may facilitate activities of daily living. Dislocation is not a concern after this procedure, in contrast to hip replacement cases. Failure to achieve adequate range of motion is a major issue. Inpatient goals on acute rehabilitation services may include attaining 90° of active knee flexion while lacking no more than 5° of extension. This allows normal sitting posture and adequate ambulation for most patients. Reaching full extension and over 100° of flexion will help performance on stairs, ramps, and curbs.

Given the importance of range of motion (ROM) goals, there has been great interest in continuous passive motion (CPM) machines. There is controversy over whether the reported initial benefits will lead to improved long-term outcomes (Naftulin & Niergarth, 1995). Some orthopedists include CPM in their post-operative clinical pathways.

Prophylaxis of deep vein blood clots is again an important issue. Risks of major bleeding events, especially at the surgical site, must be weighed against potential mortality from pulmonary emboli.

Successful outcomes are common after this procedure. Ability to walk over one mile is usually anticipated. There is about a 1% annual failure rate (Insall, 1993).

Replacement of other joints is much less common. Most of the patients who undergo those procedures have severe inflammatory arthritis involving multiple joints. Rehabilitation efforts must consider their overall condition in detail, rather than concentrating exclusively on the recent surgery.

The shoulder is another common site of orthopedic-related pain. Of the "large joints" the shoulder possesses superior mobility. With this enhanced mobility, however, also comes instability. Although various tendons cross the shoulder, the stabilizing tendon is termed the rotator cuff tendon. There are four muscles designated as the rotator cuff muscles, with their corresponding tendons joining at the shoulder to form a conjoined tendon termed the "rotator cuff tendon." Each muscle exerts forces at localized regions of the rotator cuff tendon. In unison, these forces provide shoulder stability. Complete tears within the rotator cuff tendon result in asymmetry of the rotator cuff tendon as a whole and ultimately lead to instability of the shoulder. This instability can result in improper movement of the shoulder or even dislocation during range of motion. Potential shoulder pain and other traumatic tissue/bone damage may result.

Tendon tears can be complete or incomplete. Incomplete tears seldom result in shoulder instability. They are often treated in the acute stage with physical therapy and pain control. If pain continues after a conservative trial, arthroscopic surgical interventions are then considered. Complete tendon tears typically lead to shoulder instability, with surgical repair usually being initiated early in young and active individuals.

Other common causes of shoulder pain are tendonitis (inflammation of a tendon) and impingement syndrome. Common causes of tendonitis are overuse and trauma. Many believe that tendonitis is the result of local ischemia to the affected tendon. In the acute stage, tendonitis is usually treated with rest, ice followed by heat after 48 hours, and anti-inflammatory medications (oral and/or injected). Physical therapy also plays a role in the acute stage, initially passively to maintain motion, with active exercises later on to aid in the prevention of future recurrences. Impingement syndrome occurs when a tendon is compressed between two or more objects, thus impeding its ability to glide freely. This compressive object is often the result of arthritis and osteophytes (bony overgrowths). In susceptible individuals, this decrement in space is usually associated with positioning of the shoulder. As the arms are raised over the head, the free space between the tendon and bone decreases and impingement syndrome begins. Impingement often results in tendonitis and frequently leads to "fraying" of the tendon itself with the potential for complete disruption. Treatment in the acute stage as in tendonitis is rest, anti-inflammatory medications, and physical therapy. If pain secondary to impingement persists, surgical approaches to widen the canal and provide greater room for the tendon to glide are entertained.

When range of motion of a shoulder is limited due to contracture, it is often referred to as a "frozen shoulder." Frozen shoulder is usually a late effect of shoulder pain rather than the initial cause. Although no one theory is proven, many believe that in order to minimize pain the affected shoulder is voluntarily held static. Due to inflammatory processes in association with reduced range of motion secondary to guarding, the shoulder becomes stiff and develops adhesions. These newly formed adhesions can resist voluntary motions, resulting in restriction and pain even after the pain from the initial injury has subsided. The combination of original injury in addition to pain from a frozen shoulder can result in even greater motion and functional losses than either alone. Although no formal treatment program is documented, many physicians believe that an aggressive physical therapy program along with treatment of the underlying disorder in the early stages is essential in preventing further functional deficits and reversing motion loss.

PSYCHOLOGICAL AND VOCATIONAL IMPLICATIONS

INDIVIDUALS WITH SIMILAR orthopedic impairments may have very different levels of physical disability. In some cases, this is easily predicted. A well-conditioned athlete should be able to move relatively well on crutches even if an injured leg can't bear weight. Cardiopulmonary disorders might prevent other patients with similar fractures from meeting the substantial energy demands of this abnormal way of walking. Coordination, strength of uninjured limbs, and body weight could also be critical.

Disability evaluations should take into account appropriate goals for each person. Vocational and avocational interests, family supports, social roles, and environmental factors must be noted. The athlete or manual laborer who can ambulate well with crutches may be unable to return to their usual work. Ability to care for a child may be compromised. Favorite recreational activities may be curtailed. Other people with severe physical problems may be able to continue their work effectively. Key factors include ability to travel, accessibility of the work site, specific tasks performed, and need to attend medical appointments.

Rehabilitation programs should assess travel needs. Training in car transfers or use of public transportation can be addressed. Telecommuting options can be explored.

Architectural barriers may hinder access to a building or movement once inside. Creative advice from rehabilitation professionals should include the most efficient and practical approaches to modification. Arranging access to a service entrance may be much faster than initiating construction projects. Advocacy with employers or landlords may be required.

On the macroeconomic level, the impact of orthopedic impairments is impressive. Low back pain care alone is a multibillion-dollar industry in the United States alone, and indirect costs are estimated to double the expense (Andersson, 1997). Employers face substantial compensation claims. Additional personal injury litigation may add to total expenses. Action may be taken against equipment manufacturers, landlords, or other parties not covered under compensation insurance.

At the individual level the potential for lost income is obvious. Coverage for professional health care varies significantly. Patients who require care from an attendant at home after discharge may face major out-of-pocket expenses. (Opening the home to strangers, even under the supervision of a home care agency, is also a source of anxiety to some frail individuals.) Relatives who take on direct care responsibilities may also lose income opportunities.

It is harder to quantify the social stresses that result from these conditions. Valued leadership roles in the family or community may be lost by the patient. Parents may become dependent on children. Sexuality may be affected by pain, mobility, apprehension, and altered body image. Barriers to communication about sexual issues have been noted (Gilbert, 1996), and many rehabilitation professionals are aware of this. Alteration of traditional gender roles may also be of special concern to patients and their families. Sensitivity to diverse cultural backgrounds will enhance care providers' effectiveness.

Many of the psychosocial aspects of orthopedic impairment overlap with other disabling conditions. Pain issues are of special importance. An injury may directly limit function mechanically or overwhelm pain tolerance. Fear of exacerbating the condition or causing recurrent injury may restrict activity after good physical recovery. Even after elective procedures, such as knee replacements, patients may fear the implications of pain. Understanding their specific concerns allows effective counseling. In some cases, rehabilitation emphasis is placed on functional restoration rather than pain reduction. Sustaining patient involvement requires acceptance of those priorities.

Orthopedic disorders may impact on body image. Surgical scars are not the only concern for some patients. Reduced exercise tolerance may lead to weight gain or decreased muscle bulk. Some individuals who appear to be in very good physical condition will still express concerns over changes from their baseline. This may raise questions about whether they were accustomed to excellent condition before injury, or whether they are exaggerating their current deficits. Opportunities for secondary gain are often invoked as explanations, but many factors may be involved. Other patients with extensive physical limitations may expect to achieve high levels of performance. Some cases involve some degree of denial, whereas others reflect realistic determination.

To complicate the situation even further, "referred pain" must be considered in many orthopedic cases. "Referred pain" is pain perceived in one portion of the body while originating at a distant region. Carpal tunnel syndrome (compression of a nerve at the wrist) may be felt, not as wrist pain but as elbow or shoulder pain. Herniated spinal discs often lead to arm or leg pain, without complaints of corresponding neck or back pain. In these instances, one cannot treat the symptomatic region without first addressing the asymptomatic region.

Orthopedic impairments create challenges for patients, families, providers, insurers, employers, and other agencies. Rehabilitation teams can look beyond traditional medical issues to address psychosocial issues. Complex cases warrant interdisciplinary interventions, including concerted efforts at patient education and counseling.

REFERENCES

Agnelli, G., & Sonaglia, F. (1997). Prevention of venous thromboembolism in high-risk patients. *Haematologica, 82*(4), 496–502.

Andersson, G. B. J. (1997). Guest Editorial. *Journal of Rehabilitation Research and Development, 34,* ix–x.

Andersson, G. B. J. (1999). Epidemiological features of chronic low-back pain. *Lancet, 354,* 581–585.

American College of Rheumatology. (2003). *Rheumatoid arthritis fact sheet.* Author.

American College of Rheumatology. (2004). *Systemic Lupus Erythematosis fact sheet.* Author.

Battie, M. C., Bigos, S. J., & Fisher, L. (1989). Isometric lifting strength as a predictor of industrial back complaints. *Spine, 14,* 851–856.

Battie, M. C., Bigos, S. J., & Fisher, L. (1990). Anthropometric and clinical measures as predictors of back pain complaints in industry: A prospective study. *Journal of Spinal Disorders, 3,* 195–201.

Bendix, T., & Biering-Sorensen, F. (1983). Posture of the trunk when sitting on forward reclining seats. *Scandinavian Journal of Rehabilitation Medicine, 15,* 197–203.

Bianchi, M. A. (1997). Historical view of the method according to Ilizarov. *Bulletin of the Hospital for Joint Diseases, 56*(1), 16–18.

Bigos, S. J., Bowyer, O., & Braen, G. (1994). Acute low back problems in adults. *Clinical Practice Guideline.* (AHCPR Publication 95-0642).

Brandes, V. A., Stulberg, D. S., & Chang, R. W. (1994). Rehabilitation following hip and knee arthroplasty. *Physical Medicine and Rehabilitation Clinics of North America, 5,* 815–836.

Carey, T. S., Evans, A. T., Hadler, N. M., Lieberman, G., Kalsbeek, W. D., Jackman, A. M., et al. (1996). Acute severe low back pain. *Spine, 21,* 339–344.

Cherkin, D. C., Deyo, R. A., Wheeler, K., & Ciol, M. A. (1994). Physician variation in diagnostic testing for low back pain. *Arthritis and Rheumatology, 37,* 15–22.

Cifu, D. X. (1995). Rehabilitation of fractures of the hip. *Physical Medicine and Rehabilitation: State of the Art Reviews, 9*(1), 125–140.

Cooper, C. (1997). The crippling consequences of fractures and their impact on quality of life. *American Journal of Medicine, 103*(2A), 12S–17S.

Deyo, R. A., Diehl, A. K., & Rosenthal, M. (1986). How many days of bedrest for acute low back pain? *New England Journal of Medicine, 315,* 1064–1070.

Deyo, R. A., & Weinstein, J. N. (2001). Low back pain. *New England Journal of Medicine, 344,* 363–370.

Duong, T. T. (1995). Complications of fractures. *Physical Medicine and Rehabilitation: State of the Art Reviews, 9*(1), 17–30.

Emerson, S., & Andersson, G. B. J. (1988). Ten year survival after fractures of the proximal end of the femur. *Gerontology, 34,* 186–191.

Frymoyer, J. W. (1988). Back pain and sciatica. *New England Journal of Medicine, 318,* 291–300.

Frymoyer, J. W., & Haldeman, S. (1991). Evaluation of the worker with low back pain. In M. H. Pope, G. B. J. Andersson, J. W. Frymoyer, & D. B. Chaffin (Eds.), *Occupational low back pain* (pp. 151–182). St. Louis, MO: Mosby-Year Book.

Gamburd, R. S. (1991). The use of selective injections in the lumbar spine. *Physical Medicine and Rehabilitation Clinics of North America, 2*(1), 79–96.

Gardner-Morse, M. G., & Stokes, I. A. F. (1998). The effects of abdominal muscle coactivation on lumbar spine stability. *Spine, 23,* 86–90.

Gilbert, D. M. (1996). Sexuality issues in persons with disabilities. In R. L. Braddom (Ed.), *Physical medicine and rehabilitation* (pp. 605–629). Philadelphia: W. B. Saunders.

Goh, J. C., Bose K., & Das, D. S. (1996). Pattern of fall and bone mineral density measurement in hip fractures. *Annals of the Academy of Medicine of Singapore, 6,* 820–823.

Greaves, J. D. (1997). Serious spinal cord injury due to haematomyelia caused by spinal anaesthesia in a patient treated with low dose heparin. *Anaesthesia, 52,* 150–154.

Harris, W. H., & Sledge, C. B. (1990). Total hip and total knee replacement. *New England Journal of Medicine, 323,* 725–731.

Herzog, R. J. (1991). Selection and utilization of imaging studies for disorders of the lumbar spine. *Physical Medicine and Rehabilitation Clinics of North America, 2*(1), 7–60.

Insall, J. N. (1993). *Surgery of the knee* (2nd ed.). New York: Churchill, Livingstone.

Kumar, V. N. (1995). Fracture bracing. *Physical Medicine and Rehabilitation: State of the Art Reviews, 9*(1), 11–16.

Licata, A. A. (1997). Biphosphonate therapy. *American Journal of Medical Science, 313*(1), 17–22.

Lo, T. C., & Healy, W. L. (2001). Re-irradiation for prophylaxis of heterotopic ossification after hip surgery. *British Journal of Radiology, 74*(882), 503–506.

Lyons, A. R. (1997). Clinical outcomes and treatment of hip fractures. *American Journal of Medicine, 103*(2A), 51S–63S.

Nachemson, A. L. (1992). Newest knowledge of low back pain: A critical look. *Clinical Orthopedics, 279,* 8–20.

Naftulin, S., & Niergarth, S. (1995). Continuous passive motion. *Physical Medicine and Rehabilitation: State of the Art Reviews, 9*(1), 51–65.

Philips, F. M. (2003). Minimally invasive treatments of osteoporotic vertebral compression fractures. *Spine, 28,* S45–S53.

Poss, R. (1993). Total joint replacement: Optimizing patient expectations. *Journal of the American Academy of Orthopedic Surgeons, 1,* 18–23.

Robinson, J. P., & Brown, P. B. (1991). Medications in low back pain. *Physical Medicine and Rehabilitation Clinics of North America, 2*(1), 97–126.

Saal, J. A., & Saal, J. S. (1991). Initial stage management of lumbar spine problems. *Physical Medicine and Rehabilitation Clinics of North America, 2*(1), 187–204.

Schmalzried, T. P., Szuszczewicz, E. S., Northfield, M. R., Akizuki, K. H., Frankel,

R. E., Belcher, G., et al. (1998). Quantitative assessment of walking activity after total hip or knee replacement. *Journal of Bone and Joint Surgery, 80A,* 54–59.

Sinaki, M. (1995). Rehabilitation of osteoporotic fractures of the spine. *Physical Medicine and Rehabilitation: State of the Art Reviews, 9*(1), 105–124.

Sinaki, M., & Mokri, B. (1996). Low back pain and disorders of the lumbar spine. In R. L. Braddom (Ed.), *Physical medicine and rehabilitation* (pp. 813–850). Philadelphia: W. B. Saunders.

Subbarao, J. V., & Blair, S. J. (1995). Reflex sympathetic dystrophy syndrome. *Physical Medicine and Rehabilitation: State of the Art Reviews, 9*(1), 31–50.

Triffit, P. D. (1998). The relationship between motion of the shoulder and the stated ability to perform activities of daily living. *Journal of Bone and Joint Surgery, 80A,* 41–46.

Van Tulder, M. W., Esmail, R., Bombardier, C., & Koes, B. W. (2004). Back schools for non-specific low-back pain. *Cochrane Library, 2.*

Winter, D. (1983). Energy generation and absorption at the ankle and knee during fast, natural, and slow cadences. *Clinical Orthopedics, 175,* 147–154.

Zuckerman, J. D., & Newport, M. L. (1988). Rehabilitation of fractures in adults. In J. Goodgold (Ed.), *Rehabilitation medicine* (pp. 441–456). St. Louis, MO: Mosby.

17

Ostomy Surgeries

Les Gallo-Silver, CSW-R, ACSW,
Diane Maydick-Youngberg, MS, RN, CWOCN,
and Michael Weiner, MSW

INDEPENDENCE IN TOILETING and the overall management of bowel movements and urination are considered characteristics of maturation in children and aspects of competence, health, and vibrance in adults. According to many psychodynamic theories the acquisition of bladder and bowel control is not only an aspect of physical and cortical growth but also an important emotional milestone. Some psychodynamic theories (Erickson, 1950) indicate that the overall issue of elimination is fraught with some level of shame. The oncology literature has explored this area in terms of factors that delay the detection and treatment of cancers of the bowel, rectum, bladder, kidney, and prostate. In many cultures the management of bowel movements and urination is considered a highly private matter and can often be ritualized as demonstrated by the plethora of toilet tissue products, deodorizers, and bathroom fixture styles. This mixture of developmental and psychosocial issues presents a context for understanding the impact on an individual confronted with the need to surgically alter their pattern and practice of elimination and self-care. Surgery re-routes the body's physical pattern of elimination through the creation of an abdominal opening or stoma. Numerous medical conditions, including cancer, trauma, inflammatory diseases, and certain congenital defects are ameliorated through an ostomy surgery (Hampton & Bryant, 1992).

OSTOMIES AS AN ASPECT OF SYMPTOM MANAGEMENT

A VARIETY OF MEDICAL conditions or trauma may require an ostomy. For the most part, people with diversions of the bowel or bladder can be placed in one of three general groups: those with a colostomy (large intestine), those with an ileostomy (small intestine), and those with a urostomy (urinary system). The stoma that is created by bringing a portion of the intestine to the surface of the abdomen may be characterized as permanent (unable to be closed) or temporary (ultimately to be closed). Diversions of bowel or bladder functioning occur within a dual framework of the disease or trauma as well as the psychosocial context. To separate the medical issue from the related psychological and practical issues could make even the best-intended treatment plan dehumanizing and may deny the individual the full benefits of symptom relief and healing (Colwell, Goldberg, & Carmel, 2001).

The most frequently chosen treatment for a primary adenocarcinoma of the colon is surgical resection. Genitourinary, gastrointestinal, gynecological, and other cancers may require ostomy surgery as part of tumor resection or to aggressively address life-threatening obstructions and other problems in elimination patterns and abilities. The portion of the intestine that is used to create the stoma will function according to the anatomical location (for example, an ascending colostomy will drain more liquid contents than a sigmoid colostomy which will have a more formed stool). These physically-related mechanical differences provoke diverse emotional reactions to issues of odor management, a sense of cleanliness, and feelings of worthiness and self esteem. As the surgery is an intervention to address a life-threatening illness, an individual's overall adjustment to the ostomy is framed by their understanding and ability to cope with their overall prognosis (Nugent, Daniels, Stewart, Patankar, & Johnson, 1999) Counseling encompasses the individual's adjustment to illness, changes in daily routine, alteration of life plans and expectations, as well as their changes in physical functioning (Marquis, Marrel, & Jambon, 2003).

With Brooke's creation of the "budded" stoma in 1952, many previous complications in the procedure of creating ostomies were to be avoided. At present, diversions of the small intestine are most commonly performed for inflammatory conditions of the bowel such as Crohn's disease or ulcerative colitis, although these conditions are typically treated non-surgically. An ileostomy may be performed for colorectal cancers, pseudomembranous colitis, polyposis syndromes, ischemic bowel disease, trauma radiation proctitis, toxic megacolon, and congenital anomalies. For people who require an ostomy to manage their symptoms, feelings of victimization and stigma can complicate their adjustment to their stoma. Ostomy self-help support groups can assist these individuals in feeling less socially isolated and can help normalize their sense of differentness.

Intestinal obstruction of the small or large intestine may be caused by the absence of peristalsis or a pathologic condition. The management of an obstruction initially is treated with decompression of the intestine by nasogastric suction and medical management of fluid and electrolyte balance. Treatment of the underlying cause of the obstruction may include ostomy surgery, which is either corrective or palliative in nature. Frequently, individuals with an intestinal obstruction struggle with considerable pain and anxiety. Nasogastric suction provides relief for the discomfort, but can increase anxiety and social withdrawal due to the public and visible nature of both the external mechanism and changed body functioning. Issues of sadness and of being overwhelmed about the future are areas that require counseling interventions to assist the individual with recovery and reentry into daily living. Some intestinal obstructions are caused by metastatic cancer that has spread to the intestinal tract. As this may often be a sign of progressive disease, the individual may be challenged to cope with a new ostomy as well as a worsening prognosis. This situation will often require intensive psychosocial management by the entire health care team.

Treatment of bladder cancer can require removal of the bladder and continent diversion. However, if this is not possible, the most common procedure is an ileal conduit or urostomy (Colwell et al., 2001). A urinary diversion is most often required when disease or injury require diversion of the urine away from distal structures in order to relieve an obstruction, to allow healing of a fistula, or to manage urinary incontinence. Although the urinary stream can be diverted at any level, the most common form of urinary diversion is the ileal conduit popularized by Bricker in 1950. With this procedure, the individual is required to wear a pouch for containment of the urine and for protection of the peristomal skin. Coping with an ileal conduit due to bladder cancer is framed by the individual's overall medical prognosis. Some people ultimately view the "sacrifice" of their bladder as necessary to preserve their life, while others may view the ileal conduit as the embodiment of a life change that is too difficult to accept and may struggle with receiving the self-care activities it requires. It is important to help people gain awareness of their feelings and thoughts about having a diagnosis of bladder cancer as a way of anticipating and understanding how they will react to the bladder's removal and "replacement" with an ileal conduit. As with colon and rectal cancers, the change in toileting activities is laden with complicated feelings about control, privacy, cleanliness, worthiness, and independence that are often challenging. As an example of a reaction to these complex feelings, some individuals may restrict their fluid intake as a way of controlling their urine production in order to avoid issues and concerns about their "new" urination patterns. This behavior, ancillary to the myriad of issues resulting from the ostomy, leaves these individuals vulnerable to dehydration, its vicissitudes, and its often serious symptoms. These symptoms can impair the person's quality of life by affecting energy level and blood pressure, and ultimately can be life-threatening. Identifying these and other concerns and addressing them as part of a psychosocial care plan helps to protect people from considering untoward fluid restriction as the only method of maintaining personal control. Disrupted sleep can also be an issue for people with ileal conduits due to concerns about urine collection during sleep. Fears of leakage or disruption of the urine collection bag by the natural body movements of sleep can prevent people from achieving the physical and emotional rest that sleep provides. Problem solving about night collection activities is an important part of the discharge process from the initial surgical admission. This issue requires periodic discussion with the patient to continue to evaluate the original plan's efficacy, which is to enable restful sleep.

Congenital conditions which may require an ostomy are: (a) Hirshsprungs disease, (b) anorectal malformation, and (c) cloacal exstrophy. In these cases, embryonic development does not progress as expected and a disruption of the gastrointestinal tract can occur. The treatment, considered an emergency procedure, is to relieve intestinal obstruction immediately. Once the obstruction is relieved, corrective surgery is usually deferred until the child is 9 to 12 months of age or older. Neonatal necrotizing enterocolitis (NEC) is a form of necrosis of the intestine. Prompt medical management must be initiated with the possibility of emergency surgery if a perforation or gangrene are present. During the procedure, the intestine is resected and a stoma is created. Future surgical treatment may be indicated for the infant survivor of NEC for the correction of strictured segments of the remaining intestine.

Psychosocial interventions assist parents in integrating medical information at a time of considerable anxiety, guilt, and physical stress. Parents can be empowered through instruction on managing their infant's or child's many new, complex needs. The concrete tasks related to learning these activities and the gaining of parental confidence that follows, can help absorb some of their anxiety. A major task of the multidisciplinary health care team is assisting parents in experiencing the joy of having a new baby with the ultimate goal of transmitting that joy and confidence to the infant/child being faced with surgical procedures and lengthy hospital admissions.

Serious injuries due to trauma that damages the bowel or bladder can require surgical diversion. Accepting and coping with an ostomy is one part of a comprehensive process of adjustment to the many physical and emotional challenges caused by the trauma (Rosito, Nino-Murcia, Wolfe, Kiratile, & Perkas, 2002). The mental health team that provides counseling and support to assist the individual with the psychological aspects of trauma recovery needs to be an integrated part of the surgical planning and recovery process. For some people challenged by trauma, an ostomy may help them establish more autonomy and control over their bodies than their pre-ostomy, post-injury toileting procedure. An individual's ability to successfully care for their ostomy or confidently direct the ostomy care that is provided by others, can be supportive of the overall healing process. At times, people with spinal cord injuries may elect to have an ostomy even though the bowel and bladder function. This is seen as a way of gaining more concrete control over their bodies and simplifying their care.

PSYCHOSOCIAL ADJUSTMENT TO AN OSTOMY

R ECOVERY IS COPING with and integrating the life changes caused by the ostomy and the underlying illness, as well as physical healing. Several factors influence an individual's post-surgical adjustment to an ostomy. These include: (a) the reason for the surgery, (b) the permanent or temporary nature of the stoma, (c) the individual's pre-surgical physical condition, (d) the individual's pre-surgical psychological adjustment, (e) the individual's expectations or pre-conceived notions about having an ostomy, (f) the psychosocial support and teaching available to transition to this new way of life, and (g) the fit, stability, and overall adherence of the pouch with predictable wearing time. Ongoing counseling and psychosocial support, including interventions based on support, confidence-building, validation, and empathy, need to address the emotional and practical issues involved in promoting psychological and functional adjustment to the ostomy (Schultz, 2002). For this purpose, a team approach is optimal to integrate medical, nursing, and mental health issues as part of a comprehensive ongoing treatment and rehabilitation plan. A continence nurse or an enterostomal therapist can be a crucial resource during the perioperative phase, as well as the acute and chronic rehabilitation period.

An acute or chronic illness or trauma that requires an ostomy produces a constellation of psychosocial reactions for the individual and all of those individual's interpersonal relationships. Regardless of the medical context of an ostomy's introduction, on some level most individuals experience the ostomy as emblematic of a loss of their previous life and expectations. The inclusion of family and friends is a crucial element to helping an individual adapt to a new ostomy regardless of the medical issues involved (Turnbull, 2002). Chronic illness, by its very nature, requires an on-going emotional accommodation that either assists an individual in creating a life of quality and productivity or one marked by depression and disappointment (Camilleri-Brennan & Steele, 2001). Understanding an individual's interpersonal and school/work history in the context of their ongoing struggle with a chronic medical condition is a window into their ability to manage and cope with an ostomy. Therefore, to some individuals with a chronic medical condition, an ostomy can be a tool to enhance independence, growth, and further increase the quality of their lives. Their ability to manage the necessary self-care activities and return to their typical daily routine with vitality and hope is propelled by their ability to cope effectively with their symptoms and the release of emotional energies that were previously tied to shame, frustration, and self-doubt (Gallo-Silver, 2003). For these individuals, education meetings with a stoma nurse, participation in an ostomy peer-support/education program, and continued management by their physician, provide the tools necessary to continue their own healthy adaptation to the ostomy.

For individuals with chronic conditions the ostomy may be treated as a wound that does not heal, an emblem of their differentness, their separateness, and their apartness from others and the life they want to live. When individuals undergo ostomy surgery secondary to the management of trauma, they are confronted with similar psychosocial dilemmas. The ostomy and the post-surgical activities involved in its care may serve as a means by which these individuals keep themselves isolated and keep potential caregivers and their health care team away. An individual's difficulty in coping can be frustrating for caregivers and the health care team. Social isolation and withdrawal can be the individual's maladaptive method of self-protection from further harm (Santos & Sawaia, 2001). Supportive counseling that partializes and prioritizes the individual's concerns about body image and addresses them sequentially can help the individual feel safer and more secure (Nugent et al., 1999). A psychiatric evaluation may be indicated in some cases. When the ostomy is introduced in the early acute phase of managing an injury due to trauma, the individual is often unable to separate the ostomy from the overwhelming challenge of adjusting to a profoundly and suddenly altered body image and life style. As time passes, the ostomy may serve as an ongoing physical and symbolic reminder, and at times a re-experiencing, of the original trauma suffered by the individual. For these individuals, formal ongoing counseling intervention as part of a comprehensive, integrated, medical rehabilitation and psychosocial approach is a necessary component for addressing these issues in a patient/family-centered manner.

Some individuals who are challenged by physical changes to their elimination patterns and abilities due to trauma elect to have ostomy surgery as part of their ongoing adaptation to their changed body. As the procedure is elective, these individuals may view their ostomy as an aspect of taking control over their bodies and their lives. An ostomy can be a solution to the intrusiveness of catheterization, particularly if the individual needs assistance from others, an efficient way to further protect skin integrity and overall daily hygiene, and a means to being more independent and mobile.

The proximity of the ostomy surgery to an initial diagnosis of cancer is an important factor, as a cancer diagnosis creates a reverberating psychosocial crisis that may take precedence over the individual's adjustment to a new ostomy. For these individuals, it may be too difficult for them to cognitively and emotionally concentrate on the issues presented by an ostomy without receiving comprehensive psychosocial support focused on their underlying cancer. When ostomies are part of an overall surgical resection of a tumor that results in a potentially good prognosis, the individual often has more emotional energy to adapt to the ostomy and may view the change in elimination patterns and procedures as an unavoidable "war injury" in their fight to "beat" the cancer and preserve their lives. Ostomies introduced as a form of aggressive palliation for cancer are often viewed by these individuals as another sign of their vulnerability and force them to confront their poor prognosis (Wells & Turney, 2001). After-care treatment plans need to unite patient education, practical management tools, and counseling interventions to address the complexity of adapting to an ostomy in the face of acute illness. The individual's overall adaptation and ability to cope with their cancer diagnosis and their overall prognosis are the salient features in developing the after-care counseling treatment plan.

PSYCHOEDUCATIONAL ADJUSTMENT TO AN OSTOMY

OSTOMY SURGERY IS traumatic and the uncertainty of pouch adherence can be traumatic. Resources such as the Wound, Ostomy, Continence Nurses Society, the United Ostomy Association, and manufacturers of ostomy supplies may serve as sources of information and support for the person with an ostomy. If a patient is traumatized by their pouching system leaking at unpredictable times they may begin to withdraw from usual activities, resulting in isolation and depression.

The learning and integration of self-care, which enhances the concepts of mastery and competence, is the foundation of autonomy and independence for people with ostomies (O'Shea, 2001; Schultz, 2002). People who do not have cognitive or neuromuscular/skeletal impairments that preclude self-care need to be actively engaged in regular sessions with an ostomy nurse in order to gain confidence in managing their ostomy and to shorten the learning curve. Mastering the skills to manage leaks, malfunctions and overall routine care in novel environments supports a life of quality and personal freedom. For people who struggle with emotional obstacles to learning self-care, integrating counseling interventions as a part of the visit with the ostomy nurse provides the type of comprehensive support people need to gain a sense of safety and confidence. Counseling sessions work best when conducted before the visit with the ostomy nurse and then combined with an opportunity for a brief session with the nurse present to review the visit and identify achievements. This pattern works best within an in-patient environment for people adapting to new ostomies. The ability to continue to work with the same ostomy nurse and psychosocial clinician following discharge and the sense of safety and control this continuity brings to the individual is the optimal way to assist the more fragile person to acquire an ease and comfort with their changed bodies. For people with cognitive and/or neuromuscular/skeletal impairments, self-care encompasses the acquisition of a level of comfort with the process and equipment of self-care to participate in directing health care professionals, home care workers, family members, and any other individual who will assist them in their care. All people need to be engaged in a patient education process that is appropriate for their learning, implementation, and retention abilities.

Assessment of the individual's support system and inclusion of the significant other in the process of ostomy teaching is tailored to the individual. The involvement of significant others in the management and care of an ostomy is determined by the individual in collaboration with the health care team. The individual's physical and cognitive abilities to manage their ostomy are part of an overall patient/family education assessment. Individuals determined to be independent in self-care reflect the healthy adult wish to manage their toileting needs as a private autonomous activity. It is essential to respect this important aspect of self-sufficiency while accommodating an individual's impairments and potential need for the assistance of another pair of hands. Counseling, both with the individual and jointly with the care partner, is necessary to negotiate a care contract that preserves the individual's self-esteem and sense of control while ensuring that the ostomy will be managed safely if the individual is able to do so independently. Whether the family/significant other assists in ostomy care on a temporary or permanent basis, it is important to prepare the individual and family/significant other as a natural psychosocial unit with information regarding the rationale for the surgery, the usual appearance of a stoma, the purpose of the pouching systems, and how to protect the peristomal skin. Some individuals may resist including family/significant others and their resistance requires further psychosocial assessment. Counseling may assist individuals in re-thinking this decision. In cases where the individual does not change their decision, the health care team has gained the opportunity to address special needs and circumstances.

Use of teaching materials with pictures and understandable language that explain the anatomy of the gastrointestinal and genitourinary tract may be helpful. Rehabilitation, psychosocial, and mental health professionals should thoroughly understand the procedure that was done in order to clarify accurately for the patient and significant other any information regarding post-procedure expectations and/or activities. Asking the patient/significant other what they have been told about the operation is a good starting point. Clarification of all information is crucial in helping the patient/significant other to understand what was done and what to expect. Once a clear understanding about the change in bowel or bladder function is established the teacher may proceed to other issues. Some of these issues will include the normal appearance of the stoma, the expected output from the stoma, how to care for the peristomal skin, the proper fitting of the skin barriers, the various pouches available, how to clean or empty a pouch, how to change the pouching system, the frequency of care needed, and how to go about obtaining the necessary items for self-care.

The individual is taught that the stoma is initially swollen and that it will gradually reduce in the initial post-operative period. He/she is shown how to use a measuring guide and to make a pattern to cut the proper size opening so that the peristomal skin is not exposed to the stool or urine. By using the measuring card he/she will be able to adjust the size of the opening to 1/8_ larger than the stoma. This allows just enough room for the stoma to move without constriction during peristalsis. The individual is instructed in how to select the proper type of skin barrier. If the individual has a colostomy with a pasty/semi-solid or solid output, then a standard-wear barrier may be used (i.e., Stomahesive, Flexwear, etc.). If the individual has a stoma with a liquid output such as a small bowel or urinary stoma, then a longer-lasting, extended-wear barrier must be used to provide adequate protection of the peristomal skin from the effluent (i.e., Flextend, Durahesive, etc.).

The individual is also taught that when the intact pouching system is to be removed for changing, care must be taken to remove the adherent system gently using adhesive remover or gently by hand. If the skin is damaged there is potential for non-adherence of the system as well as a plethora of other skin problems. The peristomal skin is generally washed with plain water, rinsed, and dried. The skin should be free of redness, irritation, inflammation, cuts, blisters, rashes. The skin must be completely dry before the new adhesive pouching system is applied.

If irritation is noted this should be assessed and treated before reapplication of the ostomy system.

Education interventions explain to the patient/significant other that the ostomy system may be changed once or twice weekly, depending on the type of ostomy and patient preference; that the pouch must never be reinforced if leakage occurs; that it should be changed completely to minimize irritation from the effluent; and that overfilling of the pouch should be avoided. Overfilling creates stress on the adherence of the adhesive portion of the pouch and could cause leakage. The pouch should be emptied whenever it is 1/3 to 1/2 full. In terms of allowing for full-night sleeps for the patient with a urostomy, connection to a bedside drainage collector will help manage these issues.

Additionally, patients can be educated that deodorizing sprays, drops, powders, and liquids are available over the counter wherever ostomy supplies are available, and that the pouches are made out of odor-proof materials and if closed there should be no discernible odor if the products are used as directed (i.e., changed once or twice weekly). Items such as aspirin should not be placed into the pouch to aid with odor control because the stoma may bleed easily as a result. Patients with a urinary stoma should use a pouch with an anti-reflux valve to prevent backflow of the urine.

Initially, the individual undergoing ostomy surgery may refuse to look at the stoma as a way of demonstrating their struggle with the reality of their body and its functioning. As a first step to ultimate acceptance of the ostomy, the individual and the significant other may watch the eyes and facial expressions of the nurses and doctors (functioning as a role models and educators) caring for or examining the stoma or the pouching system as a way of learning how they should experience the ostomy. The interpretation of facial expressions may be understood, interpreted, and internalized by the patient as either positive regard/acceptance or disgust/rejection. When a family member/significant other refuses to look at the ostomy, the patient may also interpret this as a rejection. Helping the family and significant others to anticipate their reactions to the stoma can provide them with the information and preparation to assist in helping the individual to cope with their new ostomy.

The individual/significant others need to be reassured that the pouching systems are odor-proof and easily concealed beneath clothing. A wide variety of pouching systems/devices exist and the system should be tailored to the individual's ability and type of ostomy. Most pouching systems are disposable after being worn for several days. They are usually emptied, but in certain instances the patient may use a pouch that is discarded one or two times daily. This is usually reserved for a patient with a low descending or sigmoid colostomy, as it would not be cost effective with a stoma that has liquid effluent because it requires more than two pouches per day.

Products are designed with features that protect the skin from the effluent, contain the odor, and provide comfort features. The choices depend on the type of ostomy. For example, a urostomy will require a spout which can be connected to bedside drainage at night, thus affording the individual a full night's rest; an ileostomy must be able to be drained due to the liquid nature of the drainage; and some colostomies have a formed stool which would allow for a non-drainable/disposable pouch to be worn. Important issues such as financial concerns also play an important part in the decision-making process when it comes to pouching choices. If the individual has insurance coverage, they need to explore what is allowed by their individual policy. If there is no insurance coverage, a pouching system that would meet the individual financial picture should be suggested.

RE-ENTRY

COUNSELING WITH PEOPLE with ostomies needs to focus on practical ways to help the individual return to work, school, and leisure activities within the context of their physical condition. Many people with ostomies can and do return to their pre-ostomy routines, as the surgery itself does not render someone disabled. This can be in contrast to the underlying injury or illness that the ostomy was used to address or ameliorate. Re-entry requires the social integration of self-care, as an individual's work, school, and leisure activities, for the most part, are outside of the home and conducted within an interpersonal context. Empowering people to learn their body's post-ostomy elimination patterns and schedule is both a practical and clinical intervention. Learning about one's elimination patterns, and how to safely modulate them when possible, increases a sense of personal control. Helping an individual learn how to prepare to be away from their home, and more specifically their bedroom or bathroom, where they manage their self-care, requires a mixture of patient education and cognitive/behavioral counseling techniques. Role play, problem solving interventions, and the use of coping statements help people gain the confidence to be able to manage their needs by identifying private areas for self-care and obtaining and anticipating the need for specific types of self-care materials. Wearing clothing with a pattern may help conceal the pouching system, and some of the newer products that are on the market are relatively flat and do not bulge. Wearing dark clothes, having a change of a potentially affected garment, and carrying items such as a mirror that has a handle for easy positioning, a rope or strap for hanging, and deodorant, are essential as specific ostomy supplies. Feeling clean and fresh is also key for people with ostomies in gaining a level of social comfort that promotes a return to work, school, and leisure activities. A travel kit with an extra pouching system, some paper towels, and a self-closing plastic bag for disposal should be carried at all times. Deodorizers are available and a few drops can be placed in the pouch after emptying. Many people prefer to wear a freshly-changed pouch, an opaque pouch, and a miniature pouch or stoma cap which could be changed back to the usual pouching system after the interlude.

PHYSICAL INTIMACY AND SEXUALITY

ALL PEOPLE BEING prepared for a new ostomy require an extensive psychosocial evaluation that includes an understanding of the individual as a sexual person (Gallo-Silver, 2003). Although some people require an ostomy on an emergent basis because of a sudden injury or unanticipated medical crisis, the vast majority of people are consented for the procedure in preparation for the aggressive management of an underlying disease. It is within this consent process that meeting with a psychosocial professional is crucial to develop a clinical plan of recovery and re-entry.

The need for closeness, affection, being touched, kissed, and hugged is not altered by ostomy surgery. The ensuing psychosocial crisis of illness and surgery can be ameliorated by love and comfort (Gallo-Silver, 2003). As important as work, school, leisure, and other daily activities are, they are no more nor less important than physical intimacy and sexuality. Nonetheless, medical, health care, and psychosocial professionals may avoid the topic of sexuality and inadvertently de-sexualize and emotionally disenfranchise people with ostomies (Gallo-Silver & Parsonnet, 2001). Learning about the intimate behavior of people prior to surgery begins to engage them in a plan of recovering and returning to this important aspect of quality of life. When medical necessity or the lack of available psychosocial support precludes a presurgical evaluation, a postsurgical psychosocial assessment should presume that the person is sexually active until the person indicates otherwise (Golis, 1996). It is the responsibility of the medical, health care, and psychosocial professionals to present the issue of sexual rehabilitation as an integrated part of the overall rehabilitation plan of care.

Helping a person become comfortable with his or her altered body image is part of learning self-care. The need to visualize the ostomy and identify signs of health and cleanliness is also preparation for physical closeness with a sexual partner. For women, some ostomy surgeries may alter the contours and size of the vagina, requiring the use of dilators to help expand the vaginal walls and to assist in gaining comfort with an appropriate level of penetration (Schover, 1997). In addition, some disease processes requiring an ostomy for best management may also alter a woman's ability to lubricate when stimulated. Vaginal lubricants and vaginal moisturizers should be included in necessary and appropriate self-care equipment. For men, some ostomy surgeries disrupt and sever the nerve bundles that control erectile function. Some men elect to have a penile implant placed at the time of their ostomy surgery or shortly thereafter as a way of addressing this difficult-to-manage side effect. Women and men both struggle with diminished libido or desire due to the impact of the overall illness and as a side effect of the fear, sadness, and sense of loss that an ostomy can represent (Gallo-Silver & Parsonnet, 2002). Although traditional counseling assists people in ventilating and exploring these important concerns, a cognitive/behavioral approach is often most helpful in promoting a return to physical intimacy and re-connecting sexually with a partner (Gallo-Silver, 2000).

Although ostomy surgery can alter a person's ability to become aroused or excited and the underlying illness can diminish desire, most people retain an ability to experience orgasmic feelings, even if the intensity of these sensations is diminished. Understanding one's changed body requires permission to explore how the body responds to stimulation during bathing and self-care activities. Self-exploration through the therapeutic use of masturbation is a basic way for an individual with a new ostomy to begin to reawaken their sexual appetite and reclaim their sexual self-esteem (Gallo-Silver, 2000). The understanding of one's new pattern and schedule of elimination, so necessary for a return to work, school, and leisure activities, is also necessary for people to resume physical intimacy (Schover & Jensen, 1988). The use of preintimacy bathing, cleaning, and deodorizing as well as strategic placement of an absorbent cotton towel and the use of decorative ostomy bag covers are important elements in reconnecting with a partner. It is most helpful for people with new ostomies to learn and practice sensate focus exercises with their partner prior to attempting coitus or other sexual activity that has orgasm as its ultimate goal. Sensate focus is a series of sensual massage techniques that provide the affected and unaffected partner an opportunity to reacquaint themselves with each other's bodies in a safe and nonpressured way (Kaplan, 1987).

Coital position change can help couples avoid putting pressure on the ostomy site. Some side-by-side positions and the female superior position are often the most advantageous in both modulating penetration, thrusting, and avoidance of the ostomy location (Schover & Jensen, 1988). Physical intimacy is a way that people with a changed body image and function can feel more alive and more connected to life.

THRIVING WITH AN OSTOMY

THE PURPOSE OF an ostomy is to improve a person's life. Helping a person connect with their ostomy as an aspect of their quality of life is an educational and psychosocial process. People with an ostomy may have several other medical and psychological problems, some due to their illness and some part of their preostomy baseline functioning. The assessment of the individual needs to include both a physical and emotional component. A treatment/rehabilitation plan of care unites and respects the mind/body connection by encouraging a biopsychosocial approach to healing. Thriving with an ostomy requires an individual to identify their physical and psychological strengths and build on them to support their quality of life. Counseling needs to focus on a strengths-based perspective, building on these qualities of the individual, as a way of bolstering and then navigating through the adjustment and integration process. The medical, nursing, rehabilitation, and mental health teams share responsibility for promoting a sense of wholeness and normalization for people with ostomies by collaborating and coordinating their respective contributions to the individual's care. Rehabilitation is a partnership among the patient, the family, and the professionals—all with the shared goal of recovery.

REFERENCES

Bloom, D. A., & Grossman, H. B. (1986). Stomal construction and reconstruction. *Urology Clinics of North America, 13,* 275–283.

Bricker, E. M. (1950). Bladder substitution after pelvic evisceration. *Surgery Clinics of North America, 30,* 1511–1521.

Brooke, B. N. (1952). The management of an ileostomy including its complications. *Lancet, 2,* 102–104.

Camilleri-Brennan, J., & Steele, R. J. (2001). Objective assessment of quality of life following panproctocolectomy and ileostomy for ulcerative colitis. *Annals of the Royal College of Surgeons of England, 85*(5), 321–324.

Colwell, J. C., Goldberg, M., & Carmel, J. (2001). The state of the standard diversion. *Journal of Wound Ostomy and Continence Nurses, 28,* 66–17.

Erickson, E. (1950). *Childhood and society.* New York: W. W. Norton.

Gallo-Silver, L. (2000). Sexual rehabilitation of persons with cancer. *Cancer Practice, 8*(1), 10–16.

Gallo-Silver, L. (2003, Fall). Physical intimacy and sexuality for people with ostomies. *Association of Oncology Social Work News, 19*(1), 10–12.

Gallo-Silver, L., & Parsonnet, L. (2002). Sexuality and fertility. In M. M. Lauria, E. J. Clark, J. F. Hermann, & N. M. Stearns (Eds.), *Social work in oncology* (pp. 27–44). Atlanta, GA: American Cancer Society.

Golis, A. M. (1996). Sexual issues for the person with an ostomy. *Journal of Wound Ostomy and Continence Nurses, 23*(1), 33–37.

Hampton, B., & Bryant, R. (1992). *Ostomies and continent diversions.* St. Louis, MO: Mosby Year Book.

Kaplan, H. S. (1987). *The illustrated manual of sex therapy.* New York: Brunner/Mazel.

Marquis, P., Marrel, A., & Jambon, B. (2003). Quality of life in patients with stomas: The Montreux Study. *Ostomy/Wound Management, 49*(2), 48–55.

Nugent, K. P., Daniels, P., Stewart, B., Patankar, R., & Johnson, C. D. (1999). Quality of life in stoma patients. *Diseases of the Colon and Rectum, 42*, 1569–1574.

O'Shea, H. (2001). Teaching the adult ostomy patient. *Journal of Wound Ostomy and Continence Nursing, 28*(1), 47–54.

Rosito, O., Nino-Murcia, M., Wolfe, V. A., Kiratile, B. J., & Perkas, T. (2002). The effects of colostomy on the quality of life in patients with spinal cord injury: A retrospective analysis. *Journal of Spinal Cord Medicine, 25*, 174–183.

Santos, V. L., & Sawaia, B. B. (2001). The pouch acting as mediator between "being a person with an ostomy," and "being a professional": Analysis of pedagogical strategy. *Journal of Wound, Ostomy and Continence Nursing, 28*, 206–214.

Schover, L. R. (1997). *Sexuality and fertility after cancer.* New York: John Wiley.

Schover, L. R., & Jensen, S. B. (1988). *Sexuality and chronic illness.* New York: Guilford Press.

Shultz, J. M. (2002). Preparing the patient for colostomy care: A lesson well learned. *Ostomy and Wound Management, 48*(10), 22–25.

Turnbull, G. The importance of coordinating ostomy care and teaching across settings. *48*(5), 12–13.

Wells, N. L., & Turney, M. E. (2001). Common issues facing adults with cancer. In M. M. Lauria, E. J. Clark, J. F. Hermann, & N. M. Stearns (Eds.), *Social work in oncology* (pp. 27–44). Atlanta, GA: American Cancer Society.

18

Pediatric Disorders: Cerebral Palsy and Spina Bifida

Joan T. Gold, MD

PHYSICALLY CHALLENGED CHILDREN present with a variety of developmental and neuromuscular disabilities that are often difficult to diagnose, harder to remediate, and impossible to cure. The restrictions imposed by such a disability may not permit the patient to have the motoric control or the experiences to acquire skills at the same rate as the typically developing child. Accordingly, secondary developmental delays may occur (Missuna & Pollack, 1991). Medical complications unique to the underlying diagnosis, with frequent hospitalizations and surgeries, social isolation, parental dependency, and financial burdens, act as stressors for patients, parents, and siblings (Worley, Rosenfeld, & Lipscomb, 1991).

It is the purpose of this chapter to discuss cerebral palsy and spina bifida, two of the more common handicapping conditions of childhood, and the strategies that allow for appropriate medical treatment and habilitation. This information permits the health professional to serve as an advocate for optimization of care, prevention of complications, referral to early intervention programs, and placement of the child in the least restrictive school setting. Additionally, potentially abusive and neglectful behaviors of parents and caretakers may be circumvented (Benedict, White, Wulff, & Hall, 1990).

CEREBRAL PALSY

CEREBRAL PALSY IS a descriptive clinical term which denotes a group of static encephalopathies of diverse etiologies that result from non-progressive lesions of the brain sustained in the pre-, peri-, or postnatal periods. The disorder is characterized by abnormalities in muscle tone, muscle control and movement, and postures, of which spasticity is the most common type of presentation, occurring in from 65 to 80% of cases. Secondary dysfunction and deformities occur, but there is not the frank regression in function seen with neurodegenerative disorders, such as the leukodystrophies. Other symptoms of cerebral dysfunction, such as learning disabilities, mental retardation, and seizures may be seen, but it is the motoric dysfunction that is essential to the diagnosis of the condition (Ingram, 1955).

INCIDENCE

THE INCIDENCE OF cerebral palsy of the past 20 years has remained at 2 cases per 1,000 births in the United States (Nelson & Ellenberg, 1986; Reddihough & Collins, 2003), with approximately 400,000 patients currently being affected. Incidence has remained stable or in some studies increased to 2.5 cases per 1,000, despite advances in intrapartum monitoring that can herald fetal distress (albeit with a false-positive rate approaching 99.8%) and in neonatal care, especially respiratory support (Grant, O'Brien, Joy, Henessy, & Mac Donald, 1989; Stanley & Blair, 1991). This implies that some of the lower-birth-weight infants are surviving unscathed, and that efforts expended at the time of delivery may be employed after the incident responsible for the disorder has occurred (Ford, Kitchen, Doyle, Richards, & Kelly, 1990). It is possible that the incidence figures may gradually increase as more infants with extremely low birth weight of less than 1,000 grams survive, as the current incidence of cerebral palsy in this population approaches 25% (Vohr & Msall, 1997). However, special services may be required in a greater percentage of this population, as from 44 to 56% in this group may require special education services.

ETIOLOGY AND RISK FACTORS

CEREBRAL PALSY WAS first described by Little in 1843 in former premature infants who developed increased tone and in-coordination primarily affecting the lower extremities, or what is now termed as spastic diplegia. With changes in medical treatment, a reduced association with dystocia (difficult labor), erythroblastosis (Rh-negative blood incompatibility), and encephalitis, and an increased association with multiple births, prematurity, acquired hydrocephalus (following intracranial hemorrhage and ante-natal infection), and trauma have been noted (Capute, Shapiro, & Palmer, 1981). Accordingly, fewer patients are affected with the writhing movement disorder of athetosis, seen with erythroblastosis and subsequent deposition of abnormal hemoglobin pigments into the basal ganglia, and a greater number of patients have diffuse cerebral dysfunction, with spasticity and cognitive dysfunction.

Etiology can be identified in up to 71% of quadriplegics (those patients with equal involvement of all four extremities), and in 40% of non-quadriplegics (Naeye & Peters, 1989). A gestational age of less than 32 out of 40 weeks is the greatest predictor for the development of cerebral palsy. Other risk factors, such as maternal mental retardation, birth weight of less than 2,001 grams, the presence of congenital malformations, and symptomatic intoxications such as fetal alcohol syndrome, support a largely prenatal etiology (Coorsen, Msall, & Duffy, 1991; Ellenberg & Nelson, 1981). Factors that result in chronic antenatal hypoxia with brain injury include maternal anemia, pre-eclampsia/gestational hypertension, a drop in third-trimester blood pressure, post-term delivery, and multiple births (Nelson, 1989). These events have a high association with the presence of congenital malformations.

A prenatal etiology for cerebral palsy has been identified in up to 50 to 60% of patients (Holm, 1982; Naeye & Peters, 1989), most presenting with hypotonia, ataxia, or hemiplegia (unilateral limb involvement). In utero infections have recently been demonstrated as one of the predisposing factors in the etiology of cerebral palsy. Inflammatory markers such as cytokines, and interferon levels of cord blood are frequently elevated in the population of patients who progress to having spastic diplegia (Nelson, 1998).

Thrombotic events in utero may also explain many cases of cerebral palsy. Analysis of cord blood levels for Protein S and Protein C deficiencies, conditions which predispose to hypercoagulability, and in utero stroke may be of value in patients who are subsequently diagnosed has having the hemiplegic variety of cerebral palsy (Gibson, Mac Lennan, Goldwater, & Dekker, 2003). Identification of a parental coagulopathy or other serological markers could potentially provide for early designation of a population at-risk, with more prompt and more effective initiation of early intervention therapeutic services and for development of a preventative protocol (Kraus, 1997).

A perinatal etiology has been identified in only about 10 to 15% of cases. Factors thought to be characteristic of birth asphyxia, such as meconium staining and fetal distress, are more often the result of non-asphyxial disorders that have been present as chronic stressors in the pregnancy, and clinically may not have a way of being identified, tracked, or ameliorated (Nelson, 1989). True perinatal asphyxia may be related to obstetrical complications such as placental abruption, nuchal cord, or meconium aspiration. Such an etiology is often accompanied by seizures in the newborn period, and evidence of other organ system dysfunction due to anoxia such as cardiac, renal, and/or hepatic dysfunction. Other perinatal etiologies include central nervous system bleeding (Williams, Lewandowski, Coplan, & D'Eugenio, 1987) and meningeal infections. Patients in this group are most likely to be spastic.

A post-natal etiology occurs in about 10% of patients (Holm, 1982). Factors include head trauma of an accidental or inflicted (abusive) nature, central nervous system infections, and cerebrovascular accidents. Such patients are likely to be hemiparetic. A mixed etiology occurs in about 7% of cases (Holm).

Neonatal indicators for the development of static encephalopathy include intracranial hemorrhage, seizures, microcephaly (small head size), hyper- or hypotonia, abnormal suck/cry/grasp reflexes, jitteriness, temperature instability, and feeding difficulties (Nelson & Ellenberg, 1979). Apgar scores that reflect immediate neonatal status are not as predictive as once thought (Nelson & Ellenberg, 1981). Periventricular hemorrhage in association with attenuation of the white matter about the ventricles (periventricular leukomalacia or P.V.L.) with formation of cysts, which can be demonstrated on head ultrasound or other neuro-imaging studies, correlates with the development of cerebral palsy (Graham, Levene, & Trounce, 1987). P.V.L. is associated with birth trauma, asphyxia and respiratory failure, cardiopulmonary defects, premature birth/low birth weight with associated immature cerebrovascular development, and lack of appropriate autoregulation of cerebral blood flow in response to hypoxic-ischemia insult. Brain cells known as oliogodendrocytes are vulnerable to exposure of free-radical chemicals which are liberated during these events, and further compromised by poor circulation and the presence of cytokines which are seen with inflammation and infection. If this process is better delineated, treatment regimens which reverse the effects of free-radicals and other inflammatory chemicals, such as the use of Interleukin-10 (Mesples, Plaisant, & Gressens, 2003), may be able to modulate the subsequent neurological outcome (Rezaie & Dean, 2002; Bell & Hallenbeck, 2002).

Delineation of an etiology may imply a specific clinical presentation and prognosis that permits parents to be supplied with an overview of the child's potential outcome. Counseling of parents that actions during the time of conception and pregnancy are most likely unrelated to the development of the cerebral palsy permits feelings of guilt to be assuaged, and promotes better acceptance of the child.

FUNCTIONAL PRESENTATION

CEREBRAL PALSY IS classified on the basis of etiology, tone, and anatomical distribution of neurological abnormalities (Perlstein, 1952). Pyramidal or spastic (clasp-knife) cerebral palsy is the most common. Resistance is noted when muscles are stretched rapidly beyond a critical point. There is associated hyperreflexia, and up-going plantar responses. Quadriplegia occurs in about 20% of these cases, with diffuse cortical involvement and, in the most disabled, widespread atrophy with cavity formation and decreased white matter density. Hemiplegia occurs in about 30% and is associated with atrophy/gliosis of the contralateral cerebral hemisphere, likely caused by a vascular disturbance. Liquifaction necrosis may occur, resulting in a porencephalic cyst (Mannino & Traunor, 1983).

Diplegics, who comprise over 50 to 65% of this population, are generally but not exclusively premature infants who have undergone significant intraventricular hemorrhages (Blair & Stanley, 1990; Hagberg & Hagberg, 1989). The periventricular areas have cortical radiations to the lower extremities, which are more involved with spasticity than the upper extremities; this differentiates these patients from quadriplegics, in whom all extremities are involved to the same degree (Banker & Larroche, 1962). Diplegia, and cerebral palsy in general, in premature infants is most correlated with periventricular leukomalacia as discussed above, and is demonstrable on head ultrasound, CT scan, and MRI studies. The severity of these findings seems to correlate with the degree of the child's sensorimotor involvement. Infants in this group, who also demonstrate thalamic lesions, are more likely to have more severe motor and cognitive dysfunction (Yokochi, 1997). Monoplegia and triplegia (affecting one and three limbs, respectively) are rare. Bilateral involvement is the most common presentation, occurring in 75% of pre-term, and 45% of term patients (Hagberg & Hagberg, 1996).

Extrapyramidal or non-spastic types of cerebral palsy are responsible for about 20% of cases. Patients who have athetosis or rigidity have basal ganglia dysfunction that accounts for their movement disorders. Ataxic patients have difficulties with balance and position sense, resulting from cerebellar pathology. Diagnostic work-up is most important with ataxias, as posterior fossa brain tumors and degenerative inherited diseases, such as ataxia telangiectasia and Friedrich's ataxia, may have similar presentations.

Hypotonic patients have widespread damage to cortical and subcortical areas, so spasticity cannot be mounted as a response, and they have the poorest prognosis for cognitive and motor function. Some hypotonic patients may become athetoid with time. The remainder of the cases have mixed features (i.e., diffuse cerebral involvement and impaired motor function).

DIFFERENTIAL DIAGNOSIS

UP TO 40% of patients with an initial diagnosis of cerebral palsy have been incorrectly diagnosed. Other disorders that present with gross motor delays, aberrant tone, and abnormal movement patterns include mental retardation, neurodegenerative disorders, hydrocephalus, subdural effusions, slowly growing brain tumors, spinal cord lesions, muscular dystrophy, spinal muscular atrophy, and congenital cerebellar ataxias. Obviously, prognosis, inheritance patterns, and treatment would vary widely in these disorders (Molnar & Taft, 1977).

Investigations that may be helpful in substantiating or excluding the diagnosis of cerebral palsy include the following: CT or MRI scans to assess for structural lesions, ultrasound of the head to exclude the possibility of intraventricular hemorrhage, lumbar puncture to exclude elevated protein in the cerebral spinal fluid that is seen in association with neurodegenerative disorders, serum uric acid and blood and urine assays for amino and organic acids to exclude congenital metabolic disorders, viral and parasitic titers (TORCH) to exclude the possibility of an intrauterine-acquired infection, and chromosomal studies to exclude such abnormalities, especially in dysmorphic children.

ASSOCIATED MEDICAL PROBLEMS

MENTAL RETARDATION CO-EXISTS in 50 to 60% of patients with cerebral palsy; communication and learning disorders in 40 to 50%; visual problems, including strabismus and myopia in 50%; deafness in 6 to 16%; seizure disorders in 33 to 38%; and orthopaedic deformities in 50% (R. O. Robinson, 1973). Generalized seizures are most common in patients with quadriplegia, and partial seizures are most common in those patients with hemiplegia (Carlson, Hagberg, & Olssom, 2003). Electroencephalograms and visual and auditory evoked potentials are helpful in delineation of such problems.

The parietal lobe syndrome is characterized by hemiplegia, limb length discrepancies (the upper extremity being more affected), and sensory deficits as manifested by reduced two-point discrimination, stereognosis, and graphesthesia (Staheli, Duncan, & Schaefer, 1960). A less common triad, seen with erythroblastosis-related disease, includes kernicterus (bilirubin deposition from red blood cell breakdown in the basal ganglia) with resultant athetosis, hearing loss, and paralysis of upward gaze.

Oropharyngeal incoordination may result in poor oral intake, with failure to thrive, occasionally necessitating placement of a gastrostomy tube for caloric supplementation (Vaughn, Neilson, & O'Dwyer, 1988). Misdirected swallowing and gastroesophageal reflux may result in aspiration pneumonias (Drvaric, Roberts, Burke, King, & Falterman, 1987; Gisel & Patrick, 1988). Poor hand function, pooling of saliva, and abnormal muscle tone can result in poor dental hygiene and malocclusion (Rosenstein, 1982). Restrictive pulmonary disease may result from hypertonicity, and scoliosis may further limit endurance (Rothman, 1978). Bladder spasticity and sphincteric incoordination, rather than cognitive limitations, may result in urinary incontinence and may be responsive to uropharmacological and behavioral management (Keating, Mc Carron, James, Gruenberg, & Lonczak, 1985; Mc Neal, Hawtrey, Wolraich, & Mapel, 1983).

Orthopaedic complications include the development of contractures and deformities, dislocations, especially at the hips, and scoliosis due to prolonged muscle imbalance. All of these conditions may require medical and therapeutic attempts at normalization of tone, and/or surgical interventions as described below. Fractures may occur in these patients as a result of osteopenia concomitant with spasm and secondary effects of anticonvulsant administration (Lingam & Joester, 1994). In non-ambulatory, quadriplegic children, lumbar spine bone mineral density may be decreased by as much as 58%, and up to 39% of the patients may suffer non-traumatic hip fractures (King, Levin, Schmidt, Oestreich, & Heubi, 2003). Initial studies are suggesting that the use of bisphosphonate infusions (Pamidronate) may be helpful in treatment of this complication (Henderson, Lark, & Kecskemethy, 2002).

CLINICAL FINDINGS AND PROGNOSTIC INDICATORS

CEREBRAL PALSY MAY be difficult to identify in a patient who is less than 1 year of age. Although gross motor milestones may be delayed, hypertonicity, movement disorders, and early hand dominance may have not yet occurred (Levine, 1980). Although the brain lesion which results in the encephalopathy is static, the child's neurological appearance may vary with growth and myelination of the brain. The infant with spastic quadriparesis is generally identified by 5 months of age; diplegics are not identified until 12 months of age, on average, and hemiplegics at 21 months (Harris, 1989). Difficulty in diagnosis is compounded by the plasticity of the immature nervous system, with compensatory branching of the corticospinal tract fibers (Farmer, Harrison, Ingram, & Stephens, 1991), allowing cerebral palsy to "disappear" in up to 55% of cases (Tardorf, 1986). Labeling an infant "high-risk" may result in over-interpretation of normal physical findings (Ashton, Piper, Warren, Stewin, & Byrne, 1991).

Motor development in the subtypes of cerebral palsy varies, but common denominators exist (B. Bobath & Bobath, 1975). Abnormal positioning of the hands, hypertonicity of the neck extensors, inability to isolate lower extremity movements (i.e., an all-flexor or all-extensor pattern), difficulty in bringing the elbows across midline suggestive of increased tone, poor head control, microcephaly, abnormal deep tendon reflexes, persistence of grasp reflexes, and up-going plantar responses beyond 12 months of age are all suspect findings. Lack of symmetrical movement and early onset of hand dominance are suggestive of a hemiparesis. Not only may gross motor activities be delayed, but when they are performed, they may be carried out in an abnormal way, often with utilization of abnormal, stereotypical primitive reflexes to initiate the movement (see below). The use of head arching to initiate rolling, and crawling on the abdomen with both legs being flexed simultaneously rather than on all fours in a reciprocal manner are two examples of these behaviors. In the absence of frankly abnormal gross motor movements or reflex abnormalities, the lack of variation of limb movements may also be a finding indicative of a static encephalopathy.

Major support for the diagnosis of cerebral palsy is given by the persistence of primitive reflexes. These subcortical reflexes are normally suppressed by 6 months of age. They can always be summoned but are modulated by more advanced learned motor activities. When these reflexes occur each time a child is placed in a position, they interfere with that child's ability to change position and to assume and maintain an anti-gravity position. These reflexes include the symmetric and asymmetric (fencer) tonic neck reflexes, the tonic labyrinthine response, positive support reaction, and the Moro (startle) response. Postural reactions such as head and neck righting responses may be delayed or absent. The persistence of more than one reflex beyond 2 years of age, in association with the child's inability to sit, is negatively associated with future ambulation (Capute, 1978; Sala & Grant, 1995). Conversely, the ability of the child to sit by 2 years correlates with a good prognosis for ambulation. More recently, identification of certain patterns of antigravity movements such as head lifting, sitting with upper extremity support, ambulation of 10 steps, and so on, may stratify the cerebral palsied population into five different types of patients where motor development can be more definitely assessed (Palisano, Rosenbaum, Walter, & Hanna, 1997). However, these studies are preliminary and should not be utilized as a way of limiting therapeutic services or other medical interventions at this time.

Children who do not ambulate by 7 to 8 years are usually unable to do so, unless limited therapeutic services have not been provided prior to this time. Ninety-eight percent of hemiplegics, 75% of diplegics, and 50% of quadriplegics will ambulate according to studies performed in the past (Molnar & Gordon, 1976). Of those patients with quadriplegia, 25% will be independent, 50% will require assistance, and 25% will utilize wheelchairs as their means of community ambulation. Most patients with the ataxia variant of cerebral palsy will ambulate. Hypotonic and rigid patients have the poorest prognosis for ambulation (Molnar, 1979). These studies were performed prior to newer interventions such as selective dorsal rhizotomy and placement of intrathecal Baclofen pumps; it is yet to be determined if such interventions will result in significant alterations of these prognostic parameters. Children ambulate abnormally because of static and dynamic muscle dysfunction (Sutherland, 1984). Gaits are energy-inefficient, resulting in fatigability and limited endurance (Mossberg, Linton, & Friske, 1990).

Fine-motor, personal-social, and language skills may also be impaired to a variable degree. The Amiel-Tison scale, Milani-Comparetti scale, Denver Developmental Screening Test, and the Bayley Scale of Infant Development are some of the tools which have been developed for documentation and tracking of these dysfunctions.

THERAPEUTIC INTERVENTIONS

DIRECT TREATMENT FOR cerebral palsy is unavailable. However, certain pharmacologic agents have been demonstrated to modulate the stressors which may result in a static encephalopathy and appear to be of statistical benefit. The use of prenatal glucocorticoid (dexathamethasone) treatment administered to mothers of pre-term infants may reduce the risk of intraventricular hemorrhage and periventricular leukomalacia. The protective effect may occur due to direct stabilization of the vasculature of the fetal brain, and to a reduction of the acid-base fluctuations which ensue with reduced/aborted respiratory distress syndrome for which these steroids are administered. The risk of the development of cerebral palsy in such a group may be reduced from 22 to 10% (Salokor et al., 1997). Research has also suggested that the use of free-radical scavengers and blockers of receptors of excitatory amino acids could limit the tissue damage that is sustained by neonates with perinatal asphyxia (Vannucci, 1990). Magnesium sulfate, which is used to protect mothers from the hypertension associated with pre-eclampsia, may also offer a protective effect by acting as a vasodilator to the fetal brain (Hirtz & Nelson, 1998), although results of some these studies are somewhat equivocal (Galvin, 1998). Other secondary treatments include therapy, tone-altering medications, provision of adaptive equipment to enhance patients' level of function, and orthopaedic and neurosurgical procedures that correct deformities and normalize tone, as discussed below (Diamond, 1986; Lord, 1984).

Therapeutic systems share the goals of maintenance of joint range, prevention of contractures, normalization of tone, improvement in interaction with the environment, postural control, assumption of anti-gravity postures, development of muscular control and coordination, and education of the family (Deaver, 1956; Kottke, Halpern, Easton, Ozel, & Burrill, 1978). Many systems are axiomatic, being based on the concept of neuroplasticity in the child, avoidance of abnormal movement patterns, and the importance of sensorimotor learning in cognitive development (Matthews, 1988). Controlled studies are difficult to design, as parents are unwilling to assign their child to a non-treatment group (Guyatt et al., 1986; Martin & Epstein, 1976; Tirosh & Rabino, 1989). It has also been problematic to document the clinical effectiveness of early intervention programs, but there is a strong sense of the clinical validity of such treatment (Palmer et al., 1990; Resnick, Eyler, Nelson, Eitman, & Bucciarelli, 1987). Meta-analyses of such interventions have revealed that when such services were initiated in at-risk infants prior to 6 months of age, an improvement of 9 to 13 points in IQ testing resulted. The developmental stimulation, rather than physical therapy alone, may be responsible for enhancement of gross motor and cognitive skills (Palmer, Shapiro, & Wachtel, 1988). This is a rationale offered by proponents of the system of conductive education (Hill, 1990). Systems have been proposed by Rood, Knott and Voss, Brunstrom, Temple Fay, and Dolman-Delacato (patterning) (Halpern, 1984), but the Bobath type of treatment generally prevails in this setting. By placing the affected child in a position in which the effects of abnormal tone and postures are de-emphasized, voluntary muscular control may develop in a proximal-to-distal fashion, paving the way for more functional activities and the use of the upper extremities for something other than support (Finnie, 1974). Secondary reductions in tone may result in improvement in oro-motor control, feeding, speech, and respiration (Nwaobi & Smith, 1986).

Other systems have been developed to deal with the visual-manual and spatial learning difficulties that may co-exist (Bachrach & Greenspun, 1990). Additional options include training the patient in age-appropriate self-care skills and behavior modification. Traditionally, strengthening programs were felt to be contraindicated in spastic conditions such as cerebral palsy, as such efforts were felt to re-enforce the patterns of spasticity that already existed. However, newer studies do not support this notion. Strengthening has been documented as resulting in improvement of strength of hip extensors, abductors, and knee extensors, in gait pattern with a reduction in crouching and improvement in speed, and in Gross Motor Functional Measurement ratings (Andersson, Grooten, Hellsten, Kaping, & Mattson, 2003). Efficacy not only exists for younger patients, but teenagers and even patients in the 5th decade have shown demonstrable improvements without negative effects or increases in Ashworth scores (a spasticity measurement scale) (Damiano, Kelly, & Vaughan, 1995; Damiano, Vaughan, & Abel, 1995). Therefore, neurologic maturation or cessation of growth is not a contraindication for continuation of services.

Abstracted from the experience with adult hemiplegic patients who have had cerebrovascular accidents, constraint therapy has been employed in a small group of hemiplegic children, but current experience is still anecdotal (Pierce, Daly, Gallaghger, Gershkoff, & Schaunburg, 2002). However, it is advisable that children selected for such treatment be chronologically/cognitively at least at the 6 to 7 year level so that these efforts are not perceived as being punitive. Although there are clinical proponents, the efficacy of other not uncommon treatments such as hyperbaric oxygenation, use of the Adeli suit for proximal stabilization, cranio-sacral therapy, massage, hippotherapy, and aquatherapy have not been substantiated in the peer-reviewed literature (Hurvitz, Leonard, Ayyangar, & Nelson, 2003).

A variety of modalities, including shaking and cold, are believed to exert effects at the level of the vestibular receptors, muscle spindles, and the Golgi tendon apparatus. Nerve and motor point blocks and biofeedback have also been employed (Halpern, 1982; Kassover, Tauber, Au, & Pugh, 1986). Nerve blocks in contrast to motor point blocks not only resulted in weakness, but concurrent, and undesirable sensory deficits/dysesthesias and therefore have been used less frequently of late.

Over the past 10 or more years, Botulinum A toxin, derived from denatured Clostridium, injected into the muscles of cerebral palsied patients has been shown to transiently reduce spasticity for a period of about 4 months, by blocking neuromuscular transmission in a controlled fashion by decreasing acetylcholine release at motor nerve endings. This temporary reduction in tone may permit reduction of dynamic deformities such as talipes equinus by reduction in tone to spastic gastrocnemius muscles, knee flexion contractures by injection into the hamstrings, and reduction in scissoring following injection into hip adductors. Strengthening of agonist muscle groups also assists in improvement of gait and function. Both upper and lower extremity muscles may be treated. Total dosage for injections at multiple sites should not exceed 6 to 10 units of Botox per kilogram. The treatment has the advantage of specifically targeting certain areas rather than globally reducing tone, so that loss or trunk and proximal control are much less of a concern. Tendon lengthening procedures may be deferred on this basis until the patient is older, but it is uncertain if such interventions will reduce the total number of surgical interventions which the patient will eventually require (Korman, Mooney, Smith, Goodman, & Mulvaney, 1993). However, studies in animal models suggest that when given early in development, it may promote growth of muscles, altering the development of contractures (Cosgrove & Graham, 1994). Other studies suggest that injection of Botox in conjunction with serial casting of lower extremity deformities may approach the results obtained from percutaneous tendon lengthenings or selective dorsal rhizotomy (Molenaers, Desloovere, & DeCat, 2001). The advantages of this treatment are the relative ease of administration, although younger children may require sedation when deeper muscles are injected, and development of usually only mild side effects which include local soreness to muscles and generalized transient myalgias. More serious but infrequent side-effects include an association with aspiration pneumonia in patients with pseudobulbar palsy and spastic quadriparesis, global muscle weakness and atrophy (Ansved, Odergren, & Borg, 1997), urinary and fecal incontinence, development of antibodies not associated with clinical disease (Goschel, Wohlfarth, Frevert, Dengler, & Bigalke, 1997), possible potentiation of weakness seen with aminoglycoside antibiotics and depolarizing agents, and acute allergic reactions (Preiss, Condie, Rowley, & Graham, 2003).

The use of oral medications to reduce tone can be tried. Some agents which can be used include Valium, Dantrolene Sodium, Baclofen, and Tizandine. Although these may be effective, Valium has central, sedative effects, is habit forming, and is relatively undesirable in patients who may already have cognitive limitations. Dantrolene, which reduces tone by modulating calcium regulation into muscles, is metabolized by the liver, and this is not a good option for children who may be concurrently prescribed anticonvulsant medications which are also metabolized by the same route, placing children at some risk for hepatic dysfunction. Baclofen may also have a sedative effect when used orally. Tizanidine is a newer drug which works on alpha-adrenergic nerve endings; it is similar to an anti-hypertensive medication from which it is derived, and therefore blood pressure needs to be monitored carefully with its introduction.

Appropriate prescription of seating devices for non-ambulatory patients permits positioning in an upright manner, improved eye contact, enhanced interaction with the environment, decreased effect of hypertonicity (which pushes the patient out of the chair and adducts the hips), and enhanced feeding, respiration, and ability to use communication devices (Bergen & Colangelo, 1982). Helmets, bed rails, and cushions are used to prevent injury.

Orthotics are prescribed to prevent progression of deformities, provide stability, and enhance function (Gold, 1991). Traditional leather and metal braces have given way to custom-molded plastic orthoses, as they are lighter and more easily control angular (varus/valgus) deformities. Full-control hip-knee-ankle-foot orthoses are generally used for positioning but are too heavy for functional ambulation. Variations of these devices exclude the medial metal uprights and thigh cuffs, and may be helpful for children with toe walking and dynamic internal rotation at the hips. Ankle-foot orthoses are indicated to improve ankle dorsiflexion and control equinus deformities. Spring-assisted devices are generally contraindicated as rapid stretch may exacerbate spasticity. Orthoses employed to maintain muscle length must be worn for at least 6 hours per day to achieve a physiological effect (Tardieu & Lespargot, 1988). The use of tone-reducing orthoses with full footplates and the toes maintained in extension (Bronkhorst & Lamb, 1987; Hinderer & Harris, 1988) may have a direct effect on muscle ultrastructure with resultant increase in sarcomere (muscle unit) length (Tardieu, de la Tour, Bret, & Tardieu, 1982). It is important to discuss these findings with parents/guardians so that compliance with the recommended wearing schedule is achieved. Ankle-foot orthoses may have hinges incorporated at the ankles to allow for active ankle dorsiflexion and to facilitate movements from sitting to standing (Wilson, Haideri, Song, & Telford, 1997). Orthoses that extend to just above the ankles (supramalleolar orthoses) can control foot alignment but do not control the ankle joints (Carlson, Vaughan, Damiano, & Abel, 1997).

For maximally involved children, the use of a walking frame with casters provides truncal alignment and support in conjunction with hip-knee-ankle orthoses. Although functional ambulation is not possible with such devices, their utilization permits tolerance of the upright posture, increased weight bearing, and a sense of movement for the child, which may be psychologically rewarding (Stallard, Major, & Farmer, 1996).

Therapeutic electrical stimulation can be utilized as an adjunct to traditional therapeutic interventions. Low-intensity transcutaneous stimulation can be applied to a variety of weak, superficial muscles nocturnally. Theoretically, the resultant increase in blood flow to these muscles at a time when growth hormone levels are highest encourages their growth. This permits the traditional strengthening efforts applied during the day to be more effective. Improvement in gait (enhanced tibialis anterior function, better balance, and improved gait pattern) has been demonstrated in a few studies (Hazelwood, Brown, Rowe, & Salter, 1994; Pape et al., 1993). However, the long-term effect of this treatment and any possible associated reduction in the subsequent need for surgical intervention have not yet been demonstrated.

Given the multiple potential interventions and confounding clinical variables which exist, truly objective research design is extremely difficult. The use of standardized testing and functional scales may serve as an adjunct in such studies, permitting the patient to be compared to his/her own pre-treatment performance. Such measurement tools include measurement of torque/resistance to passive stretch as an indicator of spasticity, the Gross Motor Function Measure, the Wee-F.I.M. or functional independence measure for patients under the age of 7 years, the Pediatric Evaluation of Disability Inventory, and the Ashworth scale for clinically reproducible measurement of spasticity.

SURGICAL OPTIONS

PREVENTION OF DEFORMITIES resulting from inequalities in muscle tone and strength in association with fixed posturing due to the influence of retained positive primitive reflexes is the best treatment option; however, orthopedic surgery should not be perceived as a failure of previous treatment, but rather as an adjunct to achievement of therapeutic goals. The muscles of spastic patients with cerebral palsy are too short, with chronic increases in tone possibly resulting in reduced sarcomere length and abnormal connectin protein (H. K. Graham & Selber, 2003). With inability of the muscles to relax, imbalances occur between the growth of the long bones and the muscle tendons resulting in secondary structural deformities (Ziv, Blackborn, Rang, & Koresk, 1984). Subluxation and early-onset osteoarthritis with regression in function not associated with an actual decline in neurological status may occur. Hence, early and efficient surgical interventions are warranted (Frieden & Lieber, 2003) and may permit less invasive soft tissue rather than bony surgery (osteotomies) to be performed. Conversely, early tendon releases may initially interfere with acquisition of motor milestones and mobility, and may increase the need for repeat surgery with growth. Psychological support services to both parent and child to cope with fears and expectations is most important. At least 6 months of extensive post-operative physical rehabilitation may be required to see signs of functional improvement because of transient deconditioning (Reimers, 1990), with reduction of muscle strength and re-adjustment of the body to a new muscle length-tension ratio. The separation of the parent from the child, and the financial burdens encountered, are other factors to be considered.

A full discussion of the orthopedic deformities and their surgical treatment may be found in several excellent texts (Bleck, 1987; Samilson, 1981). Common lower-extremity deformities include hip flexion contractures, femoral anteversion with medial rotation of the legs, hip adduction with subluxation, pelvic asymmetry with secondary scoliosis, hamstring spasticity with knee flexion contractures, and equinovarus or equinovalgus deformities with hemiplegia and diplegia, respectively. Typical upper-extremity deformities include internal rotation contractures of the shoulders, flexion contractures at the elbows, wrist flexion contractures, ulnar deviation, finger flexion contractures, and thumb-in-palm deformities. For dependent patients, surgery may be performed to facilitate perineal care, reduce pain associated with dislocation, and correct pelvic asymmetry that may exacerbate a scoliosis and reduce supported sitting tolerance (Carr & Gage, 1987; Cooperman, Bartucci, Dietrick, & Millar, 1987). For children with better gross motor function, surgery is indicated to improve lower-extremity alignment and correct a progressively crouched gait, scissoring, and other gait abnormalities which result in poor balance and easy fatigability due to excessive energy expenditure.

Procedures include adductor tenotomies and varus derotation osteotomies of the femurs (Bleck, 1990). Previously, these patients were confined in extensive plaster casts post-operatively, but this is less commonly employed resulting in fewer cases of secondary skin breakdown and earlier mobilization and rehabilitation. Hamstring lengthenings are performed to correct knee flexion contractures, avoiding overlengthening which could result in hyperextension at the knees (Gage, 1990), requiring a secondary procedure, rectus femoris transfers, to be performed. Achilles tendon lengthenings are the most commonly performed procedure; with correction of the equninus deformity, toe walking is corrected, a stable base of support on a flat foot is established, and walking speed and stride length are increased (Shapiro & Susa, 1990). A posterior tibialis tendon transfer may be indicated to correct equinovarus and to elevate the foot when walking; the indication may be supported by results of computerized gait analysis (Perry & Hoffer, 1976). For more resistant deformities at the foot, an extra-articular (Grice) procedure or other arthrodesis may be required (Fulford, 1990).

Surgery for the upper extremities is performed less frequently, as results may be limited by cognitive and sensory impairments. Procedures include release of the internal rotators of the shoulder, release of the biceps tendon and anterior capsulotomy to correct elbow flexion contractures, transfer of wrist flexors to function as wrist extensors, and release of the thumb-in-palm deformity (Mital & Sakellarides, 1981). Spinal fusion may be required to control scoliosis. Luque and other newer spinal instrumentations permit some patients to forgo prolonged immobilization in a body jacket (Lonstein & Akbamia, 1983).

Neurosurgical procedures to restore function and to control associated intractable seizures by resection of localized focus of electrical abnormalities are newer adjuncts in the care of the cerebral palsied patient. Implantation of a cerebellar pacemaker had been utilized in the past but is not currently employed in any large numbers (Penn, Mykleburst, Gottlieb, Agarwal, & Etzel, 1980).

The selective dorsal rhizotomy procedure to decrease lower-extremity tone and to secondarily permit development of isolated lower-extremity tone and improvement in gait has recently been implemented. Spinal nerve rootlets that have been determined as being electrically abnormal (Cahan & Kundi, 1987) are surgically lesioned in purely spastic children without clinical evidence of a progressive neurological disorder. With modulation of abnormal sensory input, there is a resetting of muscle spindle sensitivity with a reduction in tone. Electromyographic monitoring is employed intra-operatively to assess which of the spastic rootlets should be lesioned, although responses may be less consistent than previously thought. In conjunction with a well-delineated postoperative program, improvements in tone, range, posture, sitting balance, and gait occur in 85 to 90% of appropriate selected candidates (Abbott, Johann-Murphy, & Gold, 1991; Peacock & Staudt, 1991) to a greater extent than would be anticipated on the basis of physical therapy intervention alone (Steinbok, Reiner, Beauchamp, Armstrong, & Cochrane, 1997). Improvement in gait is characterized by increased dynamic range of motion at the hips, improved velocity of ambulation, and improved stride length (Thomas, Aiona, Pierce, & Piatt, 1996). Over time, this may result in a decreased need for Achilles tendon lengthenings, adductor releases, and hamstring releases but may not affect the subsequent rates of ankle-foot operations, femoral osteotomies, and ilipsoas releases in these patients (Chicoine, Park, & Kaufman, 1997). An improvement of 12.1 versus 4.4 points in children treated with physical therapy alone has been documented on the GMFM (Gross Motor Functional Assessment) (Wordmark, Janlo, & Hagglund, 2000) at 6 to 12 months postoperatively. Although not a specific indication for performance of the procedure, secondary improvements in upper-extremity function and reduction in bladder spasticity may also result (Sweetser, Badell, Schneider, & Badlin, 1995). Complications may include dysesthesias, sensory deficits, and on long-term follow-up, spinal stenosis (Gooch & Walker, 1996). Despite the documented improvements, 66 to 75% of patients undergoing rhizotomy will still require additional orthopedic surgery.

The effect of anoxia on the spinal cord has been described (Clancy, Sladsky, & Rorke, 1989; Harrison, 1988). This lends credence to the use of Baclofen, as noted above, an inhibitor of the neurotransmitter gamma-aminobutyric acid at the spinal cord level (Young & Delwaide, 1981). This medication may also be administered by the intrathecal route (Albright, Cervi, & Singletary, 1991) via a surgically implantable and by the programmable pump, allowing for titration and reversal of dosage with reduced risk of side-effects (Albright, 1996). The implementation of this treatment is more suitable in patients with less satisfactory underlying strength, who may require some spasticity for antigravity/ambulatory activities, and in older patients. Documented benefits in hamstring motion, upper-extremity function, ambulation (Gerszten, 1997), and activities of daily living have been associated with this treatment (Albright, Barron, Fascik, Polinko, & Janosky, 1993), as well as possibly a reduction in the need for subsequent orthopedic surgical interventions from 58 to 21% in one population studied (Armstrong, Steinbok, & Cochrane, 1997). Complications of this device include long-term reliance upon the device with need for approximately monthly refills of the reservoir in which the medication is housed, risk of catheter breakage and infection, risk of acute Baclofen withdrawal, risk of exacerbation of seizure disorders, loss of ability to assume and maintain anti-gravity positions, and possibly an increased risk of aspiration pneumonia when utilized in the most physically involved of the patients (Sgoros & Seri, 2002). Selective dorsal rhizotomy, which reduces tone by surgical lesioning of sensory input at the spinal cord level (Fasano, Barolat-Romana, Zeme, & Squazzi, 1979), may also be utilized to this goal, as detailed above.

PSYCHOLOGICAL, VOCATIONAL, AND MEDICAL PROBLEMS OF ADULTS

THERAPEUTIC SERVICES MAY enhance acquisition of gross motor skills, but cognitive improvement and emotional maturity are more elusive to treat. The severity of the physical disability does not correlate with the physical or psychological health of the parents (Wallender, Varni, et al., 1989). Sibling and spousal support are pertinent predictors of achieving mental health and improvement in physical performance (Craft, Lakin, Oppliger, Clancy, & Vanderlinder, 1990). Lives of 50 to 90% of adolescents with cerebral palsy (and spina bifida) may be characterized by dependence on parents for personal care, lack of responsibility for home chores, lack of information about sexuality, and limited participation in social activities and sexual relationships (Blum, Resnick, Nelson, & St. Germaine, 1991; Hirst, 1989; Murphy, Molnar, & Lankasky, 2000). This does not encourage independent living, marriage, or employment. Only 30 to 50% of cerebral palsy patients are employed full-time at maturity; diplegics and hemiplegic patients are more successful (Bleck, 1987). Other positive factors relating to employability include independence in activities of daily living, ability to ambulate, being female, and enrollment in a non-restrictive high school setting (Sillanpaa, Piekkala, & Pisiria, 1982; Magill-Evans & Restall, 1991; Tobimatsu & Nakamura, 2000). Therefore, it is important to asses the ability for adult patients to perform instrumental activities of daily living which include money management, travel training, and meal planning (van der Dussen, Nieuwstraten, Roebroeck, & Stam, 2001).

It has not been established what therapeutic services are necessary for adult cerebral palsy patients to maintain their function. It is sobering to acknowledge that deterioration in gait in the presence of a static encephalopathy may begin prior to 14 years of age, and is manifested by an increase in double-support time and a decrease in knee, ankle, and pelvic motion (Johnson, Damiano, & Abel, 1997). Due to this probable deterioration, only 20% of patients with cerebral palsy will be independent ambulators, 40% will ambulate with assistance, and 40% will be non-ambulatory, although 75% of these patients will retain their independence in activities of daily living (Brown, Bontempo, & Turk, 1992; Andersson & Mattson, 2001). Medical complications in an aging population (Bachrach & Greenspun, 1990), include cervical and lumbar radiculopathies (Ebura et al., 1990; Fuji et al., 1987; Reese, Msall, & Owens, 1991), carpal tunnel syndrome (Alvarez, Larkin, & Roxborough, 1981), and arthritis at major joints, each of which may require surgical intervention for restoration of function. Specifically, cervical disc disease is eight times more frequent in the adult athetoid patient than in the general patient (Harade et al., 1996). There is an overall 63% incidence of degenerative arthritis, especially at the hips, in cerebral palsy patients under the age of 50 years. Chronic pain may occur in up to 84% of the adult population, and this may require direct and indirect management, including treatment of increased spasticity (Engel, Kartin, & Jensen, 2002). Seizure disorders persist into adulthood. Neurogenic bladder and unrecognized problems with toileting accessibility also may be problematic. Referral sources for provision of gynecological care, especially in provision of mammograms to non-ambulatory patients, may be sorely lacking. Little in the way of organized and proactive treatment is available for this population (Murphy, Molnar, & Lankasky, 1995). As activity decreases, there may be a greater mortality in this population due to ischemic heart disease, compounded by difficulty with communication and lack of family supervision once placement options have been sought (Strauss, Cable, & Shavelte, 1999), and an increased incidence of deep vein thromboses also related to inactivity (Rapp & Torres, 2000).

Despite potential complications, 90% survival into adulthood is seen with cerebral palsy (Evans, Evans, & Alberman, 1990). Earlier demise occurs in patients who have severe mental deficiency, are totally dependent, have poorly controlled seizures, require gastrostomy feeding, have no means of communication, and whose secondary illnesses are primarily respiratory in nature (Evans & Alberman, 1990; Maudsley, Hultor, & Pharoah, 1999). Recently, the poor prognostic implication of gastrostomy tube placement has come under review, and does not appear to auger quite as dire a prognosis when placed in the elderly. One study indicated that 83% of the pediatric population in whom gastrostomy placement occurs survive 2 years, 75% survive 7 years, and there is family satisfaction with quality of life in 90% (Smith, Camfield, & Camfield, 1999). Some studies suggest that an increased susceptibility to infection exists not only on a neuromuscular basis but on a biological basis as well. Some patients have been noted to have decreased soluble interleukin-2 receptors and lymphocyte proliferative and lytic responses which would reduce resistance to an infectious agent. Demise is often co-incident with the "aging-out" of parents and relocation from the home to an institutional facility (Eyman & Grossman, 1990). These findings should prompt the reexamination of public policies for provision of medical benefits to handicapped adults whose parents wish them to retain the family domicile and other financial assets that would permit home-based care.

SPINA BIFIDA

SPINA BIFIDA, OR myelomeningocele, denotes a condition in which there are congenital abnormalities of the vertebral elements in association with extrusion of abnormally formed neural elements. Patients present with various lower-extremity motor and sensory deficits concomitant with variable bowel and bladder control, hydrocephalus, and other medical problems. The resultant condition impinges on normal motor development and may alter fine-motor, perceptual, linguistic, and cognitive function. A discussion of treatment strategies reflects not only technical advancements but the changes in the advocacy for the treatment of the physically challenged child. This is a congenital but not a static disorder, in which progressive neurological and other organ system dysfunctions may occur over time in up to 40% of the patients (Spindel, Bauer, & Dyron, 1987).

ANATOMICAL ABNORMALITIES

FAILURE OF FUSION of the posterior elements of the lumbosacral spine without associated neurological abnormalities is known as spina bifida occulta and occurs in 20% to 25% of the general population (without overt or open spina bifida). Should such findings be noted in a patient with incontinence, cavus (high-arched) feet, and/or a hairy tuft or hemangioma over the lower spine, an associated malformation of the spinal cord may be present which can be readily documented on magnetic resonance (MRI) study. A terminal myelocystocele is a closed defect which presents with a lumbosacral fat-containing mass with cerebrospinal fluid and neural tissue which will require surgical intervention. It may be associated with abnormal development of the lower spine, genitalia, bowel, bladder, kidneys, and the abdominal wall, such as omphalocele. It is not generally associated with hydrocephalus. Ambulatory compromise may require interventions similar to those in the more typical form of spinal dysraphism (Choi & Mc Comb, 2000).

In its most severe or manifest form, spina bifida is associated with exposure of the neural plaque, leakage of cerebrospinal fluid, and susceptibility of the meninges to infection (Brocklehurst, 1976). Abnormally formed neural elements with cystic structures within the spinal cord result in a picture of both upper and lower motor neuron deficits (Stark & Baker, 1967). Defects at the lumbosacral level are the most common; thoracic and cervical lesions occur less frequently. Due to the resultant lack of normal innervation, paralysis/paresis of the lower extremities occurs and there are secondary and often severe orthopedic deformities which occur due to the imbalance of muscular forces.

THE LORBER CRITERIA AND THEIR ABANDONMENT

IN THE PAST, severely deformed infants with myelomeningocele succumbed, without treatment, to meningitis, hydrocephalus, and/or renal failure in the interest of not prolonging the lives of children who would be cognitively subnormal, non-ambulatory, and chronically ill. The mortality rate within the 1st month of life was 63% and it was 89% by the 6th month. Lorber (1981) advised no treatment for those infants who would be totally plegic in the lower extremities, had severe hydrocephalus, had severe kyphoscoliosis that would not permit an erect posture, and/or had severe congenital malformations such as extrophy of the bladder or congenital heart disease. He felt that only 18% of the population would be ambulatory, cognitively normal, and able to earn an income. It was not recognized that the survivors would be more compromised than necessary (Mc Laughlin & Shurtleff, 1979), nor that there was inability to predict which of the cognitively normal patients would be sacrificed by the lack of treatment. Adoption of these criteria implied that life in a wheelchair was one without quality. Other assumptions have recently proved invalid with more advanced treatments, as noted below (Khoury, Erickson, & James, 1982; Mc Clone, Dias, Kaplan, & Sommers, 1985).

Neurosurgery in the neonate to drain the collection of excessive cerebrospinal fluid associated with hydrocephalus can result in restoration of a relatively normal head circumference and re-expansion of the cerebral mantle. With appropriate treatment, a 5-year survival rate of 86% has been reported; however, patients with brain stem dysfunction had a greater mortality (Worley, Schuster, & Oakes, 1996). The severe gibbus deformity associated with kyphoscoliosis may be surgically corrected (Linter & Lindseth, 1994), as may other congenital abnormalities. Mental retardation is not intrinsic to spina bifida nor to the Arnold-Chiari malformation, which results in hydrocephalus. Up to 75% of patients with spina bifida manifesta may have normal intelligence (Mc Clone, Czyzewski, Raimondi, & Sommers, 1982), but the incidence of learning disabilities will be high, with arithmetic and design copying skills frequently being compromised (Wills, Holmbeck, Dillon, & Mc Clone, 1990). Functional bowel and bladder continence may ideally be achieved in

80% of school-age children. Eight percent of school-age children will be community ambulators. Only 10 to 15% of patients will require supportive care. The emotional and psychological costs for delaying treatment are high. Hence, early and aggressive treatment of these infants is now the rule.

INCIDENCE, EMBRYOLOGY, AND ETIOLOGY

THE INCIDENCE OF spina bifida manifesta in the United States is approximately 2 cases per 10,000 births, which represents a decline of over 27% during the past decade (Lary & Edmonds, 1996; Meyer & Siega-Riz, 2002). This is largely attributable to the supplementation of grain products such as cereal with folic acid. The decline has been greatest in mothers over the age of 30 years, who had a high-school education, whose medical care was not Medicaid funded, and who were non-Hispanic Caucasians.

Although folic acid supplementation plays a role in prevention, the etiology for neural tube defects is likely multifactorial and has a genetic basis The undefined insult to the embryo occurs at 21 to 26 days of gestation, when the neural tube that will become the central nervous system is invaginating. Early theories suggested that there was a failure of fusion or disruption of the tissue column caused by abnormalities in the cerebrospinal fluid pressure (Streeter, 1942). More recently, studies from animal models have revealed a group of developmental genes, termed homeobox genes, which direct the segmental development of the nervous system. In mammals, the Hox genes have been demonstrated to encode positions from the top of the brain to the lower spinal cord. Another similar group of genes has been described as assisting in differentiation of the ventral from the dorsal spinal cord. Mechanisms which damage gene function may effect the process of nervous system development, resulting in myelomeningocele and the related Chiari II malformation responsible for hydrocephalus; clinically this may explain the mechanism in at least 15% of patients with spina bifida (Mc Clone, 1998).

The incidence of neural tube defects can be reduced by up to 86% by the intake of folic acid in the periconceptual period at a dosage of 0.4 mg/day. Decreased folate and increased total homocysteine levels have been documented in the mothers of such patients. This metabolically may result in a decrease in methionine formation, which results in abnormal gene transcription and impairment of neural tube differentiation and closure (Botto & Yang, 2000; Veland, Hustad, Schneede, Refsum, & Vollset, 2001).

Control of obesity (maternal weight less than 31 kg/M^2) prior to the onset of pregnancy also may reduce the risk of neural tube defects (Waller et al., 1995). There is an increased familial tendency toward the disorder, with a 5% chance of recurrence with subsequent pregnancies and in patients with spina bifida who sire offsprings. Other, non-familial etiologies proposed include exposure to potato blight which might retrospectively be related to folate deficiency, other vitamin B and mineral deficiencies (Holmes, 1988), maternal fever/infection, hormonal exposures, zinc deficiencies, subfertility, twinning, high sound-intensity exposure, ethanol, and use of phenytoin and valproic acid (Khoury et al., 1982; Leck, 1974).

Prenatal diagnosis can be made by ultrasound (Robinson, Hood, Adam, Gibson, & Ferguson-Smith, 1980). Prenatal anatomic level as determined on high-resolution ultrasound can reliably be utilized to discuss functional motor outcome with the parents (Coniglio, Anderson, & Ferguson, 1996). Analysis of amniotic fluid and/or maternal serum for elevated alpha-fetoprotein, a substance that is liberated by fetal blood vessels of the uncovered neural elements, is also indicative of the disorder. Analyses are performed in the second trimester so that termination of pregnancy, if desired, is possible. False-positive results may occur in association with gastrointestinal malformations (Milunsky & Alpert, 1976a, 1976b). Anencephaly and skin-covered lesions cannot be identified by chemical analysis, so ultrasound is very important. These tests were not consistently performed in pregnancy so that in previous decades, the majority of cases were not diagnosed in utero. Of all neural tube defects so identified, 39.9% result in termination of pregnancy (Bower, Raymond, Lumley, & Bury, 1993). For those pregnancies that go to completion, a caesarian section is indicated in fetuses with functional lower-extremity movements to lessen the risk of trauma to the exposed neural elements and hydrocephalic head.

ANTENATAL AND NEONATAL TREATMENT

IN UTERO REPAIR of myelomeningocele is still a very experimental option for attempting to reduce subsequent neurological dysfunction. Interposition of latissimus dorsi flaps over the neurologic lesion may prevent further in utero damage to the spinal cord and nerve roots or damage that occurs at the time of delivery (Meuli et al., 1997; Meuli-Simmen, Meuli, Adzick, & Harrison, 1997). In utero treatment of hydrocephalus has also been attempted. Both of these treatment options may result in premature delivery, so there is a risk of trading one developmental disability for another given the current state of the art (Chervenak & Mc Cullough, 2002).

The deformities of spina bifida manifesta are obvious at birth. The spinal defect is closed at 24 to 48 hours, and a ventriculoperitoneal shunt is placed in the 80% of patients in whom it is required at that time or at a variable time thereafter. In the period proceeding surgical intervention, the infant should be transferred to a tertiary care facility where a multidisciplinary team is available, kept abdomen-down in a warmer, and placed on prophylactic intravenous antibiotics to prevent central nervous system infection. The patient should be assessed for other congenital abnormalities and should have urological and orthopedic assessments (Alexander & Steg, 1989). The hiatus from birth to the surgical treatment permits parents to be supplied with information about their child's condition, which will facilitate their ability to select suitable treatment options (Charney, 1990). Pediatricians who are unfamiliar with the diagnosis may offer an unnecessarily dire prognosis (Siperstein, Wolraich, Reed, & O'Keefe, 1988). Parents should handle the infant as soon as possible and be familiarized with range-of-motions techniques, learn how to deal with the infant's insensate skin, and be instructed in intermittent urinary catheterization (Boytim, Davidson, Charney, & Melchionne, 1991).

THE ARNOLD-CHIARI MALFORMATION AND HYDROCEPHALUS

THE ARNOLD-CHIARI II malformation, seen in up to 90% of patients with spina bifida (Badell-Ribera, Swinyard, Greenspan, & Deaver, 1964), is characterized by a downward displacement of a portion of the cerebellum through the foramen magnum into the spinal canal, with secondary compression of the fourth ventricle and development of hydrocephalus (Lemire, 1988). Untreated, this condition results in progressive expansion of the ventricles, with compression of cerebral tissue, spasticity, retardation, blindness, dysphagia, apnea, and death (Charney, Rorke, Sutton, & Schut, 1991). A shunt is placed from the ventricles into the peritoneal space to decompress the hydrocephalus. Shunted patients and those in whom shunting is not required have normal intelligence quotients (IQ of 95 and 102, respectively). However, for each episode of bacterial ventriculitis, there is a 10 to 15 point decrement in the IQ, with an average score of 72 (Hunt & Holmes, 1976). Shunt surgery may also be complicated by breakage, distal blockage, nephritis, and hydrocele. Patients requiring shunt revision after the age of 2 years may have a poorer prognosis for cognitive function (Hunt, Oakesholt, & Kerry, 1999).

A newly developed alternative for the management of hydrocephalus is endoscopic third ventriculostomy. At present, its application may best be suited for patients over the age of 6 months. Long-term shunt dependence with late complications may thereby be avoided (Teo & Jones, 1996).

Seizures may occur in up to 21% of patients with spina bifida. All of these patients have shunted hydrocephalus (Noetzel & Blake, 1991). However, most also have evidence of other central nervous system pathology, such as encephalomalacia, agenesis of the corpus callosum, and/or other malformations or calcifications (Talwar, Baldwin, & Horbatt, 1995).

NEUROLOGICAL LEVEL: FUNCTIONAL IMPLICATIONS

THE PERFORMANCE OF a neurological examination in the neonate is challenging because of lack of cooperation and existence of spinal shock (Chiaramonte, Horowitz, Kaplan, & Brook, 1986). Stimulation of the arms and the upper trunk rather than of the lower extremities may more reliably evoke volitional rather than reflexogenic movements (Stark & Baker, 1967). Somatosensory-evoked potentials also may be performed to document the level of innervation. This determination is crucial, as it will indicate, with good reliability, ambulatory status and risk for the development of orthopedic deformities, those patients with the lowest levels of spinal involvement having the best prognosis (De Souza & Carroll, 1976; Hoffer, Feiwell, Perry, Perry, & Bonnett, 1973). Further delineation of prognosis involves the determination of strength of the musculature at a given level (Mc Donald, Jaffe, Mosca, Shurtleff, & Menelaus, 1991), especially the strength of the hip flexors and knee extensors and the presence of scoliosis, which may occur in up to 50% of the population (Drennan, 1976). Factors of lesser importance include age, sitting balance, height, sex, motivation, presence of spasticity, adequacy of bracing, appropriateness of orthopedic surgery, and motor planning abilities (Asher & Olsen, 1983). Infants with a thoracic level lesion will have no voluntary movements in their lower extremities. With training and correction of lower-extremity contractures, 50% of this group become therapeutic or community ambulators in childhood, with extensive bracing (Charney, Melchionni, & Smith, 1991; Shafer & Dias, 1983). With age, increasing weight, upward displacement of the center of gravity, and underlying trunk and respiratory muscle dysfunction, energy expenditure increases (Findley & Agre, 1988). By adulthood, this group is usually reliant on wheelchairs for mobility but is capable of independent transfers, dressing, bowel and bladder management, and employment (Carroll, 1977). Despite the transient nature of their ambulation, walking should be attempted to provide patients with a vertical orientation, to permit performance of tabletop activities in standing, to improve respiratory excursion and urinary drainage, and to lessen the possibilities of skin breakdown, contractures, and osteoporosis-related fractures.

Patients with innervation at the lumbar 1, 2, and 3 levels have motor power in hip flexors and adductors (which bring the legs to midline), and to a variable degree in the knee extensors. There is no ability to extend or abduct the hips or to move the feet. At this level, there is the highest risk of hip dislocation, given the imbalance of muscle pull. Hip dislocation may be an impediment to continued ambulation, especially if the hips are stiff or if the dislocation is unilateral resulting in leg length discrepancy, pelvic obliquity, and progressive scoliosis (Crandall, Birkeback, & Wintor, 1989; Curtis, 1973). Iliopsoas transfers (Sharrard, 1964) were routinely performed in the past in order to prevent hip flexion contractures, but this limited patients' abilities to flex at hips and ascend stairs, and currently it is rarely performed. Osteotomies of the femoral heads for treatment of subluxation are performed to restore symmetry about the hips, but are not obligatory for ambulation to be achieved (Sherk, Uppal, Lane, & Melchionnni, 1991). Release of hip flexion contractures of greater than 30° also can be considered in this group (Frawley, Broughton, & Menelaus, 1996). Infants may be provided with foot drop splints to prevent progressive equinus deformities and may require hip abduction devices to maintain stability at those joints.

In non-ambulatory children with high-level lesions, unilateral hip dislocations may cause little functional disability, and surgical intervention is less frequently indicated than in years past. In ambulatory patients with lower-level lesions, leg-length discrepancy and its effect on functional problems mandates surgical correction (Fraser, Bourke, Broughton, & Menelaus, 1995). Patients with higher-level lesions are generally braced with full-control devices necessitated not only by their lower-extremity weakness, but by their hydrocephalus-related hypotonia. They can be supplied with a standing device known as a parapodium at about 18 months (Letts, Fulford, Eng, & Robson, 1976). A spina bifida cart also can be provided for independent mobility (Charney, Rorke, et al., 1991). By 2 to 3 years, hip-knee-ankle-foot orthoses can be provided and gait training with a rollator commenced (Lough & Nielsen, 1986). Alternatively, an Orlau parawalker can be considered (Major, Stollard, & Farmer, 1997). Depending on praxis and eye-hand coordination, crutches may be supplied at 4 to 5 years, with household and some community ambulation anticipated. Reciprocating gait (cable) orthoses may help to facilitate ambulation and reduce energy consumption by up to 50% in this group when compared with the use of traditional knee-ankle-foot orthoses used with a four-point gait (Cuddleford et al., 1997).

With full innervation at the lumbar 4 level, knee extensors are stronger, and patients may be advanced to knee-ankle-foot orthoses. Some patients may have imbalance between knee flexors and extensors, requiring surgical release of the hamstrings to improve gait (Marshall, Broughton, Menelaus, & Graham, 1996). With innervation at the lumbar 5 level, muscle power about the hips is more balanced. The ankle dorsiflexors, but not the plantar flexors, are functioning, usually resulting in calcaneal deformities, with ambulation occurring on insensate heels. Bilateral transfer of the tibialis anterior muscles, which dorsiflex the feet, may be required to achieve a stable standing position; this is generally performed at about 5 years. A variety of other foot deformities,

including planovalgus, may occur at this and other levels. Triple arthrodesis (subtalar fusions to stabilize inversion/eversion) may be performed
at about 12 years of age, when the feet are relatively grown. Other surgical procedures considered for correction of valgus deformities include
extra-articular subtalar fusion or Grice procedures, talectomy, calcaneal-
lengthening osteotomy, fibula-Achilles tendon tenodesis, distal medial
tibial epiphysiodesis, and supramalleolar osteotomy (Abraham, Lubicky,
Sanger, & Millar, 1996).

Patients with such lower-lumbar lesions can be anticipated to pull to
standing by 1 year and ambulate in the community with or without
orthoses despite gait deviations. For patients with sacral level lesions, only
minor foot deformities would be anticipated. These patients may require
shoe modifications or ankle-foot orthoses, but would be able to ambulate without them. They would be expected to have bowel and bladder
incontinence. It is very important to follow patients with such low
lesions as almost one third may show a decline in ambulatory abilities
over time, declines being related to skin breakdown, osteomyelitis, and
the need for amputations in association with under-recognized tethering of the spinal cord and syringomyelia, as discussed below (Brinker et
al., 1994).

SCOLIOSIS AND TETHERING OF THE SPINAL CORD

MANAGEMENT OF A paralytic spinal curvature is difficult. As posterior vertebral elements are lacking, surgical fixation with metal rods
usually has to be performed anteriorly and posteriorly (Banta & Park,
1983). Surgical procedures require a period of immobilization, with the
risk of further neurological compromise and development of
pseudoarthroses. Unchecked, scoliosis causes restrictive pulmonary disease with decreased endurance. The uneven posture which results dis-
turbs sitting balance, the upper extremities being used as tripods. The
listing to one side, especially in tandem with hip dislocation, may result
in formation of intractable decubiti due to asymmetries of pressure distribution.

Scoliosis may occur in response to unequal innervation of the
paraspinal muscles and may be compounded by vertebral abnormalities, but rapid progression may herald the development of neurological complications. Prior to the development of MRI, many of these
conditions went undetected, and many childhood ambulators were
using wheelchairs by adolescence. Other factors that may negatively
affect ambulatory performance include obesity, joint stiffness with
arthritic changes, and lack of motivation.

The two primary conditions responsible for the deterioration in
function and often seen with progression of scoliosis are tethering of

the spinal cord and syringomyelia. With tethering, the spinal cord is subject to repeat microtrauma with flexion/extension, to which it is predisposed by scar tissue that keeps the cord firmly adherent at lower-lumbar levels (Yamada, Zinke, & Saunders, 1981). Patients exhibit decreased lower-extremity strength, spasticity frequently associated with a crouched gait, dysesthesias or progressive sensory deficits, pain over the neural placode, and/or decompensation of a previously well-managed neurogenic bowel and bladder (Peacock, Arens, & Berman, 1987). MRI studies and somatosensory-evoked potentials may be helpful in providing objective evidence of the changes noted on physical examination (Li, Albright, Sclabassi, & Pang, 1996). Urodynamics and perineal-evoked potentials are also useful diagnostic tools in demonstrating change in neurological function (Torre et al., 2002). Surgical release of the tether can result in restoration of function or can stop further neurological progression in most cases (Clancy et al., 1989; Reigel, 1983). Surgical techniques should permit the neural elements to remain free in the cerebrospinal fluid, preventing the risk of retethering (Zide, Constantini, & Epstein, 1995). An expanding fluid-filled cyst may distend the cord at any level, and may be associated with increasing weakness and sensory deficits, frequently involving the upper extremities. This is known as syringomyelia; it can be treated by surgical drainage of the cyst and placement of a shunt.

THERAPEUTIC ASSESSMENT AND INTERVENTION

ASSESSMENT SHOULD INCLUDE evaluation and description of joint contractures and deformities, neurological level and muscle power, presence, location and extent of pressure sores, mobility, and self-care skills. Treatment includes gentle, active, assistive range-of-motion exercises for the lower extremities, strengthening of innervated musculature, transfer training, gait training, and instruction in self-care skills (U.K. Collaborative Study, 1977). Physical activity programs aimed at improving cardiovascular fitness and strength may improve the self-image of this disabled child (Andrade, Kramer, Garber, & Longmuir, 1991).

In general, infants with myelomeningocele are less active (Morrow, 1995). This coupled with low tone, weakness, and upper-extremity dysfunction, is a compelling reason for referral to an early intervention program. Initial studies of patients so referred suggest subsequent enhancement of functional ambulatory abilities and cognitive abilities so that educational mainstreaming is more apt to occur.

Hypo- or hypertonia may exist in the trunk and upper extremities in association with hydrocephalus. Even children with sacral lesions may have delays in performance of erect activities, integration of primitive reflexes, and acquisition of automatic reactions (Wolf & Mc

Laughlin, 1992). The infant should be encouraged to assume antigravity positions, such as quadruped with weight bearing on extended forearms. These attempts may have to be augmented by placing the child over a bolster in prone position and/or by provision of a scooter board. As the child progresses, he/she can be set on a bolster to work on trunk and abdominal strengthening and sitting balance. Later, a standing table can be utilized. Depending on the neurological level, the child can then progress to rising from sitting to half-kneeling, and from half-kneeling to standing, utilizing adaptive equipment as needed.

Appropriate orthoses are either of metal and leather or of the newer custom-molded plastic variety (Krebs, Edelstein, & Fishman, 1988). Ambulation, especially with hip-knee-ankle-foot orthoses, is energy-inefficient; caloric expenditures are about six times normal. The use of reciprocating gait orthoses should therefore be considered to reduce energy consumption and improve endurance (Mc Call & Schmidt, 1986). More recently, it has been felt that these devices are a trade-off, and more conventional bracing might permit for rapid increases in speed which may be required in some circumstances, such as when crossing the street.

Upper-extremity dysfunction and perceptual-motor problems correlate with the severity of the hydrocephalus and the level of the lesion. With the development of increased intracranial pressure, there is stretching of the motor and sensory fibers which surround the enlarged ventricles seen with the Arnold-Chiari malformation, and this may be compounded by abnormalities of the cervical nerve roots (Hwang, Kentish, & Burns, 2002). Hand function should be assessed in terms of preference, tactile discrimination and kinesthetic awareness, ability to conform to certain positions and to perform activities including page turning, stacking of blocks and checkers and the speed with which these activities are carried out, grasp, manipulation of small objects, handling of feeding utensils, graphesthesias, and two-point discrimination (Brunt, 1980; Grimm, 1976; Wallace, 1973). Older children must be assessed in terms of figure copying, graphomotor skills, and academic difficulties. Letter reversals and difficulty in sequencing tasks are not uncommon. Visual problems of astigmatism, nystagmus, and hyperopia seen in association with hydrocephalus may be contributory factors (Mankinen-Heikkinen & Mustonene, 1987). Remediation of perceptual motor difficulties may require use of occupational therapy and special education services (Gluckman & Barling, 1980). Upper-extremity dysfunction may adversely affect the ability to use crutches (Radke & Gosky, 1981; Wallace, 1973), accounting for the discrepancies in ambulation that occur among patients of the same neurological level.

Activities of daily living skills in spina bifida patients are likely to be below age-level (Sousa, Gordon, & Shurtleff, 1976). This may be related to praxis and motor planning and to parental overprotection and time constraints. Preparation for adulthood and independent living may be restricted by these factors rather than by lack of intelligence. The development of standardized assessments of self-care, such as the Functional Independence Measure for Children (Wee-FIM) (Granger, Hamilton, & Kayton, 1987) and the Pediatric Evaluation of Disability Inventory (PEDI) (Feldman, Haley, & Coryell, 1990), will help to clarify the specific areas of training required.

Up to 61% of spina bifida patients may have strabismus. There is a high incidence of amblyopia as well, likely related to the presence of hydrocephalus. Such deficits require treatment, and their amelioration may permit better upper-extremity and perceptual-motor function (Biglan, 1995).

Respiratory problems may occur as a result of brainstem dysfunction, either on the basis of a congenital malformation or as a result of repeated traction on that area. Loss of central ventilatory function may present with stridor, intermittent loss of consciousness, and apnea. Sleep studies with analysis of respiratory gases document the lack of chemoregulatory ability, which can result in hypercarbia and anoxia (Swaminathan et al., 1989). Positive pressure or frank respiratory support may be required, in association with a tracheostomy necessitated by vocal cord paralysis; some children gradually improve over time. Some centers advocate a posterior decompression of the cervical spine, although ultimate survival may not be improved with this intervention (Worley, Schuster, & Oakes, 1991). Similarly, brainstem dysfunction may lead to oro-motor incoordination, feeding difficulties, and aspiration.

Speech and language dysfunction arise from the various central structural abnormalities associated with spina bifida. Developmental as well as acquired lesions of the cerebellum result in a disruption of motor speech skills. There is resultant dysfluency, ataxic dysarthria, and abnormality in the rate of speech or prosody, and alternation of intelligibility and vocal intensity. Abnormalities of the corpus callosum may result in difficulty in comprehension and in pragmatic speech and language skills with relative preservation of grammar and lexicon (Fletcher, Barnes, & Dennis, 2002). More specifically, these abnormalities are characterized by echolalia/repetition, excessive use of social phrases in conversation, and overfamiliarity, in what has been termed the "cocktail party syndrome" (Tew, 1979). The patients may appear to function on a superficial basis better than they actually perform. Therapeutic efforts are indicated in these children to develop pragmatic, step-by-step verbal skills. These skills are pre-requisites for instruction in dressing, learning the sequencing required to master self-catheterization, and other ADL skills. Without development of such skills, subsequent academic skills and employment potential may be compromised.

Bowel and bladder incontinence results from lack of innervation at the sacral 2, 3, and 4 levels, with paralysis and incoordination of the bladder and urinary sphincter on the basis of upper and lower motor neuron involvement. Urinary incontinence, stasis, and reflux of urine back into the kidneys may result in chronic infections with a potential for urosepsis, chronic renal acidosis, hypertension, renal failure, and death (Mundy, Shah, Borzyskowski, & Saxton, 1985). Until about 25 years ago, upper-tract deterioration was felt to be inevitable, resulting in surgical correction of an ileal conduit. Currently, intermittent urinary catheterization is the mainstay of treatment, decreasing the risk of infection and stasis and permitting functional urinary continence (Petersen, 1987) and maintenance of good renal function (Pecker, Damber, Hjalmas, Sjodin, & Von Zweigbergk, 1997). Catheterization may be required in infancy to prevent hydronephrosis, which can be present in up to 81% of patients by 5 years of age (Charney, Snyder, & Melchionni, 1991). Earlier initiation of catheterization also may prevent irreversible bladder dysfunction and reduce the number of children indicated for bladder augmentation from 27 to 11% (Iwu, Baskin, & Kogan, 1997). Depending on sitting balance, hand function, and cognitive skills, self-catheterization can begin as early as 5 years (K. A. Smith, 1991). Perceptual problems may make the technique difficult; anatomically correct dolls on which the child can practice may facilitate training.

Continence can be further enhanced by use of uropharmacologic agents that relax bladder tone to prevent voiding or improve contraction of the urinary sphincter to prevent leakage. Low-dose oral antibiotic therapy may be required to prevent recurrent infections. In males, external collecting devices can be used as a back-up measure, but females must rely on diapers or pads. Attention should be paid to the development of latex allergies in up to 35% of such patients, possibly because of prolonged and repeated exposures to the material from multiple surgeries and intermittent catheterization regimens (Slater, 1989). Allergic manifestations are not only those of reactive airway disease, but those patients so affected may present with urticaria and IgE-mediated intraoperative anaphylaxis. The average time from exposure to development of symptoms is from 1.5 to 9 years, with an average of 5.6 years, with the incidence being proportionate to the number of prior surgical procedures (Obojski et al., 2002). The mainstay of current recommendations is the avoidance of latex-containing items, including the maintenance of a latex-free operating room in major medical centers. Patients should be provided with emergency identification bracelets which notes their latex allergy in addition to their other multiple medical problems. Under circumstances in which procedures need to be performed under less than optimal conditions, premedication with steroids and gastrointestinal prophylaxis should occur.

Yearly renal ultrasound studies and blood tests to monitor renal function are mandatory. Surgical techniques which have been developed include bladder augmentation to increase bladder capacity between catheterizations and the placement of an artificial urinary sphincter (Kaplan, 1985). In patients with some residual sensation, biofeedback techniques also may be successful (Kaplan & Richards, 1988). Low-intensity transcutaenous therapeutic electrical stimulation may be a method for achieving urinary and fecal continence (Balcom, Wiatrak, Biefield, Rauen, & Langenstroer, 1997). Bowel continence is generally managed by the use of stool softeners, diet, and suppositories or enemas given at a consistent time. The olfactory stigma of an incontinent child may result in ostracism; this is a compelling reason for the early implementation of an effective bowel and bladder program.

Until recently, endocrinologic dysfunction has been overlooked in this population. Up to 15% of patients may have reduction in growth hormone as manifested by a decrease in longitudinal height and arm span. This is likely hydrocephalus-related, with secondary pressure effects being exerted on the hypothalamus and/or pituitary gland (Hochhaus, Butenandl, Schwarz, & Ring-Mrozik, 1997). Higher-level spina bifida lesions may result in a greater degree of growth impairment (Rotenstein & Riegel, 1996). Not only are such reductions in height stigmatizing, but the associated changes in bony maturation may alter the standard surgical timetable. Supplementation of growth hormone is a treatment option; its long-term effect in terms of accentuating linear growth, elevating the center of gravity, and increasing the incidence of symptomatic tethering of the spinal cord has not yet been determined (Gold, 1996).

General pediatric care may be compromised in this group given the 20-fold increase in frequency of hospitalizations for surgery, acute, intercurrent infections, and other medical problems. Up to 25% of pediatric patients may be deficient in routine immunizations despite provision of multiple sub-specialty medical services, augmented by parental concern in regard to pertussis vaccine administration due to co-existent neurological dysfunction. Accordingly, an immunization history is an important part of each clinic visit (Raddish, Goldman, Kaplan, & Perrin, 1998).

Given the increased longevity of the spina bifida patient and the possibility of late complications, it is essential that team management is continued throughout the adult years. Without such services, well over half of the patients might not receive any specialized services, and some might receive no medical care at all (Kaufman et al., 1994). With ongoing care, potentially preventable complications, including pyelonephritis, renal calculi, decubitus formation with an underlying infection of the bone, and occult, late shunt malfunctions, can be avoided (Kinsman

& Doehring, 1996). In this setting, patients also can be monitored for a possible increased risk of colorectal cancer (Tomlinson & Sugarman, 1995). Instead of treating complications, proactive procedures such as release of a tethered spinal cord, tendon releases, and bladder augmentation can be considered (Begeer & Staal-Schreinemachers, 1996).

PSYCHOLOGICAL AND VOCATIONAL IMPLICATIONS

IN THE SETTING of multiple physical and medical problems, it is admirable that patients with spina bifida can function as well as has been described. Acknowledgement of psychological differences in myelomeningocele patients may be seen as early as in the preschool period. Figure drawings by such children reveal fewer portrayals of lower extremities than in the general population. Children tend to rate themselves as significantly different in terms of physical and cognitive competence, but not on maternal or peer acceptance (Mobley, Harless, & Miller, 1996).

The secondary disability of social isolation results from the time allocated to medical care and hospitalization, augmented by parental overprotectiveness, with mothers exhibiting this tendency to a greater extent than fathers (Holmbeck et al., 2002). Thus, by mid-childhood, children so afflicted have up to a fourfold risk of developing a psychiatric disorder, primarily neurotic in nature. Hence, early intervention, socialization, and family counseling are warranted (Connell & Mc Connel, 1981). Dorner (1976, 1977) detailed the social dysfunction of the group. Teenagers were found to be lonely and unhappy, and to have limited exposure to the typically developing population, sexual experiences, and community resources. Despite attempts at comprehensive interventions and care, newer studies reflect similar findings (Buran, Mc Daniel, & Bree, 2002; Cate, Kennedy, & Stevenson, 2002). Academic achievement may be somewhat improved on the basis of mainstreaming (Borjeson & Logergren, 1990; Lord, Varzos, Behrman, Wicks, & Wicks, 1990).

Adult males with spina bifida have decreased understanding of sexual function, decreased fertility, and difficulty in maintaining erections. Conversely, females often achieve fertility early because of their hydrocephalus. Pregnant females may be predisposed to premature labor due to a contracted pelvis and urinary tract abnormalities. Ventriculoperitoneal shunts may have an increased incidence of dysfunction during this period. If a C-section is indicated for delivery, then prophylactic antibiotics should be given and peritoneal irrigation should be performed (Rietberg & Lindhout, 1993). Sexual education in either circumstance is exceedingly important.

Despite good cognitive skills and educational opportunities, it is not uncommon for patients to remain in the homes of their parents past

maturity. This may not only be a sign of prolonged emotional dependence, but may be an economic necessity, as only 20% of adults are likely
to be employed (Castree & Walker, 1981). Functional numeracy but not
functional literacy skills appear to be correlated with a better chance
for employment (Dennis & Barnes, 2002). The survival rate for the majority of patients with spina bifida now exceeds 90%. This provides the
medical community with a mandate to expand the range of services
available to such adults.

REFERENCES

Abbott, R., Johann-Murphy, M., & Gold, J. T. (1991). Selective functional rhizotomy
for the treatment of spasticity in children. In M. Sindou (Ed.), *Neurosurgery
for spasticity* (pp. 149–157). New York: Springer-Verlag.

Abraham, E., Lubicky, J. P., Sanger, M. N., & Millar, E. A. (1996). Supramalleolar
osteotomy for ankle valgus in myelomeningocele. *Journal of Pediatric
Orthopedics, 16,* 774–781.

Albright, A. L. (1996). Baclofen in the treatment of cerebral palsy. *Journal of Child
Neurology, 11,* 77–83.

Albright, A. L., Barron, W. B., Fascik, D., Polinko, P., & Janosky, J. (1993). Continuous
intrathecal Baclofen infusion for spasticity of cerebral origin. *Journal of
the American Medical Association, 270,* 2475–2477.

Albright, A. L., Cervi. A., & Singletary, J. (1991). Intrathecal Baclofen for spasticity in cerebral palsy. *Journal of the American Medical Association, 265,*
1418–1422.

Alexander, M. A., & Steg, N. L. (1989). Myelomeningocele: Comprehensive treatment. *Archives of Physical Medicine and Rehabilitation, 70,* 637–641.

Alvarez, N., Larkin, C., & Roxborough, J. (1981). Carpal-tunnel syndrome in
athetoid-dystonic cerebral palsy. *Archives of Neurology, 39,* 311–326.

Andersson, C., Grooten, W., Hellsten, M., Kaping, K., & Mattson, E. (2003). Adults
with cerebral palsy: Walking ability after progressive strength training.
Developmental Medicine and Child Neurology, 45, 220–228.

Andersson, C., & Mattson, E. (2001). Adults with cerebral palsy: Survey describing problems, needs, and resources with special emphasis on locomotion. *Developmental Medicine and Child Neurology, 43,* 76–82.

Andrade, C. K., Kramer, J., Garber, M., & Longmuir, P. (1991). Changes in self-
concept, cardiovascular endurance, and muscle strength of children with
spina bifida aged 8 to 13 years in response to a 10-week physical activity
programme: A pilot study. *Child: Care and Health Development, 17,* 183–196.

Ansved, T., Odergren, T., & Borg, K. (1997). Muscle fiber atrophy in leg muscles
after botulinum toxin type A treatment of cervical dystonia. *Neurology,
48,* 1440–1442.

Armstrong, R. W., Steinbok, P., & Cochrane, D. D. (1997). Intrathecally administered Baclofen for the treatment of children with spasticity of cerebral origin. *Journal of Neurosurgery, 87,* 409–414.

Asher, M., & Olsen, J. (1983). Factors affecting the ambulatory status of patients with spina bifida cystica. *Journal of Bone and Joint Surgery, 65-A,* 350–356.

Ashton, B., Piper, M. C., Warren, S., Stewin, L., & Byrne, P. (1991). Influence of medical history of assessment of at-risk infants. *Developmental Medicine and Child Neurology, 33,* 412–418.

Bachrach, S., & Greenspun, B. (1990). Care of the adult with myelomeningocele. *Del. Medical Journal, 62,* 1287–1295.

Badell-Ribera, A., Swinyard, C. A., Greenspan, L., & Deaver, G. G. (1964). Spina bifida with myelomeningocele: Evaluation of rehabilitation potential. *Archives of Physical Medicine and Rehabilitation, 45,* 443–453.

Balcom, A. H., Wiatrak, M., Biefeld, T., Rauen, K., & Langenstroer, P. (1997). Initial experience with home therapeutic electrical stimulation for continence in the myelomeningocele population. *Journal of Urology, 158,* 1272–1276.

Banker, B., & Larroche, J. C. (1962). Periventricular leukomalacia of infancy: A form of neonatal anoxic encephalopathy. *Archives of Neurology, 7,* 386–410.

Banta, J. V., & Park, S. M. (1983). Improvement in pulmonary function in patients having combined anterior and posterior spine fusion for myelomeningocele scoliosis. *Spine, 8,* 765–770.

Begeer, I. H., & Staal-Schreinemachers, A. L. (1996). The benefits of team treatment and control of adult patients with spinal dysraphism. *European Journal of Pediatric Surgery, 6,* 15–16.

Bell, M. J., & Hallenbeck, E. Effects of intrauterine inflammation on developing rat brain. (2002). *Journal of Neuroscience Research, 70,* 570–579.

Benedict, M. I., White, R. B., Wulff, L. M., & Hall, B. J. (1990). Reported maltreatment in children with multiple disabilities. *Child Abuse and Neglect, 14,* 207–217.

Bergen, A. F., & Colangelo, C. (1982). *Positioning of the client with central nervous system deficits: The wheelchair and other adaptive equipment.* Valhalla, NY: Valhalla Rehabilitation.

Bigan, A. W. (1995). Strabismus associated with meningomyelocele. *Journal of Pediatric Ophthalmology and Strabismus, 32,* 309–314.

Blair, E., & Stanley, F. (1990). Intrauterine growth retardation and spastic cerebral palsy: 1. Association with birth weight for gestation age. *American Journal of Obstetrics and Gynecology, 162,* 229–237.

Bleck, E. E. (1987). Orthopedic management of cerebral palsy. In *Clinical developmental medicine* (vol. 99/100). Oxford, England: MacKeith.

Bleck, E. E. (1990). Management of the lower extremities in children with cerebral palsy. *Journal of Bone and Joint Surgery, 72-A,* 140–144.

Blum, R. W., Resnick, M. D., Nelson, R., & St. Germaine, A. (1991). Familial and peer issues among adolescents with spina bifida and cerebral palsy. *Pediatrics, 88,* 280–285.

Bobath, B., & Bobath, K. (1975). *Motor development in the different types of cerebral palsy*. London: Heineman.

Bobath, K. (1980). *A neurophysiologic basis to the treatment of cerebral palsy*. Laveham, UK: Spastics International.

Borjeson, M. C., & Logergren, J. (1990). Life conditions of adolescents with myelomeningocele. *Developmental Medicine and Child Neurology, 32,* 698–706.

Botto, L. D., & Yang, Q. (2000). Ethylene tetrahydrofolate reductase gene variants and congenital anomalies, a HuGE review. *American Journal of Epidemiology, 151,* 862–877.

Bower, C., Raymond, M., Lumley, J., & Bury, G. (1993). Trends in neural tube defects 1980–1989. *Medical Journal of Australia, 158,* 152–154.

Boytim, M. J., Davidson, R. S., Charney, E., & Melchionne, J. B. (1991). Neonatal fractures in myelomeningocele patients. *Journal of Pediatric Orthopedics, 11,* 28–30.

Brinker, M. R., Rosenfeld, S. R., Feiwell, E., Granger, S. P., Mitchell, D. C., & Rice, J. C. (1994). Myelomeningocele at the sacral level. *Journal of Bone and Joint Surgery, 76-A,* 1293–1300.

Brocklehurst, G. (Ed.). (1976). *Spina bifida for the clinician*. Philadelphia: J. B. Lippincott.

Bronkhorst, A. J., & Lamb, G. A. (1987). Orthosis to aid in the reduction of lower extremity spasticity. *Orthotics and Prosthetics, 41,* 23–28.

Brown, M. C., Bontempo, A., & Turk, M. A. (1992). *Secondary consequences of cerebral palsy: Adults with cerebral palsy in New York State*. Albany, NY: New York State.

Brunt, A. (1980). Characteristics of upper limb movements in a sample of myelomeningocele children. *Perceptual Motor Skills, 51,* 431–437.

Buran, C. F., Mc Daniel, A., & Bree, T. J. (2002). Needs assessment in a spina bifida program: A comparison of the perceptions by adolescents with spina bifida and their parents. *Clinical Nurse Specialist, 16,* 256–262.

Cahan, L. D., & Kundi, M. S. (1987). Electrophysiological studies in selective dorsal rhizotomy for spasticity in children with cerebral palsy. *Applied Neurophysiology, 50,* 459–460.

Capute, A. J. (1978). *Primitive reflex profile*. Baltimore: University Park Press.

Capute, A. J., Shapiro, B. K., & Palmer, F. B. (1981). Spectrum of developmental disabilities. *Orthopedic Clinics of North America, 12,* 3–22.

Carlson, W. E., Vaughn, C. L., Damiano, D. L., & Abel, M. F. (1997). Orthotic management of gait in spastic diplegia. *American Journal of Physical Medicine and Rehabilitation, 76,* 216–225.

Carlsson, M., Hagberg, G., & Olssom, I. (2003). Clinical and etiological aspects of epilepsy in children with cerebral palsy. *Developmental Medicine and Child Neurology, 45,* 371–376.

Carr, C., & Gage, J. R. (1987). The fate of the non-operated hip in cerebral palsy. *Journal of Pediatric Orthopedics, 7,* 262–267.

Carroll, N. C. (1977). The orthotic management of spina bifida children: Present status, future goals. *Prosthetics and Orthotics International, 1,* 39–42.

Castree, B. J., & Walker, J. H. (1981). The young adult with spina bifida. *British Medical Journal, 283,* 1040–1042.

Cate, I. M. P., Kennedy, C., & Stevenson, J. (2002). Disability and quality of life in spina bifida and hydrocephalus. *Developmental Medicine and Child Neurology, 44,* 317–322.

Charney, E. B. (1990). Parental attitudes toward management of newborns with myelomeningocele. *Developmental Medicine and Child Neurology, 32,* 14–19.

Charney, E. B., Melchionni, J. B., & Smith, D. R. (1991). Community ambulation by children with myelomeningocele and high-level paralysis. *Journal of Pediatric Orthopedics, 11,* 579–582.

Charney, E. B., Rorke, L. B., Sutton, L. N., & Schut, L. (1991). Management of Chiai II complications in infants with myelomeningocele. *Journal of Pediatrics, 111,* 374–371.

Charney, E. B., Snyder, H. M., & Melchionni, J. B. (1991). Upper urinary tract deterioration with myelomeningocele. *Developmental Medicine and Child Neurology, 33*(Suppl. 64), 18–37.

Chervenak, R. A., & Mc Cullough, L. B. (2002). A comprehensive ethical framework for fetal research and its application to fetal surgery for spina bifida. *American Journal of Obstetrics and Gynecology, 187,* 10–14.

Chiaramonte, R. M., Horowitz, R. M., Kaplan, G. M., & Brook, W. A. (1986). Implications of hydronephrosis in newborns with myelodysplasia. *Journal of Urology, 136,* 427–429.

Chicoine, M. R., Park, T. S., & Kaufman, B. A. (1997). Selective dorsal rhizotomy and rates of orthopedic surgery in children with spastic cerebral palsy. *Journal of Neurosurgery, 86,* 34–39.

Choi, S. H., & Mc Comb, J. G. (2000). Long-term outcome of terminal myelocystocele patients. *Pediatric Neurosurgery, 32,* 86–91.

Clancy, R. R., Sladsky, J. T., & Rorke, L. B. (1989). Hypoxic-ischemic spinal cord injury following perinatal asphyxia. *Annals of Neurology, 25,* 185–189.

Coniglio, S. J., Anderson, S. M., & Ferguson, J. E. (1996). Functional motor outcome in children with myelomeningocele. Correlation with anatomic prenatal ultrasound. *Developmental Medicine and Child Neurology, 38,* 675–680.

Connell, H. M., & Mc Connel, T. S. (1981). Psychiatric sequelae in children treated operatively for hydrocephalus in infancy. *Developmental Medicine and Child Neurology, 23,* 505–517.

Cooperman, D. R., Bartucci, E., Dietrick, E., & Millar, E. A. (1987). Hip dislocation in spastic cerebral palsy: Long-term consequences. *Journal of Pediatric Orthopedics, 7,* 268–276.

Coorsen, E. A., Msall, M. E., & Duffy, L. C. (1991). Multiple minor manifestations as a marker for prenatal etiology of cerebral palsy. *Developmental Medicine and Child Neurology, 33,* 730–736.

Cosgrove, A. P., & Graham, H. K. (1994). Botulinum toxin A prevents the development of contractures in the hereditary spastic mouse. *Developmental Medicine and Child Neurology, 36,* 379–385

Craft, M. J., Lakin, J. A., Oppliger, R. A., Clancy, G. M., & Vander linden, D. W. (1990). Siblings as change agents for promoting the functional status of children with cerebral palsy. *Developmental Medicine and Child Neurology, 32,* 1049–1057.

Crandall, R. C., Birkeback, C. R., & Wintor, B. R. (1989). The role of hip location and dislocation in the functional status of the myelodysplastic patient. *Orthopedics, 12,* 675–683.

Cuddeford, T. J., Freeling, R. P., Thomas, S. S., Aniona, M. D., Rex, D., Sirolli, H., et al. (1997). Energy consumption in children with myelomeningocele: A comparison between reciprocating gait orthosis and hip-knee-ankle-foot orthosis ambulators. *Developmental Medicine and Child Neurology, 39,* 239–242.

Curtis, B. H. (1973). The hip in the myelomeningocele child. *Clinical Orthopedics, 90,* 11–21.

Damiano, D. L., Kelly, L. E., & Vaughan, C. L. (1995). Effects of quadriceps femoris muscle strengthening on crouch gait in children with spastic diplegia. *Physical Therapy, 75,* 658–667.

Damiano, D. L., Vaughan, C. L., & Abel, M. F. (1995). Muscle response to heavy resistance exercise in children with spastic cerebral palsy. *Developmental Medicine and Child Neurology, 37,* 731–739.

De Souza, L. L., & Carroll, N. (1976). Ambulation of the braced myelomeningocele patient. *Journal of Bone and Joint Surgery, 58-A,* 1112–1118.

Deaver, G. (1956). Cerebral palsy: Methods of beating the neuromuscular disability. *Archives of Physical Medicine and Rehabilitation, 37,* 363–378.

Dennis, M., & Barnes, M. (2002). Math and numeracy in young adults with spina bifida and hydrocephalus. *Developmental Medicine and Child Neurology, 41,* 141–155.

Diamond, M. (1986). Rehabilitation strategies for the child with cerebral palsy. *Pediatric Annals, 15,* 230–236.

Dorner, S. (1976). Adolescents with spina bifida: How they view their situation. *Archives of Diseases of Childhood, 51,* 439–444.

Dorner, S. (1977). Sexual interest and activity in adolescents with spina bifida. *Journal of Child Psychology, 18,* 229–237.

Drennan, J. C. (1976). Orthotic management of the myelomeningocele spine. *Developmental Medicine and Child Neurology, 18,* 97–103.

Drvaric, D. M., Roberts, J. M., Burke, S. W., King, A. G., & Falterman, K. (1987). Gastroesophageal evaluation in totally involved cerebral palsy patients. *Journal of Pediatric Orthopedics, 7,* 187–190.

Ebura, S., Yamazaki, Y., Harada, T., Hosono, N., Morimoto, Y., Tang, L., et al. (1990). Motion analysis of the cervical spine in athetoid cerebral palsy. *Spine, 15,* 1097–1103.

Ellenberg, J. H., & Nelson, K. B. (1981). Early recognition of infants at risk for cerebral palsy. Examination at age 4 months. *Developmental Medicine and Child Neurology, 23,* 705–714.

Engel, J. M., Kartin, D., & Jensen, M. D. (2002). Pain treatment in persons with cerebral palsy. Frequency and helpfulness. *Journal of Physical Medicine and Rehabilitation, 81,* 291–296.

Evans, D. M., & Alberman, E. (1990). Certified cause of death in children and young adults with cerebral palsy. *Archives of Diseases of Childhood, 66,* 325–329.

Evans, D. M., Evans, J. W., & Alberman, E. (1990). Cerebral palsy: Why we must plan for survival. *Archives of Diseases of Childhood, 65,* 1329–1333.

Eyman, R. K., & Grossman, H. J. (1990). The life expectancy of profoundly handicapped people with mental retardation. *New England Journal of Medicine, 323,* 584–589.

Farmer, S. F., Harrison, L. M., Ingram, D. A., & Stephens, J. A. (1991). Plasticity of central motor pathways in children with hemiplegic cerebral palsy. *Neurology, 41,* 1505–1510.

Fasano, V. A., Barolat-Romana, G., Zeme, S., & Squazzi, A. (1979). Electrophysiological assessment of spinal circuits in spasticity by direct dorsal root stimulation. *Neurosurgery, 4,* 146–151.

Feldman, A. B., Haley, S. M., & Coryell, J. (1990). Concurrent and construct validity of the Pediatric Evaluation of Disability Inventory. *Physical Therapy, 70,* 602–610.

Findley, T. W., & Agre, J. C. (1988). Ambulation in the adolescent with spina bifida: Oxygen cost of mobility. *Archives of Physical Medicine and Rehabilitation, 69,* 855–861.

Finnie, N. R. (1974). *Handling the young cerebral palsied child at home.* New York: E. P. Dutton.

Fletcher, J. M., Barnes, M., & Dennis, M. (2002). Language development in children with spina bifida. *Semiars in Pediatric Neurology, 9,* 201–208.

Ford, G. W., Kitchen, W. H., Doyle, L. W., Richards, A. L., & Kelly, E. (1990). Changing diagnosis of cerebral palsy in very low birth weight children. *American Journal of Perinatology, 7,* 178–181.

Fraser, R. K., Bourke, H. M., Broughton, N. S., & Menelaus, M. B. (1995). Unilateral dislocation of the hip in spina bifida: A long-term follow-up. *Journal of Bone and Joint Surgery, 77-B,* 615–619.

Frawley, P. A., Broughton, N. S., & Menelaus, M. B., (1996). *Journal of Bone and Joint Surgery, 78-B,* 299–302.

Frieden, J., & Lieber, R. (2003). Spastic muscle cells are shorter and stiffer than normal cells. *Muscle and Nerve, 26,* 157–164.

Fuji, T., Yoonebu, K., Fujiwara, K., Yamashita, K., Ebara, S., Ono, K., et al. (1987). Cervical radiculopathy or myelopathy secondary to athetoid cerebral palsy. *Journal of Bone and Joint Surgery, 69-A,* 815–821.

Fulford, G. E. (1990). Surgical management of ankle and foot deformities in cerebral palsy. *Clinical Orthopaedics, 253,* 55–61.

Gage, J. R. (1990). Surgical treatment of knee dysfunction in cerebral palsy. *Clinical Orthopaedics, 253,* 45–54.

Galvin, K. A. (1998). Postinjury magnesium sulfate treatment is not markedly neuroprotective for striatal medium spiny neurons after perinatal hypoxic/ischemia in the rat. *Pediatric Research, 44,* 740–745.

Gerszten, P. C. (1997). Effect on ambulation of continuous intrathecal baclofen infusion. *Pediatric Neurosurgery, 27,* 40–44.

Gibson, C. S., Mac Lennan, A. H., Goldwater, P. N., & Dekker, G. A. (2003). Antenatal causes of cerebral palsy: Association between inherited thrombophilias, viral, and bacterial infections, and inherited susceptibilities to infection. *Obstetrics, Gynecology, and Surgery, 58,* 209–220.

Gisel, E. G., & Patrick, J. (1988). Identification of children with cerebral palsy unable to maintain a normal nutritional state. *Lancet, 1,* 283–286.

Gluckman, S., & Barling, J. (1980). Effect of remedial program on visual-motor perception in spina bifida children. *Journal of General Psychology, 136,* 195–200.

Gold, J. T. (1991). Orthotic management and rehabilitation of the foot and ankle in the neurologically impaired child. In M. H. Jahss (Ed.), *Disorders of the foot and ankle.* Philadelphia: W. B. Saunders.

Gold, J. T. (1996). Growth hormone treatment of children with neural tube defects [Letter; comment]. *Journal of Pediatrics, 129,* 771.

Gooch, J. L., & Walker, M. L. (1996). Spinal stenosis after total lumbar laminectomy for selective dorsal rhizotomy. *Pediatric Neurosurgery, 25,* 28–30.

Gosechel, H., Wohlfarth, K., Frevert, J., Dengler, R., & Bigalke, T. T. (1997). Botulinum A toxin therapy: Neutralizing and non-neutralizing antibodies—therapeutic consequences. *Experimental Neurology, 147,* 96–102.

Graham, H. K., & Selber, P. (2003). Musculoskeletal aspects of cerebral palsy. *Journal of Bone and Joint Surgery, 85-B,* 157–166.

Graham, L., Levene M. I., & Trounce, J. Q. (1987). Prediction of cerebral palsy in very low birth weight infants: Prospective ultrasound study. *Lancet, 2,* 593–596.

Granger, C. V., Hamilton, B. B., & Kayton, R. (1987). *Guide for the use of the Functional Independence Measure for Children (WeeFIM) of the Uniform Data Set for medical rehabilitation.* Buffalo, NY: Research Foundation, State University of New York.

Grant, A., O'Brien, N., Joy, M. T., Hennessy, E., & Mac Donald, D. (1989). Cerebral palsy among children born during the Dublin randomized trial of intrapartum monitoring. *Lancet, 2,* 1233–1236.

Grimm, R. A. (1976). Hand preference and tactile perception in a group of children with myelomeningocele. *American Journal of Occupational Therapy, 30,* 234–250.

Guyatt, G., Sackett, D., Taylor, D. W., Chong, J., Roberts, R., & Dugsley, S. (1986). Determining optimal therapy: Randomized trials in individual patients. *New England Journal of Medicine, 314,* 889–892.

Hagberg, B., & Hagberg, G. (1989). The changing panorama of cerebral palsy in Sweden: 5. The birth year period 1979–82. *Acta Paediatrica Scandinavica, 78,* 283–290.

Hagberg, B., & Hagberg, G. (1996). The changing panorama of cerebral palsy: Bilateral spastic forms in particular. *Acta Paediatrica Scandinavica, 416,* 48–52.

Halpern, D. (1982). Duration of relaxation after intramuscular neurolysis with phenol. *Journal of the American Medical Association, 247,* 1473–1476.

Halpern, D. (1984). Therapeutic exercises for cerebral palsy. In J. V. Basmajian (Ed.), *Therapeutic exercises* (pp. 118–143). Baltimore: Williams & Wilkins.

Harade, T., Ebara, S., Anwar, M. M., Okawa, A., Kajiura, I., Hiroshima, K., et al. (1996). The cervical spine in athetoid cerebral palsy: A radiological study of 180 patients. *Journal of Bone and Joint Surgery, 78-B,* 613–619.

Harris, S. R. (1989). Early diagnosis of spastic diplegia, spastic hemiplegia and quadriplegia. *American Journal of Diseases of Childhood, 143,* 1356–1360.

Harrison, A. (1988). Spastic cerebral palsy: Possible spinal interneuronal contributions. *Developmental Medicine and Child Neurology, 30,* 769–780.

Hazlewood, M. I., Brown, J. K., Rowe, P. J., & Salter, P. M. (1994). The use of therapeutic electrical stimulation in the treatment of hemiplegic cerebral palsy. *Developmental Medicine and Child Neurology, 36,* 661–673.

Henderson, R. C., Lark, R. K., & Kecskemethy, H. (2002). Bisphosphonates to treat osteopenia in children with quadriplegic cerebral palsy: A randomized clinical trial. *Journal of Pediatrics, 141,* 644–651.

Hill, A. E. (1990). Conductive education for physically handicapped children. *Ulster Medical Journal, 59,* 41–45.

Hinderer, K. A., & Harris, S. R. (1988). Effects of tone reducing versus standard plaster casts on gait improvement in children with cerebral palsy. *Developmental Medicine and Child Neurology, 30,* 370–377.

Hirst, M. (1989). Patterns of impairment and disability related to social handicap in young people with cerebral palsy and spina bifida. *Journal of Biosocial Science, 21,* 1–12.

Hirtz, D. G., & Nelson, K. (1998). Magnesium sulfate and cerebral palsy in premature infants. *Current Opinions in Pediatrics, 10,* 131–137.

Hochhaus, F., Butenandl, O., Schwarz, H. P., & Ring-Mrozik, E. (1997). *European Journal of Pediatrics, 156,* 597–601.

Hoffer, M. M., Feiwell, E., Perry, R., Perry, J., & Bonnett, C. (1973). Functional ambulation in patients with myelomeningocele. *Journal of Bone and Joint Surgery, 55-A,* 137–148.

Holm, V. A. (1982). The causes of cerebral palsy. *Journal of the American Medical Association, 247,* 1473–1475.

Holmbeck, G. N., Johnson, S. Z., Wills, K. E., Mc Kernon, W., Rose, B., Erklin, S., et al. (2002). Observed and perceived parental overprotection in relation to psychosocial adjustment in preadolescents with a physical disability: The mediational role of behavioral autonomy. *Journal of Consultation in Clinical Psychology, 70,* 96–110.

Homes, L. B. (1988). Does taking vitamins at the time of conception prevent neural tube defects? *Journal of the American Medical Association, 260,* 3181–3183.

Horn, D. G., Lorch, R. F., & Culatta, B. (1985). Distractability and vocabulary deficits in children with spina bifida and hydrocephalus. *Developmental Medicine and Child Neurology, 27,* 713–720.

Hunt, G. M., & Holmes, A. E. (1976). Factors relating to intelligence in treated cases of spina bifida cystica. *American Journal of Diseases of Childhood, 130,* 823–827.

Hunt, G. M., Oakesholt, P., & Kerry, S. (1999). Link between the CSF shunt and achievement in adults with spina bifida. *Journal of Neurology, Neurosurgery and Psychiatry, 67,* 591–595.

Hurvitz, E. A., Leonard, C., Ayyangar, R., & Nelson, V. S. (2003). Complementary and alternative medicine use in families of children with cerebral palsy. *Developmental Medicine and Child Neurology, 45,* 364–370.

Hwang, R., Kentish, M., & Burns, Y. (2002). Hand positioning sense in children with spina bifida myelomeningocele. *Australian Journal of Physiotherapy, 48,* 17–22.

Ingram, T. S. S. (1955). Early manifestations and course of diplegia in childhood. *Archives of Diseases of Childhood, 30,* 244–250.

Iwu, H. Y., Baskin, L. S., & Kogan, B. A. (1997). Neurogenic bladder dysfunction due to myelomeningocele: Neonatal versus childhood treatment. *Journal of Urology, 157,* 2295–2297.

Johnson, D. C., Damiano, D. L., & Abel, M. F. (1997). The evolution of gait in childhood and adolescent cerebral palsy. *Journal of Pediatric Orthopaedics, 17,* 392–296.

Kaplan, W. E. (1985). Management of myelomeningocele. *Urology Clinics of North America, 12,* 93–101.

Kaplan, W. E., & Richards, I. (1988). Intravesical bladder stimulation in myelodysplasia. *Journal of Urology, 140,* 1282–1284.

Kassover, M., Tauber, C., Au, J., & Pugh, J. (1986). Auditory biofeedback in spastic diplegia. *Journal of Orthopaedic Research, 4,* 246–249.

Kaufman, B. A., Terbrock, A., Winters, N., Ito, J., Klosterman, A., & Park, T. S. (1994). Disbanding a multidisciplinary clinic: Effects on health care of myelomeningocele patients. *Pediatric Neurology, 21,* 36–44.

Keating, J. C., McCarron, K., James, J., Gruenberg, J., & Lonczak, R. S. (1985). Urobehavioral intervention in the rehabilitation of lower urinary tract dysfunction: A case report. *Journal of Manipulative Physiologic Therapy, 8,* 185–189.

Khoury, M. J., Erickson, J. D., & James, L. M. (1982). Etiologic heterogenicity of neural tube defects: Clues from epidemiology. *American Journal of Epidemiology, 115,* 538–548.

King, W., Levin, R., Schmidt, R., Oestreich, A., & Heubi, J. E. (2003). Prevalence of reduced bone mass in children and adults with spastic quadriplegia. *Developmental Medicine and Child Neurology, 45*, 12–16.

Kinsman, S. L., & Doehring, M. C. (1996). The cost of preventable conditions in adults with spina bifida. *European Journal of Pediatric Surgery, 6*, 17–20.

Korman, L. A., Mooney, J. F., Smith, B., Goodman, A., & Mulvaney, T. (1993). Management of cerebral palsy with botulinum-A toxin: Preliminary investigation. *Journal of Pediatric Orthopaedics, 13*, 489–495.

Kottke, F. J., Halpern, D., Easton, J. K. M., Ozel, A. T., & Burrill, C. A. (1978). The training of coordination. *Archives of Physical Medicine and Rehabilitation, 59*, 567–578.

Kraus, F. T. (1997). Cerebral palsy and thrombi in placental vessels of the fetus: Insights from litigation. *Human Pathology, 28*, 246–248.

Krebs, D. E., Edelstein, J. E., & Fishman, S. (1988). Comparison of plastic/metal and leather/metal knee-ankle-foot orthoses. *American Journal of Physical Medicine, 67*, 175–185.

Lary, J. M., & Edmonds, L. D. (1996). Prevalence of spina bifida at birth—United States, 1983–1990: A comparison of two surveillance systems. *Morbidity and Mortality Weekly Report CDC Surveillance Summaries, 45*, 15–26.

Leck, I. (1974). Causation of neural tube defects: Clues from epidemiology. *British Medical Bulletin, 30*, 158–163.

Lemire, R. J. (1988). Neural tube defects. *Journal of the American Medical Association, 259*, 558–562.

Letts, R. M., Fulford, D., Eng, B., & Robson, D. A. (1976). Mobility aids for the paraplegic child. *Journal of Bone and Joint Surgery, 58-A*, 38–41.

Levine, M. S. (1980). Cerebral palsy diagnosis in children over 1 year of age: Standard criteria. *Archives of Physical Medicine and Rehabilitation, 61*, 385–392.

Li, V., Albright, A. L., Sclabassi, R., & Pang, D. (1996). The role of somatosensory evoked potentials in the evaluation of spinal cord retethering. *Pediatric Neurosurgery, 24*, 126–133.

Ligam, S., & Joester, J. (1994). Lesion of the week: Spontaneous fractures in children and adolescents with cerebral palsy. *British Medical Journal, 309*, 265–268.

Lintner, S. A., & Lindseth, R. E. (1994). Kyphotic deformity in patients who have a myelomeningocele: Operative treatment and long-term follow-up. *Journal of Bone and Joint Surgery, 76-A*, 1301–1307.

Lonstein, J. E., & Akbamia, B. (1983). Operative treatment of spinal deformities in patients with cerebral palsy or mental retardation. *Journal of Bone and Joint Surgery, 63-A*, 43–57.

Lorber, J. (1971). Results of treatment of myelomeningocele: An analysis of 524 selected cases with special reference to possible selection for treatment. *Developmental Medicine and Child Neurology, 13*, 279–303.

Lord, J., Varzos, N., Behrman, B., Wick, J. G., & Wicks, D. (1990). Implications of mainstream classrooms for adolescents with spina bifida. *Developmental Medicine and Child Neurology, 32,* 20–29.

Lord, J. P. (1984). Cerebral palsy: A clinical approach. *Archives of Physical Medicine and Rehabilitation, 65,* 542–556.

Lough, L. K., & Nielsen, D. H. (1986). Ambulation of children with myelomeningocele: Parapodium versus parapodium with Orlau swivel modification. *Developmental Medicine and Child Neurology, 28,* 489–497.

Magill-Evans, J. E., & Restall, G. (1991). Self-esteem of persons with cerebral palsy: From adolescence to adulthood. *American Journal of Occupational Therapy, 45,* 819–825.

Major, R. E., Stollard, J., & Farmer, S. E. (1997). A review of 42 patients of 16 years and over using the Orlau Parawalker. *Prosthetics and Orthotics International, 21,* 147–152.

Mankinen-Heikkinen, A., & Mustonene, E. (1987). Ophthalmologic changes in hydrocephalus. *Acta Ophthalmology, 65,* 81–86.

Mannino, F. L., & Traunor, D. (1983). Stroke in neonates. *Journal of Pediatrics, 102,* 605–609.

Marshall, P. D., Broughton, N. S., Menelaus, M. B., & Graham, H. K. (1996). Surgical release of knee flexion contractures in myelomeningocele. *Journal of Bone and Joint Surgery, 78-B,* 912–916.

Martin, J. E., & Epstein, L. H. (1976). Evaluating treatment effectiveness in cerebral palsy. *Physical Therapy, 56,* 285–293.

Matthews, D. (1988). Controversial therapies in the management of cerebral palsy. *Pediatric Annals, 17,* 762–765.

Maudsley, G., Hultor, J. L., & Pharoah, P. (1999). Cause of death in cerebral palsy: A descriptive study. *Archives of Diseases of Childhood, 81,* 390–394.

McCall, R. E., & Schmidt, W. T. (1986). Clinical experience with the reciprocating gait orthosis in myelodysplasia. *Journal of Pediatric Orthopaedics, 16,* 157–161.

McClone, D. G. (1998). The biological resolution of malformations of the central nervous system. *Neurosurgery, 43,* 1375–1380.

McClone, D. G., Czyzewski, D., Raimondi, A., & Sommers, M. (1985). Central nervous system infections as a limiting factor in the intelligence of children with myelodysplasia. *Pediatrics, 70,* 338–342.

McClone, D. G., Dias, L., Kaplan, W., & Sommers, R. (1985). Concepts in the management of spina bifida. *Concepts in Pediatric Neurosurgery, 5,* 97–106.

McDonald, C. M., Jaffe, K. M., Mosca, V. S., Shurtleff D. B., & Menalaws, M. B. (1991). Ambulatory outcome of children with myelomeningocele: Effect of lower extremity strength. *Developmental Medicine and Child Neurology, 33,* 482–490.

McDonald, C. M., Jaffe, K. M., Mosca, V. S., Shurtleff, D. B., & Menelaus, M. B. (1991). Modifications to the traditional description of neurosegmental innervation in myelomeningocele. *Developmental Medicine and Child Neurology, 33,* 473–481.

McLaughlin, J. F., & Shurtleff, D. B. (1979). Management of the newborn with myelodysplasia. *Clinical Pediatrics, 18,* 463–476.

McNeal, D., Hawtrey, C. E., Wolraich, M. L., & Mapel, J. R. (1983). Symptomatic neurogenic bladder in a cerebral palsy population. *Developmental Medicine and Child Neurology, 25,* 612–621.

Menelaus, M. B. (1980). *Orthopedic management of spina bifida cystica* (2nd ed.). Edinburgh, Scotland: Churchill-Livingstone.

Mesples, B., Plaisant, F., & Gressens, P. (2003). Effects of interleukin-10 on neonatal excitotoxic brain lesions in mice. *Brain Research, 141,* 25–32.

Meuli, M., Meuli-Simmen, C., Hutchins, G. M., Seiler, M. J., Harrison, M. R., & Adzick, N. S. (1997). The spinal cord lesion in human fetuses with myelomeningocele. Implications for fetal surgery. *Journal of Pediatric Surgery, 32,* 448–452.

Meuli-Simmen, C., Meuli, M., Adzick, N. S., & Harrison, M. R. (1997). Latissimus dorsi flap procedures to cover myelomeningocele in utero: A feasibility study in human fetuses. *Journal of Pediatric Surgery, 32,* 1154–1156.

Meyer, R. E., & Siega-Riz, A. M. (2002). Sociodemographic patterns in spina bifida with prevalence trends—North Carolina, 1995–1999. *Morbidity Mortality Weekly Report, 51,* 12–15.

Milunsky, A., & Alpert, E. (1976a). Prenatal diagnosis of neural tube deficits: 1. Problems and pitfalls: Analysis of 2495 cases using the alpha-fetoprotein assay. *Journal of Obstetrics and Gynecology, 48,* 1–5.

Milunsky, A., & Alpert, E. (1976b). Prenatal diagnosis of neural tube deficit: 2. Analysis of false positive and false negative alpha-fetoprotein results. *Journal of Obstetrics and Gynecology, 48,* 6–12.

Missuna, C., & Pollack, N. (1991). Play deprivation in children with physical disabilities: The role of the occupational therapist in preventing secondary disability. *American Journal of Occupational Therapy, 45,* 882–888.

Mital, M. A., & Sakellarides, H. (1981). Surgery of the upper extremity in the retarded individual with spastic cerebral palsy. *Orthopedic Clinics of North America, 12,* 127–136.

Mobley, C. E., Harless, L. S., & Miller, K. L. (1996). Self-perception of preschool children with spina bifida. *Journal of Pediatric Nursing, 11,* 217–224.

Molenaers, G., Desloovere, K., & DeCat, J. (2001). Single event multi-level botulinum toxin type A treatment and surgery: Similarities and differences. *European Journal of Neurology, 8,* 88–97.

Molnar, G. E. (1979). Cerebral palsy prognosis and how to judge it. *Pediatric Annals, 8,* 10–24.

Molnar, G. E., & Gordon, S. U. (1976). Cerebral palsy: Predictive value of selective clinical signs for early prognostication of motor function. *Archives of Physical Medicine and Rehabilitation, 57,* 153–159.

Molnar, G. E., & Taft, L. T. (1977). Pediatric rehabilitation: Part I. Cerebral palsy and spinal cord injuries. *Current Problems in Pediatrics, 7,* 6–11.

Morrow, J. D. (1995). Temperament in the infant with myelomeningocele. *Journal of Pediatric Nursing, 10,* 99–104.

Mossberg, K. A., Linton, K. A., & Friske, K. (1990). Ankle-foot orthoses: Effect on energy expenditure of gait in spastic diplegic children. *Archives of Physical Medicine and Rehabilitation, 71,* 490–494.

Mundy, A. R., Shah, P. J. R., Borzyskowski, M., & Saxton, H. M. (1985). Sphincter behavior in myelomeningocele. *British Journal of Urology, 57,* 647–651.

Murphy, K. P., Molnar, G. E., & Lankasky, K. (1995). Medical and functional status of adults with cerebral palsy. *Developmental Medicine and Child Neurology, 37,* 1075–1084.

Murphy, K. P., Molnar, G. E., & Lankasky, K. (2000). Employment and social issues in adults with cerebral palsy. *Archives of Physical Medicine and Rehabilitation, 81,* 807–811.

Naeye, R. L., & Peter, E. C. (1989). Origins of cerebral palsy. *American Journal of Diseases of Childhood, 143,* 1154–1160.

Nelson, K. B. (1989). Relationship of intrapartum and delivery events to long-term neurologic outcome. *Clinics in Perinatology, 16,* 995–1007.

Nelson, K. B. (1998). Neonatal cytokines and coagulation factors in children with cerebral palsy. *Annals of Neurology, 44,* 665–675.

Nelson, K. B., & Ellenberg, J. H. (1979). Neonatal signs as predictors of cerebral palsy. *Pediatrics, 64,* 2–14.

Nelson, K. B., & Ellenberg, J. H. (1981). Apgar scores as predictors of chronic neurologic disability. *Pediatrics, 68,* 36–46.

Nelson, K. B., & Ellenberg, J. H. (1986). Antecedents of cerebral palsy. *New England Journal of Medicine, 315,* 81–86.

Noetzel, M. J., & Blake, J. N. (1991). Prognosis for seizure control and remission in children with myelomeningocele. *Developmental Medicine and Child Neurology, 33,* 803–810.

Nwaobi, O. M., & Smith, P. D. (1986). Effects of adaptive seating on pulmonary function in children with cerebral palsy. *Developmental Medicine and Child Neurology, 28,* 351–354.

Obojski, A., Chodorski, J., Borg, W., Medrala, W., Fal, A. M., & Malolepsz, Y. (2002). Latex allergy and sensitization in children with spina bifida. *Pediatric Neurosurgery, 37,* 262–266.

Palisano, R. J., Rosenbaum, P. L., Walter, S. D., & Hanna, S. (1997). Development and reliability of a system to classify gross motor function in children with cerebral palsy. *Developmental Medicine and Child Neurology, 39,* 214–223.

Palmer, F. B., Shapiro, B. K., Allen, M. C., Mosher, B. S., Bilker, S. A., Harryman, S. E., et al. (1990). Infant stimulation curriculum for infants with cerebral palsy: Effects on infant temperament, parent infant interaction and home environment. *Pediatrics, 85,* 411–415.

Palmer, F. B., Shapiro, B. K., & Wachtel, R. C. (1988). Effects of physical therapy on cerebral palsy. *New England Journal of Medicine, 318,* 803–808.

Pape, K. E., Kirsch, S. E., Galil, A., Boulton, J. E., White, M. A., & Chipman, M. (1993). Neuromuscular approach to the motor deficits of cerebral palsy: A pilot study. *Journal of Pediatrics Orthopaedics, 13,* 628–633.

Park, T. S., Cail, W. S., & Maggio, W. M. (1985). Progressive spasticity and scoliosis in children with myelomeningocele. *Journal of Neurosurgery, 62,* 367–375.

Peacock, W. J., Arens, L. J., & Berman, B. (1987). Cerebral palsy spasticity: Selective posterior rhizotomy. *Pediatric Neuroscience, 13,* 61–66.

Peacock, W. J., & Staudt, L. A. (1991). Functional outcomes following selective posterior rhizotomy for children with cerebral palsy. *Journal of Neurosurgery, 74,* 380–385.

Pecker, R., Damber, J. E., Hjalmas, K., Sjodin, J. G., & Von Zweigbergk, M. (1997). The urological fate of young adults with myelomeningocele: A three decade follow-up study. *European Urology, 32,* 213–217.

Penn, R. D., Mykleburst, B. M., Gottlieb, G. L., Agarwal, G. C., & Etzel, M. E. (1980). Chronic cerebellar stimulation for cerebral palsy. *Journal of Neurosurgery, 53,* 160–169.

Perlstein, M. A. (1952). Infantile cerebral palsy: Classification and clinical correlations. *Journal of the American Medical Association, 149,* 30–37.

Perry, J., & Hoffer, M. M. (1976). Pre-operative and post-operative dynamic electromyography as an aid in planning tendon transfer in children with cerebral palsy. *Journal of Bone and Joint Surgery, 58-A,* 531–543.

Petersen, T. (1987). Management of urinary incontinence in children with myelomeningocele. *Acta Neurologica Scandinavica, 75,* 52–55.

Pierce, S. R., Daly, K., Gallagher, K. G., Gershkoff, A. M., & Schaumburg, S. W. (2002). Constraint-induced therapy for a child with hemiplegic cerebral palsy: A case report. *Archives of Physical Medicine and Rehabilitation, 83,* 1462–1463.

Preiss, R. A., Condie, D. N., Rowley, D. I., & Graham, H. K. (2003). The effects of Botulinum Toxin (BTX-A) on spasticity of the lower limb and gait in cerebral palsy. *Journal of Bone and Joint Surgery, 85-B,* 943–948.

Raddish, M., Goldman, D. A., Kaplan, D. C., & Perrin, J. M. (1998). The immunization status of children with spina bifida. *American Journal of Diseases of Childhood, 147,* 849–853.

Radke, J., & Gosky, G. A. (1981). Hearing and speech screening in a hydrocephalus myelodysplasia population. *Spina Bifida Therapy, 3,* 25–26.

Rapp, C. E., & Torres, M. M. (2000). The adult with cerebral palsy. *Archives of Family Medicine, 9,* 466–472.

Reddihough, D. S., & Collins, K. J. (2003). The epidemiology and causes of cerebral palsy. *Australian Journal of Physiotherapy, 49,* 7–12.

Reese, M. E., Msall, M. E., & Owens, S. (1991). Acquired cervical spine impairment in young adults with cerebral palsy. *Developmental Medicine and Child Neurology, 33,* 153–156.

Reigel, D. H. (1983). Tethered spinal cord. *Concepts in Pediatric Neurosurgery, 4,* 142–164.

Reimers, J. (1990). Functional changes in the antagonists after lengthening of the agonists in cerebral palsy. *Clinics in Orthopaedics, 253,* 30–37.

Resnick, M. B., Eyler, F. D., Nelson, R. M., Eitman, D. V., & Bucciarelli, R. L. (1987). Developmental intervention for low birth weight infants: Improved early developmental outcome. *Pediatrics, 80,* 68–74.

Rezaie, P., & Dean, A. (2002). Periventricular leukomalacia, inflammation and white matter lesions within the developing nervous system. *Neuropathology, 22,* 106–132.

Rietberg, C. C., & Lindhout, D. (1993). Adult patients with spina bifida cystica. *European Journal of Obstetrics, Gynecology and Reproductive Biology, 52,* 63–70.

Robinson, H. P., Hood, V. D., Adam, A. H., Gibson, A. A. M., & Ferguson-Smith, M. A. (1980). Diagnostic ultrasound: Early detection of fetal neural tube defects. *Obstetrics and Gynecology, 56,* 705–710.

Robinson, R. O. (1973). The frequency of other handicaps in children with cerebral palsy. *Developmental Medicine and Child Neurology, 15,* 305–316.

Rosenstein, S. N. (1982). *Dentistry in cerebral palsy and related handicapping conditions.* Springfield, IL: Charles C Thomas.

Rotenstein, D., & Riegel, D. H. (1996). Growth hormone treatment of children with neural tube defects: Results from 6 months to 6 years. *Journal of Pediatrics, 128,* 184–189.

Rothman, J. G. (1978). Effects of respiratory exercises on the vital capacity and forced volume in children with cerebral palsy. *Physical Therapy, 58,* 421–425.

Sala, D. A., & Grant, A. D. (1995). Prognosis for ambulation in cerebral palsy. *Developmental Medicine and Child Neurology, 37,* 1020–1026.

Salakor, P. T., Sajaniemi, N., Hallback, H., Kari, A., Rila, H., & von Wendt, L. (1997). Randomization study of the effects of antenatal dexamethasone on growth and development of premature children at the corrected age of two years. *Acta Paediatrica, 86,* 294–298.

Samilson, R. L. (1981). Current concepts of surgical management in the lower extremities in cerebral palsy. *Clinical Orthopaedics, 158,* 99–113.

Sgoros, S., & Seri, S. (2002). The effect of intrathecal Baclofen on muscle co-contraction in children with spasticity of cerebral origin. *Pediatric Neurosurgery, 37,* 225–230.

Shafer, M. F., & Dias, L. S. (1983). *Myelomeningocele: Orthopedic treatment.* Baltimore: Williams & Wilkins.

Shapiro, A., & Susa, K. Z. (1990). Pre-operative and post-operative gait evaluation in cerebral palsy. *Archives of Physical Medicine and Rehabilitation, 71,* 236–240.

Sharrard, W. J. W. (1964). Posterior iliopsoas transplantation in the treatment of paralytic dislocation of the hip. *Journal of Bone and Joint Surgery, 46-B,* 426–444.

Sherk, H. H., Uppal, G. S., Lane, G., & Melchionni, J. (1991). Treatment versus non-treatment of hip dislocations in ambulatory patients with myelomeningocele. *Developmental Medicine and Child Neurology, 33,* 491–494.

Sillanpaa, M., Piekkala, P., & Pisira, H. (1982). The young adult with cerebral palsy and his chances of employment. *International Journal of Rehabilitation Research, 5,* 467–476.

Siperstein, G. N., Wolraich, M. L., Reed, D., & O'Keefe, P. (1988). Medical decisions and prognostications of pediatricians for infants with myelomeningocele. *Journal of Pediatrics, 113,* 835–840.

Slater, J. E. (1989). Rubber anaphylaxis. *New England Journal of Medicine, 320,* 1126–1129.

Smith, K. A. (1991). Bowel and bladder management of the child with myelomeningocele in the school setting. *Journal of Pediatrics Health Care, 4,* 175–180.

Smith, S., Camfield, C., & Camfield, D. (1999). Living with cerebral palsy and tube feeding: A population-based follow-up study. *Journal of Pediatrics, 135,* 307–310.

Sousa, J. C., Gordon, L. H., & Shurtleff, D. B. (1976). Assessing the development of daily living skills in patients with spina bifida. *Developmental Medicine and Child Neurology, 37*(Suppl. 18), 134–143.

Spindel, M. R., Bauer, S. B., & Dyron, I. M. (1987). The changing lesion in myelodysplasia. *Journal of the American Medical Association, 258,* 1630–1633.

Staheli, L. T. L., Duncan, W. R., & Schaefer, E. (1960). Growth alterations in the hemiplegic child. *Clinical Orthopaedics, 60,* 205–212.

Stallard, J., Major, R. E., & Farmer, S. E. (1996). The potential for ambulation by severely handicapped cerebral palsy patients. *Prosthetics and Orthotics International, 20,* 122–128.

Stanley, F., & Blair, E. (1991). Why have we failed to reduce the frequency of cerebral palsy? *Medical Journal of Australia, 154,* 623–626.

Stark, G. D., & Baker, G. C. W. (1967). The neurological involvement of the lower limb in myelomeningocele. *Developmental Medicine and Child Neurology, 9,* 732–743.

Steinbok, P., Reiner, A. M., Beauchamp, R., Armstrong, R. W., & Cochrane, D. D. (1997). A randomized clinical trial to compare selective posterior rhizotomy plus physiotherapy with physiotherapy alone in children with spastic diplegic cerebral palsy. *Developmental Medicine and Child Neurology, 39,* 178–184.

Strauss, D., Cable, W., & Shavelte, R. (1999). Causes of excess mortality in cerebral palsy. *Developmental Medicine and Child Neurology, 41,* 580–585.

Streeter, G. L. (1942). Developmental horizons in human embryos: Description of age group XI, 13 to 20 somites, and age group XII, 21-29 somites. *Contributions to Embryology, 30,* 211–245.

Sutherland, D. H. (1984). *Gait disorders of childhood and adolescence.* Baltimore: Williams & Wilkins.

Swaminathan, S., Patton, J. Y., Ward, S. D. L., Jacobs, R. A., Sargent, C. W., & Keens, T. G. (1989). Abnormal control of ventilation in adolescents with myelodysplasia. *Journal of Pediatrics, 115,* 898–903.

Sweetser, P. M., Badell, A., Schneider, S., & Badlin, G. H. (1995). Effects of sacral dorsal rhizotomy on bladder function in patients with spastic cerebral palsy. *Neuroradiology and Urodynamics, 14,* 57–64.

Talwar, D., Baldwin, N. A., & Horbatt, C. (1995). Epilepsy in children with meningomyelocele. *Pediatric Neurology, 13,* 29–32.

Tardieu, C., de la Tour, H., Bret, M. D., & Tardieu, G. (1982). Muscle hypoextensibility in children with cerebral palsy. *Archives of Physical Medicine and Rehabilitation, 63,* 97–110.

Tardieu, C., & Lespargot, A. (1988). For how long must the soleus muscle be stretched each day to prevent contracture? *Developmental Medicine and Child Neurology, 30,* 3019.

Tardoff, K. (1986). Spontaneous remission in cerebral palsy. *Neuropediatrics, 17,* 19–22.

Teo, C., & Jones, R. (1996). Management of hydrocephalus by endoscopic third ventriculostomy in patients with myelomeningocele. *Pediatric Neurosurgery, 25,* 57–63.

Tew, B. (1979). The "cocktail party syndrome" in children with hydrocephalus and spina bifida. *British Journal of Disorders of Community, 14,* 89–101.

Thomas, S. S., Aiona, M. D., Pierce, R., & Piatt, J. H. (1996). Gait changes in children with spastic diplegia after selective dorsal rhizotomy. *Journal of Pediatric Orthopaedics, 16,* 474–752.

Tirosh, E., & Rabino, S. (1989). Physiotherapy for children with cerebral palsy. *American Journal of Diseases of Childhood, 143,* 551–553.

Tobimatsu, Y., & Nakamura, R. (2000). Retrospective study of factors affecting employability of individuals with cerebral palsy in Japan. *Tohoku Journal of Experimental Medicine, 192,* 291–299.

Tomlinson, P., & Sugarman, I. D. (1995). Complications in shunts in adults with spina bifida. *American Journal of Diseases of Childhood, 143,* 551–553.

Torre, M., Planche, D., Louis-Borrione, C., Sabiani, F., Lena, G., & Guys, J. M. (2002). Value of electrophysiological assessment after surgical treatment of spinal dysraphism. *Journal of Urology, 168,* 1759–1763.

U.K. collaborative study on alpha-fetoprotein measurement in antenatal screening for anencephaly and spina bifida in early pregnancy. (1977). *Lancet, 1,* 1323–1332.

van der Dussen, L., Nieuwstraten, W., Roebroeck, M., & Stam., H. J. (2001). Functional level of young adults with cerebral palsy. *Clinical Rehabilitation, 15,* 84–91.

Vannucci, R. C. (1990). Experimental biology of cerebral hypoxic ischemia: Relationship of perinatal brain damage. *Pediatric Research, 27,* 317–326.

Vaughn, C. W., Neilson, P. D., & O'Dwyer, N. J. (1988). Motor control deficits in oro-facial muscles in cerebral palsy. *Journal of Neurology, Neurosurgery and Psychiatry, 51,* 534–539.

Veland, P. M., Hustad, S., Schneede, J., Refsum, H., & Vollset, S. (2001). Biological and clinical implications of MTHFR C677T polymorphism. *Trends in Pharmacological Science, 22,* 195–201.

Vohr, B. R., & Msall, M. E. (1997). Neuropsychological and functional outcomes of very low birth weight infants. *Seminars in Perinatology, 21,* 202–220.

Wallace, S. J. (1973). The effect of upper-limb function on mobility of children with myelomeningocele. *Developmental Medicine and Child Neurology, 15,* 84–91.

Wallander, J. L., Babani, L., Varni, J. W., Banis, H. T., & Wilcox, K. T. (1989). Family resources as resistance factors for psychological maladjustment in chronically ill and handicapped children. *Journal of Pediatric Psychology, 14,* 157–173.

Wallender, J. L., Feldman, W., & Varni, J. W. (1989). Physical status and psychological adjustment in children with spina bifida. *Journal of Pediatric Psychology, 14,* 89–102.

Wallender, J. L., Varni, J. W., Babani, L., Deltaan, C. B., Wilcox, K. T., & Banis, H. T. (1989)The social environment and the adaptation of mothers of physically handicapped children. *Journal of Pediatric Psychology, 14,* 371–387.

Waller, D. K., Mills, J. L., Simpson, J. L., Cunningham, G. C., Conley, M. R., Lassman, M. R., et al. (1995). Are obese woman at greater risk for producing malformed offspring? *American Journal of Obstetrics and Gynecology, 172,* 245–247.

Williams, M. D., Lewandowski, L. J., Coplan, J., & D'Eugenio, D. B. (1987). Neurodevelopmental outcome of preschool children born preterm with and without intracranial hemorrhage. *Developmental Medicine and Child Neurology, 29,* 243–249.

Wills, K. E., Holmbeck, G. N., Dillon, K., & McClone, D. G. (1990). Intelligence and achievement in children with myelomeningocele. *Journal of Pediatrics Psychology, 15,* 161–176.

Wilson, H., Haideri, M. E., Song, K., & Telford, D. (1997). Ankle foot orthosis for perambulatory children with spastic diplegia. *Journal of Pediatric Orthopaedics, 17,* 370–376.

Wolf, L. S., & McLaughlin, J. F. (1992). Early motor development in infants with meningomyelocele. *Pediatric Physical Therapy, 3,* 12–17.

Wordmark, E., Janlo, G. B., & Hagglund, G. (2000). Comparison of the Gross Motor Function Measure and Paediatric Evaluation of Disability Inventory in assessing motor function in children undergoing selective dorsal rhizotomy. *Developmental Medicine and Child Neurology, 42,* 245–252.

Worley, G., Rosenfeld, L. R., & Lipscomb, J. (1991). Financial counseling for families of children with chronic disabilities. *Developmental Medicine and Child Neurology, 33,* 679–689.

Worley, G., Schuster, J. M., & Oakes, W. J. (1991). The influence on survival of cervical laminectomy for children with meningomyelocele who have potentially lethal brainstem dysfunction due to the Chiari II malformation. *Developmental Medicine and Child Neurology, 33*(Suppl. 64), 19–26.

Worley, G., Schuster, J. M., & Oakes, W. J. (1996). Survival at 5 years of a cohort of newborn infants with myelomeningocele. *Developmental Medicine and Child Neurology, 38,* 816–822,

Yamada, S., Zinke, D. E., & Saunders, D. (1981). Pathophysiology of tethered cord syndrome. *Journal of Neurosurgery, 54,* 494–503.

Yokochi, K. (1997). Thalamic lesions revealed by M. R. I. associated with periventricular leukomalacia and clinical profiles of suspect. *Acta Paediatrica, 86,* 493–496.

Young, R. R., & Delwaide, P. J. (1981). Drug therapy: Spasticity. *New England Journal of Medicine, 304,* 28–43.

Zide, B., Constantini, S., & Epstein, F. J. (1995). Prevention of recurrent tethered spinal cord. *Pediatric Neurosurgery, 22,* 111–114.

Ziv, I., Blackborn, N., Rang, M., & Koresk, J. (1984). Muscle growth in normal and spastic mice. *Developmental Medicine and Child Neurology, 26,* 94–99.

19

Peripheral Vascular Disorders

GLENN R. JACOBOWITZ, MD

PERIPHERAL VASCULAR DISEASE encompasses not only diseases of arteries and veins, but also multiple underlying medical conditions such as coronary artery disease, diabetes, and renal insufficiency which are associated with, and are often the cause of, the vascular pathology. Such a broad range of diseases involves the entire body, literally from head to toe. The brain, abdominal viscera, lungs, and upper and lower extremities are all end organs affected by vascular disease. It is not uncommon for one patient to manifest different aspects of vascular disease. There are various functional presentations which must be recognized. After treatment of peripheral vascular disease, patients are often left with disabilities which require extensive rehabilitation, both physical and psychological. Ambulation and activities of daily living must often be re-learned following either revascularization or amputation of an extremity. Cerebrovascular disease may lead to central cognitive and/or motor deficits. A wide range of services may be required for these patients, including physical therapy, occupational therapy, and psychosocial support services. In addition, rehabilitation physicians and staff must be aware of the chronic nature of peripheral vascular disease. In the rehabilitation phase of recovery, these patients may have recurrence of their disease (e.g., leg ischemia, transient ischemic attack) which must be recognized and expeditiously treated. Therefore, it is critical for the rehabilitation physician to have an understanding of the functional presentation and treatment of peripheral vascular disease.

The broad scope of peripheral vascular disease may be separated into several areas. A practical organization should include: (a) lower-extremity peripheral arterial occlusive disease, (b) cerebrovascular disease, (c) venous disease, and (d) peripheral and abdominal arterial aneurysmal disease. All of these entities are associated with specific medical presentations, indications for operation, treatment modalities, recovery regimens, and disabilities which warrant separate attention, and will therefore be reviewed individually.

FUNCTIONAL PRESENTATION

LOWER EXTREMITY PERIPHERAL ARTERIAL OCCLUSIVE DISEASE

THERE ARE SEVERAL disease processes, associated disorders, and degrees of disability related to lower extremity peripheral vascular disease (PVD). The most common is atherosclerotic occlusive disease. Patients with chronic lower extremity ischemia have been divided into two groups. The first includes patients with intermittent claudication, who are considered to have a good prognosis, benign course, and low rate of amputation or need for surgical intervention. The second group, in contrast, includes patients with limb-threatening ischemia. These patients have been thought to have a poor prognosis with almost certain amputation if no intervention could be performed. The definition of limb-threatening ischemia is rest pain or the presence of gangrene in the extremity.

In the past, the presence of limb-threatening ischemia was the primary indication for surgical intervention and the appropriate angiographic studies. However, as the diagnostic and interventional armamentarium has expanded in recent years, previous indications for intervention and imaging have been re-evaluated. The advent of balloon angioplasty, intra-arterial stenting, thrombolytic agents, and endovascular prostheses have revolutionized the treatment of PVD. Imaging techniques, including both conventional angiography and magnetic resonance angiography (MRA), have greatly improved. There is now a multitude of treatment options for vascular disease, and physicians caring for patients with vascular disease should be aware of these options and the indications for their use.

The term claudication is derived from the latin verb "to limp." Intermittent claudication is defined as the inability to mount an appropriate augmentation of blood supply in response to exercise. It consists of three essential features: the pain is in a functional muscle unit, it is reproducibly precipitated by a consistent amount of exercise, and it is promptly relieved by a cessation of exercise. At least 10% of the population above the age of 70 as well as 1%–2% of younger patients have intermittent claudication (Peabody, Kannel, & McNamara, 1974). However, the vast majority of these patients can be treated non-operatively. A thorough understanding of the natural history of lower extremity ischemia and the available treatment options form the basis of sound clinical decision-making.

The most important studies on the natural history of intermittent claudication have focused not only on patient history, but also on objective evidence of arterial obstruction by arteriography or non-invasive means, such as ankle-brachial blood pressure indices. Some of these studies document up to 80% of such patients remaining stable or improving over 2.5–6 years (Imparato, Kim, Davidson, & Crowley, 1975; Jonason & Ringquiest, 1985). Other studies have shown only 40%–60% of claudication improvement over time (Cronenwett et al., 1984; Rosenbloom et al., 1988). Risk factors of worsening ischemia include cigarette smoking and diabetes. The single worst prognostic factor is the severity of arterial occlusive disease at the time of initial presentation (Imparato et al.; Jonason & Ringquiest; Cronenwett et al.; Rosenbloom et al.).

Limb-threatening ischemia occurs when resting blood flow is unable to meet baseline metabolic demands due to arterial occlusion. Clinically this presents as rest pain (typically in the most distal portion of the extremity, such as the forefoot or toes), ulceration, or gangrene. The pain is typically exacerbated by elevation of the extremity and alleviated by placing the leg in a dependent position from which arterial pressure is increased by gravity. Ischemic ulceration may occur when minor traumatic lesions fail to heal due to inadequate blood flow. Gangrene occurs when arterial blood flow is so poor that areas with the least perfusion undergo spontaneous necrosis (see Figure 19.1).

The assumption that rest pain or tissue loss results in uniform limb loss is not entirely valid, as shown by several studies using non-operative therapy (Rivers, Veith, Ascer, & Gupta, 1986; Schuler et al., 1984). Chronic ischemia represents a spectrum of levels of disease from fairly benign, mild intermittent claudication to gangrene in the extremity. The likelihood of limb loss remains related to the severity of the ischemia at initial presentation, as measured both angiographically and via arterial Doppler signals. Absent Doppler signals carry a poor prognosis for the limb in question if no intervention is performed (Felix, Siegel, & Gunther, 1987).

The success of exercise and cessation of smoking makes this non-operative therapy the first treatment option in patients with intermit-

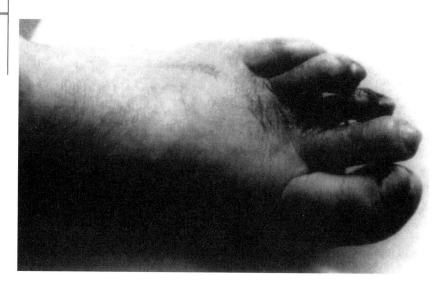

FIGURE 19.1   Gangrene of the left third toe resulting from ischemia.

tent claudication. An addition reason is the observation (although controversial) that a failed bypass graft may acutely induce limb-threatening ischemia or ultimately necessitate a higher level of amputation than a non-operated limb (Schlenker & Wolkoff, 1975; Dardik, Kahn, Dardik, Sussman, & Ibrahim, 1982). Operative management is thus reserved for threatened limb loss as determined by clinical and angiographic parameters.

EXTRACRANIAL CEREBROVASCULAR DISEASE

CEREBROVASCULAR DISEASE MAY include disease of the aortic arch, carotid arteries, or the vertebrobasilar system. Functional presentation of extracranial cerebrovascular disease may be asymptomatic, a transient ischemic attack (e.g., amaurosis fugax or other neurologic deficit resolving within 24 hours), or following a completed stroke. Depending on the degree of disability, patients may require varying degrees of rehabilitation and support services. It is extremely important to evaluate the extracranial circulation in patients presenting for rehabilitation after strokes so that further strokes may be prevented when possible by surgical or medical intervention.

The diagnosis and treatment of extracranial cerebrovascular disease begins at the aortic valve. The decrease in annual stroke rate in the United States has paralleled the increase in the frequency of carotid endarterectomy (Lamparello & Riles, 1975). Currently more than 100,000 carotid endarterectomies are performed annually in this country. Over the last 40 years, the safety of carotid surgery has progressed, with most large centers reporting perioperative morbidity and mortality rates of less than 2%. Indications for extracranial cerebral revascularization have been well defined for both symptomatic and asymptomatic patients in large prospective, randomized trials. The North American Symptomatic Carotid Endarterectomy Trial (NASCET) established that symptomatic patients with greater than 70% diameter reduction of the internal carotid artery have a significant reduction in the incidence of stroke with surgery when compared to medical management alone (NASCET, 1991). Similarly, the Asymptomatic Carotid Atherosclerosis Study (ACAS) demonstrated better stroke prevention in patients with greater than 60% stenosis treated with endarterectomy versus those treated medically (ACAS, 1995). As noted above, these patients may present after completed strokes, with a history of a transient ischemic attack, or they may be asymptomatic, with carotid stenoses detected on duplex examinations performed as part of a work-up for a bruit heard on physical exam or for non-specific neurological symptoms.

Upper extremity ischemia is also often related to aortic arch disease. Emboli to the hands or fingers may originate in the chambers of the heart, aortic arch, or axillary and subclavian arteries. Transesophageal echocardiography (TEE) and aortic arch and upper extremity angiography are the tests of choice for identifying a potential source of emboli. Magnetic resonance angiography may also be useful. Functional presentation is similar to that in the lower extremity with the sudden onset of pain and cyanosis of the distal hand or fingers. Pulses may be absent. Collateral circulation of the upper extremity is usually excellent, often allowing the hand to remain viable during work-up.

In the last decade, significant advancements have been made in the technology and efficacy of carotid artery stenting. This is a less invasive procedure that can be performed under local anesthesia via a femoral arterial puncture. Long-term results are still not available, but there appears to be a benefit from carotid stenting, particularly for high-risk surgical patients (Yaday, 2002). This includes patients with significant medical comorbidities, anatomically inaccessible lesions, and radiation induced carotid stenosis (Veith et al., 2001). It is not uncommon for patients undergoing rehabilitation to have significant medical comorbidities, and the risks and benefits of carotid stenting versus carotid endarterectomy should be considered. Early results of carotid stenting had higher rates of periprocedural strokes, but this complication has been significantly reduced with the advent of balloon and umbrella type cerebral protection devices which are temporarily deployed during the procedure to prevent distal embolization of plaque material.

VENOUS DISEASE

PATIENTS WITH VENOUS disorders frequently exhibit a chronic course and are not often dramatically improved by surgical procedures. Chronic venous insufficiency is the most common form of venous disease, and non-operative therapy remains the mainstay of treatment. The other form of venous disease seen commonly, especially in the non-ambulatory patient, is acute deep venous thrombosis. This is more sudden in onset and requires systemic anticoagulation or occasionally placement of a vena caval filter. These two forms of venous disease will be discussed separately.

Chronic Venous Insufficiency

The functional presentation of chronic venous insufficiency (CVI) includes swelling, pain, and ulceration of the lower extremity. This is due to valvular incompetence of the venous system resulting in increased hydrostatic pressure. Typically, CVI presents as swelling of the distal lower extremity with thickening of the subcutaneous tissue in the perimalleolar "gaiter" distribution. Mild CVI is associated with mild to moderate ankle edema. Often the patients complain of a feeling of heaviness or pain in the legs. This mild form of insufficiency is usually limited to the superficial veins. Moderate CVI presents with hyperpigmentation of the skin, moderate brawny edema, and subcutaneous fibrosis without ulceration. Severe CVI is associated with ulceration, eczemoid skin changes (stasis dermatitis), and severe edema. Extensive involvement of the deep venous system and diffuse loss of valvular function are present.

The venous anatomy consists of a superficial and a deep system. In the lower extremity, the longest superficial vein, the greater saphenous vein, is located anterior to the medial malleolus and courses along the medial aspect of the leg until it reaches the sapheno-femoral junction in the medial aspect of the proximal thigh. Connecting the superficial system to the deep system are the perforating veins.

The perforating veins are variable in location. However, the most important set is in the medial aspect of the lower leg, called Cockett's perforators. Insufficiency of the valves in these perforators leads to the characteristic physical findings of CVI in the postero-medial malleolar area. Blood flow in the leg is from the superficial to the deep system via the perforating veins. Blood is propelled to the heart via the deep veins. Failure of any of the venous valves, perforators, or calf muscle pump (which acts to force blood against gravity) will create a situation where the lower leg is exposed to the pressure created by a column of blood. The sustained venous hypertension is felt to be the cause of CVI. The venous hypertension is transmitted to the skin causing dermal proliferation. Eventually, lymphatic destruction occurs with the subsequent accumulation of colloid materials in the subcutaneous tissue. The resulting edema and fibrin deposition causes cellular damage and eventual ulceration.

Bed rest and limb elevation have universally been accepted as effective therapy for CVI. However, they are impractical for most patients, particularly those in a rehabilitation program promoting ambulation. Effective therapy must control the symptoms of CVI, promote healing, and prevent recurrence of venous stasis ulcers while allowing for normal ambulation.

Several studies have shown the benefits of compression stockings in the treatment of CVI and venous ulceration (Dinn & Henry, 1992; Mayberry, Moneta, & Taylor, 1991). Cellulitis may be associated with CVI and often requires oral or intravenous antibiotic therapy. Hydrocortisone cream may help surround stasis dermatitis. Typical compression stockings have 30 to 40 torr of elastic compression at the level of the ankle, which gradually decreases more proximally. This type of stocking may be used with normal arterial circulation. If arterial circulation is compromised, a stocking with less compression must be used. In addition, Ace bandages may be used. There are multiple brands of compression stockings on the market, with different designs to make application possible for the patient with disability.

Acute Deep Venous Thrombosis

Acute deep venous thrombosis may occur in the upper or (more commonly) the lower extremity. In the upper extremity, thrombus may occur in the axillo-subclavian vein, and the most common causes are thoracic outlet syndrome and catheter-related thrombosis. Under most circumstances, one or more of the features of Virchow's triad for venous thrombosis is present. The triad includes endothelial injury (as by a catheter), stasis (as by thoracic outlet obstruction), or a hypercoagulable state (as with some malignancies).

Functional presentation of upper extremity deep venous thrombosis includes swelling of the extremity, usually to the level of the axilla, and prominence of the subcutaneous veins over the shoulder girdle and the anterior chest wall, which become engorged with collateral venous flow due to obstruction of the deep vein (see Figure 19.2). Pain of an aching or stabbing type may be felt in the shoulder and axilla but can also be felt in the arm. These classic symptoms are particularly common in patients who thrombose acutely due to thoracic outlet compression. This can occur after weight-lifting or similar exertional activity with the upper extremity. Axillo-subclavian vein thrombosis may also present after sleeping, probably due to sleeping with the arm overhead (with the thoracic outlet partially obstructed).

Initial diagnosis of axillo-subclavian vein thrombosis is by venous

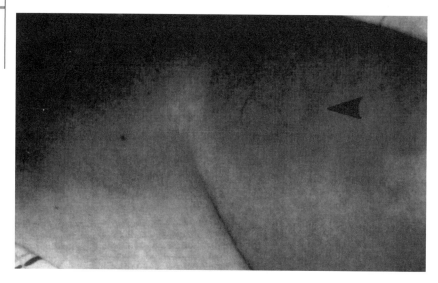

FIGURE 19.2   Swollen proximal left upper arm in patient with axillosubclavian thrombosis. Arrow shows engorged subcutaneous veins over anterior shoulder.

duplex examination. If this is negative but there is a high clinical index of suspicion, then a venogram should be performed. Similarly, if the duplex is positive and thrombolytic therapy is being considered, venography is indicated. The reported incidence of pulmonary embolism with untreated upper extremity deep venous thrombosis is about 9%–12% (Becker, Philbrick, & Walker, 1991). Patients should be treated with heparin anticoagulation followed by a 3 to 6 month course of Coumadin. Persistent symptoms are least likely in patients with catheter-related thrombosis. Chronic symptoms (arm swelling with exercise) occur in about 38% of patients treated with anticoagulation and 15% receiving thrombolytic therapy (intra-arterial urokinase infusion), compared with 64% receiving no therapy (Becker et al.). When axillo-subclavian vein thrombosis is recognized, a vascular surgeon should be consulted to further direct therapy. Unless contraindicated, anticoagulation should be started promptly to prevent further propagation of thrombus.

The signs and symptoms of lower extremity deep venous thrombosis are similar to that of the upper extremity. They include swelling of the limb, prominence of superficial veins, and pain which is usually dull in character. Unfortunately, physical examination is falsely negative in approximately 50% of patients with acute deep venous thrombosis, as well as falsely positive in patients with symptoms related to conditions other than deep venous thrombosis.

The acute complication of deep venous thrombosis is pulmonary embolism and the late complication is the post-thrombotic syndrome. This syndrome is that of chronic swelling and venous insufficiency due to valvular damage which occurs from the thrombus. Anticoagulation will reduce the risk of pulmonary embolus from approximately 25% if left untreated to less than 5% (Hyers, Hull, & Weg). In patients with a contraindication to anticoagulation, a vena-caval filter may be placed (usually percutaneously). Such a device will lower the incidence of pulmonary embolus to 2%–4%.

ABDOMINAL AORTIC AND PERIPHERAL ARTERIAL ANEURYSMAL DISEASE

ABDOMINAL AORTIC ANEURYSM (AAA) is defined as a focal dilation of the aorta of at least 50% greater than the expected normal diameter (Imparato et al., 1975) (see Figure 19.3). The main complication of AAA is rupture, for which the mortality rate may exceed 90%. The 5-year risk of rupture for AAA 5 cm or greater in diameter ranges from 25%–40%. This may be as high as 20% per year for aneurysms greater than 7 cm in diameter. Aneurysms measuring between 4 and 5 cm in diameter have lower

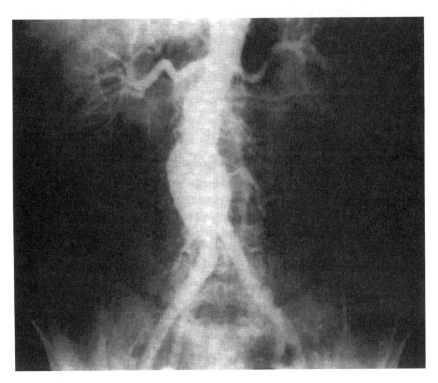

FIGURE 19.3   Angiogram of an infrarenal abdominal aortic aneurysm.

5-year rupture rates of about 3%–12% (Brown, Pattenden, & Gutelius, 1992). Aneurysms less than 4 cm in diameter have about a 2% rate of rupture. Overall elective surgical mortality is about 2%–4% (Ernst, 1993). Therefore, repair of AAA is reserved for asymptomatic aneurysms greater than 5 cm in diameter, symptomatic aneurysms (abdominal or back pain), or a ruptured AAA. Rarely, a laminated thrombus from the inner lining of an aneurysm sac may embolize to the lower extremities. This is also an indication for repair regardless of aneurysm diameter. Standard surgical repair is by replacement of the aneurysmal segment with a synthetic graft, usually of Dacron. Recent technological advances have included the successful usage of transfemorally placed vascular endografts which exclude the aneurysmal segment from arterial pressure. This method of endovascular repair has been shown to be effective in preventing AAA rupture with reduced patient morbidity and mortality (Arko et al., 2002; Zarins et al., 1999). Debilitated patients who were prohibitive risks for standard surgical repair are now often considered for the less invasive endovascular repair. Hospital stay is often as short as 2 days, and patients can resume oral intake within 1 day. Long-term complications include endoleaks, which occur when the endovascular graft does not completely seal off the aneurysm sac. These endoleaks can often be treated with additional endovascular maneuvers, but they require continued follow-up imaging with CT or duplex scanning.

AAA usually presents as a finding on routine physical examination (pulsatile abdominal mass) or as an incidental finding on a radiologic study (abdominal ultrasound, CT scan, or magnetic resonance image) obtained for other reasons. Any aneurysm greater than 3 cm in diameter should be brought to the attention of an internist or vascular surgeon who can follow the patient with yearly ultrasound examinations to monitor the aneurysm size. Average annual growth of AAA is about 0.4 cm in diameter per year.

Popliteal artery aneurysms (PAA) are the most common peripheral artery aneurysm. There is a strong association of PAA with AAA. A patient with a unilateral PAA has a 50% chance of having a contralateral PAA and a 30% chance of having an AAA. More than 90% of PAAs occur in men (Szilagyi, Schwartz, & Reddy, 1981).

A popliteal artery is considered aneurysmal if its diameter exceeds 2 cm or 1.5 times the diameter of the proximal, nonaneurysmal segment. The clinical presentation is variable. Almost 30% of PAAs are symptomatic. They are usually found on physical examination (pulsatile mass or wide pulse at popliteal fossa), or incidentally on ultrasound, CT scan, or magnetic resonance imaging of the popliteal fossa. Results of surgical management in this group of patients are excellent. Symptomatic PAAs usually present with distal embolization to the tibial arteries. Rupture is rare. This embolization is often severe, with lower limb ischemia occurring in up to 70% of patients and amputation rates as high as 20% (Reilly, Abbott, & Darling, 1983). Elective repair of all PAAs is recommended because of the high rate of limb loss once these aneurysms become symptomatic.

PSYCHOLOGICAL AND VOCATIONAL IMPLICATIONS

PERIPHERAL VASCULAR DISEASE can leave patients with severe vocational impairment and psychological stress. Partial or complete amputation of a limb and the ramifications of strokes can be tremendously disabling, both physically and psychologically.

Two thirds of all lower-extremity amputations are currently performed as a result of complications of peripheral vascular disease or diabetes. As a result, a majority of lower-extremity amputations are being performed by vascular surgeons. The purpose of amputation is to remove gangrenous tissue, relieve pain, obtain primary healing of the most distal amputation possible, and obtain maximum rehabilitation after amputation.

It has been shown that the greatest chance of successful ambulation is with expeditious rehabilitation, either by immediate postoperative prosthesis or accelerated conventional programs utilizing a temporary prosthesis until a permanent prosthesis can be made (Folsum, King, & Rubin, 1992). Advantages of early ambulation include decreased hospital time, increased rates of rehabilitation, a reduction in the complications of amputation, and an improvement in the psychological outcome of the patient after amputation (Bradway, Racy, & Malone, 1984). Early ambulation alleviates a sense of loss and inadequacy experienced by many amputees. It is clear that a full rehabilitation team provides the best outcome. This should include the rehabilitation physician, prosthetist, physical and occupational therapists, social services, the patient's family, and community services.

Peripheral vascular disease is present in many patients who have had strokes, and it is commonly the underlying cause of those strokes. Fortunately, the perioperative stroke rate for carotid endarterectomy in most major centers is less than 3%. However, many patients present with a completed stroke prior to carotid endarterectomy, and the operation serves only to prevent further infarction. As a result, many patients with peripheral vascular disease, particularly those with extracranial cerebrovascular disease, may require rehabilitation from stroke.

Major factors affecting rehabilitation of stroke victims include motivation and family support (Evans & Northwood, 1983). In addition, depression may be a significant complication of stroke, and it can inhibit patient motivation (Parikh, Lipsey, & Robinson, 1987). Anxiety and fear are also common among stroke victims. This distress can be eased by an empathetic rehabilitation team. The recovery of physical function and motor skills is often enhanced by emotional stability of the patient. In turn, the return of function enhances psychosocial functioning. Thus, psychosocial, recreational, and vocational interventions must all be provided. Peer support may also be extremely helpful. All of these services should be provided in the setting of a directed stroke rehabilitation program, which has been shown to enhance functional ability beyond that of natural recovery (Kalra, 1994).

Age alone probably does not play a major role in determining the recovery of a patient with stroke. However, it may be associated with significant medical comorbidities (such as peripheral vascular disease) which may make recovery more difficult. Consequently, older patients may have longer recovery times and require increased psychosocial support.

CONCLUSIONS

PATIENTS WITH PERIPHERAL vascular disease usually have multiple medical problems, and the nature of their disease may be chronic and involve multiple organ systems. The high incidence of limb surgery, limb loss, and stroke make patients with peripheral vascular disease in particular need of rehabilitation medicine and services. The chronic nature of peripheral vascular disease requires the rehabilitation team to be keenly aware of its functional presentation, as recurrences or progression of disease are not uncommon. It is only with a full range of physical and psychological rehabilitation services that patients with peripheral vascular disease may be completely treated.

REFERENCES

Arko, F. W., Lee, W. A., Hil, B. B., Olcott, C., Dalman, D. L., Harris, E. J., et al. (2002). Aneurysm-related death: Endpoint analysis for comparison of open and endovascular repairs. *Journal of Vascular Surgery, 36,* 297–304.

Asymptomatic Carotid Atherosclerosis Study. Executive Committee. (1995). Endarterectomy for asymptomatic carotid artery stenosis. *Journal of the American Medical Association, 273,* 1421–1428.

Becker, D. M., Philbrick, J. T., & Walker, F. B. (1991). Axillary and subclavian venous thrombosis: Prognosis and treatment. *Archives of Internal Medicine, 151,* 1934–1943.

Bradway, J. P., Racy, J., & Malone, J. M. (1984). Psychological adaptation to amputation. *Orthotics and Prosthetics, 38,* 46–50.

Brown, P. M., Pattenden, R., & Gutelius, J. R. (1992). The selective management of small abdominal aortic aneurysms: The Kingston study. *Journal of Vascular Surgery, 15*, 21–27.

Cronenwett, J. L., Warner, K. G., Zelenock, G. B., Whitehouse, W. M., Graham, L. M., Lindenhauser, S. M., et al. (1984). Intermittent claudication: Current results of non-operative management. *Archives of Surgery, 119*, 430–436.

Dardik, H., Kahn, M., Dardik, I., Sussman, B., & Ibrahim, I. (1982). Influence of failed bypass procedures on conversion of below-knee to above-knee amputation levels. *Surgery, 91*, 64–69.

Dinn, E., & Henry, M. (1992). Treatment of venous ulceration by injection sclerotherapy and compression hosiery. *Phlebology, 7*, 23–26.

Ernst, C. B. (1993). Abdominal aortic aneurysm. *New England Journal of Medicine, 328*, 1167–1173.

Evans, R. L., & Northwood, L. (1983). Social support needs in adjustment to stroke. *Archives of Physical Medicine and Rehabilitation, 64*, 61–64.

Felix, W. R. Jr., Siegel, B., & Gunther, N. L. (1987). The significance for morbidity and mortality of Doppler-absent pedal pulses. *Journal of Vascular Surgery, 5*, 849–855.

Folsum, D., King, T., & Rubin, J. (1992). Lower extremity amputation with immediate postoperative prosthetic placement. *American Journal of Surgery, 164*, 320–323.

Hyers, T. M., Hull, R. D., & Weg, J. G. (1992). Antithrombotic therapy for venous thromboembolic disease. *Chest, 102*(Suppl.), 408–425.

Imparato, A. M., Kim, G. E., Davidson, T., & Crowley, J. G. (1975). Intermittent claudication: Its natural course. *Surgery, 78*, 795–799.

Johnston, K. W., Rutherford, R. B., Tilson, M. D., Shah, D. M., Hollier, L., & Stanley, C. (1991). Suggested standards for reporting on arterial aneurysms. Subcommittee on Reporting Standards for Arterial Aneurysms, Ad Hoc Committee in Reporting Standards, Society for Vascular Surgery and North American Chapter, International Society for Cardiovascular Surgery. *Journal of Vascular Surgery, 13*, 452–458.

Jonason, T., & Ringquiest, I. (1985). Factors of prognostic importance for subsequent rest pain in patients with intermittent claudication. *Acta Medicin Scandinavia, 218*, 27–33.

Kalra, L. (1994). The influence of stroke unit rehabilitation on functional recovery from stroke. *Stroke, 25*, 821–825.

Lamparello, P. J., & Riles, T. S. (1975). MR angiography in carotid stenosis: A clinical perspective. *MRI Clinics of North America, 3*, 455–465.

Mayberry, J. C., Moneta, G. L., & Taylor, L. M. (1991). Fifteen-year results of ambulation compression therapy for chronic venous ulcers. *Surgery, 109*, 573–581.

North American Symptomatic Carotid Endarterectomy Trial Collaborators. (1991). Beneficial effect of carotid endarterectomy in symptomatic patients with high-grade stenosis. *New England Journal of Medicine, 325*, 445–453.

Parikh, R. M., Lipsey, J. R., & Robinson, R. G. (1987). Two-year longitudinal study of post-stroke mood disorders: Dynamic changes in correlates of depression at one and two years. *Stroke, 18,* 579–584.

Peabody, C. N., Kannel, W. B., & McNamara, P. M. (1974). Intermittent claudication—surgical experience. *Archives of Surgery, 109,* 693–697.

Reilly, M. K., Abbott, W. M., & Darling, R. C. (1983). Aggressive surgical management of popliteal artery aneurysms. *American Journal of Surgery, 145,* 498–502.

Rivers, S. P., Veith, F. J., Ascer, E., & Gupta, S. K. (1986). Successful conservative therapy of severe limb-threatening ischemia: The value of nonsympathectomy. *Surgery, 99,* 759–762.

Rosenbloom, M. S., Flanigan, D. P., Schuler, J. J., Meyer, J. P., Durham, J. P., Edrup-Jorgensen, J., et al. (1988). Risk factors affecting the natural history of claudication. *Archives of Surgery, 123,* 867–870.

Schlenker, J. D., & Wolkoff, J. S. (1975). Major amputation after femoropopliteal bypass procedures. *American Journal of Surgery, 129,* 495–499.

Schuler, J. J., Flanigan, D. P., Holcroft, J. W., Ursprung, J. J., Mohrland, J. S. A., & Pyke, J. (1984). Efficacy of prostaglandin E1 in the treatment of lower extremity ischemic ulcers secondary to peripheral vascular occlusive disease: Results of a prospective randomized double-blind multicenter clinical trial. *Journal of Vascular Surgery, 1,* 160–170.

Szilagyi, D. E., Schwartz, R. I., & Reddy, D. L. (1981). Popliteal arterial aneurysms. *Archives of Surgery, 116,* 724–728.

Veith, F. J., Amor, M., Ohki, T., Beebe, H. G., Bell, P. R., Bolia, A., et al. (2001). Current status of carotid bifurcation angioplasty and stenting based on a consensus of opinion leaders. *Journal of Vascular Surgery, 33*(2 suppl.), S111–S116.

Yadav, J., for the SAPPHIRE Investigators. (2002). Stenting and angioplasty with protection in patients at high risk for endarterectomy: The SAPPHIRE study. *Circulation, 106,* 2986–2989.

Zarins, C. K., White, R. A., Schwarten, D., Kinney, K., Dietrich, E. B., Hodgson, K. J., et al. for the Investigators of the Medtronic AneuRx Multicenter Clinical Trial. (1999). AneuRx stent graft vs. open surgical repair of abdominal aneurysm: Multicenter prospective clinical trial. *Journal of Vascular Surgery, 29,* 292–308.

20

Psychiatric Disabilities

GARY R. BOND, PhD, KIKUKO CAMPBELL,
AND NATALIE DELUCA

THE TERM "PSYCHIATRIC" *disability* has been used by the vocational rehabilitation (VR) system to describe a range of psychiatric disorders interfering with the capacity to work and function successfully in the community. The VR disability coding system distinguishes three types of psychiatric disability: psychotic disorders, psychoneurotic disorders, and other character disorders. Derived from the psychiatric diagnostic system in practice 5 decades ago, these categories are now archaic. Currently, the diagnostic standards in the mental health field are codified in the Diagnostic and Statistical Manual Version IV Text Revision (DSM-IV-TR) (American Psychiatric Association, 2000a). This compendium of mental disorders is the culmination of work by the American Psychiatric Association (APA) begun in 1952 and updated periodically.

Unlike earlier diagnostic systems, DSM-IV-TR has adopted a descriptive, atheoretical stance toward classifying disorders. It attempts to define symptoms of psychiatric disorders based on observable criteria. To increase specificity, DSM-IV-TR uses a *multiaxial system* of diagnosis, with assessment on five distinct dimensions: clinical syndromes (Axis I), personality disorders and mental retardation (Axis II), general medical conditions (Axis III), psychosocial stressors (Axis IV), and current level of functioning (Axis V). Most pertinent to psychiatric disability are clinical syndromes and personality disorders; substance use disorders (on Axis I) and mental retardation (on Axis II) are grouped separately from the psychiatric disabilities not only by VR but also by most state mental health systems.

Proper assessment requires a trained diagnostician who administers a structured interview and has access to records of the patient's psychiatric history (First, Spitzer, Gibbon, & Williams, 1994). In practice, however, diagnoses are often given based on far less rigorous assessment procedures. Not only is the VR disability coding system archaic, it also does not reflect the limited role of psychiatric diagnoses in rehabilitation. Although important for treatment planning, particularly medication decisions, diagnosis is less relevant to rehabilitation planning than is a functional assessment of the individual's strengths and weaknesses in specific environments (Anthony, Cohen, Farkas, & Gagne, 2002). This chapter will first briefly describe the major psychiatric syndromes and then address the associated functional impairments that define the degree to which a psychiatric disorder can be disabling.

KEY PSYCHIATRIC DIAGNOSES

INFORMATION ON PSYCHIATRIC diagnosis is widely available in many sources, ranging from technical manuals (APA, 1994) to less technical but detailed sources such as abnormal psychology textbooks and guides for the general public (Andreasen, 1984; Bernheim, Lewine, & Beale, 1982; Mueser & Gingerich, 1994; Torrey, 2001). Space does not permit more than a general description of only a few of the major psychiatric classifications.

SCHIZOPHRENIA & RELATED DISORDERS

GIVEN ITS DEBILITATING symptoms and profound impact on the person, the family, and society, schizophrenia is the most severe of all psychopathologies. It is a complex disorder, affecting individuals in diverse ways, including the ability to think clearly, to sort out and interpret incoming sensations, and to act decisively. Difficulties in relating to others is perhaps the most common characteristic of schizophrenia (Mueser & Tarrier, 1998). Schizophrenia is a *psychotic* disorder that typically is punctuated by episodes of impaired reality testing, as indicated by disorientation and confusion, odd sensory experiences, false beliefs, and/or severe disturbances of mood. The course of the illness is highly individualized. For some, psychotic episodes are brief and nonrecurrent (as in brief reactive psychosis); in other individuals, there are acute episodes interspersed with normal or near-normal adjustment. In still other instances, the disturbance is relatively continuous, punctuated by periods of temporary improvement and deterioration.

A commonly accepted prevalence rate for schizophrenia is that it affects approximately 1% of the population at any time, but epidemiological studies differ (Andreasen, 1984; Torrey, 2001). A review of recent major epidemiological studies concluded that schizophrenia occurs in all populations with a prevalence rate in the range of 1.4 to 4.6 per 1000 (Jablensky, 2000). The peak age of onset of schizophrenia is 15–30; however, approximately 15% of persons with the disorder may experience initial symptoms after age 45 (Harris & Jeste, 1988). Males are as likely as females to develop schizophrenia, but males are more likely to have their first psychiatric hospitalization before the age of 25, whereas the opposite is true after the age of 25. Related diagnoses in the DSM-IV include *schizophreniform disorder*, which applies when all the symptoms of schizophrenia are present, but the duration of the disorder is less than 6 months, and *schizoaffective disorder*, where symptoms of schizophrenia are accompanied by prominent affective symptoms (depression and/or mania).

Positive symptoms of schizophrenia comprise hallucinations (sensory experiences in the absence of any environmental stimuli), delusions (false and often bizarre beliefs, usually held firmly even in the face of disconfirming evidence), and disorganized speech. Hallucinations in schizophrenia are most often auditory, frequently in the form of hearing voices. In a major study of schizophrenia, 74% of the sample reported auditory hallucinations (Sartorius, Shapiro, & Jablonsky, 1974). Delusions range from innocuous confusions to extensive paranoid delusions involving perceived threats from conspiracies of seemingly unrelated people and events. Delusions often involve *ideas of reference*, where one attaches personal significance to unrelated activities of others (e.g., concluding that an overheard conversation between strangers refers to oneself). *Paranoid delusions* may be combined with *delusions of grandeur*, an exaggerated belief in one's own powers and sometimes the assumption of the identity of a famous person. *Thought broadcasting* (belief in the ability to transmit thoughts directly from one's mind to another person) and *thought insertion* (belief in the reception of thoughts in this fashion) are also positive symptoms of schizophrenia.

Other common symptoms relate to peculiar patterns of speech, such as *loose associations* (odd juxtaposition of topics and ideas), *neologisms* (invented words with private meanings), and poverty of speech (conversation conveying little information). Persons with schizophrenia have difficulty with words that have more than one meaning; a word they interpret with the wrong meaning may lead them off on a tangent. They are also often baffled by simple analogies, as suggested by their poor performance in diagnostic tests requiring that they interpret common proverbs. Green (1996) concluded that deficits in verbal memory and vigilance are common in people with schizophrenia, and that these neurocognitive deficits affect their everyday functioning.

Negative symptoms of schizophrenia consist of patterns of nonresponsivity: passivity, a lack of spontaneity, *flat affect* (a lack of emotional expression), social withdrawal, a lack of motivation, and *anhedonia* (an inability to experience pleasure). Flat affect is especially common, present in about two thirds of individuals with schizophrenia (Sartorius et al., 1974). The negative symptom of *ambivalence* (difficulty making decisions) may perpetuate a pattern of inaction. Negative symptoms usually interfere more with psychosocial functioning than do positive symptoms. Family members often find negative symptoms the most distressing aspect of schizophrenia, and more burdensome than positive symptoms (Mueser & Glynn, 1995).

MOOD DISORDER

THE TWO MAJOR types of mood disorders (also known as "affective disorders") are depressive disorders and bipolar disorders. Mood disorders are very common. The 1-year prevalence rates of mood disorders are 10.3% for *major depression*, 2.5% for *dysthymic disorder* (a chronic dysphoria or anhedonia not severe enough to meet the full criteria for major depression), and 1.3% for *bipolar disorder* (Kessler et al., 1994). During a lifetime, roughly 20% of women and 10% of men will suffer a *major depressive episode*; about a third of them will be hospitalized (Maxmen & Ward, 1995). Bipolar disorders affect men and women equally (APA, 1994). The age of onset for depression is highly variable, while the average age of onset of bipolar disorder is in the late 20s (APA).

The cognitive symptoms of depression include negative, pessimistic beliefs; distorted, negative self-image (including feelings of guilt and worthlessness); suicidal thoughts; and trouble concentrating. Whereas disordered thought in schizophrenia is often bizarre and puzzling, the distortions accompanying major depression are usually coherent, albeit often magnifying difficulties and jumping to distorted conclusions from incomplete information or selective attention to details. Beck (1967) has termed these distortions *faulty logic*. Depression also includes physical symptoms such as lethargy, insomnia or hypersomnia, loss of appetite or overeating, and lack of sexual interest. Severe depression can be termed psychotic when it includes hallucinations or delusions (e.g., "I am dead"). Depression is probably the widest-ranging psychiatric disorder in terms of severity and duration. There are vexing diagnostic problems, for example, in deciding if depressed feelings accompanying a physical disability or recent bereavement qualify as a separate psychiatric diagnosis.

Bipolar disorder (also known as "manic depression") differs symptomatically from major depression primarily by the presence of *mania*, an episode of elevated or irritable mood. Manic episodes last from several days to several months. In its most severe form, bipolar disorder involves frequent alternation between manic and depressive episodes (*rapid cycling*), but there are many different patterns including those in which either mania or depression rarely occurs. Persons experiencing a manic episode are expansive, unrealistically happy (although they can also be irritable when thwarted), impulsive, and easily distracted. They often have an exaggerated belief in their own abilities and make reckless decisions (e.g., extravagant purchases). Another common symptom is nonstop talking (*pressured speech*), even when others try to break in, or when no one is listening. Their conversation may show *flight of ideas* in which they quickly shift from one unfinished topic to another.

ANXIETY DISORDERS

AFFECTING 12.6% OF the population in any given 12-month period, anxiety disorders are the most prevalent of all psychiatric diagnoses (Narrow, Regier, Rae, Manderscheid, & Locke, 1993). In contrast to psychotic disorders, persons with anxiety disorders usually recognize their symptoms and are not out of touch with reality. These conditions, however, can be severely debilitating and frequently co-occur with other psychiatric disorders (Regier, Rae, Narrow, Kaelber, & Schatzberg, 1998).

One of the most debilitating anxiety disorders is *panic disorder*, characterized by sudden and unanticipated attacks of an imminent sense of doom, accompanied by symptoms such as increased heart rate, difficulty breathing, dizziness, and terror. In DSM-IV-TR, panic disorders are diagnosed as with or without *agoraphobia*, which may take the form of a fear of leaving home, even to do simple errands or to be employed outside the home. *Generalized anxiety disorder* is a condition of constant worry and fretting across many situations. *Phobic disorders* are characterized by an intense fear of an object or situation representing no real danger. Phobic disorders run the gamut from childhood fears (e.g., of the dark), which often disappear spontaneously, to more pervasive and enduring conditions such as a social phobia, involving exaggerated shyness. *Obsessive-compulsive disorder* (OCD) involves intrusive and recurring thoughts and impulses, known as *obsessions*, and ritualistic repetitions of illogical behaviors in response to these obsessions, known as *compulsions*. Lastly, *post-traumatic stress disorder* (PTSD) is an extreme emotional reaction to a life trauma, such as combat, rape, or an accident, in which the individual re-experiences the feared event in nightmares and flashbacks. Symptoms include a reduced interest in previous activities, estrangement from others, poor concentration, and an inability to recall aspects of the trauma.

PERSONALITY DISORDERS

PERSONALITY DISORDERS ARE defined by the presence of inflexible and maladaptive personality traits that cause significant functional impairment or subjective distress. Severe cases of personality disorders may be accompanied by brief psychotic symptoms.

Personality disorders are grouped into three clusters in DSM-IV-TR. The Odd/Eccentric Cluster consists of *paranoid personality disorder* (marked by pervasive and unwarranted suspiciousness and mistrust of others), *schizoid personality disorder* (marked by detachment from social relationships and a restricted range of expression of emotions), and *schizotypal personality disorder* (marked by social/interpersonal deficits due to eccentricities of cognition and/or behavior). The Dramatic/ Emotional/Erratic Cluster consists of *antisocial personality disorder* (marked by violation of the rights of others without remorse), *borderline personality disorder* (marked by impulsivity and a pervasive pattern of instability of interpersonal relationships, self-image, and affects), *narcissistic personality disorder* (marked by exaggerated sense of self-importance and need for admiration), and *histrionic personality disorder* (marked by excessive emotionality and attention seeking). The Anxious/Fearful Cluster consists of *avoidant personality disorder* (marked by extreme social discomfort because of a pervasive fear of negative evaluation), *dependent personality disorder* (marked by submissive behavior due to an excessive need to be taken care of), and *obsessive-compulsive personality disorder* (marked by pervasive orderliness, perfectionism, and mental and interpersonal control).

Except for the antisocial personality, the diagnostic reliability for personality disorders is poor (Beck, Ward, Mendelson, Mock, & Erbaugh, 1962). Furthermore, frequent comorbidity of personality disorders (Marinangeli et al., 2000; Widiger, Frances, & Trull, 1987) suggests that the current categorical diagnostic system may not be ideal for classifying personality disorders.

FUNCTIONAL PRESENTATION OF PSYCHIATRIC DISABILITY

PSYCHIATRIC DISABILITIES INCLUDE a heterogeneous group of disorders. Even within a single diagnosis there are wide variations in the severity of the illness and the success in coping with the symptoms; however, the pattern of symptoms within any one individual tends to be quite consistent. One further distinction is the difference between *disabling* psychiatric disorders and those in which individuals are still relatively capable of functioning in major life roles. Of most interest to the rehabilitation field, then, is *severe (and persistent) mental illness* (abbreviated as SMI; previously referred to as chronic mental illness), as defined by three criteria: diagnosis, disability, and duration (Goldman, 1984). These criteria have been widely accepted within the mental health field, although the specific operational definitions developed by state mental health authorities have varied (Schinnar, Rothbard, Kanter, & Jung, 1990). At a minimum, the SMI classification requires a DSM-IV diagnosis. The majority of persons with SMI have a diagnosis of schizophrenia, while a sizable minority have mood disorders. Severe cases of personality disorder or anxiety disorder also may fulfill this criterion. Disability is defined by role impairment, typically in several of the following areas of functioning: employment, self-care, self-direction, interpersonal relationships, learning and recreation, independent living, and economic self-sufficiency. The criterion for sufficient duration is usually met by at least one admission to a psychiatric hospital or other restrictive setting (e.g., group home) within a 5-year period. The comments in the remainder of this chapter apply to an estimated 4.8 million Americans (3% of the population) who meet the criteria for SMI (Federal Register, 1999). Some of the functional impairments associated with severe mental illness are described below.

DIFFICULTIES RELATING TO OTHERS

MANY PERSONS WITH SMI are withdrawn and avoid contact with others; one study reported that 75% were moderately to very isolated (Minkoff, 1978). They may lack assertiveness in even routine social transactions (e.g., receiving correct change at a store). They often are not inclined to initiate or continue conversations. Lack of spontaneity and other negative symptoms interfere with the formation and maintenance of intimate relationships. In most studies of SMI, the rate of those currently married is 20% or less (Rogers, Anthony, & Jansen, 1988), with particularly low rates reported for men with schizophrenia.

Not surprisingly, persons with SMI have impoverished social networks, sometimes dominated by professional helpers. If asked to name whom they depend on, they may mention someone they just met. Often an immediate family member or case manager provides the only continuous social contact. Such relationships tend to be nonreciprocal. A person with SMI may show little gratitude or awareness of the effort put forth by the caregiver even under conditions of extreme dependency (Torrey, Erdman, Wolfe, & Flynn, 1990).

Individuals with SMI are vulnerable to exploitation, often a result of poor judgment in selecting friendships. Sexually active individuals with SMI display increased human immunodeficiency virus (HIV) risk behaviors indicated by multiple sexual partners, sex for money or barter, drug use associated with sexual activity, and infrequent condom use, placing individual with SMI at much higher risk for HIV than the general adult population (Gordon, Carey, Carey, Maisto, & Weinhardt, 1999; McKinnon, 1996).

COGNITIVE DIFFICULTIES

INDIVIDUALS WITH SMI, especially those with schizophrenia, may have functional difficulties related to cognition. Persons with schizophrenia range widely in their intelligence, following a distribution similar to that in the general population. Their capacity to apply their intellectual abilities, however, is impaired by the disorder. After the onset of schizophrenia, they often do not attain or regain the level of accomplishment expected by their premorbid educational achievement. When the onset occurs in adolescence, not only is the individual's peer group affiliation disrupted, but also the educational process.

Persons with SMI may be concrete and literal (e.g., "Do you think you could take out the trash?" "I don't think about the trash at all"). Transfer of training from one context to another (e.g., applying skills learned in a hospital setting to a community setting) is often poor (Stein & Test, 1980).

Treatment is difficult when clients act uncooperatively, e.g., by refusing to share personal information. However, secretive or suspicious attitudes are characteristic of approximately two thirds of all persons with schizophrenia (Sartorius et al., 1974). Moreover, this same survey found that 97% of the sample lacked insight about their illness. Indeed, people with schizophrenia often have little or no awareness that they have a mental illness or even that they have any problems at all. This pervasive denial of illness often leads to non-adherence to recommended treatment, e.g., refusing to take medications.

VULNERABILITY TO STRESS

PERSONS WITH SMI often have limited tolerance for stress of any kind, e.g., noise, inclement weather, and everyday hassles. They tend to function poorly in emotionally charged, critical social situations. In particular, persons with schizophrenia are much more likely to have an exacerbation of psychotic symptoms if they live in families with high expressed emotion, that is, those that are hostile and critical (Brown, Birley, & Wing, 1972). Similar findings have been reported for major depression and bipolar disorder (Mueser & Glynn, 1995).

SUBSTANCE ABUSE

SUBSTANCE USE DISORDER is the most common and clinically significant co-occurring disorder in SMI, affecting 50% of people with SMI at some time during their lifetime (Regier et al., 1990). Substance use is a complicating factor in SMI because of its interaction with the mental illness and with psychotropic medications. Presence of a dual disorder of substance use with SMI has consistently been associated with negative outcomes including increased relapses and hospitalizations, housing instability and homelessness, violence, economic burden on the family, serious infections such as HIV and hepatitis, and treatment non-adherence (Drake & Brunette, 1998).

UNEMPLOYMENT

ALTHOUGH THE MAJORITY of adults with SMI desire to work and feel that work is an important goal in their recovery (McQuilken et al., 2003), less than 15% of them are competitively employed at any time (Rogers et al., 1988). Those who work often do so at the risk of losing the entitlements. Most persons with SMI do not have access to any vocational programs, partly because VR counselors and mental health professionals often regard persons with SMI as poor prospects for employment (Noble, Honberg, Hall, & Flynn, 1997). The barriers to access to the VR system are substantial (Drake, Becker, Xie, & Anthony, 1995). Moreover, people with SMI have far more difficulty than persons with physical disabilities in obtaining any VR services (Marshak, Bostick, & Turton, 1990). Reviews of the literature indicate that traditional vocational rehabilitation approaches (e.g., job clubs, sheltered workshops, transitional employment) are not effective in helping people with SMI achieve permanent jobs in the community (Bond, 1992).

POVERTY

POVERTY IS another common consequence of SMI. Among persons with SMI attending mental health programs, 80% or more typically have government entitlements as their main source of support (Rogers et al., 1988).

LIVING SITUATION

THE LARGE MAJORITY of people with SMI are not well integrated in community life. Fortunately, relatively few spend years in psychiatric hospitals, as was the case a half-century ago. However, only a minority are in independent living. For example, among individuals with schizophrenia, about 31% are living independently, 28% are living with a family member, 17% are in supervised living (e.g., halfway houses), and 24% are in hospitals, nursing homes, jails/prisons, shelters, or on the streets (Torrey, 2001). Among those counted as "living in the community" are many who are leading isolated, barren lives, often without social or recreational outlets (Segal & Aviram, 1978). Unfortunately, "successful discharges" from psychiatric hospitals often include individuals transferred to nursing homes and supervised group home settings. Some observers have suggested that in this process, many consumers have not been deinstitutionalized but are *transinstitutionalized* (Geller, 2000). The Supreme Court ruling in *Olmstead vs. L.C.* (1999) underscored the fact that many people with SMI are continuing to be unnecessarily segregated in institutions when community living would be possible if the proper supports were in place. Studies of homelessness further document the grim realities of severe mental illness. An estimated 28% to 37% of the homeless population have a psychiatric disability (Dennis, Buckner, Lipton, & Levine, 1991).

INCARCERATION

THE RATE OF major mental illness in the incarcerated population is double that in the general population (Teplin, 1990). Of the 1.1 million individuals held in state and federal prisons in 1995, the 1-year prevalence rates were 5% for schizophrenia, 6% for bipolar disorder, and 9% for major depression (Substance Abuse and Mental Health Services Administration [SAMHSA], 1997). In 1998, of those incarcerated in American prisons and jails on any given day, approximately 284,000 (16%) were individuals with SMI (Ditton, 1999). This was four times the number of people in state mental hospitals throughout the country. Furthermore, offenders with SMI were more likely than other offenders to have a history of substance use disorder and higher rates of homelessness and unemployment prior to incarceration (Ditton).

The belief that mental illness leads to increased risk of violent behavior is a popular and damaging stereotype, reinforced by dramatic examples (e.g., the assassination attempt on President Reagan by John Hinkley, who has a diagnosis of schizophrenia). Although rates of self-reported violent behaviors in adults with SMI are higher than those with no psychiatric diagnosis (Arseneault, Moffitt, Caspi, Taylor, & Silva, 2000; Swanson, Holzer, Ganju, & Jono, 1990), the vast majority of individuals with SMI do not commit violent acts, and when violence does occur, it is often associated with substance abuse, medication non-adherence, past violent victimization, and violence in the surrounding environment (Steadman et al., 1998; Swanson et al., 2002; Swartz et al., 1998). Therefore, usually it is not the SMI *per se* that leads to assaultiveness, but its convergence with other risk factors that, together, significantly increase the likelihood of violent behavior.

VICTIMIZATION AND TRAUMA

PERSONS WITH SMI are at far greater risk to be victimized by violence and crime than to be perpetrators. Between 43% and 81% of those with SMI report some type of victimization over their lifetime (Rosenberg et al., 2001). In a recent large-scale survey, one third of men and women with schizophrenia reported severe physical or sexual assault in the past year (Goodman et al., 2001). In addition, up to 53% of persons with SMI report childhood sexual or physical abuse (Rosenberg et al., 2001). Given the high prevalence, especially among homeless women, interpersonal violence can be considered a normative experience for people with SMI (Goodman, Dutton, & Harris, 1997).

Although often overlooked, PTSD is a common comorbid diagnosis in SMI. Research suggests that the *current* rates of PTSD in persons with SMI (29%–43%) far exceed the *lifetime* rates reported in community studies (Mueser, Goodman, et al., 1998; Rosenberg et al., 2001). Exposure to trauma and the presence of PTSD are associated with poorer functioning in people with SMI, including more severe symptoms, poorer health, and higher rates of psychiatric and medical hospitalization (Switzer et al., 1999).

INCREASED RISK FOR SUICIDE

FEELINGS OF WORTHLESSNESS and self-hatred are very common in persons with SMI and are associated with suicidal ideation and attempts (E. C. Harris & Barraclough, 1997). The lifetime suicide rate for mood disorders is approximately 15%, over 30 times the rate in the general population (Maxmen & Ward, 1995). The suicide rate for persons with schizophrenia has been estimated to be 10%–13% (Caldwell & Gottesman, 1990).

Environmental Influences

Although many of the characteristics described previously are directly related to psychiatric symptoms, they are also influenced by external factors (e.g., institutionalization and societal attitudes). For example, the stultifying effects of hospitals and nursing homes undoubtedly reinforce the passivity and withdrawal so prominent in SMI (Goffman, 1961). At the societal level, the labeling process in mental illness is demoralizing and discriminatory (Estroff, 1989). Due to diagnostic preconceptions, the label of schizophrenia is "sticky." Once obtained, even normal behavior cannot easily eradicate it (Rosenhan, 1973). Moreover, employers attach more stigma to psychiatric disabilities than to physical disabilities (Berven & Driscoll, 1981; Hazer & Bedell, 2000). In the housing domain, the NIMBY (Not In My Back Yard) prejudice against persons with SMI is intense; group homes are especially likely to meet with community resistance if located in conservative, middle-class neighborhoods (Segal & Aviram, 1978). Stigma and discrimination continue to be significant barriers to community integration (Hall, Graf, Fitzpatrick, Lane, & Birkel, 2003; Wahl, 1997). Some have expressed hope that prominent individuals with mental illness can help combat stigma by public disclosure (Corrigan, 2003).

PROGNOSIS

THE PROGNOSIS FOR schizophrenia is generally worse than for most other major psychiatric disorders. For many, it is a lifelong, disabling condition. However, contrary to an early misconception, schizophrenia does not follow a relentlessly downward course; rather, decline in psychosocial functioning typically plateaus approximately 5 to 10 years after onset (McGlashan, 1988). Traditionally, the prognostic rule of thumb for schizophrenia has been that one third are expected to show a sharp decline in functioning, one third to achieve a marginal adjustment, and one third to recover to essentially former levels of functioning. With appropriate community support and rehabilitation, a substantially larger percentage may approach former levels of functioning (Harding, Brooks, Ashikaga, Strauss, & Breier, 1987). Among persons with schizophrenia, approximately half (and two thirds of their families) recognize the prodromal symptoms (i.e., the warning signs of an impending psychotic episode specific to each individual) prior to their decompensation (Herz, 1984). Psychoeducational groups are designed to assist clients to recognize these symptoms and to employ coping strategies (e.g., reducing stress, seeking additional support).

Most people with major depression recover with or without treatment. In a longitudinal study by Coryell et al. (1994), about 60% and 80% of both clinical and non-clinical populations who developed a major depressive episode recovered by 6 months and 1 year, respectively. Roughly half of all patients recover with no recurrence (Maj, Veltro, Pirozzi, Lobrace, & Magliano, 1992). However, a substantial minority experience recurrent and chronic depression: the 2- and 6-month relapse rates are 20% and 30%, respectively (Belsher & Costello, 1988), and 22% of patients experience an episode persisting more than 1 year (Thornicroft & Sartorius, 1993). Between episodes, persons with major depression may be highly functional and productive, as illustrated by the historical examples of Winston Churchill and Abraham Lincoln. With proper treatment, the prognosis is good for the majority of those who suffer from major depression. By contrast, bipolar disorder is generally far more debilitating; untreated, it has a poor prognosis.

Personality disorders are, by definition, pervasive and enduring patterns of thinking, feeling, and behaving that typically remain quite stable over time. As such, we do not yet have many effective treatment strategies to help such individuals "recover" from a personality disorder, although with targeted interventions, promising functional improvements have been shown for some diagnoses such as borderline personality disorder (Linehan & Armstrong, 1991).

TREATMENT AND REHABILITATION

HISTORY OF TREATMENT APPROACHES

PRIOR TO THE 1950s, there were numerous somatic treatments for SMI (Isaac & Armat, 1990). With the exception of electroconvulsive therapy, none of these proved to be effective and many were harmful. In the case of electroconvulsive therapy, its demonstrated effectiveness has been limited to accelerating improvement in some major depressions (Crow & Johnstone, 1986), although it was once widely used for schizophrenia as well. Psychiatric hospitalization providing little more than custodial care (and often neglect) was standard practice.

Beginning in the 1950s, a combination of economic, legal, and humanitarian factors, in addition to the widespread use of psychotropic medications, led to *deinstitutionalization*, the process of releasing patients from state hospitals (Talbott, 1978). The resident population of state and county mental hospitals, which peaked at 558,922 in 1955, declined to fewer than 60,000 by 1998 (Lamb & Bachrach, 2001). In 1963, the Community Mental Health Centers Act authorized the creation of a network of community mental health centers (CMHCs) with a broad mission to address the mental health needs of the nation including the care and treatment of discharged patients with mental disorders (U.S. Congress, 1963). Altogether, 789 CMHCs were eventually funded, providing the bulk of public mental health services for people with SMI (Torrey, 2001).

Initially, most CMHCs were unprepared to serve people with SMI for several reasons. First, many professionals incorrectly assumed that antipsychotic medications by themselves would be sufficient to enable people with SMI to return to the community. Second, CMHCs typically were limited to office-based services based on the assumption that discharged patients would seek their services as necessary. This assumption also proved wrong: a 1986 national survey found that 937,000 (78%) of 1.2 million persons with schizophrenia living outside of institutions were not receiving any CMHC-based outpatient treatment (Torrey, 1988).

Other studies showed that clients with SMI receiving outpatient treatment had high dropout rates (Axelrod & Wetzler, 1989). Finally, CMHCs failed to address a wide range of needs relating to housing, employment, socialization, and other areas of functioning discussed above. The phenomenon of *revolving-door* clients—those who return frequently to psychiatric hospitals—was one consequence of this limited treatment focus. Over half of all psychiatric patients released from state hospitals return within 2 years (Anthony, Cohen, & Vitalo, 1978). Even today, the problem of revolving-door clients still has not been fully solved, with 250,000 short-term psychiatric hospitalizations in the U.S. annually (Weiden & Olfson, 1993). These trends suggested the need for new, comprehensive psychosocial approaches to augment traditional CMHC services (Talbott, 1978) and to compliment pharmacological treatments.

PHARMACOLOGICAL TREATMENTS

Medications for Schizophrenia

About two thirds of people with schizophrenia benefit from a group of *traditional* antipsychotic medications (also called "neuroleptics"), including chlorpromazine (Thorazine), thioridazine (Mellaril), and haloperidol (Haldol). The efficacy of these traditional neuroleptics in reducing the relapse rate and the positive symptoms of schizophrenia is well established (Davis, 1980). Unfortunately, traditional neuroleptics have troubling side effects, summarized by the mnemonic, THE SEA: Tardive dyskinesia, Hypotension, Extrapyramidal symptoms, Sedation, Endocrine disturbances, and Anticholinergic symptoms (Wittlin, 1988). *Tardive dyskinesia*, the most serious of the side effects, involves stereotyped, involuntary movements of the mouth and face. Occurring more commonly after long use of antipsychotic drugs, it is usually irreversible. *Hypotension* refers to abnormally low blood pressure, which may be experienced as dizziness. *Extrapyramidal* symptoms, prominent during the first week of drug treatment, include tremors of the arms, rigidity of extremities, *akinesia* (listlessness), and *akathisia* (internal restlessness). *Sedation* is experienced as drowsiness. *Endocrine disturbances* include sexual dysfunction and weight gain. *Anticholinergic* symptoms include dry mouth and blurred vision. Treatment of side effects includes reducing dosage levels, changing medications, and, in the case of extrapyramidal symptoms, the use of antiparkinsonian drugs such as benztropine (Cogentin). Another limitation to traditional antipsychotics is their lack of impact on negative symptoms.

Recently, a number of new *atypical* neuroleptics have been developed. Five of these newer drugs and their year of approval by the Food and Drug Administration for use in the U.S. are clozapine (Clozaril),

1990; risperidone (Risperdal), 1994; olanzapine (Zyprexa), 1996; quetiapine (Seroquel), 1997; and ziprasidone (Geodon), 2001. With advantages of lower rates of extrapyramidal symptoms (Tamminga, 1997) and equal effectiveness in reducing positive symptoms of schizophrenia, the atypical neuroleptics are rapidly replacing traditional neuroleptics as the most prescribed and also increasingly as the *"first line"* (i.e., prescribed at first diagnosis) medications for schizophrenia (Wang, West, Tanielian, & Pincus, 2000). One major drawback is that they are priced many times higher than traditional neuroleptics. Some atypical neuroleptics (especially clozapine and olanzapine) have also been associated with clinically significant bodyweight gain (Allison et al., 1999), increasing the risk of medical comorbidity including diabetes, hypertension, cardiovascular disease, and high cholesterol (Alao, Malhotra, & Dewan, 2002; Henderson, 2002; Nasrallah, 2002). Clozapine is regarded as the most effective of the atypicals. Often prescribed to people with schizophrenia not helped by other medications (Safferman, Lieberman, Kane, Szymanski, & Kinon, 1991), clozapine requires that patients have frequent blood tests because of the risk of life-threatening *agranulocytosis* (a significant decrease in white blood cell counts).

Medications for Mood Disorders

A range of drugs have been used in the treatment of mood disorders. Lithium is used to treat bipolar disorder, particularly during the manic phases, although it is also used by patients who have never had manic episodes. It is effective in 63%–90% of all cases of mania (Noll, Davis, & DeLeon-Jones, 1985). Lithium is lethal in high doses; thus, patients require careful blood monitoring. Various antidepressant drugs have been used for major depression. Before the 1990s, the most common were the tricyclics including amitriptyline (Elavil) and imipramine (Tofranil). The side effects of the tricyclics include anticholinergic effects, sedation, and irregularities in the cardiovascular system. A group of newer antidepressants known as *selective serotonin reuptake inhibitors* (SSRIs) including fluoxetine (Prozac), paroxetine (Paxil), and sertraline (Zoloft) are relatively free of side effects (Glod, 1996; Möller & Volz, 1996) and have become enormously popular in a short period of time. They are widely prescribed for major depression and a wide array of other psychiatric disorders.

Medications for Anxiety Disorders

Persons with anxiety disorders are often prescribed antianxiety drugs (also called *"anxiolytics"*), including diazepam (Valium), which at one time was the most frequently prescribed medication in the U.S. (Lickey & Gordon, 1991). Research on the psychopharmacology of anxiolytics has been rapidly expanding in recent years with the attempt to find specific agents to reduce the symptoms of specific disorders. For example, alpra-zolam (Xanax) has been used in the treatment of panic and phobic dis-orders. Major drawbacks of some anxiolytics are that they are addictive and dangerous if taken in combination with alcohol (Brunette, Noordsy, Xie, & Drake, 2003). Buspirone (BuSpar), which is often used to treat gen-eralized anxiety disorder, appears to avoid both of these problems.

Medication Nonadherence

Medication nonadherence is a major barrier to effective treatment of psy-chotic disorders, with as many as 50% of patients not taking drugs as prescribed (Streicker, Amdur, & Dincin, 1986). One review concluded that patients on neuroleptics took an average of 58% of the recommended amount, with higher adherence rates for patients on antidepressants (Cramer & Rosenheck, 1998). Nonadherence in SMI has serious conse-quences, often resulting in higher rates of relapse and rehospitalization and poorer community adjustment. Medication education (Wallace, Liberman, MacKain, Blackwell, & Eckman, 1992) and *behavioral tailoring* (i.e., fitting medication-taking into daily routines) (Mueser et al., 2002) are strategies used to increase adherence. A strategy to ensure adher-ence to antipsychotic medication is to substitute long-acting injectable forms of medications such as fluphenazine decanoate (Prolixin) for the usual oral administration (Kane, Woerner, & Sarantakos, 1986). Another strategy is to reduce dosage levels. Some research has suggested that with careful monitoring, the use of much lower dosage levels than usu-ally prescribed can reduce side effects while retaining the positive effects of neuroleptics (Hogarty et al., 1988). Finally, because of fewer side effects, atypical neuroleptics may result in superior adherence to their tradi-tional counterparts.

Evidence-Based Medication Management

In recent years, *practice guidelines* and *algorithms* have been developed to systematize knowledge about "best practices" in the pharmacological treatment of psychiatric disorders (APA, 1997, 2000b, 2002; Miller et al., 1999). These guidelines incorporate evidence from clinical trials and expert consensus. Principles of evidence-based medication manage-ment include: respecting and incorporating client preferences, accu-rate diagnosis and specification of target symptoms, choosing medication and dosage range supported by the research evidence, ongoing evalua-tion of changes in symptoms and side effects and modification recom-mended by the illness-specific guidelines (e.g., raising dosage, changing to another efficacious medication, using an augmentation strategy), treatment of co-occurring syndromes, and patient and family involve-ment in treatment planning (Mellman et al., 2001). Research evidence indicates that following appropriate medication guidelines can reduce symptoms and hospitalizations in persons with SMI (Rush et al., 1999). Medication practice guidelines for psychiatric disorders are evolving.

Psychotherapy

There is no single "best" therapeutic approach for persons with psychiatric disabilities given the heterogeneity of the population. Moreover, most psychosocial interventions with individuals with SMI are not formal clinic-based counseling sessions, but are embedded in psychiatric rehabilitation practices described below. The foundation for all successful interventions is a therapeutic relationship. This principle applies to people with SMI (McGrew, Wilson, & Bond, 1996) as well as to individuals with less severe psychiatric disorders. The helper should be energetic, supplying "dynamic hopefulness" especially when the client appears unresponsive (Dincin, 1975). Psychotherapeutic approaches emphasizing insight and self-examination are most helpful for individuals who are least disabled. The literature demonstrating the efficacy of psychotherapy for relieving distress in persons with mild anxiety and depression is substantial (Lipsey & Wilson, 1993). Both cognitive-behavioral therapy and interpersonal therapy have been used successfully in the treatment of depression (Elkin et al., 1989). Insight-oriented psychotherapy, however, is of limited use in treating schizophrenia and is sometimes harmful (Drake & Sederer, 1986). Effective interventions for people with SMI entail direct, unambiguous communication; supportive, noncritical attitudes; and a focus on problem-solving and skills training (Mueser & Gingerich, 1994). *Motivational interviewing*, a set of techniques that tailors interventions to the client's readiness to change, has received increasing recognition as an important therapeutic tool (W. R. Miller & Rollnick, 2002).

PSYCHIATRIC REHABILITATION

IT IS WIDELY accepted that pharmacological treatment of SMI works best in conjunction with practical psychosocial interventions (Bond & Meyer, 1999). *Psychiatric rehabilitation* (also referred to as "psychosocial rehabilitation") tackles the psychosocial correlates of SMI not adequately addressed by medication alone, such as unemployment, isolation, vulnerability to stress, substandard living conditions, homelessness, and the heavy burden of caregiving on relatives. Research substantially supports the view that people with SMI (to be referred to as *"consumers"* for the rest of the chapter) can, with the right type of support, achieve successful normal adult roles in the community.

Though psychiatric rehabilitation approaches vary, they embrace a common set of guiding principles (Bond & Resnick, 2000; Dincin, 1975; Pratt, Gill, Barrett, & Roberts, 1999). These principles include but are not limited to: *individualized and comprehensive assessment, planning, and intervention; community integration* (helping consumers exit patient roles, treatment centers, segregated housing arrangements, and/or sheltered work); *pragmatism* (helping consumers with the practical problems in everyday life, with services organized around specific, tangible goals); *consumer choice* (as experts of their own illness, consumers are empowered to set their own goals and make informed decisions in their treatment and rehabilitation, and services are shaped to their preferences); *sense of hope* (focusing on consumer strengths, building their self-confidence, and instilling hope for recovery through a rehabilitation relationship); and *integration of treatment and rehabilitation.*

In the 1970s, a national conference of mental health experts culminated in the conceptualization of a *community support program* (CSP) (Turner & TenHoor, 1978). The concept assumes that nontraditional roles for mental health providers are necessary for successful interventions for consumers with SMI, including outreach to those not receiving services, assistance in housing and other basic needs, development of permanent support networks, vocational rehabilitation, and advocacy. For nearly 30 years, the CSP model has had a dramatic impact on the way systems planners conceptualize organizing services, supports, and opportunities to help consumers with SMI reach their full potential in the society. A number of approaches compatible with CSP principles have been developed including the *clubhouse model, skills training, self-help activities* associated with the consumer movement, and a group of *evidence-based practices.*

Clubhouse Model

The psychosocial approach known as the clubhouse originated with the Fountain House program in New York City (Beard, Propst, & Malamud, 1982). In the 1940s, the precursor to Fountain House was a self-help group for patients discharged from the state psychiatric hospital. Subsequently, the group sought a professional to serve as their center director. Under his direction, the group evolved into an innovative program for helping consumers with SMI adjust to community living. Operating outside of the mental health system, the program became known as a clubhouse because its identity revolved around a central meeting place for "members" to socialize. Fountain House pioneered many innovations including two key vocational concepts: the *work-ordered day* and *transitional employment*. As part of the work-ordered day, members participate in prevocational work crews doing chores around the clubhouse. Transitional employment consists of temporary, part-time community jobs secured by the clubhouse staff. The clubhouse model emphasizes informal and experiential learning as opposed to more structured approaches found in skills training.

Skills Training

The rationale for skills training is based on the findings that consumers with SMI often experience difficulties in interpersonal situations ranging from intimate relationships to everyday contacts in public settings. The goal of social skills training is to systematically teach the component skills necessary for effective social interactions. Typically, the steps in skills training are as follows: (a) give a rationale for learning the skill, (b) role-play the skill, (c) provide an exercise for the client to role-play the skill, (d) give specific positive and corrective feedback on client's role-play, (e) practice the skill, and (f) give a homework assignment in a real-life situation (Mueser, Drake, & Bond, 1997). Although skills training typically focuses on social skills, it also has been used for a range of other skills needed for independent living. There is little doubt that well-defined skills including social skills can be taught to consumers with SMI (Wallace et al., 1992). However, most of the extensive research on skills training suffers from a failure to show whether the skills taught in classroom settings generalize to everyday settings (Dilk & Bond, 1996).

Consumer Movement

In the last 2 decades, the consumer movement has prompted major changes in the conception of mental health services. Advocates have insisted that individuals with mental illness should have equal access to societal and environmental resources, equal access to options and opportunities, and equal "location of life," that is, places where people live, work, play, and pray are the same regardless of the presence of mental illness (Ralph, 2000). President Bush's New Freedom Initiative echoes these same themes (New Freedom Commission on Mental Health, 2003). Nationally there is widespread interest in receiving training in the Wellness Action Recovery Plan (Copeland, 1997), a manual providing systematic tools for coping with symptoms and developing relapse prevention plans.

Over 500 mental health self-help groups have formed nationwide (Chamberlin, Rogers, & Sneed, 1989). These groups have been active in developing drop-in centers, which provide friendship, social and recreational activities, and concrete assistance (Mowbray, Chamberlain, Jennings, & Reed, 1988). Since its inception in 1979, the National Alliance for the Mentally Ill (NAMI), an organization for families, has grown to 1,200 state and local affiliates in the U.S. and a membership of 210,000 (NAMI, 2003).

Evidence-Based Practices

One of the most significant advances in the psychiatric rehabilitation field in recent years is the movement toward *evidence-based practices*, defined as a set of well-delineated interventions that have demonstrated effectiveness in rigorous empirical research (Drake, Goldman, et al., 2001). Six evidence-based practices have been endorsed by a national consensus panel of leading mental health researchers, advocates, and program directors for widespread adoption for the treatment and rehabilitation of SMI: *assertive community treatment, family psychoeducation, illness management and recovery, integrated dual disorders treatment, medication management,* and *supported employment* (Mueser, Torrey, Lynde, Singer, & Drake, 2003). Controlled trials on these practices suggest specific benefits in the areas of reductions in rates of relapse, hospitalization, and substance use; better control of symptoms; and improvements in housing stability, employment, and overall quality of life. Medication management was discussed previously in the section "Pharmacological Treatments"; each of the remaining five evidence-based practices is briefly described below.

Assertive Community Treatment (ACT).   Developed in the 1970s by Stein and Test (1980), ACT is an intensive approach most appropriate for consumers with SMI whose needs have not been adequately met by more traditional, less intensive programs of treatment. ACT services are provided by a group of professionals representing various disciplines (e.g., psychiatry, nursing, case management, vocational and substance abuse specialists) who work as a team. They serve clients on an individual basis, with most contact occurring in consumers' homes and neighborhoods, rather than in agency offices. The ACT team keeps in frequent contact with clients, typically averaging two visits per week. The nature of the contacts depends on the needs of a client on a given day. ACT teams help in such things as budgeting money, shopping, finding housing, and taking medications. ACT teams attempt to anticipate crises, for example, by paying attention to the warning signs of a relapse. It is common for ACT staff to provide service outside the traditional workday, often with 24-hour crisis coverage and weekend staffing. ACT programs exemplify assertive outreach in that staff members actively initiate contact with clients, rather than depending on clients to keep appointments. Another feature of ACT is its emphasis on continuity and consistency. Clients are not discharged from ACT teams but continue to receive services on a time-unlimited basis (Test, 1992). The effectiveness of the ACT model has been well-established; a review of 25 randomized controlled studies concluded that ACT clients experienced reduced psychiatric hospitalization, increased housing stability, improvement of symptoms and subjective quality of life (Bond, Drake, Mueser, & Latimer, 2001).

Family Psychoeducation.   Family psychoeducation aims to achieve the best possible outcome for consumers with SMI, alleviate the stress in the family, and improve functioning of all family members through collaborative treatment. Controlled studies have shown a 25%–75% reduction in relapse and rehospitalization rates among consumers with SMI whose families received psychoeducation. Although the existing models of family interventions vary, effective family psychoeducation programs share the following elements: basic psychoeducation about SMI and its management; communication and problem solving skills training; provision of emotional support, empathy, and hope; development of social support networks; and long-term, flexible interventions tailored to the needs of individual families (Dixon et al., 2001). In family psychoeducation, the term "family" is interpreted broadly to including anyone in the consumer's natural support system who is functioning as family.

Illness Management and Recovery (IMR). The primary aim of IMR is to empower consumers with SMI to manage their illness, find their own goals for recovery, and make informed decisions about their treatment by teaching them the necessary knowledge and skills. IMR involves a variety of interventions designed to help consumers improve their ability to overcome the debilitating effects of their illness on social and role functioning. The evidence-based components of IMR are psychoeducation, behavioral tailoring for medication, relapse prevention training, and coping skills training (Mueser et al., 2002). To effectively teach these components and to ensure that knowledge is put into practice, practitioners use a variety of techniques including motivational, educational, and cognitive-behavioral strategies.

Integrated Dual Disorders Treatment (IDDT). As noted previously, about 50% of individuals with SMI have a comorbid substance use disorder; these consumers are said to have dual disorders, which are associated with a variety of negative outcomes. In IDDT, the same clinicians or teams of clinicians working in one setting provide psychiatric and substance abuse interventions in a coordinated fashion. IDDT aims to help the consumer learn to manage both illnesses so that he/she can pursue meaningful life goals. The critical ingredients of IDDT include assertive outreach, motivational interventions, and a comprehensive, long-term, staged and individualized approach to recovery (Drake, Essock, et al., 2001). Contrary to traditional treatments for people with dual disorders, abstinence is not a prerequisite to assisting with consumer goals for stable housing or meaningful activity such as employment. Controlled studies have shown IDDT's effectiveness in reducing substance abuse, which in turn leads to improvement in other outcomes including symptoms, general functioning, housing stability, and treatment retention.

Supported Employment. Defined as paid work that takes place in normal work settings with ongoing support services, supported employment was developed originally for people with developmental disabilities as a more effective, humane, and cost-effective alternative to sheltered workshops (Wehman & Moon, 1988). The evidence-based principles of supported employment for individuals with SMI include the following principles: eligibility based on consumer choice, integration with mental health treatment, competitive employment as the goal, attention to consumer preferences, rapid job search (i.e., no requirements for completing extensive pre-employment assessment and training), and continuous follow-along support (Becker & Drake, 2003). Nine experimental studies and four quasi-experimental studies comparing supported employment to traditional vocational approaches (e.g., skills training preparation, sheltered workshops, transitional employment, and day treatment) suggest that between 40% and 60% of clients with SMI enrolled in supported employment programs obtain jobs in the competitive employment market, compared to less than 20% of clients not receiving supported employment (Bond, Becker, et al., 2001; Crowther, Marshall, Bond, & Huxley, 2001; Twamley, Jeste, & Lehman, 2003).

One key limitation of supported employment is that in practice it is limited mostly to entry-level jobs (Bond, Drake, Mueser, & Becker, 1997). Educational programs are one option for higher-functioning consumers who may not be challenged sufficiently by traditional psychiatric rehabilitation programs (Hatfield, 1989). Many people with SMI attempt college but are frequently unable to complete the course work due to the nature of their illness and its treatment. The concept of *supported education* refers to helping consumers with psychiatric disabilities obtain education and training in order to have the skills and credentials necessary for obtaining jobs with career potential (Moxley, Mowbray, & Brown, 1993). A few quantitative studies of the impact of supported education have begun to appear in the literature (Carlson, Eichler, Huff, & Rapp, 2003).

Starting in the late 1980s, supported education has also been applied to training consumers to work as mental health providers (Sherman & Porter, 1991). This concept has been widely emulated (Mowbray, Moxley, Jasper, & Howell, 1997).

ACCESS

CONSUMERS WITH SMI continue to have problems accessing effective services (Drake, Goldman, et al., 2001; Torrey, 2001). Despite extensive evidence and expert agreement on effective practices, most mental health centers do not provide them (Lehman & Steinwachs, 1998). The number of exemplary programs in the U.S. is dwarfed by the size of the population in need. For example, Meisler (1997) identified 397 ACT programs in 14 states serving an estimated 24,000 consumers, which falls far short of the estimated 20% of consumers with SMI who could benefit from ACT (Bond, Drake, et al., 2001). Underfunding of mental health services is one major factor in this disparity between need and program capacity. In an effort to disseminate the best practices of psychiatric rehabilitation, a national project is underway to develop standardized guidelines, training materials, and fidelity scales in the form of toolkits, and to demonstrate that the toolkits can facilitate faithfully implementing each of the six evidence-based practices in routine mental health service settings (Drake, Goldman, et al.).

CONCLUSIONS

PSYCHIATRIC DISORDERS CAN look very different from one another in terms of symptom presentation, course, and treatment. An encouraging shift in the collective mindset regarding the treatment of SMI has occurred, with an emphasis on recovery and the right and ability to pursue meaningful goals comparable to those held by nondisabled individuals.

Like individuals with other types of long-term illnesses, people with SMI want to manage their own illnesses, work with and relate to a range of other people, and live in normal housing situations. The goal of psychiatric rehabilitation is not just to keep consumers stable and out of the hospital but to assist and empower them in pursuing their own goals for recovery, management of their illnesses, independence, and self-fulfillment. Progress has been made toward realizing these goals, although many changes are needed in the mental health system before exemplary services are available to everyone who could benefit from them.

REFERENCES

Alao, A. O., Malhotra, K., & Dewan, M. J. (2002). Comparing the side effect profile of the atypical antipsychotics. *West African Journal of Medicine, 21*(4), 313–315.

Allison, D. B., Mentore, J. L., Heo, M., Chandler, L. P., Cappelleri, J. C., Infante, M. C., et al. (1999). Antipsychotic-induced weight gain: A comprehensive research synthesis. *American Journal of Psychiatry, 156,* 1686–1696.

American Psychiatric Association. (1994). *Diagnostic and statistical manual of mental disorders* (4th ed.). Washington, DC: Author.

American Psychiatric Association. (1997). APA: Practice guideline for the treatment of patients with schizophrenia. *American Journal of Psychiatry. Special Issue: Practice Guideline for the Treatment of Patients with Schizophrenia, 154*(4 Suppl.), 1–63.

American Psychiatric Association. (2000a). *Diagnostic and Statistical Manual of Mental Disorders: Fourth Edition, Text Revision* (4th ed.). Washington, DC: Author.

American Psychiatric Association. (2000b). APA: Practice guideline for the treatment of patients with major depressive disorder (revision). *American Journal of Psychiatry, 157*(4 Suppl.), 1–45.

American Psychiatric Association. (2002). APA: Practice guideline for the treatment of patients with bipolar disorder (revision). *American Journal of Psychiatry, 159*(4 Suppl.), 1–50.

Andreasen, N. C. (1984). *The broken brain.* New York: Harper & Row.

Anthony, W. A., Cohen, M., Farkas, M. D., & Gagne, C. (2002). *Psychiatric rehabilitation* (2nd ed.). Boston: Center for Psychiatric Rehabilitation.

Anthony, W. A., Cohen, M. R., & Vitalo, R. (1978). The measurement of rehabilitation outcome. *Schizophrenia Bulletin, 4,* 365–383.

Arseneault, L., Moffitt, T. E., Caspi, A., Taylor, P. J., & Silva, P. A. (2000). Mental disorders and violence in a total birth cohort: Results from the Dunedin Study. *Archives of General Psychiatry, 57*(10), 979–986.

Axelrod, S., & Wetzler, S. (1989). Factors associated with better compliance with psychiatric aftercare. *Hospital and Community Psychiatry, 40,* 397–401.

Beard, J. H., Propst, R. N., & Malamud, T. J. (1982). The Fountain House model of rehabilitation. *Psychosocial Rehabilitation Journal, 5*(1), 47–53.

Beck, A. T. (1967). *Depression: Clinical, experimental, and theoretical aspects.* New York: Harper & Row.

Beck, A. T., Ward, C. H., Mendelson, M., Mock, J. E., & Erbaugh, J. K. (1962). Reliability of psychiatric diagnosis: II. A study of consistency of clinical judgments and ratings. *American Journal of Psychiatry, 119,* 351–357.

Becker, D. R., & Drake, R. E. (2003). *A working life for people with severe mental illness.* New York: Oxford Press.

Belsher, G., & Costello, C. G. (1988). Relapse after recovery from unipolar depression: A critical review. *Psychological Bulletin, 104*(1), 84–96.

Bernheim, K. F., Lewine, R. R., & Beale, C. T. (1982). *The caring family: Living with chronic mental illness.* Chicago: Contemporary Books.

Berven, N. L., & Driscoll, J. H. (1981). The effects of past psychiatric disability on employer evaluation of a job applicant. *Journal of Applied Rehabilitation Counseling, 12,* 50–55.

Bond, G. R. (1992). Vocational rehabilitation. In R. P. Liberman (Ed.), *Handbook of psychiatric rehabilitation* (pp. 244–275). New York: Macmillan.

Bond, G. R., Becker, D. R., Drake, R. E., Rapp, C. A., Meisler, N., Lehman, A. F., et al. (2001). Implementing supported employment as an evidence-based practice. *Psychiatric Services, 52*(3), 313–322.

Bond, G. R., Drake, R. E., Mueser, K. T., & Becker, D. R. (1997). An update on supported employment for people with severe mental illness. *Psychiatric Services, 48,* 335–346.

Bond, G. R., Drake, R. E., Mueser, K. T., & Latimer, E. (2001). Assertive community treatment for people with severe mental illness: Critical ingredients and impact on patients. *Disease Management & Health Outcomes, 9,* 141–159.

Bond, G. R., & Meyer, P. S. (1999). The role of medications in the employment of people with schizophrenia. *Journal of Rehabilitation, 65*(4), 9–16.

Bond, G. R., & Resnick, S. G. (2000). Psychiatric rehabilitation. In R. G. Frank & T. Elliott (Eds.), *Handbook of rehabilitation psychology* (pp. 235–258). Washington, DC: American Psychological Association.

Brown, G. W., Birley, J. L., & Wing, J. K. (1972). Influence of family life on the course of schizophrenic disorders: A replication. *British Journal of Psychiatry, 121,* 241–258.

Brunette, M. F., Noordsy, D. I., Xie, H., & Drake, R. E. (2003). Benzodiazepine use and abuse among patients with severe mental illness and co-occurring substance use disorders. *Psychiatric Services, 54,* 1395–1401.

Caldwell, C. B., & Gottesman, I. I. (1990). Schizophrenics kill themselves too: A review of risk factors for suicide. *Schizophrenia Bulletin, 16,* 571–589.

Carlson, L., Eichler, M. S., Huff, S., & Rapp, C. A. (2003). *A tale of two cities: Best practices in supported education.* Lawrence, KS: University of Kansas School of Social Welfare.

Chamberlin, J., Rogers, J. A., & Sneed, C. S. (1989). Consumers, families, and community support systems. *Psychosocial Rehabilitation Journal, 12*(3), 93–106.

Copeland, M. E. (1997). *Wellness Recovery Action Plan.* Brattleboro, VT: Peach Press.

Corrigan, P. W. (2003). Beat the stigma: Come out of the closet. *Psychiatric Services, 54,* 1313.

Coryell, W., Akiskal, H. S., Leon, A. C., Winokur, G., Maser, J. D., Mueller, T. I., et al. (1994). The time course of nonchronic major depressive disorder. Uniformity across episodes and samples. National Institute of Mental Health Collaborative Program on the Psychobiology of Depression— Clinical Studies. *Archives of General Psychiatry, 51*(5), 405–410.

Cramer, J. A., & Rosenheck, R. (1998). Compliance with medication regimens for mental and physical disorders. *Psychiatric Services, 49,* 196–201.

Crow, T. J., & Johnstone, E. C. (1986). Controlled trials of electroconvulsive therapy. In S. Malitz & H. A. Sackeim (Eds.), *Electroconvulsive therapy: Clinical and basic research issues* (pp. 12–29). New York: New York Academy of Sciences.

Crowther, R. E., Marshall, M., Bond, G. R., & Huxley, P. (2001). Helping people with severe mental illness to obtain work: Systematic review. *British Medical Journal, 322,* 204–208.

Davis, J. M. (1980). Antipsychotic drugs. In H. I. Kaplan, A. M. Freedman, & B. J. Sadock (Eds.), *Comprehensive textbook of psychiatry* (vol. 3, pp. 2257–2289). Baltimore: Williams & Wilkins.

Dennis, D. L., Buckner, J. C., Lipton, F. R., & Levine, I. S. (1991). A decade of research and services for homeless mentally ill persons. *American Psychologist, 46,* 1129–1138.

Dilk, M. N., & Bond, G. R. (1996). Meta-analytic evaluation of skills training research for individuals with severe mental illness. *Journal of Consulting and Clinical Psychology, 64*, 1337–1346.

Dincin, J. (1975). Psychiatric rehabilitation. *Schizophrenia Bulletin, 1*, 131–147.

Ditton, P. J. (1999). *Bureau of Justice Statistics Special Report: Mental Health Treatment of Inmates and Probationers.* Washington, DC: U.S. Department of Justice.

Dixon, L., McFarlane, W. R., Lefley, H., Lucksted, A., Cohen, M., Falloon, I., et al. (2001). Evidence-based practices for services to families of people with psychiatric disabilities. *Psychiatric Services, 52*(7), 903–910.

Drake, R. E., Becker, D. R., Xie, H., & Anthony, W. A. (1995). Barriers in the brokered model of supported employment for persons with psychiatric disabilities. *Journal of Vocational Rehabilitation, 5*, 141–149.

Drake, R. E., & Brunette, M. F. (1998). Complications of severe mental illness related to alcohol and drug use disorders. In Galanter (Ed.), *Recent developments in alcoholism, vol. 14: The consequences of alcoholism* (pp. 285–299). New York: Plenum Press.

Drake, R. E., Essock, S. M., Shaner, A., Carey, K. B., Minkoff, K., Kola, L., et al. (2001). Implementing dual diagnosis services for clients with severe mental illness. *Psychiatric Services, 52*(4), 469–476.

Drake, R. E., Goldman, H. H., Leff, H. S., Lehman, A. F., Dixon, L., Mueser, K. T., et al. (2001). Implementing evidence-based practices in routine mental health service settings. *Psychiatric Services, 52*(2), 179–182.

Drake, R. E., & Sederer, L. I. (1986). The adverse effects of intensive treatment of chronic schizophrenia. *Comprehensive Psychiatry, 27*, 313–326.

Elkin, I., Shea, T., Watkins, J. T., Imber, S. D., Sotsky, S. M., Collins, J. F., et al. (1989). National Institute of Mental Health Treatment of Depression Collaborative Research Program: General effectiveness of treatment. *Archives of General Psychiatry, 46*, 971–982.

Estroff, S. E. (1989). Self, identity, and subjective experiences: In search of the subject. *Schizophrenia Bulletin, 15*, 189–196.

Federal Register. (1999). Estimation methodology for adults with serious mental illness, *Federal Register* (vol. 64, pp. 33890–33897). Washington, DC: Center for Mental Health Services, Substance Abuse and Mental Health Services Administration, Health and Human Services.

First, M. B., Spitzer, R. L., Gibbon, M., & Williams, J. B. (1994). *Structured Clinical Interview for Axis I DSM-IV Disorders—Patient Edition (SCID-I/P, Version 2.0).* New York: Biometric Research Department, New York State Psychiatric Institute.

Geller, J. L. (2000). The last half-century of psychiatric services as reflected in Psychiatric Services. *Psychiatric Services, 51*, 41–67.

Glod, C. A. (1996). Recent advances in the pharmacotherapy of major depression. *Archives of Psychiatric Nursing, 10*, 355–364.

Goffman, E. (1961). *Asylums: Essays on the social situation of mental patients and other inmates.* Chicago: Aldine.

Goldman, H. H. (1984). Epidemiology. In J. A. Talbott (Ed.), *The chronic mental patient: Five years later* (pp. 15–31). Orlando, FL: Grune & Stratton.

Goodman, L. A., Dutton, M. A., & Harris, M. (1997). The relationship between violence dimensions and symptom severity among homeless, mentally ill women. *Journal of Traumatic Stress, 10*(1), 51–70.

Goodman, L. A., Salyers, M. P., Mueser, K. T., Rosenberg, S. D., Swartz, M., Essock, S. M., et al. (2001). Recent victimization in women and men with severe mental illness: Prevalence and correlates. *Journal of Traumatic Stress, 14*(4), 615–632.

Gordon, C. M., Carey, M. P., Carey, K. B., Maisto, S. A., & Weinhardt, L. S. (1999). Understanding HIV-related risk among persons with a severe and persistent mental illness: Insights from qualitative inquiry. *Journal of Nervous & Mental Disease, 187*(4), 208–216.

Green, M. F. (1996). What are the functional consequences of neurocognitive deficits in schizophrenia? *American Journal of Psychiatry, 153,* 321–330.

Hall, L. L., Graf, A. C., Fitzpatrick, M. J., Lane, T., & Birkel, R. C. (2003). *Shattered lives: Results of a national survey of NAMI members living with mental illness and their families.* Arlington, VA: NAMI/TRIAD (Treatment/Recovery Information and Advocacy Data Base).

Harding, C. M., Brooks, G. W., Ashikaga, T., Strauss, J. S., & Breier, A. (1987). The Vermont longitudinal study of persons with severe mental illness: II. Long-term outcome of subjects who retrospectively met DSM-III criteria for schizophrenia. *American Journal of Psychiatry, 144,* 727–735.

Harris, E. C., & Barraclough, B. (1997). Suicide as an outcome for mental disorders: A meta-analysis. *British Journal of Psychiatry, 170,* 205–228.

Harris, M. J., & Jeste, D. V. (1988). Late-onset schizophrenia: An overview [Comment]. *Schizophrenia Bulletin, 14*(1), 39–55.

Hatfield, A. B. (1989). Serving the unserved in community rehabilitation programs. *Psychosocial Rehabilitation Journal, 13*(2), 71–82.

Hazer, J. T., & Bedell, K. V. (2000). Effects of seeking accommodation and disability on preemployment evaluations. *Journal of Applied Social Psychology, 30,* 1201–1223.

Henderson, D. C. (2002). Diabetes mellitus and other metabolic disturbances induced by atypical antipsychotic agents. *Current Diabetes Reports, 2*(2), 135–140.

Herz, M. I. (1984). Recognizing and preventing relapse in patients with schizophrenia. *Hospital and Community Psychiatry, 35,* 344–349.

Hogarty, G. E., McEvoy, J. P., Munetz, M., DiBarry, A. L., Bartone, P., Cather, R., et al. (1988). Dose of fluphenazine, familial expressed emotion, and outcome in schizophrenia. *Archives of General Psychiatry, 45,* 797–805.

Isaac, R. J., & Armat, V. C. (1990). *Madness in the streets: How psychiatry and the law abandoned the mentally ill.* New York: Free Press.

Jablensky, A. (2000). Epidemiology of schizophrenia: The global burden of disease and disability. *European Archives of Psychiatry & Clinical Neuroscience, 250*(6), 274–285.

Kane, J. M., Woerner, M., & Sarantakos, S. (1986). Depot neuroleptics: A comparative review of standard, intermediate, and low-dose regimens. *Journal of Clinical Psychiatry, 47*(5 Suppl.), 30–33.

Kessler, R. C., McGonagle, K. A., Zhao, S., Nelson, C. B., Hughes, M., Eshleman, S., et al. (1994). Lifetime and 12-month prevalence of DSM-III-R psychiatric disorders in the United States. Results from the National Comorbidity Survey. *Archives of General Psychiatry, 51*(1), 8–19.

Lamb, H. R., & Bachrach, L. L. (2001). Some perspectives on deinstitutionalization. *Psychiatric Services, 52*(8), 1039–1045.

Lehman, A. F., & Steinwachs, D. M. (1998). Patterns of usual care for schizophrenia: Initial results from the Schizophrenia Patient Outcomes Research Team (SPORT) Client Survey. *Schizophrenia Bulletin, 24*(1), 11–20; discussion 20–32.

Lickey, M. E., & Gordon, B. (1991). *Medicine and mental illness.* New York: W. H. Freeman.

Linehan, M., & Armstrong, H. (1991). Cognitive-behavioral treatment of chronically parasuicidal borderline patients. *Archives of General Psychiatry, 48,* 1060–1064.

Lipsey, M. W., & Wilson, D. B. (1993). The efficacy of psychological, educational, and behavioral treatment: Confirmation from meta-analysis. *American Psychologist, 48,* 1181–1209.

Maj, M., Veltro, F., Pirozzi, R., Lobrace, S., & Magliano, L. (1992). Pattern of recurrence of illness after recovery from an episode of major depression: A prospective study. *American Journal of Psychiatry, 149*(6), 795–800.

Marinangeli, M. G., Butti, G., Scinto, A., Di Cicco, L., Petruzzi, C., Daneluzzo, E., et al. (2000). Patterns of comorbidity among DSM-III-R personality disorders. *Psychopathology, 33*(2), 69–74.

Marshak, L. E., Bostick, D., & Turton, L. J. (1990). Closure outcomes for clients with psychiatric disabilities served by the vocational rehabilitation system. *Rehabilitation Counseling Bulletin, 33,* 247–250.

Maxmen, J. S., & Ward, N. G. (1995). *Essential psychopathology and its treatment* (2nd ed.). New York: W. W. Norton.

McGlashan, T. H. (1988). A selective review of recent North American long-term followup studies of schizophrenia. *Schizophrenia Bulletin, 14,* 515–542.

McGrew, J. H., Wilson, R., & Bond, G. R. (1996). Client perspectives on helpful ingredients of assertive community treatment. *Psychiatric Rehabilitation Journal, 19*(3), 13–21.

McKinnon, K. (1996). Sexual and drug-use risk behavior. In F. Corrnos & N. Bakalor (Eds.), *AIDS and people with severe mental illness: A handbook for mental health professionals* (pp. 17–46). New Haven, CT: Yale University Press.

McQuilken, M., Zahniser, J. H., Novak, J., Starks, R. D., Olmos, A., & Bond, G. R.

(2003). The Work Project Survey: Consumer perspectives on work. *Journal of Vocational Rehabilitation, 18,* 59–68.

Meisler, N. (1997). Assertive community treatment initiatives: Results from a survey of selected state mental health authorities. *Community Support Network News, 11*(4), 3–5.

Mellman, T. A., Miller, A. L., Weissman, E. M., Crismon, M. L., Essock, S. M., & Marder, S. R. (2001). Evidence-based pharmacologic treatment for people with severe mental illness: A focus on guidelines and algorithms. *Psychiatric Services, 52*(5), 619–625.

Miller, A. L., Chiles, J. A., Chiles, J. K., Crismon, M. L., Rush, A. J., & Shon, S. P. (1999). The Texas Medication Algorithm Project (TMAP) schizophrenia algorithms. *Journal of Clinical Psychiatry, 60*(10), 649–657.

Miller, W. R., & Rollnick, S. (2002). *Motivational interviewing: Preparing people for change* (2nd ed.). New York: Guilford.

Minkoff, K. (1978). A map of chronic mental patients. In J. A. Talbott (Ed.), *The chronic mental patient* (pp. 11–37). Washington, DC: American Psychiatric Association.

Möller, H., & Volz, H. (1996). Drug treatment of depression in the 1990s: An overview of achievements and future possibilities. *Drugs, 52,* 625–638.

Mowbray, C. T., Chamberlain, P., Jennings, M., & Reed, C. (1988). Consumer-run mental health services: Results from five demonstration projects. *Community Mental Health Journal, 2,* 151–156.

Mowbray, C. T., Moxley, D. P., Jasper, C. A., & Howell, L. L. (Eds.). (1997). *Consumers as providers in psychiatric rehabilitation.* Columbia, MD: International Association of Psychosocial Rehabilitation Services.

Moxley, D. P., Mowbray, C. T., & Brown, K. S. (1993). Supported education. In R. W. Flexer & P. L. Solomon (Eds.), *Psychiatric rehabilitation in practice* (pp. 137–153). Boston: Andover Medical Publishers.

Mueser, K. T., Corrigan, P. W., Hilton, D. W., Tanzman, B., Schaub, A., Gingerich, S., et al. (2002). Illness management and recovery: A review of the research. *Psychiatric Services, 53*(10), 1272–1284.

Mueser, K. T., Drake, R. E., & Bond, G. R. (1997). Recent advances in psychiatric rehabilitation for patients with severe mental illness. *Harvard Review of Psychiatry, 5,* 123–137.

Mueser, K. T., & Gingerich, S. (1994). *Coping with schizophrenia: A guide for families.* Oakland, CA: New Harbinger Publications.

Mueser, K. T., & Glynn, S. M. (1995). Families as members of the treatment team. In K. Mueser & S. M. Glynn (Eds.), *Behavioral family therapy for psychiatric disorder* (pp. 1–29). Needham Heights, MA: Allyn & Bacon.

Mueser, K. T., Goodman, L. B., Trumbetta, S. L., Rosenberg, S. D., Osher, F. C., Vidaver, R., et al. (1998). Trauma and posttraumatic stress disorder in severe mental illness. *Journal of Consulting and Clinical Psychology, 66,* 493–499.

Mueser, K. T., & Tarrier, N. (Eds.). (1998). *Handbook of social functioning in schizophrenia.* Needham Heights, MA: Allyn & Bacon.

Mueser, K. T., Torrey, W. C., Lynde, D., Singer, P., & Drake, R. E. (2003). Implementing evidence-based practices for people with severe mental illness. *Behavior Modification, 27*(3), 387–411.

National Association for the Mentally Ill. (2003). *NAMI mission & history.* Retrieved 2003 from http://www.nami.org/history.htm

Narrow, W. E., Regier, D. A., Rae, D. S., Manderscheid, R. W., & Locke, B. Z. (1993). Use of services by persons with mental and addictive disorders. Findings from the National Institute of Mental Health Epidemiologic Catchment Area Program. *Archives of General Psychiatry, 50*(2), 95–107.

Nasrallah, H. A. (2002). Pharmacoeconomic implications of adverse effects during antipsychotic drug therapy. *American Journal of Health-System Pharmacy, 59*(22 Suppl. 8), S16–21.

New Freedom Commission on Mental Health. (2003). *Achieving the promise: Transforming mental health care in America. Final Report. DHHS Pub. No. SMA-03-3832.* Rockville, MD: Substance Abuse and Mental Health Services Administration.

Noble, J. H., Honberg, R. S., Hall, L. L., & Flynn, L. M. (1997). *A legacy of failure: The inability of the federal-state vocational rehabilitation system to serve people with severe mental illness.* Arlington, VA: National Alliance for the Mentally Ill.

Noll, K. M., Davis, J. M., & DeLeon-Jones, F. (1985). Medication and somatic therapies in the treatment of depression. In E. E. Beckham & W. R. Lebe (Eds.), *Handbook of depression: Treatment, assessment and research* (pp. 220–315). Homewood, IL: Dorsey Press.

Olmstad vs. L. C. (1999). 527 U.S. 581 (138 F. 3d 893) (98-536).

Pratt, C. W., Gill, K. J., Barrett, N. M., & Roberts, M. M. (1999). *Psychiatric rehabilitation.* New York: Academic Press.

Ralph, R. O. (2000). *A synthesis of a sample of recovery literature 2000.* Alexandria, VA: National Technical Center for State Mental Health Planning, National Association for State Mental Health Program Directors.

Regier, D. A., Farmer, M. E., Rae, D. S., Locke, B. Z., Keith, S. J., Judd, L. L., et al. (1990). Comorbidity of mental disorders with alcohol and other drug abuse. Results from the Epidemiologic Catchment Area (ECA) Study [Comment]. *Journal of the American Medical Association, 264*(19), 2511–2518.

Regier, D. A., Rae, D. S., Narrow, W. E., Kaelber, C. T., & Schatzberg, A. F. (1998). Prevalence of anxiety disorders and their comorbidity with mood and addictive disorders. *British Journal of Psychiatry, 34*(Suppl.), 24–28.

Rogers, E. S., Anthony, W. A., & Jansen, M. A. (1988). Psychiatric rehabilitation as the preferred response to the needs of individuals with severe psychiatric disability. *Rehabilitation Psychology, 33*, 5–14.

Rosenberg, S. D., Mueser, K. T., Friedman, M. J., Gorman, P. G., Drake, R. E., Vidaver, R. M., et al. (2001). Developing effective treatments for posttraumatic disorders among people with severe mental illness. *Psychiatric Services, 52*(11), 1453–1461.

Rosenhan, D. L. (1973). On being sane in insane places. *Science, 179*, 250–258.

Rush, A. J., Rago, W. V., Crismon, M. L., Toprac, M. G., Shon, S. P., Suppes, T., et al. (1999). Medication treatment for the severely and persistently mentally ill: The Texas Medication Algorithm Project. *Journal of Clinical Psychiatry, 60*(5), 284–291.

Safferman, A., Lieberman, J. A., Kane, J. M., Szymanski, S., & Kinon, B. (1991). Update on the clinical efficacy and side effects of clozapine. *Schizophrenia Bulletin, 17,* 247–261.

Sartorius, N., Shapiro, R., & Jablonsky, A. (1974). The international pilot study of schizophrenia. *Schizophrenia Bulletin, 2,* 21–35.

Schinnar, A., Rothbard, A., Kanter, R., & Jung, Y. (1990). An empirical literature review of definitions of severe and persistent mental illness. *American Journal of Psychiatry, 147,* 1602–1608.

Segal, S. P., & Aviram, U. (1978). *The mentally ill in community-based sheltered care: A study of community care and social integration.* New York: Wiley-International.

Sherman, P. S., & Porter, R. (1991). Mental health consumers as case management aides. *Hospital and Community Psychiatry, 42,* 494–498.

Steadman, H. J., Mulvey, E. P., Monahan, J., Robbins, P. C., Appelbaum, P. S., Grisso, T., et al. (1998). Violence by people discharged from acute psychiatric inpatient facilities and by others in the same neighborhoods. *Archives of General Psychiatry, 55,* 393–404.

Stein, L. I., & Test, M. A. (1980). An alternative to mental health treatment. I: Conceptual model, treatment program, and clinical evaluation. *Archives of General Psychiatry, 37,* 392–397.

Streicker, S. K., Amdur, M., & Dincin, J. (1986). Educating patients about psychiatric medications: Failure to enhance compliance. *Psychosocial Rehabilitation Journal, 9*(4), 15–28.

Substance Abuse and Mental Health Services Administration (SAMHSA). (1997). *Just the Facts: The prevalence of co-occurring mental and substance disorders in the criminal justice system.* Rockville, MD: National GAINS Center, SAMHSA.

Swanson, J. W., Holzer, C. E. 3rd, Ganju, V. K., & Jono, R. T. (1990). Violence and psychiatric disorder in the community: Evidence from the Epidemiologic Catchment Area surveys [Erratum appears in *Hospital Community Psychiatry* (1991), *42*(9), 954–955]. *Hospital & Community Psychiatry, 41*(7), 761–770.

Swanson, J. W., Swartz, M. S., Essock, S. M., Osher, F. C., Wagner, H. R., Goodman, L. A., et al. (2002). The social-environmental context of violent behavior in persons treated for severe mental illness. *American Journal of Public Health, 92*(9), 1523–1531.

Swartz, M. S., Swanson, J. W., Hiday, V. A., Borum, R., Wagner, H. R., & Burns, B. J. (1998). Violence and severe mental illness: The effects of substance abuse and nonadherence to medication. *American Journal of Psychiatry, 155*(2), 226–231.

Switzer, G. E., Dew, M. A., Thompson, K., Goycoolea, J. M., Derricott, T., & Mullins, S. D. (1999). Posttraumatic stress disorder and service utilization among urban mental health center clients. *Journal of Traumatic Stress, 12*(1), 25–39.

Talbott, J. A. (Ed.). (1978). *The chronic mental patient.* Washington, DC: American Psychiatric Association.

Tamminga, C. A. (1997). The promise of new drugs for schizophrenia treatment. *Canadian Journal of Psychiatry, 42,* 265–273.

Teplin, L. A. (1990). The prevalence of severe mental disorder among male urban detainees: Comparison with the epidemiologic catchment area program. *American Journal of Public Health, 80,* 663–669.

Test, M. A. (1992). Training in community living. In R. P. Liberman (Ed.), *Handbook of psychiatric rehabilitation* (pp. 153–170). New York: Macmillan.

Thornicroft, G., & Sartorius, N. (1993). The course and outcome of depression in different cultures: 10-year follow-up of the WHO Collaborative Study on the Assessment of Depressive Disorders. *Psychological Medicine, 23*(4), 1023–1032.

Torrey, E. F. (1988). *Nowhere to go.* New York: Harper and Row.

Torrey, E. F. (2001). *Surviving schizophrenia: A manual for families, consumers, and providers* (4th ed.). New York: Harper-Collins.

Torrey, E. F., Erdman, K., Wolfe, S. M., & Flynn, L. M. (1990). *Care of the seriously mentally ill: A rating of state programs* (3rd ed.). Arlington, VA: National Alliance for the Mentally Ill.

Turner, J. C., & TenHoor, W. J. (1978). The NIMH community support program: Pilot approach to a needed social reform. *Schizophrenia Bulletin, 4,* 319–348.

Twamley, E. W., Jeste, D. V., & Lehman, A. F. (2003). Vocational rehabilitation in schizophrenia and other psychotic disorders: A literature review and meta-analysis of randomized controlled trials. *Journal of Nervous and Mental Disease, 191,* 515–523.

U.S. Congress. (1963). *P.L. 88-164—Mental Retardation Facilities and Community Mental Health Centers Construction Act of 1963,* Washington, DC: U.S. Government Printing Office.

Wahl, O. (1997). *Consumer experience with stigma: Results of a national survey.* Alexandria, VA: NAMI.

Wallace, C. J., Liberman, R. P., MacKain, S. J., Blackwell, G., & Eckman, T. A. (1992). Effectiveness and replicability of modules for teaching social and instrumental skills to the severely mentally ill. *American Journal of Psychiatry, 149,* 654–658.

Wang, P. S., West, J. C., Tanielian, T., & Pincus, H. A. (2000). Recent patterns and predictors of antipsychotic medication regimens used to treat schizophrenia and other psychotic disorders. *Schizophrenia Bulletin, 26,* 451–457.

Wehman, P., & Moon, M. S. (Eds.). (1988). *Vocational rehabilitation and supported employment.* Baltimore: Paul Brookes.

Weiden, P. J., & Olfson, M. (1993). The cost of relapse in schizophrenia. *Schizophrenia Bulletin, 21*, 419–428.

Widiger, T. A., Frances, A., & Trull, T. J. (1987). A psychometric analysis of the social-interpersonal and cognitive-perceptual items for the schizotypal personality disorder. *Archives of General Psychiatry, 44*(8), 741–745.

Wittlin, B. J. (1988). Practical psychopharmacology. In R. P. Liberman (Ed.), *Psychiatric rehabilitation of chronic mental patients* (pp. 117–145). Washington, DC: American Psychiatric Association.

21

Pulmonary Disorders

FREDERICK A. BEVELAQUA, MD, FACP, FCCP

C HRONIC OBSTRUCTIVE PULMONARY disease (COPD) encompasses a spectrum of disorders from asthmatic bronchitis and
chronic obstructive bronchitis, which are largely diseases of the
airways, to emphysema, which affects both the airways and the alveoli.
The economic effect of these disorders can be estimated in terms of the
cost of treatment, reduced productivity because of morbidity and
reduced productivity in terms of mortality. However, with proper treatment and rehabilitation many individuals may achieve a degree of comfort and physical capability that will allow hem to return to work.
Although bronchial asthma may be considered a separate disorder from
COPD, it is also a disease of the airways and has many features that are
similar to COPD.

Other chronic pulmonary disorders such as occupational lung diseases, interstitial lung diseases, and cystic fibrosis have some characteristics in common with COPD. Therefore, an understanding of the
clinical characteristics, pathology, and physiology of COPD is crucial to
an understanding of these other disorders. In this chapter we will discuss these points in detail and review the management, prognoses of
these disorders. We will also discuss the vocational and psychological
implications involved in the care of these patients.

CHRONIC OBSTRUCTIVE PULMONARY DISEASE

DISEASE DESCRIPTION AND DEFINITIONS

CHRONIC OBSTRUCTIVE PULMONARY disease (COPD) is characterized by decreased airflow during expiration. Reduction in airflow during expirations has two causes: decreased expiratory airflow pressure
(decrease in driving pressure) and increased resistance to expiratory airflow. In the lung the driving pressure for expiratory airflow is primarily
caused by the elastic recoil pressure of the lung. Increased resistance to
airflow results from narrowing of the airways. COPD patients seldom
have only one type of lesion, but often one may predominate. In chronic
bronchitis, the obstruction to airflow is predominately due to disease
of the airways, which results in increased resistance to airflow. In emphysema, the obstruction to airflow results primarily from loss of the elastic recoil pressure, which decreases the airflow driving pressure. The
anatomical changes in the lung associated with the loss of alveoli in
emphysema also result in premature compression or closure of the bronchioles on exhalation, which contributes to airflow obstruction. In
chronic bronchitis, obstruction to airflow is caused primarily by chronic
inflammation of the bronchial passageways which results in increased
mucus production, smooth muscle hyperplasia, increased bronchial
smooth muscle tone, and thickening of the bronchial wall.

The term "asthmatic bronchitis" is sometimes used to refer to a variation of chronic bronchitis in which there is a variable degree of airflow obstruction superimposed on a chronic, fixed degree of obstruction.
This variable portion of airway obstruction is reminiscent of asthma in
that there is some reversibility of airflow obstruction with the use of
bronchodilator drugs. However, although in this respect there is some
similarity to asthma, which will be discussed in more detail later in this
chapter, there is unlikely to be the major reversibility in airflow obstruction with the use of bronchodilator therapy that is seen in most forms
of asthma. The pathophysiology of asthmatic bronchitis is quite similar to that of chronic bronchitis and is characterized by varying degrees
of airflow obstruction due to inflammation of the airways and increased
bronchial smooth muscle tone. Indeed, asthmatic bronchitis is essentially
a form of chronic bronchitis, and the distinction between the two may
be truly irrelevant. However, in emphysema the primary pathological
process is the loss of alveoli with subsequent loss of alveolar surface
area. This results in hyperinflation of the lung, but airflow obstruction
during expiration occurs because anatomical changes in the lung associated with the loss of alveoli also predispose to collapse of the smaller
airways during expiration which impairs expiratory flow.

Emphysema and chronic bronchitis are often considered together under the term COPD because most such patients have a combination of chronic bronchitis (or asthmatic bronchitis) and emphysema. In other words they have both airway disease and alveolar disease. The classic textbook criterion for chronic bronchitis, namely, a chronic productive cough for at least 3 months of the year for 2 consecutive years, is really not adequate. The underlying pathophysiology must also be considered. By the time the patient has advanced to irreversible airflow obstruction, particularly at an older age, there is little point in seeking a more specific diagnosis than COPD. However, there is a great deal of importance in identifying those patients who have a major potential for reversibility in response to therapy, because they often have much better prognosis than those with more fixed or progressive airflow obstruction.

There are other disease states also characterized by chronic airflow obstruction, such as cystic fibrosis, bronchiectasis, bronchiolitis obliterans, and some interstitial lung diseases. However, they should not be designated as COPD because they have different prognoses, etiologies, and treatments. Because these disorders are not as common as COPD, they will be discussed separately and in less detail later in this chapter.

Etiology, Pathophysiology, and Clinical Features

Several factors are involved in pathogenesis of COPD, but smoking is the most important. Inflammation of the respiratory tract produced by smoking promotes bronchoconstriction and interferes with the protective antibacterial function of the alveolar macrophages. Smoking also inhibits the normal clearance mechanism of the tracheobronchial tree. Occupational exposure to dust and fumes also promotes inflammation, bronchospasm, and edema of the airways. Epidemiological data also suggest a close relationship between air pollution and COPD, but these factors are usually less significant than smoking as a cause of COPD. Inflammation, hypersecretion, and bronchoconstriction increase susceptibility to subsequent infection. This in turn leads to further bronchial obstruction, alveolar destruction, and emphysema. Bronchial obstruction creates a mismatch of ventilation to perfusion that may lead to hypoxia and hypercapnia. If the hypoxia is severe enough and chronic, it may lead to pulmonary hypertension because hypoxia leads to pulmonary vasoconstriction. Chronic hypoxia also induces secondary polycythemia. If pulmonary hypertension is severe enough right heart failure may ensue. Hypercapnia causes respiratory acidosis, which further worsens pulmonary vasoconstriction and bronchoconstriction. A cycle is thereby set up that may eventually lead to respiratory failure.

In addition to all of the above, the development and progression of COPD is largely related to genetic predisposition. In one particular form of COPD, the development of emphysema is associated with an inherited deficiency of a proteolytic enzyme inhibitor, alpha 1-antitrypsin. Severe alpha 1-antitrypsin deficiency is associated with emphysema beginning at a relatively early age, usually under 40. The mechanism accounting for this type of familial emphysema is thought to be due to breakdown or lysis of elastic lung tissue by enzymes released from blood leukocytes, alveolar macrophages, and bacteria. In the presence of normal levels of this inhibitor the enzymes are prevented from causing lung damage, but when the levels are insufficient, the lung issue is unprotected from the destructive forces of these enzymes.

There are many factors that combine to produce airway obstruction in COPD. Spasm of the smooth muscles of the respiratory tract, edema of the airways, excess mucus production, and compression or collapse of bronchial walls are all involved in producing obstruction to airflow. With the loss of alveoli in emphysema, there is a decrease in the supporting framework in which the terminal bronchioles are suspended. Therefore, during expiration, pressure in the alveoli exceeds the pressure in the bronchioles, so the bronchioles are exposed to a compressive force that overwhelms the traction forces of the remaining alveoli that tend to keep the bronchioles open. This compression of the airways during exhalation leads to premature airway collapse and obstruction to expiratory airflow. In chronic bronchitis, inflammation of the bronchial mucosa is the primary pathologic process. The inflammation may be caused by a variety of infections or irritants, resulting in damage to the mucus lining the respiratory tract. As a result of this damage excess amounts of mucus are secreted. The mucosa and the smooth muscles lining the respiratory tract become hypertrophic or enlarged. The mucociliary system that moves mucus upward and out of the respiratory tract is impaired, and the normal protective function of the mucus, which is to trap bacteria and irritants, is therefore compromised.

In addition to damaging the mucosa and causing excess mucus production, this inflammation stimulates the parasympathetic nervous system, which in turn enhances spasm of the smooth muscle lining the respiratory tract. Thus there are two basic types of airway obstruction in chronic bronchitis. One involves direct blockage of the airway due to inflammation and swelling of the mucosa, with subsequent accumulation of mucus in the bronchial tubes and smooth muscle hypertrophy. The other involves narrowing of the bronchial lumen by smooth muscle spasm resulting from inflammation and irritation. Both types of bronchial obstruction also occur in patients with asthma, which will be discussed later, and contribute to the airflow obstruction in emphysema as well.

Although the clinical and pathophysiological features of chronic bronchitis and emphysema often overlap, some patients with COPD have characteristics that more clearly place them in one category or the other. The reason why some patients develop a predominantly bronchitis pattern whereas others develop a predominantly emphysematous pattern is unclear. As mentioned previously, overlap is so common that it is difficult to consider emphysema and chronic bronchitis as completely separate entities. However, for the sake of simplicity patients are often labeled as having one or the other. The patients who have predominantly chronic bronchitis are characterized by a more prominent cough and sputum production. They are more likely to be hypoxic and hypercapneic and to develop cor pulmonale (enlargement of the right ventricle of the heart) secondary to pulmonary hypertension, which occurs because of chronic vasoconstriction of the pulmonary arterioles associated with hypoxia and hypercapnea. Pathologic changes in the large airways are more extensive in chronic bronchitis, including mucus gland hyperplasia, smooth muscle hypertrophy, and increased mucus production. Disease in the smaller airways is even more important in limiting airflow since these smaller airways may undergo obliteration, resulting in a decrease in the total cross-sectional area of the airways.

Clinically, the patients who predominantly have emphysema have less cough and sputum production. The loss of alveoli is more pronounced. They also tend to be less hypoxic and hypercapneic until the disease is very far advanced. In emphysema the loss of alveoli results in decreased elastic recoil of the lung, which in turn results in hyperinflation of the lung. This tends to flatten the diaphragm, placing it at a mechanical disadvantage so that it does not contract properly. Loss of elastic recoil also results in limitation of airflow because it facilitates compression of the airways during expiration. In severe cases, airflow is limited even during quiet breathing because of this collapsibility of the airways during exhalation. Such a severely compromised patient would have marked dyspnea even at rest.

Airflow limitation in emphysema is also affected by pathologic changes in the small airways themselves. Small airways are normally responsible for 10%–20% of the airway resistance in the respiratory tract. In obstructive lung disease, the resistance to airflow in the small airways resulting from these pathologic changes can increase tremendously. In patients with emphysematous lung disease, such small airway disease can also greatly increase the airflow limitation caused by the easy compressibility of the airways described above. Thus, in patients with emphysema, airflow limitation has two causes. First, the loss of elastic recoil (due to loss of alveoli) causes easy collapsibility or compressibility of the airways during expiration. Second, the pathologic changes in the small airways themselves produce an increase in airway resistance.

In patients with COPD the loss of alveoli is associated with loss of alveolar capillaries, so emphysematous lungs contain many areas with higher than normal ratios of ventilation to blood perfusion. This results in increased physiological "dead space," which means that areas of the lung are being ventilated but not perfused so that gas exchange with the atmosphere is impaired. As this happens, the minute ventilation (liters per minute of air moved in and out of the lung) required to produce adequate levels of alveolar ventilation (liters per minute of air actually involved with gas exchange in functioning alveoli) increases, and therefore the total work of breathing increases as well. As the disease progresses, the patient becomes less able to compensate even with increased work of breathing. An even more severe impairment in gas exchange may occur in areas of the lung where there is underventilation in relation to perfusion, or so-called "shunting." This is the major cause of hypoxia in COPD.

Patients with emphysema also have areas of low ventilation-to-perfusion match-up and resultant hypoxia because of obstructive inflammatory changes in the airways. This is usually most striking in patients who present clinically with features of both chronic bronchitis and emphysema. Patients who predominantly have emphysema usually maintain an arterial oxygen level remarkably close to normal, despite a marked degree of airflow limitation, until the disease is very far advanced. Such preservation of arterial oxygen is unusual in patients with severe chronic bronchitis, bronchiectasis, or cystic fibrosis. For an equivalent degree of airflow limitation, the patient who predominantly has emphysema is less likely to develop a low blood-oxygen level and high carbon dioxide (CO_2) level than is the patient who predominantly has chronic bronchitis. This also reflects the relatively intact ventilatory response to CO_2 in the emphysema patient. The reasons for the preservation of CO_2 responsiveness in emphysema patients and the apparently impaired responsiveness in chronic bronchitis patients are not well understood. Although the patient with emphysema tends to have less severe hypoxemia than does the patient with chronic bronchitis, hypercapnia often becomes a feature late in the course of even relatively pure emphysema, and once again the distinctions between emphysema and chronic bronchitis become blurred.

When emphysema exists in a relatively pure form (i.e., no major pathologic changes in the airways), there is dyspnea on minimal exertion, but the patient is generally free from productive cough or bronchospasm. Cyanosis and clubbing are usually absent. Use of accessory muscles of respiration and pursed-lip breathing occur. By restricting the airway opening, pursed-lip breathing serves to maintain pressure within the airway itself and helps to minimize the external compression of the airways during expiration that is characteristic of emphysema. In classic chronic bronchitis there is also dyspnea with minimal exertion, but the patient usually has a more productive cough, often associated with bronchospasm, and cyanosis is more common. Use of accessory muscles and pursed-lip breathing may also occur, but it is less pronounced than in the more emphysematous type patient. On physical examination the emphysematous lung is hyperresonant. Diaphragmatic excursion and breath sounds are diminished. Wheezes and rhonchi are the result of turbulence associated with obstructive airway pathology and not of the emphysema (loss of alveoli) per se.

When chronic bronchitis predominates, the wheezes and rhonchi are often much more noticeable. Inspection of the thorax and chest x-rays of patients with emphysema usually give the impression of an increased front-to-back diameter of the chest. Clinicians often diagnose pulmonary emphysema from chest-x-rays based on findings of low, flat diaphragms, increased retrosternal airspace, elongated mediastinum, enlarged hilar vessels, and bullous lung changes. However, these are relatively insensitive findings, and in general the clinician should place much more emphasis on physical examination and pulmonary function testing when evaluating patients with suspected airflow obstruction of any type.

OTHER TYPES OF COPD

ASTHMA, BRONCHIECTASIS, AND cystic fibrosis are other forms of COPD in which the major pathology involves the airways. Asthma and cystic fibrosis will be discussed in more detail later in this chapter because they are important disorders, with characteristic features deserving special attention.

Bronchiectasis is characterized pathologically by chronic and irreversible dilation and distortion of the bronchi. These changes usually follow some sort of inflammatory insult to the respiratory tract (e.g., severe pneumonia or respiratory tract infection) and may be more likely seen if the infection or inflammation occurs in early childhood or infancy, before the development of the respiratory tract has been completed. Anatomical bronchial abnormalities that are congenital in nature may also lead to the development of bronchiectasis. The clinical manifestations depend on the severity of the pathology and the degree of vascularity associated with the anatomical distortion of the bronchi. Patients usually have a chronic cough that is productive of mucopurulent sputum and often have hemoptysis, which at times may be severe and life-threatening. Chronic sinusitis and clubbing of the fingers are also common clinical characteristics.

FUNCTIONAL DISABILITIES

THE EARLIEST MANIFESTATIONS of COPD may be relatively mild, but as time goes on, dyspnea becomes the most important limiting factor.

Years may pass before the degree of dyspnea is severe enough to limit routine daily activities such as walking. As time progresses, activities such as dressing, bathing, speech, and even eating cannot be accomplished without severe shortness of breath. Until disease is extremely far advanced, relatively sedentary activities may be accomplished without too much difficulty. Driving may be possible, but walking even limited distances may not be, particularly if an incline or stairs are involved. Nonetheless, there are some patients even with severe lung disease who maintain a good level of activity despite reduced oxygen levels and elevated CO_2 levels. Such individuals may be able to remain at work in a sedentary capacity, although physical activity such as walking more than a few feet on a level plane or stair climbing may be totally beyond their capabilities. Therefore, assessment of a given patient's functional capability may be difficult to determine based on pulmonary function studies and blood gases alone. Depression, fear, and anxiety are potent factors that may further exacerbate the patient's physical limitations. Many such patients are unaware that medical treatment and rehabilitation may greatly improve their functional capacities. Recurrent respiratory tract infections and continuation of smoking greatly enhance the progress of the disease. Preparation for a sedentary occupation would be wise even at the time of relatively mild disease because the rate of progression is variable.

MEDICAL EVALUATION

IN GENERAL, PATIENTS with symptomatic respiratory disease should be examined and evaluated by a specialist in internal medicine or pulmonary disease. Appropriate therapy can sometimes make a tremendous difference in a patient's functional capacity. A chest x-ray should be obtained to rule out cancer and infections such as tuberculosis. Although a chest x-ray may often show the changes characteristic of emphysema, often there is not a very close correlation between x-ray findings and the patient's functional capacity or rehabilitation potential.

Pulmonary function studies are particularly important. The forced vital capacity (FVC), which is the maximum amount of air that can be inspired and expired, and the forced expired volume in 1 second (FEV_1) are important parameters to follow in COPD. The volume exhaled with a forced expiratory maneuver during the 1st, 2nd, and 3rd seconds (FEV_1, FEV_2, FEV_3) is often measured. The FVC, FEV_1, FEV_2, and FEV_3 are all reduced in obstructive lung disease, but restrictive lung diseases (see "Interstititial Lung Disease," below) can also reduce them. However, in obstructive lung disease the ratios of FEV_1, FEV_2, and FEV_3 to FVC are reduced, whereas in the restrictive lung diseases these ratios tend to be normal or above normal. The maximum voluntary ventilation (MVV) is another parameter that is sometimes used in evaluating physical capacity. This maneuver records the maximal volume of air the patient can breathe in 12 seconds while breathing in and out as rapidly and forcefully as possible.

Pulmonary function studies are useful in evaluating patient performance only when patient cooperation is complete and a competent technician is performing the study. Arterial blood gas determinations and lung volume measurements are often helpful in the evaluation. On occasion the blood gases are significantly worse than would be expected based on pulmonary function abnormalities alone. The reverse is also sometimes true. Knowing the arterial oxygen and carbon dioxide levels, particularly with exercise, may be quite helpful in evaluating the patient's functional capacity. Motivation and conditioning are also extremely important in assessing the patient. Highly motivated and well-conditioned patients may be much more capable of physical activity than poorly motivated, deconditioned patients even though their pulmonary function studies are comparable.

TREATMENT

MANY PATIENTS WITH chronic pulmonary disorders may have a potential for some reversibility, which can be achieved with proper medical management. Periodic exacerbations caused by a variety of factors, including infection, may also occur. Such exacerbations may cause an acute deterioration in function that will improve as the acute process is treated. A wide variety of antibiotics are available to treat respiratory tract infections. There are also a number of medications that can help to alleviate the bronchospasm found in many patients with COPD. Theophylline-type drugs were commonly used in the past to relieve bronchospasm, but they have been largely replaced by other more effective medications. Inhaled B-adrenergic type drugs such as albuterol and salbutamol, either as aerosols or dry powder inhalations, can also help to alleviate bronchospasm. Ipatropium bromide is an atropine derivative that is also used in an aerosol form. It has significant bronchodilating effects and can be used in conjunction with other bronchodilators such as the B-adrenergic type drugs to enhance bronchodilating effect.

Glucocorticoid steroids have marked anti-inflammatory effects that can be extremely useful in the management of severe bronchospasm. However, when given orally or parenterally these drugs are difficult to use on a long-term basis because of associated side effects, including osteoporosis, weight gain, muscle weakness, worsening of diabetes mellitus, cataract formation, peptic ulcer disease, and others. Inhaled glucocorticoid steroids such as beclomethasone, budesonide, fluticasone, and others may be particularly useful for long-term management of steroid-responsive bronchospasm because of their minimal side effects. However, they are not very useful for acute severe bronchospasm. Newer medications such as the antileukotrienes, although primarily developed to reduce inflammation in asthma, may be helpful in reducing the inflammatory response in patients who have chronic obstructive lung disease with a bronchospastic component.

Preventing dehydration in patients with chronic obstructive pulmonary disease is important since dehydration will tend to dry out respiratory secretions, making it much more difficult for the patient to clear the airways. Chest physical therapy and pulmonary rehabilitation programs are very useful in a variety of ways. The physical therapist can assist the patient, through postural drainage and percussion, to expel mucus from the respiratory tract. Breathing exercises and relaxation techniques may help the patient in activities of daily living. Exercise reconditioning can help to increase endurance and improve work capacity even though conventional lung function tests may change little if at all.

Patients in graded exercise programs should be monitored closely because oxygen desaturation can occur during exercise, along with arrhythmia and myocardial ischemia. Supplemental oxygen may be necessary during such programs. Nocturnal oxygen supplementation may also be useful in patients who have arterial oxygen desaturation at night. Improved oxygen saturation may have beneficial effects on the pulmonary circulation and cardiac function. Continuous oxygen therapy may be needed in patients who are chronically hypoxic. Judicious use of oxygen therapy may help such patients remain active. However, oxygen use requires careful monitoring and supervision. Arterial blood gases should be obtained periodically to assess the efficacy of the oxygen administration and to make sure patients are not developing excessive levels of CO_2 retention in response to the elevated oxygen levels.

VOCATIONAL IMPLICATIONS

IT IS EXTREMELY important that patients and their families develop an understanding of the illness in order to deal with it effectively. In many instances patients may be inadequately treated or may not be taking their medications properly. Frequently, with the proper use of medications, patients can derive significant relief of their symptoms and may be able to resume some if not all of their routine activities. Smoking cessation may be crucial in helping to delay the progression of the disease. Proper nutrition, exercise reconditioning, and chest physical therapy sometimes prove invaluable in helping the patient to resume a more active and normal life. Psychological counseling often helps the patient deal with the anxiety and stress associated with diseases that can cause frightening shortness of breath and marked limitation of activity. Learning to deal effectively with these problems and to make satisfactory adaptations in lifestyle may mean the difference between a productive life and a desperate one. Patients may have to change their employment goals. Cough and expectoration can preclude some occupations requiring close personal interaction. For patients who are severely compromised (e.g., FEV_1 of 1 liter or less), slow walking on the level is often possible, whereas stair climbing is impossible. Likewise, resting hypoxemia (PaO_2 of 60 torr or lower) can be adequate for a sedentary job, but even minimal strenuous activity can cause a significant decrease in oxygen level that would preclude employment. Access to supplemental oxygen can often allow the chronically hypoxemic patient or the patient who desaturates with minimal exertion to remain employed at a sedentary activity. However, even sedentary activities may periodically require greater levels of activity than are feasible. Traveling to and from work sometimes poses a level of exertion beyond the patient's capability.

Most methods employed in assessing disability or impairment from respiratory disease consider several factors, including a clinical examination and diagnostic tests. The nature of the underlying disease is extremely important. For example, patients with asthma may be terribly incapacitated during acute attacks but quite functional between attacks. On the other hand, patients with severe chronic bronchitis or emphysema are much less likely to have dramatic remissions of their symptoms. The progressive deterioration of lung function in COPD produces a progressive disability. Some diseases, on the other hand, are acute but non-progressive. For example, the patient who has lung cancer and undergoes a lung resection may develop impairment of lung function, but the resultant disability remains relatively stable providing the remaining lung stays healthy. Pulmonary function studies are particularly important in evaluating pulmonary impairment, and criteria for impairment based on pulmonary function testing have been established by the Social Security Administration. The degree of impairment based on pulmonary function testing may be divided into mild, moderate, and severe. Mild impairment is usually not correlated with diminished ability to perform most jobs. Moderate impairment is correlated with a decreased ability to meet the demands of many jobs. Severe impairment prevents the patient from meeting the demands of most jobs. Exercise testing may also be very helpful in estimating a patient's physical capacity to do work, and may be very important in the evaluation of the patient's degree of disability.

ASTHMA

DISEASE DESCRIPTION, ETIOLOGY, PATHOPHYSIOLOGY, AND CLINICAL FEATURES

ASTHMA IS AN inflammatory disease of the airways that is characterized by reversible airway obstruction and bronchial hyperreactivity. Asthma is often divided into either an allergic, or extrinsic, type, which commonly has its onset in childhood, and an adult-onset, or intrinsic, type. In extrinsic asthma, exposure to an allergen (pollen, dust, animal dander, mold, foods, medication) may clearly precipitate an attack. Intrinsic asthma attacks are more often precipitated by infection. However, there is considerable overlap between the two groups, with the majority of patients demonstrating clinical features of both. Because bronchial hyperreactivity or hyperresponsiveness is present in all asthma attacks, they may be precipitated by environmental stimuli of many types (air temperature, humidity, ozone levels, particulate levels, cigarette smoke, cooking odors, insecticides, etc.). Exercise has been demonstrated to produce bronchoconstriction in many asthmatic patients, as can a simple cough or laugh. Aspirin and food additives such as sulfites are also well-known potential triggers of asthma attacks for some patients.

In an asthma attack there is constriction of bronchial smooth muscle, mucus hypersecretion, and plugging of small airways with mucus. The end result is obstruction of airflow. The frequency, duration, and severity of the attacks vary markedly from patient to patient. Asthmatic attacks are sometimes divided into early phase and late phase. The late-phase may develop hours after the initial onset. This late phase reaction may explain why asthma attacks may last for days or weeks in some patients.

Although there are differences from patient to patient, the asthma attack is typically characterized by shortness of breath and wheezing. Cough and mucus production are usually also present. In some patients cough may be the only symptom of asthma. During an asthma attack the patient demonstrates a rapid rate of respiration, often requiring use of accessory muscles of respiration in the neck and chest. Severe attacks may lead to exhaustion with slowing of the respiratory rate and eventually arrest of breathing.

FUNCTIONAL DISABILITY

DURING ASTHMA ATTACK the patient is totally disabled. Even talking may be impossible because of severe breathlessness. The patient may be totally consumed by the effort to breath and unable to eat or dress. The patient is restless and unable to lie flat. Severe cough may produce musculoskeletal pain that aggravates the condition. Depending on the severity of the patient's disease, the attack may be totally or partially reversible, allowing the patient to resume normal activity between episodes. Patients with very severe asthma remain symptomatic chronically and resemble chronic bronchitis and emphysema patients with similar levels of disability.

MEDICAL EVALUATION

THE STANDARD EVALUATION is similar to that of the COPD patient. In addition, an allergy evaluation is also required regardless of the age of onset. As in the COPD patient, pulmonary function testing is used in diagnosis and in follow-up of patients. Laboratory evaluation should also include consideration of immunodeficiency and cystic fibrosis, especially in children and young adults. Psychological evaluation may be important because emotional factors can precipitate attacks. In children and young adults, social service evaluation may be helpful in identifying developmental and environmental factors.

TREATMENT

THERAPY IS FOCUSED on the treatment and prevention of an asthma attack. The emphasis on prevention stems from the view of asthma as an inflammatory process and has been aided by the development of anti-inflammatory agents.

Asthma medications are divided into "controllers" (primarily anti-inflammatory agents or long-acting bronchodilators), which are taken on a regular basis, and "relievers" (short-acting bronchodilators), which are used as needed. Patients with mild, intermittent asthma may be treated with rapid-acting bronchodilators alone, taken infrequently. Patients with more frequent symptoms that define mild, moderate, and severe asthma are treated with an anti-inflammatory agent such as inhaled steroid sprays in combination with a bronchodilator. Patients with severe asthma may require oral bronchodilator medications or oral corticosteroids given intermittently or, in the most severe cases, continuously.

Self-monitoring with a home peak-flow meter can aid in determining the degree of airway obstruction, allowing the patient and the physician to recognize the severity of an attack and adjust medication accordingly. In this way emergency room treatment or hospitalization maybe avoided. Severe asthma attacks often require hospitalization despite appropriate outpatient treatment. Some patients with allergic asthma may be helped by desensitization with specific allergens. Careful avoidance of environmental allergens should be practiced at home and at work. New treatments involving the injection of antibodies to block or inactivate allergic antibodies may prove to be quite helpful to individuals with an allergic or extrinsic type of asthma.

VOCATIONAL IMPLICATIONS

THE DEGREE OF disability secondary to asthma will, of course, vary from patient to patient, depending on the severity of the disease and the frequency of attacks. The vocational counselor should confer with the client's physician to determine the severity of the disease. This information should be used as a guide to determine the suitability of various occupations. In general, the asthma patient should avoid adverse environmental conditions such as outdoor work, temperature changes, fumes, cigarette smoke, and the like. Physical labor is not absolutely contraindicated, but should be limited to patients with mild disease who are well-controlled on medications and under medical supervision. The counselor also should interact with employers to attempt to ensure the avoidance of environmental irritants and to achieve recognition of the client's illness and potential for absenteeism.

Asthma may also develop as a result of exposure to certain occupational materials. This occupational asthma has been documented in meat packers, woodworkers, and agriculture workers and can occur in virtually any industry that creates exposure to organic dusts, fibers, or fungal spores. Industrial asthma also can occur where workers are exposed to chemical fumes or powders. A change of vocation or workplace may clearly be necessary for the asthmatic patient. The counselor must consider the client's potential for retraining and additional education. The asthmatic population is usually a younger age group, compared to COPD patients, and therefore has more potential for career changes.

INTERSTITIAL LUNG DISEASE

INTERSTITIAL LUNG DISEASES (ILD) are those that involve the supporting structure (interstitium) of the gas-exchanging units (alveoli) of the lung. Although ILD represents a heterogeneous group of diseases in which there may be inflammation and fibrosis of alveolar walls (alveolitis), vascular components, and small airways, there are many common features. One striking common feature is loss of lung volume, which is often described as "restrictive" lung disease in contrast to the "obstructive" pattern of COPD and asthma.

DISEASE DESCRIPTION

INHALATION OF ORGANIC dusts may result in hypersensitivity pneumonitis. These dusts originate from animal proteins, agricultural products, or bacteria or fungi that contaminate food, wood, or detergents. These illnesses are often named after the occupation in which they occur. For example, "farmer's lung" results from exposure to fungi in moldy hay and "bird breeder's lung" results from inhalation of avian proteins.

Inhalation of inorganic dusts results in another form of occupational lung disease, termed pneumoconiosis ("dusty lungs"). Silica (silicosis) and silicates (asbestosis) are two examples of dusts that may produce pulmonary fibrosis. Other potential offenders are aluminum, beryllium, and cobalt. In pneumoconiosis the duration and intensity of exposure to the offending material, as well as smoking history, are important factors in determining etiology. It should be noted that pulmonary fibrosis in pneumoconiosis often occurs 10 to 20 years after exposure began, and symptoms frequently occur after the patient has left the occupation in which he or she was exposed.

Idiopathic pulmonary fibrosis is a well-described ILD in which the cause of the fibrosis is unknown. At times an identical form of pulmonary fibrosis will coexist with a systemic disease such as rheumatoid arthritis ("rheumatoid lung"). Sarcoidosis is another idiopathic inflammatory disease that may result in pulmonary fibrosis. Although often a benign disease of young adults that may present with eye or skin lesions, the pulmonary involvement may result in severe fibrosis and disability.

Functional Disability

The common clinical feature of patients with interstitial lung disease is dyspnea or shortness of breath. Depending on the severity of the fibrosis or inflammation, the patient may be symptomatic at rest or only on exertion. Difficulty in walking will often be noted, first with increased distress on stair climbing. Simple daily activities such as eating, dressing, and bathing may become difficult. Patients with severe disease demonstrate striking "air hunger," with rapid respiratory rates and obvious respiratory distress. Cough also may be a predominate feature. Patients with hypersensitivity pneumonitis may present with constitutional symptoms such as fever or with wheezing. The patient with rheumatoid arthritis and pulmonary fibrosis will typically have severe joint disease. The patient with severe pulmonary fibrosis secondary to sarcoidosis will typically have extra pulmonary disease involving the skin, eyes, and bones.

AS IN the COPD patient, significant psychosocial disabilities may result from severe breathlessness. Anxiety and depression are common, not only as a result of the air hunger but also from the drastic change in lifestyle and activities. Household family members are often affected by concern over the patient's health and by financial and social problems that stem from the patient's inability to function. Spouses often have specific concerns regarding sexual activity.

MEDICAL EVALUATION

THE MEDICAL EVALUATION will resemble that of the COPD patient, as detailed above. A thorough and detailed occupational history will be necessary and is essential to the diagnosis of hypersensitivity pneumonitis and pneumoconiosis. Diagnosis will also depend on patterns of chest x-ray abnormality in many of these disease entities. In pneumoconiosis the chest x-ray may be used to grade severity and intensity of exposure, whereas in silicosis and asbestosis it can form the basis of the diagnosis. The roentgenographic manifestations of pulmonary fibrosis may be nonspecific in terms of etiology but yet reflect the severity of the disease.

As with the COPD patient and the asthma patient, pulmonary function testing is essential in determining disability. As noted above, the characteristic pattern in patients with ILD is restrictive, with a loss of vital capacity (VC) and lung volumes (functional residual capacity [FRC], residual capacity [RC], and total lung capacity [TLC]). In early stages of inflammation and fibrosis and occasionally in patients with more advanced disease, little change in lung volume may be noted but more significant reduction will be seen in diffusion capacity and blood gases. Resting arterial oxygen tensions, however, may be within normal limits in patients with significant functional limitations. In these patients, and in patients with interstitial disease in general, an exercise evaluation can be extremely helpful in demonstrating a marked reduction in oxygen tension on minimal exertion and may clearly demonstrate the functional disability.

In view of the large number of disease entities that comprise the category of ILD, a lung biopsy is often necessary to establish a definite diagnosis. As in the COPD patient, a psychological evaluation may be useful to assess anxiety and depression. Social service evaluation of the patient's family is also helpful in determining the extent of support mechanisms in the home. Family members may require psychosocial evaluation and treatment.

TREATMENT

KNOWLEDGE OF THE natural history of each disease entity is essential in its management. In this heterogeneous group of diseases the ability to reverse the disease process will vary considerably according to the nature of the injury (e.g., inhalation of organic dust) and the stage at which the disease is detected. In hypersensitivity pneumonitis, withdrawal of the offending material is necessary and may have dramatic results. In pneumoconiosis, reduction of intensity and duration of exposure will reduce the severity of the disease.

For a disease that may be reversible, introduction of drug therapy during the earliest inflammatory stage is essential. In general, the decision to treat is often based on the presence of symptomatology (e.g., dyspnea). Because immunologically mediated inflammation is characteristic of many of the interstitial diseases, corticosteroids are considered the drug of choice. Other immunosuppressive agents also have been used, either in conjunction with corticosteorids or alone.

VOCATIONAL IMPLICATIONS

IN THE OCCUPATIONAL lung diseases, the counselor should work with the physician and employer in determining the offending substances that must be avoided. Retraining and extension of education will be necessary for those with occupationally induced disease.

As in the COPD patient, dyspnea will reduce functional ability. Pulmonary function testing should provide guidance in the determination of disability. Patients with lung volumes and or diffusion capacities reduced to 50% or less of predicted values are usually totally disabled. Those with less severe disease may perform sedentary activities but may require shortened workdays or workweeks. Again, the counselor may have to work with employers to obtain these adjustments in the workplace. Supplemental oxygen and rehabilitation programs can increase functional abilities, although the results of these measures are not as helpful as they are in the COPD group.

CYSTIC FIBROSIS

DISEASE DESCRIPTION

CYSTIC FIBROSIS (CF) is a genetic deficiency disease that is characterized by recurrent respiratory tract infections and progressive respiratory insufficiency. It is estimated that 1 of every 20 people is a carrier of the defect. It occurs more often in Caucasians (1 in 2,500 births) than in other racial groups. The disease is usually diagnosed by age 6 and limits life expectancy to 29 years. However, more prolonged survival is increasingly common with better medical treatment and lung transplantation, and as such has created a need for increased social and psychosocial support for these patients.

The specific gene responsible for CF was discovered in 1989. Scientists have now discovered hundreds of mutations in this gene. Because of these varied abnormalities, the severity of CF may vary from person to person. The genetic defect in CF affects the mechanism by which chemicals such as sodium and chloride pass out of cells. In CF, the epithelial cells that line the surface passages of many organs, such as the lung and pancreas, retain increased amounts of sodium and chloride. The high concentration of these chemicals draws water from the airways of the lung (or pancreatic ducts), producing thick, dehydrated mucus. This highly viscous mucus obstructs and plugs the passageways, producing secondary infection and destruction of tissue. Although pulmonary involvement is the most striking feature of CF, multiple organs may be affected, including the pancreas, liver, intestine, and genitalia.

FUNCTIONAL DISABILITY

RECURRENT RESPIRATORY TRACT infection (including infection in the sinuses) is characteristic of the disease. In children, poor nutrition, slow growth, and delayed puberty are common. The patient has a chronic cough, with wheezing and recurrent bronchitis, pneumonitis, and sinusitis. Hemoptysis and bronchiectasis are evident, and as a result dyspnea is present and progressive. Pancreatic and intestinal involvement create malabsorption and abdominal discomfort. Hepatic involvement creates jaundice and cirrhosis. Sodium loss in sweat may lead to circulatory collapse. There is considerable variation in time of presentation of these symptoms. Although 75% of patients with CF are diagnosed before age 6, they may not exhibit symptoms until adolescence or later in life.

MEDICAL EVALUATION

THE DIAGNOSIS OF CF is usually made clinically by the presence of pancreatic insufficiency and recurrent respiratory tract infection. The laboratory finding of elevated sodium in sweat has been the diagnostic standard for CF for many years, but genetic testing (DNA analysis) has replaced the sweat test.

The chest x-ray typically reflects the disease with evidence of cystic bronchiectasis, fibrosis, mucus plugging, and hyperinflation. Pulmonary function studies are useful in documenting the progress of the disease. As in patients with COPD or asthma, there is evidence of airway obstruction and ultimately "air trapping" which results in hyperinflation. Blood gases reveal a decrease in oxygen tension early in the disease, with elevation of CO_2 tension being noted later. Progressive pulmonary disease ultimately leads to cardiac failure as well.

TREATMENT

ADVANCES IN ANTIBIOTIC therapy, nutritional support, and chest physiotherapy have markedly increased survival in patients with CF. Heart-lung transplants are also being used in patients with CF with increasing success. Genetic engineering may offer another approach that will ultimately increase survival.

Patients with CF require daily chest physiotherapy to loosen secretions and prevent stagnation and secondary infections. Antibiotics are essential in treating infection and usually must be given intravenously for prolonged periods. Newer techniques for intravenous therapy now permit treatment outside the hospital and frequently permit the patient to remain functional and at home. Inhaled antibiotic therapy may also be quite useful in treating patients with CF. Nutritional support is critical in these often malnourished patients.

VOCATIONAL AND PSYCHOLOGICAL IMPLICATIONS

PATIENTS WITH CF often have excellent educational success and are typically productive individuals. The counselor will have to work with employers to provide the support mechanisms that will allow the patient to remain in the workplace as long as possible. This might include the provision of time for chest physiotherapy or antibiotic therapy during the workday. Also, the work environment must be reviewed to ensure the absence of irritants that might exacerbate the disease. Supplemental oxygen may be necessary to allow the patient to continue to remain productive and ambulatory.

Psychological outcome in CF patients appears to depend on factors such as the altered physical appearance, loneliness, and family strife that the patients attribute to their illness. Faced with these factors and concerns over their sexual function, individuals may develop anxiety and/or depression. Psychological evaluation and treatment will often be necessary. The counselor may also have to work with patients' families to improve support at home that will allow the patient to increase social and vocational activities.

REFERENCES

Albert, R., Spiro, S., & Jet, J. (2001). *Comprehensive respiratory medicine.* London: Mosby.

American Thoracic Society. (1982). Evaluation of impairment/disability secondary to respiratory disease. *American Review of Respiratory Disease, 126,* 945–951.

American Thoracic Society. (1986). Evaluation of impairment/disability secondary to respiratory disorders. *American Review of Respiratory Disease, 133*, 1205–1209.

American Thoracic Society. (1993). Guidelines for the evaluation of impairment/disability in patients with asthma. *American Review of Respiratory Disease, 147*, 1056–1061.

Braunwald, E., Fauci, A., Kasper, D., Hauser, S., Longo, D., & Jameson, J. L. (Eds.). (2001). *Harrison's principles of internal medicine.* New York: McGraw-Hill.

Carey, T. S., & Hadler, N. M. (1986). The role of the primary care physician in disability determination for Social Security insurance and worker's compensation. *Annals of Internal Medicine, 104*, 706–710.

Hadler, N. M. (1982). Medical ramifications of the federal regulation of the Social Security Disability Insurance Program. *Annals of Internal Medicine, 96*, 665–669.

Murray, J. F., Nadel, J. A., Mason, R. J., & Boushey, H. A. (2000). *Textbook of respiratory medicine* (3rd ed.). Philadelphia: W. B. Saunders Company.

Respiratory system. (1992). In Disability evaluation under social security (SSA Publication No. 64-039, pp. 1–103). Baltimore: U.S. Department of Health and Human Services.

Richman, S. I. (1980). Meanings of impairment and disability. *Chest, 78*(Suppl. 2), 367–371.

22

Chronic Kidney Disease

KOTRESHA NEELAKANTAPPA, MD, AND
JEROME LOWENSTEIN, MD

CHRONIC RENAL FAILURE poses a singular challenge for health professionals who deal with illness-related disability and rehabilitation. The course of progressive chronic kidney disease (CKD) leading to renal failure often spans many years; during the period before dialysis or renal transplantation is undertaken, the patient may experience disabilities related to cardiovascular disease, anemia, malnutrition, metabolic bone disease, neuropathy, muscle wasting, and acid-base and electrolyte disturbances. Dialysis treatment and transplantation significantly prolong the lives of patients with renal failure, but often allow some of the most disabling features of renal disease to persist or progress. Better understanding of the pathophysiologic basis for many of the disabling aspects of chronic renal failure has led to therapies which may reduce the frequency and/or severity of these aspects of the disease. Prevention of disability and rehabilitation have become increasingly important as dialysis therapy and renal transplantation have become more common. United States Renal Data System's (USRDS) 2003 Annual Data Report (ADR) shows that the prevalence rate of end stage renal disease (ESRD) has quintupled from 271 to almost 1,400 per million population since 1980.

DISEASE DESCRIPTION

CHRONIC KIDNEY DISEASE AND ITS PROGRESSION

MOST RENAL PARENCHYMAL diseases, regardless of the etiology of the underlying disease, exhibit progressive scarring and loss of function over a period of many years (see Table 22.1). In some instances, progression occurs because of persistent disease or repeated recurrences of the primary disease, but more frequently progression occurs without evidence of residual activity of the primary disease. Surgical ablation of a critical mass of renal tissue in rats and in dogs results in progressive loss of nephrons in the remaining, previously healthy tissue (the "remnant kidney model"). Glomerular sclerosis and obsolescence of some nephrons and hypertrophy of the remaining nephrons characterize this form of progression. Studies of the mechanisms underlying this "non-immunologic" progression have provided therapeutic strategies for delaying the onset of renal failure.

Micropuncture studies in the remnant kidney model have shown that after ablation of a critical mass of renal tissue, single nephron plasma flow and glomerular capillary hydrostatic pressure are increased in the remaining nephrons. The factors responsible for glomerular hemodynamic alterations and glomerular hypertrophy are not well understood. Increased levels of growth hormone, certain dietary amino acids, vasodilator renal prostaglandins, increased local concentrations of angiotensin II, and autoregulation of glomerular blood flow leading to glomerular hypertension have all been implicated. The increase in glomerular hydrostatic pressure may occur in the absence of systemic hypertension. Increased surface area of the glomerular filtering bed and glomerular hypertension, while maintaining overall GFR close to normal, appear to lead to accelerated glomerular injury and fibrosis of the

TABLE 22.1 National Kidney Foundation K/DOQI (Kidney Disease Outcome Quality Initiative) Classification of Chronic Kidney Disease

Stage	Description	GFR (ml/min/m²)
1	Kidney damage with normal or ↑ GFR	≥ 90
2	Kidney damage with mild ↓ in GFR	60–89
3	Moderate ↓ in GFR	30–59
4	Severe ↓ in GFR	15–29
5	Renal failure	< 15 (or on dialysis)

Chronic Kidney Disease is defined as either kidney damage or glomerular filtration rate (GFR) of < 90 ml/min/1.73 m2 for ≥ 3 months.

remaining nephrons. Treatment with antihypertensive agents is beneficial in slowing the rate of progression in a variety of renal diseases in both experimental animals and humans. Angiotensin converting enzyme (ACE) inhibitors and angiotensin receptor blocker (ARBs) appear to exert a protective effect in CKD, which may be independent of the reduction in systemic blood pressure. It has been suggested that this may result from blocking the mitogenic effects of angiotensin II (Wolf & Neilson, 1993). Low-protein diet prevents the compensatory increase in glomerular plasma flow, hypertension, and hypertrophy and leads to marked attenuation of sclerosis in rats with the remnant kidney model of progressive renal disease. Most studies of protein restriction in humans with both diabetic and nondiabetic chronic renal disease also demonstrated a similar benefit. However, the largest study to date (Klahr et al., 1994), which examined the effect of protein restriction on progression of nondiabetic renal disease in 585 patients, did not show a statistically significant benefit. This finding was surprising and it has been suggested that the beneficial effects of good control of hypertension and the use of angiotensin converting enzyme inhibitor (ACEi) may have masked the effects of dietary protein restriction on disease progression.

FUNCTIONAL ADAPTATION TO NEPHRON LOSS

Adaptive changes in residual nephrons permit the kidney to retain much of its function despite marked reduction in the number of nephrons. Systemic and intrarenal hemodynamic changes, hormonal stimuli, and possibly structural changes along the nephron lead to increase in single nephron GFR and to changes in tubular reabsorption and tubular secretion of various metabolites in the surviving nephrons. With further nephron loss, compensatory changes in the residual nephrons fail to maintain normal total renal function and abnormalities in blood composition become evident.

Minute changes in the body composition resulting from retention of some substances trigger mechanisms which result in compensatory increase in their excretion with little change in the internal milieu. These mechanisms themselves are associated with varying degrees of untoward but less harmful effects than those of retention of the substance in question. This is referred to as the "trade-off hypothesis." It is well illustrated by the compensatory responses that maintain external balance of sodium, potassium, hydrogen ion, calcium, and phosphate.

SODIUM

Under normal circumstances, approximately 25,000 mEq of Na^+ are filtered daily. All except about 150 mEq (average daily intake) are reabsorbed. As the glomerular filtration rate and the filtered load of sodium decline with progressive renal disease, there is a reciprocal increase in the fraction of filtered sodium that escapes reabsorption. Despite marked reduction in filtered sodium in advanced renal failure, overt sodium retention and edema in the absence of heart failure or the nephritic syndrome are not usually observed before the most advanced (oliguric) stage. The mechanism responsible for rejection of an increased fraction of the filtered sodium may directly or indirectly be related to an increased systemic blood pressure. Hypertension may be the price to be paid for maintaining sodium balance in the face of declining GFR. The same mechanisms that maintain sodium excretion when GFR is reduced may be responsible for impaired sodium conservation when dietary sodium intake is reduced or extrarenal losses of sodium occur. Under such conditions, the compensatory mechanism may become a liability.

POTASSIUM

Filtered potassium is completely reabsorbed before the glomerular filtrate reaches the distal convoluted tubule. Potassium balance is maintained mainly by secretion by the principal cells in the late distal convoluted tubule and cortical collecting duct. Hyperkalemia is usually not seen until GFR declines to less than 10%–15% of normal. Tubular secretion of potassium is dependent on the negative electrical charge in the lumen created by sodium reabsorption and sodium conductance across the epithelium of the collecting duct, which in turn are dependent on aldosterone. Although plasma aldosterone concentration is not usually elevated in chronic renal disease, patients with moderately advanced renal failure are prone to develop hyperkalemia if drugs which antagonize aldosterone (spironolactone) or reduce angiotensin II production (ACEis and non-steroidal anti-inflammatory drugs) or block angiotensin II receptors (ARB) are given.

HYDROGEN ION

Daily metabolism leads to generation of fixed acids (predominantly sulfuric acid) which dissociate into their respective anions (e.g., sulfate) and the cation, H^+ (protons). Daily metabolic production averages about 1mEq/kg/day. The protons titrate the body buffers, predominantly bicarbonate. The kidney excretes the anions of the acids and regenerates the bicarbonate (and other body buffers). The regeneration of bicarbonate stores and the "back titration" of other body buffers (predominantly proteins) are accomplished by the renal tubular secretion of H^+ and by renal ammoniagenesis. The renal secretion of H^+, formed from the breakdown of H_2CO_3 ($H_2CO_3 \leftrightarrow H^+ + HCO_3$) generates an equimolar quantity of bicarbonate, which is absorbed across the basolateral membrane of the renal tubule. Renal ammoniagenesis results in the formation of NH_4^+ and glutamate or α-ketoglutarate. The NH_4^+ is excreted and the organic anion is metabolized to yield bicarbonate.

Renal acid excretion is only modestly reduced despite marked reduction in nephron number as renal disease progresses. This is the result of an increase in proton secretion and renal ammonia production per residual nephron. Although total ammonia generation is reduced, increased ammonia generation in remaining nephrons leads to an increase in local NH_4^+ concentration. In experimental animals this has been shown to cause activation of complement components and to the generation of reactive oxygen species and superoxides, which contribute to tubulointerstitial damage. Prevention of increased local ammonia concentration by bicarbonate administration ameliorates tubulointerstitial damage (Nath, Hostetter, & Hostetter, 1985). One can view tubulointerstitial damage as another example of "trade-off" in which adaptation, i.e., increased ammonia genesis, which provides "new buffer" per residual nephron, results in higher renal ammonia concentration leading to complement activation and tissue injury.

Calcium and Phosphorus

Calcium and phosphorus metabolism are markedly altered in progressive renal disease. The concentration of $1,25(OH)_2$ vitamin D_3, the active form of vitamin D, is governed by the enzymatic hydroxylation of $25(OH)$ vitamin D_3 by the kidneys. The concentration of $1,25(OH)_2$ vitamin D_3 is reduced in advanced renal failure and calcium absorption by the intestine decreases, resulting in hypocalcemia. The filtration of phosphorus decreases as the glomerular filtration rate falls. Normally 80%–90% of the filtered phosphorus is reabsorbed. In renal failure, even though the filtered load of phosphorus declines steadily, the serum phosphorus level does not rise, since the daily intake can be excreted by reduction in reabsorption down to nearly 50%. Beyond this point, steady state is achieved by a combination of further reduction in reabsorption and a relative increase in the filtered load achieved by a rise in the plasma level. Phosphate retention contributes to hypocalcemia both by deposition of calcium phosphate in tissues and by reduced synthesis of $1,25 (OH)_2$ vitamin D_3. Despite these perturbations in calcium and phosphorus balance, serum calcium and phosphorus concentrations are maintained within the normal range until GFR is markedly reduced. In large part this is attributable to increased parathyroid hormone (PTH) secretion. PTH not only reduces tubular reabsorption of phosphate, but also mobilizes calcium from the skeletal system. The pathogenesis of this "secondary hyperparathyroidism" involves several mechanisms. Hypocalcemia stimulates PTH release from parathyroid cells. Reduced vitamin D concentration leads to parathyroid hyperplasia by removing

a normal suppressive effect it exerts on the parathyroid and a concomitant down regulation of vitamin D receptors on parathyroid cells.
The "trade off" for maintenance of calcium and phosphorus concentrations is the development of bone disease secondary to hyperparathyroidism characterized by osteomalacia and osteitis fibrosa cystica.

TREATMENT OF CHRONIC RENAL FAILURE

MANAGEMENT OF CHRONIC renal disease involves both delaying progression of the renal disease and correcting the metabolic
abnormalities.

HYPERTENSION

ALTHOUGH HYPERTENSION IS almost always a result rather than a
cause of renal disease, it leads to accelerated progression of the underlying disease, creating a vicious circle. The control of hypertension in
renal disease is directed at both a reduction in cardiovascular morbidity and the slowing of progression of the underlying renal disease.
Antihypertensive drugs have selective actions on afferent or efferent
arterioles and differ in their ability to reduce glomerular hypertension.
Angiotensin converting enzyme inhibitors (ACEi) and angiotensin receptor blockers (ARB), which lower glomerular capillary pressure (P_{GC}), have
been shown to reduce proteinuria and delay progression in both diabetic and non-diabetic renal diseases. Calcium channel blockers differ
in their effect on the kidney. Dihydropyridines, which are potent
vasodilators, lead to an increase in proteinuria, perhaps because afferent arteriolar dilatation leaves P_{GC} unchanged or increased.
Nondihydropyridines have been shown to result in reduction in proteinuria, which is additive to that brought about, by ACEi.

METABOLIC ACIDOSIS

METABOLIC ACIDOSIS IN chronic renal disease is generally well tolerated and is usually not treated unless it is severe. The arguments against
treatment have included the risk of sodium overload associated with
sodium bicarbonate therapy, reduction in ionized calcium concentration resulting in tetany and seizures and perhaps diminished O_2 delivery to tissues due to reversal of an adaptive change in the O_2 dissociation
curve. More recent evidence suggests that the benefits of treatment outweigh these objections. Treatment of metabolic acidosis with bicarbonate or with a metabolizable anion, which can act as a substitute for
bicarbonate (e.g., citrate or lactate), has been shown to prevent growth

retardation in children with renal tubular acidosis. It has been shown that correction of metabolic acidosis by increasing dialysate bicarbonate concentration in patients with end stage renal disease improves bone mineralization, diminishes bone resorption, and reduces the severity of secondary hyperparathyroidism.

Chronic metabolic acidosis is associated with muscle weakness and decreased lean body mass. Forearm muscle studies in patients with chronic renal disease, utilizing phenylalanine appearance rate as a measure of protein degradation and its disposal rate as a measure of protein synthesis, have demonstrated that protein catabolic rate is directly related to the degree of acidosis and to plasma cortisol levels; plasma cortisol levels in turn, are directly related to the degree of acidosis. Further, albumin synthesis is diminished and negative nitrogen balance increased in patients with chronic renal disease made acidotic by the administration of ammonium chloride. The down-regulation of protein catabolic rate seen in patients with chronic renal disease placed on a protein restricted diet is impaired in those who also have metabolic acidosis; this can be corrected by treatment of acidosis with bicarbonate.

ANEMIA

ALTHOUGH THERE ARE many causes of anemia in chronic renal disease, reduced erythropoietin (EPO) production seems to be the most important factor. Both type I renal interstitial cells and proximal tubular epithelial cells are known to produce EPO. A heme protein acts as the oxygen sensor in the kidney. When stimulated by diminished oxygen delivery, this sensor leads to synthesis of a protein (hypoxia-inducible factor 1, HIF-1α) (Semenza, 2000), which binds to the enhancer region of the EPO gene leading to an increase in the production of EPO. EPO levels are markedly reduced in patients with anemia of chronic renal disease. Administration of recombinant human erythropoietin (rHuEPO) corrects the anemia of renal disease in a dose-dependent manner. Ninety percent of patients on dialysis in the United States and many patients with chronic renal disease who are not yet on dialysis receive rHuEPO therapy. The target hematocrit of 33%–36% is reached in a majority of patients at a dose of 50–100 U/kg given 3 times a week (TIW). 70% of patients respond to a dose of 50 U/kg TIW and 90% respond to 100 U/kg TIW. More recently, a longer acting preparation, darbipoetin alpha, has made administration and compliance more convenient for patients not yet receiving dialysis. The most common cause of resistance to rHuEPO is iron deficiency. Other causes of resistance to EPO include bone marrow fibrosis, inflammatory conditions, poor nutrition, and underdialysis.

Anemia has been found to be an independent predictor of the de novo occurrence of congestive heart failure and increased mortality in ESRD. Left ventricular hypertrophy also has been found to be associated with increased mortality in ESRD. Successful treatment of anemia with rHuEPO has been shown to reverse cardiovascular and hemodynamic abnormalities such as left ventricular hypertrophy, increased cardiac output, and decreased peripheral vascular resistance. Patients report improved vitality and exercise tolerance; amelioration of angina, congestive heart failure, and fatigue have been observed. Other beneficial effects of EPO therapy include improvement in platelet dysfunction of uremia, uremic pruritus, impaired carbohydrate and cortisol metabolism, and sexual function in male patients.

RENAL OSTEODYSTROPHY

ALTHOUGH SYMPTOMATIC RENAL osteodystrophy, for example, bone pain and fractures, seldom occurs prior to the onset of ESRD, altered mineral metabolism is present early is the course of renal failure. The two classic forms of renal osteodystrophy are osteitis fibrosa, characterized by an increased rate of bone turnover secondary to hyperparathyroidism, and osteomalacia in which bone turnover is diminished and there is an increased volume of unmineralized bone (osteoid). Although osteomalacia was initially thought to result from vitamin D deficiency in patients with ESRD, it is now believed that the major cause is aluminum toxicity. More recently, a third entity called adynamic bone disease or aplastic bone disease has been described. Low levels of PTH, diminished skeletal turnover, and reduced rate of osteoid formation characterize this condition. In some cases, it may result from excessive suppression of PTH by synthetic $1,25(OH)_2$ vitamin D_3 or its analogs.

The management of renal osteodystrophy involves both suppression of hyperparathyroidism and control of hyperphosphatemia. Although the administration of $1,25(OH)_2$ vitamin D_3 has been extremely useful in the suppression of hyperparathyroidism, hypercalcemia has been a limiting factor. This has led to the development of other vitamin D analogs with better ability to suppress parathyroid hormone for a given calcium level. Most recently, the first of a new generation of products, cinacalcet HCl (Sensipar®), referred to as calcimimetic agents, has been approved by the FDA. These drugs mimic the suppressive effect of calcium on the parathyroid gland.

Aluminum containing antacids have been replaced by calcium carbonate and calcium acetate as dietary phosphate binders, which avoid the risk of aluminum toxicity. Even calcium-containing compounds have come under scrutiny because of the positive calcium balance and soft tissue calcification such as coronary and other vascular calcification in dialysis patients. Sevelamer (Renagel®) is a cationic polymer, which binds negatively charged phosphates without the risk of aluminum toxicity or positive calcium balance. Ability to control hyperparathyroidism and hyperphosphatemia has resulted in a marked reduction in the incidence of renal osteodystrophy.

In certain instances, the nodular parathyroid hyperplasia is so severe that it is not possible to suppress it medically, a condition referred to as "tertiary hyperparathyroidism"; this may necessitate surgical parathyroidectomy.

UREMIC NEUROPATHY

UREMIC NEUROPATHY CAN present as either a polyneuropathy or a mononeuropathy involving both sensory and motor fibers. It generally occurs in advanced renal failure and is an indication to start dialysis for ESRD. When it occurs in patients who are already on dialysis, one needs to consider inadequate dialysis as a cause. Pathologically, uremic polyneuropathy is associated with demyelination and axonal degeneration and the involvement is directly proportional to axonal length, affecting longer axons first. It is usually symmetrical in nature. The metabolic and chemical defects leading to these changes are not well understood. Clinically, it first presents as paresthesias, burning sensation, and pain in distal areas such as feet. Sensory symptoms usually precede motor symptoms. The onset of motor symptoms reflects advanced disease which, unlike the sensory neuropathy, may not reverse with the institution of dialysis. Electrophysiologic studies are very useful in detecting subclinical neuropathy. Uremic mononeuropathy usually involves median and ulnar nerves. Other nerves involved include seventh and eighth cranial nerves and peroneal nerves. Carpal tunnel syndrome is common in ESRD. It results from compression of median nerve at the wrist between carpal bones and transverse carpal ligament. Deposition of β2-microglobulin-related amyloid fibrils in the carpal tunnel plays an important role in the pathogenesis of the syndrome. Early initiations of dialysis, the use of better dialysis membranes with higher clearance for β_2 microglobulin, and close attention to the adequacy of dialysis have reduced the incidence of uremic neuropathy. The extent of recovery is inversely related to the degree of dysfunction prior to initiation of dialysis. Restoration of renal function with renal transplantation results in remarkable recovery from even the most severe sensory and motor neuropathy.

SEXUAL DYSFUNCTION

ERECTILE DYSFUNCTION AND a decrease in libido and frequency of intercourse are present in over half the men with uremia. This is organic in nature as evidenced by a decline in nocturnal penile tumescence. The decline in nocturnal penile tumescence is more marked than in normal controls and in patients with other chronic illness, suggesting that it is the effect of uremia and yet does not improve with hemodialysis. The factors other than uremia which can contribute to erectile dysfunction include peripheral neuropathy, autonomic dysfunction, and peripheral vascular disease. Psychological and physical stress may also play a role.

Lack of ovulation and scant menstruation are common in women with chronic renal failure. Some women may have menorrhagia leading to worsening of anemia. Pregnancy can rarely occur with chronic renal failure but fetal loss is the rule. Elevated prolactin levels are also seen in women with chronic renal disease. Although suppression of very high prolactin levels with bromocriptine in women with normal renal function improves the clinical syndrome of amenorrhea and galactorrhea, it fails to restore normal menstruation or correct galactorrhea in uremic women. Successful renal transplantation, however, leads to restoration of fertility and sexual function in most patients.

TREATMENT OF END STAGE RENAL FAILURE

WHEN WILHELM KOLPH introduced hemodialysis a little over 60 years ago, it was restricted to treatment of patients with acute reversible renal failure. Today, hemodialysis and peritoneal dialysis serve to support and rehabilitate patients with end stage, irreversible renal failure. The United States Renal Data System's 2003 Annual Data Report (USRDS's 2003 ADR) shows that 406,000 patients were being treated for ESRD in 2001. Approximately 65% of these were treated with hemodialysis, 7% with peritoneal dialysis, and 28% had a successful renal transplantation. Forty-five percent of patients on hemodialysis were 65 years and older and 41.5% were diabetics. Total cost of treatment of ESRD for the year 2001 was $22.8 billion. A major part of this (15.4 billion) was borne by Medicare.

HEMODIALYSIS

HEMODIALYSIS IS TYPICALLY performed 3 times a week. The procedure involves diffusion of solutes between the plasma and the dialysis bath (dialysate) across the semipermeable dialyzer membrane down a concentration gradient. Fluid (usually equal to the volume retained from one dialysis to the next) is removed by ultra-filtration by regulating the dialyzer transmembrane hydrostatic pressure. Blood flow rates through the dialyzers in excess of 200 ml/min are necessary in order to obtain sufficient clearance of solutes over a reasonably short period of time. Since the normal blood flow rates in peripheral veins are insufficient for this purpose, it is necessary to have some form of access to the circulation where the blood flow rate is of this magnitude. A simple catheter placed in a central vein and an arteriovenous fistula/shunt, with or without the interposition of a synthetic tubular graft, serve as the most common forms of hemodialysis access.

PERITONEAL DIALYSIS

IN THIS TECHNIQUE, the patient's peritoneum substitutes for the dialyzer membrane. When the peritoneal cavity is filled with dialysate solution, diffusion of solutes occurs between the plasma flowing in the capillaries supplying the peritoneum and the dialysate until concentration equilibrium is reached. In 1976, Popovich and Moncrief described the basic concept of Continuous Ambulatory Peritoneal Dialysis (CAPD). They made use of the fact that some solute transfer continued to occur for as long as 4–5 hours and one could achieve sufficient solute clearance with 4–5 2-liter exchanges of dialysis fluid a day. This led the way to the use of peritoneal dialysis as a treatment option for patients with ESRD. The incidence of peritonitis as a complication of this procedure has been markedly reduced by improvements in techniques and the design of catheters, connections, and the use of automated cyclers which can be used at night when the patients are asleep.

SURVIVAL OF ESRD PATIENTS

ALTHOUGH MAINTENANCE DIALYSIS prevents death from uremia, patient survival is still limited. USRDS's 2003 ADR data show a mean expected remaining lifespan of 7.3 years for patients beginning dialysis between the ages of 40–44 and 3.85 years for those beginning between the ages of 60–64 years. These are roughly 1/5th the expected lifespan for the general U.S. population of comparable age groups. Understandably, survival depends on comorbid conditions. For the year 1994, diabetics had a death rate of 27 per 100 patient years compared to 18.1 per 100 patient years in patients with glomerulonephritis as the etiology of ESRD. Although most of these data are from patients on hemodialysis (60% of the ESRD population in 1994), similar observations hold true for the peritoneal dialysis population.

Although all-cause mortality has declined steadily since 1988, cardiovascular events (strokes and heart attack) account for about 50% of deaths in ESRD. The other important causes of death in ESRD are infections, most often stemming from hemodialysis access sites or peritonitis in those on peritoneal dialysis. About 5%–10% of deaths are due to withdrawal from dialysis.

ADEQUACY OF DIALYSIS

THE NATIONAL COOPERATIVE Dialysis Study (NCDS), a prospectively randomized and controlled study, demonstrated that the "dose of dialysis" as measured by urea clearance correlated with morbidity (Lowrie, Laird, Parker, & Sargent, 1981). The dose of dialysis therapy can be expressed as the virtual volume of plasma completely cleared of urea during dialysis, relative to the volume of distribution. The formula Kt/V expresses this, where K is urea clearance, t is duration of dialysis and V is volume of distribution. The urea reduction ratio (URR) is also a correlate of Kt/V. The Work Group of the National Kidney Foundation-Dialysis Outcomes Quality Initiative (NKF-DOQI) (1997) recommended a prescribed minimum of 1.3 for Kt/V and 70% for URR. Several studies (Hakim, Breyer, Ismail, & Schulman, 1994; Parker, Husni, Huang, Lew, & Lowrie, 1994; Held et al., 1996) have shown that increasing the dose of dialysis reduces the mortality, which in one study (Held et al.) was 7% for each 0.1 unit increment in Kt/V. However, increasing URR and Kt/V to higher levels (75% and 1.7) does not seem to be associated with further reduction in morbidity and mortality (Eknoyan et al., 2002). A target URR of $\geq$ 65% set by K/DOQI (Kidney Disease Outcome Quality Initiative) was met by 83.5% of patients on hemodialysis in 2000. Similar observations have been made regarding adequacy of dialysis and mortality and morbidity for patients on maintenance peritoneal dialysis. The Canada-USA (CANUSA) Peritoneal Dialysis Study Group (1996), in a prospective cohort study, found that a decrease in 0.1 unit Kt/V was associated with a 5% increase in the relative risk of death. A weekly Kt/V of 2.1 and a weekly creatinine clearance of 70 L/1.73 m^2 were each associated with a 2-year survival of 78%. Nearly half the patients on peritoneal dialysis in 2000 had a weekly Kt/V of $\geq$ 2.3 (USRDS 2003 ADR).

NUTRITION

MALNUTRITION IS COMMON in chronic renal disease. It results not only from protein restriction in an attempt to slow the progression of renal disease, but also as a function of advancing renal disease. Analysis of the data from the Modification of Diet in Renal Disease (MDRD) study showed that body mass index, anthropometric measurements, and urinary creatinine excretion (an index of muscle mass) were lower than expected in patients with moderately advanced renal disease entering the study (Klahr et al., 1994). Several indices of nutrition, such as dietary protein intake, serum cholesterol, transferrin, insulin-like growth factor-1 (IGF-1), percent body weight, and urinary creatinine excretion, decline as the renal function deteriorates (Ikizler, Greene, Wingard, Parker, & Hakim, 1995).

Mild to moderate protein-calorie malnutrition is present in a third of the patients on maintenance dialysis. Concentrations of plasma proteins such as albumin, prealbumin, transferrin, and IGF-1 as well as markers of tissue protein stores are already reduced in patients when dialysis is instituted. Factors contributing to malnutrition in the dialysis population include poor nutrient intake, intercurrent illness, and dialysis itself. Although several markers of malnutrition such as low blood urea, serum cholesterol, creatinine, potassium, and phosphorus have been associated with increased risk of mortality, low serum albumin concentration seems to be the strongest predictor of mortality. The odds ratio for the risk of death is inversely related, exponentially, to serum albumin concentration in patients maintained on either hemo- or peritoneal dialysis. Nearly half the patients with ESRD starting dialysis have serum albumin concentration below the normal range. Even though peritoneal losses contribute to hypoalbuminemia in CAPD patients, Lowrie, Huang, and Lew (1995) found that the relative risk of death was the same for hemodialysis and CAPD patients with hypoalbuminemia, suggesting that regardless of the mechanism, hypoalbuminemia carried the same risk. Various interventions ranging from simple nutritional supplements to administration of intra-dialytic parenteral nutrition may be of value in correcting malnutrition in patients with ESRD. Experimentally, recombinant human growth hormone (rhGH) and recombinant human insulin-like growth factor-1 (rhIGF-1) have been shown to lead to positive nitrogen balance.

PHYSICAL REHABILITATION

A S IN ANY other chronic illness, rehabilitation is extremely important if patients with ESRD are to live as "normal" a life as possible. Even though hemodialysis and peritoneal dialysis provide means to sustain life in the absence of kidney function, patients are generally weak and disabled to a variable extent. The trend in favor of institution of dialysis before severe debility is incurred has made rehabilitation more effective.

The availability of synthetic $1,25(OH)_2$ vitamin D_3 and vitamin D_3 analogs and better understanding of the pathophysiology of renal osteodystrophy, including the importance of aluminum toxicity, have reduced the incidence of severe skeletal disease to a great extent. The incidence of dialysis-related amyloidosis, causing carpal tunnel syndrome and arthropathy, has markedly decreased since the introduction of synthetic dialysis membranes with better β^2 microglobulin clearance. In addition to these advances in medical care, flexibility and range of movement exercises will help improve patients' abilities to perform activities of daily living, such as stooping, bending, and reaching. Although strengthening (isometric) exercises such as weight lifting have been shown to increase blood pressure, well-selected exercises, such as lifting and carrying objects, in moderation help maintain muscle strength, which is also important for activities of daily living.

Preliminary studies in patients with chronic kidney disease indicate that resistance training reduces markers of inflammation such as C-reactive protein and interleukin-6 as well as leads to skeletal muscle hypertrophy (Castaneda et al., 2004).

Maximal aerobic capacity as measured by peak oxygen uptake (VO_2 peak) is reduced in patients with ESRD to roughly half of what is seen in normal sedentary individuals. The determinants of VO_2 peak are (a) oxygen delivery to the muscles, which is dependent on arterial oxygen content and blood supply to the muscle, and (b) oxygen extraction by the muscle. Hemodialysis patients demonstrate a limitation in both cardiac output (mainly as a blunted response of heart rate to exercise) and diminished ability to extract oxygen at the muscle level. These abnormalities continue to worsen because of disease progression, development of comorbid conditions, and deconditioning. Correction of anemia with rHuEPO results in an increase in the arterial oxygen content and improves VO_2 peak by an average of 28%, but the change in VO_2 peak is much smaller than that expected for the change in hemoglobin and arterial oxygen content. The resultant VO_2 peak is only 65% of that of age-matched sedentary controls. Painter and Moore (1994) have analyzed the available data and compared the improvement in VO_2 peak relative to the rise in hemoglobin in dialysis patients and normal subjects whose hemoglobin was varied by phlebotomy and reinfusion of packed cells. They concluded that normal subjects get nearly twice the VO_2 change per change in hemoglobin as compared to dialysis patients. They suggested that there may be an underlying limitation in maximal oxygen extraction by skeletal muscles in dialysis patients. Skeletal muscle abnormalities described in dialysis patients have included reduced oxidative enzyme activity, decreased type I to type II muscle fiber ratio, atrophy of fibers, low capillary density, mitochondrial dysfunction, low carnitine content and accumulation of acylated metabolites of carnitine. Utilizing phosphorus[31] magnetic resonance spectroscopy (^{31}PMRS) measurements of pH and the ratio of phosphocreatine to phosphocreatine + inorganic phosphorus have revealed that the intrinsic metabolic capacity of muscles during static hand grip, when blood flow through capillaries and O_2 delivery cease, is similar in hemodialysis patients, successful transplant recipients, and normal controls. However, rhythmic hand grip, which is dependent on both intrinsic muscle function and oxygen delivery, led to increased intracellular acidosis and phosphocreatine depletion in hemodialysis patients. These studies suggest a reduction in oxidative generation of ATP, a need for more ATP for the same amount of muscle function, or the utilization of more ATP for non-muscular activity such as ion pumping. Exercise training alone has been shown to improve VO_2 peak by 25%. Two dialysis athletes who participated in the 1991 California Transplant Games (Noakes, 1991) exemplify the remarkable effects of exercise training combined with EPO treatment. One had diabetes and had been on peritoneal dialysis for 4 years and the other had glomerulonephritis and had been on hemodialysis for 8 years. They finished in the top two places in the one-mile run and had VO_2 max of 40.2 and 36.1 ml/kg/min, respectively. These values were better than those of age- and sex-matched normal sedentary individuals. Although these are exceptional examples, they serve as reminders of what can be achieved by training. The mechanisms by which aerobic exercise training leads to improved oxygen utilization in normal individuals (Saltin & Rowell, 1980) include increased oxidative enzyme number and activities, increased type I fibers, increased capillary to fiber ratio, and increased total muscle blood flow. Moore et al. (1993) reported that 5 of 11 hemodialysis patients increased VO_2 peak by 26% after exercise training. This change was due to an increase in a–vO_2 difference (oxygen extraction); there was no change in cardiac output, stroke volume, heart rate, or hemoglobin concentration. Even patients who did not show an increase in VO_2 peak showed an increase in peak workload achieved, suggesting that exercise training improves efficiency of work at a given VO_2.

As is well appreciated in the general population, exercise training offers other health benefits in dialysis patients. Endurance exercise training in hemodialysis patients offers cardiovascular risk benefits, including lowering of both systolic and diastolic blood pressure sufficient to decrease or withdraw anti-hypertensive therapy in a number of patients, and a decline in plasma triglycerides and VLDL levels while increasing HDL level (Harter & Goldberg, 1985; Hagberg et al., 1983; Miller et al., 2002). Plasma insulin declines and glucose tolerance improves. Exercise training has also been shown to improve hemoglobin concentration. Psychosocial functioning, including Beck Depression Score, the frequency of pleasant activities, and participation in enjoyable events, are reported to improve after exercise training (Harter & Goldberg). Although psychosocial function is better with exercise, improvement in vocational rehabilitation, which is dependent on many other issues such as economic incentives, needs to be demonstrated.

Although the best time for exercise in relation to hemodialysis is not clear, exercising training during dialysis sessions has the advantages of supervision and encouragement by the staff as well as a productive use of dialysis time. One can expect an improved compliance to exercise program. Flexibility, strengthening, and aerobic exercises can all be performed effectively during dialysis. Because of the likelihood of hypotension and muscle cramps during the latter part of dialysis, exercise is best performed in the first hour of dialysis. It has been suggested that exercise during dialysis might improve efficiency of the latter. Although there are some risks of musculoskeletal injury associated with participation in an exercise program for a patient with ESRD, proper patient selection makes this risk negligible.

CARNITINE

CARNITINE IS AN important intermediary in fat metabolism. It not only combines with toxic acyl-CoA to form acylcarnitine, but also transports long chain fatty acids such as acylcarnitine into mitochondria for β-oxidation, providing energy. Carnitine is synthesized by the liver, kidney, and brain and derived from dietary red meat and dairy products. About 95% of carnitine is stored in the muscle. Free carnitine is filtered readily at the glomerulus but is reabsorbed almost totally by the renal tubule. On the other hand, acylcarnitine is also filtered but is not reabsorbed. Renal clearance of acylcarnitine is 4–8 times greater than that of free carnitine. Although the levels of both free and acylcarnitine are elevated in chronic renal failure, the ratio of free to acyl form is markedly reduced. Hemodialysis removes free carnitine preferentially and leads to very high levels of acylcarnitine relative to free carnitine. Low plasma levels of free carnitine are also reported in patients on CAPD. Because many of the manifestations of carnitine deficiency mimic those of uremia and do not correlate with plasma carnitine profiles, the clinical response to carnitine supplementation has been used to define its effective deficiency. A multicenter double-blind placebo-controlled study (Ahmad et al., 1990) of L-carnitine administration in hemodialysis patients involving 82 patients found that intradialytic hypotension and muscle cramps were significantly reduced in the carnitine group. This group also showed a decline in the predialysis urea, creatinine, and phosphorus levels, suggesting a decreased muscle catabolism. Measurement of mid-arm circumference and triceps skin-fold thickness showed an increase in the calculated mid-arm muscle area in the carnitine group. VO_2 peak also increased in the carnitine group. Other uncontrolled studies have shown that L-carnitine supplementation improves plasma lipid profile, muscle strength, exercise capacity, cardiac function, anemia, response to rHuEPO, and a sense of well-being. An interdisciplinary consensus panel convened by National Kidney Foundation in 2002 recommended the use of intravenous L-carnitine to patients with dialysis-related carnitine disorder (DCD) presenting with anemia with decreased response to rHuEPO, intradialytic hypotension, cardiomyopathy, and skeletal muscle weakness. Stopping L-carnitine therapy was recommended if there was no improvement after 9–12 months (Eknoyan, Latos, & Lindberg, 2003).

PSYCHOLOGICAL AND VOCATIONAL REHABILITATION

In addition to the appropriate management of the gamut of abnormalities resulting from chronic renal failure outlined above, one must also address the issue of the patient returning to living a full life. For some, this may not mean returning to work, but feeling well enough to enjoy one's family and surroundings. The goal should be to help the patient to resume all the duties, responsibilities, and benefits he/she enjoyed prior to the illness. Psychological problems stemming from chronic illness, dependence on dialysis, sexual dysfunction, and change in status from an earning and supporting member of the family to a dependent person need to be identified and addressed. Gainful employment is extremely important for an adult in the earning period of his/her life to regain self-esteem and to interact with the society he/she lives in with confidence. However, the fear of losing financial benefits such as Social Security Disability Insurance (SSDI) and Social Security Income (SSI) may deter some patients from seeking employment, even if they are able to return to work. In several states, there are work incentive programs whereby the state agencies waive the termination of financial benefits to persons with disabilities if they seek employment (Renal Rehabilitation Report, 1997). Assistance by a knowledgeable social worker in the field is extremely helpful in this regard. The USRDS Dialysis Morbidity and Mortality Study: Wave 2 conducted in 1996 (USRDS 2003 ADR) found that 37% of younger (18–54 years) and 16% of older (55+ years) patients reported that they were able to work at the start of therapy for ESRD. Of these, only 60% of the younger and 40% of the older group were actually employed. Patients' educational level correlated with reported ability to work and with employment status. Consistent with the association of lower educational level and increased risk of chronic disease in the general population, dialysis patients with lower educational status were more likely to be diabetic. Rasgon and others (1993, 1995) have shown that multidisciplinary predialysis intervention leads to maintenance of employment in a larger number of patients starting dialysis, both in the in-center setting as well as in the home hemodialysis and CAPD population. The quality of life is significantly better after a successful transplantation. A long-term study (Matas et al., 1996) showed that more than 40% of transplant recipients were employed part-time or full-time 8 years after transplantation.

The Life Options Rehabilitation Advisory Council (LORAC), which was formed in 1993 by a group of patients, health care providers, researchers, government representatives and private business persons, has played a major role in bringing the rehabilitation and quality of life issues into focus. The *Renal Rehabilitation Report* (www.lifeoptions.org), its newsletter for patients and professionals, has been an important publication devoted to all issues concerning rehabilitation for the ESRD patient.

REFERENCES

Ahmad, S., Robertson, H. T., Golper, T. A., Wolfson, M., Kurtin, P., Katz, L. A., et al. (1990). Multicenter trial of L-carnitine in maintenance hemodialysis patients. II. Clinical and biochemical effects. *Kidney International, 38*, 912–918.

Canada-USA (CANUSA) Peritoneal Dialysis Study Group. (1996). Adequacy of dialysis and nutrition in continuous peritoneal dialysis: Association with clinical outcomes. *Journal of the American Society of Nephrology, 7*, 198–207.

Castaneda, C., Gordon, P., Parker, R., Uhlin, K. L., Rubenoff, R., & Levy, A. S. (2004). Resistance training to reduce the malnutrition-inflammation complex syndrome of chronic kidney disease. *American Journal of Kidney Disease, 43*, 607–616.

Eknoyan, G., Beck, G. J., Cheung, A. K., Dougirdas, J. T., Greene, T., Kusek, J. W., et al. (2002). Effect of dialysis dose and membrane flux in maintenance hemodialysis. *New England Journal of Medicine, 347*, 2010–2019.

Eknoyan, G., Latos, D. L., & Lindberg, J. (2003). Practice recommendations for the use of L-Carnitine in dialysis-related carnitine disorder. National Carnitine Consensus Conference. *American Journal of Kidney Diseases, 41*, 868–867.

Hagberg, J. M., Goldberg, A. P., Ehsani, A. A., Heath, G. W., Delmez, J. A., & Harter, H. R. (1983). Exercise training improves hypertension in hemodialysis patients. *American Journal of Nephrology, 3*, 209–212.

Hakim, R. M., Breyer, J., Ismail, N., & Schulman, G. (1994). Effect of dose of dialysis on mortality and morbidity. *American Journal of Kidney Diseases, 2*, 661–669.

Harter, H. R., & Goldberg, A. P. (1985). Endurance exercise training: An effective therapeutic modality for hemodialysis patients. *Medical Clinics of North America, 69*, 159–175.

Held, P. J., Port, F. K., Wolfe, R. A., Stannard, D. C., Carroll, C. E., Daugirdas, J. T., et al. (1996). The dose of hemodialysis and patient mortality. *Kidney International, 50*, 550–556.

Ikizler, T. A., Greene, J., Wingard, R. L., Parker, R. A., & Hakim, R. M. (1995). Spontaneous dietary protein intake during progression of chronic renal failure. *Journal of American Society of Nephrology, 6*, 1386–1391.

Klahr, S., Levy, A. S., Beck, G. J., Caggiula, A. W., Hunsicker, L., Kusek, J. W., et al. (1994). The effects of dietary protein restriction and blood pressure control on the progression of chronic renal disease. Modification of Diet in Renal Disease Study Group. *New England Journal of Medicine, 330*, 877–884.

Lowrie, E. G., Huang, W. H., & Lew, N. L. (1995). Death risk predictors among peritoneal dialysis and hemodialysis patients: A preliminary comparison. *American Journal of Kidney Diseases, 26,* 220–228.

Lowrie, E. G., Laird, N. M., Parker, T. F., & Sargent, J. A. (1981). Effect of the hemodialysis prescription on patient morbidity. *New England Journal of Medicine, 305,* 1176–1180.

Matas, A. J., Lawson, W., McHugh, L., Gilligham, K., Payne, W. D., Dunn, D. L., et al. (1996). Employment patterns after successful kidney transplantation. *Transplantation, 61,* 729–733.

Moore, G. E., Parsons, D. B., Stray-Gundersen, J., Painter, P. L., Brinker, K. R., & Mitchell, J. H. (1993). Uremic myopathy limits aerobic capacity in hemodialysis patients. *American Journal of Kidney Diseases, 22,* 277–287.

Miller, B. W., Cress, C. L., Johnson, M. E., Nichols, D. H., & Schnitzler, M. A. (2002). Exercise durign hemodialysis decreases the use of antihypertensive medications. *American Journal of Kidney Diseases, 39,* 828–833.

Nath, K. A., Hostetter, M. K., & Hostetter, T. H. (1985). Pathophysiology of chronic tubulo-interstitial disease in rats. Interaction of dietary acid load, ammonia and complement component C3. *Journal of Clinical Investigation, 76,* 667–675.

National Kidney Foundation-Dialysis Outcomes Quality Initiative (NKF-DOQI). (1997). Clinical practice guidelines for hemodialysis adequacy. *American Journal of Kidney Diseases, 30*(Suppl. 2), S32–S37.

Noakes, T. (1991). *Lore of running: The science and spirit of running.* Champaign, IL: Oxford University Press.

Painter, P. L., & Moore, G. E. (1994). The impact of recombinant human erythropoietin on exercise capacity in hemodialysis patients. *Advances in Renal Replacement Therapy, 1,* 55–65.

Papovich, R. P., Moncrief, J. W., Decherd, J. F., et al. (1976). The definition of a novel portable-wearable equilibrium peritoneal technique. *Transactions of American Society of Artificial Internal Organs, 5,* 64.

Parker, T. F. III, Husni, L., Huang, W., Lew, N., & Lowrie, E. G. (1994). Survival of hemodialysis patients in the United States is improved with a greater quantity of dialysis. *American Journal of Kidney Diseases, 23,* 670–680.

Rasgon, S., Schwankovsky, L., James-Rogers, A., Widrow, L., Glick, J., & Butts, E. (1993). An intervention for employment maintenance among blue-collar workers with end-stage renal disease. *American Journal of Kidney Diseases, 22,* 403–412.

Rasgon, S. A., Chemleski, B. L., Ho, S., Widrow, L., Yeoh, H. H., Schwankovsky, L., et al. (1996). Benefits of a multidisciplinary predialysis program in maintaining employment among patients on home dialysis. *Advances in Peritoneal Dialysis, 12,* 132–135.

Saltin, B., & Rowell, L. B. (1980). Functional adaptations to physical activity and inactivity. *Federation Proceedings, 39,* 1506–1513.

Semenza, G. L. (2000). Surviving ischemia: Adaptive responses mediated by hypoxia-inducible factor 1. *Journal of Clinical Investigation, 106*, 809–812.

United States Renal Data System 2003 Annual Data Report. (2003). *American Journal of Kidney Diseases, 42*(6) Suppl. 5.

Wolf, G., & Neilson, E. G. (1993). Angiotensin II as a renal growth factor. *Journal of the American Society of Nephrology, 3*(9), 1531–1540.

Work incentives: Thoughts from an expert. (1997). *Renal Rehabilitation Report, 5*(5), 3.

23

Rheumatic Diseases

SICY H. LEE, MD, AND
STEVEN B. ABRAMSON, MD

RHEUMATIC DISEASES ENCOMPASS all disorders in which some portion of the musculoskeletal system, including synovial joints, periarticular structures, or muscles, is involved. Arthritis is the general term used when the joint disease predominates in the patient's illness. Examples of some inflammatory arthritides include rheumatoid arthritis, Reiter's syndrome, and psoriatic arthritis. In other conditions, the periarticular soft tissue or muscle disease is the primary concern, and the joint complaints are only a minor component. Some examples of these diseases include fibomyalgia, polymyositis, polymyalgia rheumatica, and scleroderma.

The classification of rheumatic diseases established by the American College of Rheumatology (ACR), the professional medical organization of the subspecialty of rheumatology, lists 116 rheumatic diseases under 10 major general classes of disorders. The current classification is based on known pathological changes induced in affected tissues, clinical patterns, and/or causative agents of each disease. The classification of the rheumatic diseases is a dynamic process that undergoes periodic review as important new information and concepts concerning pathophysiological mechanisms of these diseases are discovered.

According to the latest estimates derived from numerous surveys, there are over 43 million persons suffering from some form of arthritis or related diseases in the United States. This number will reach 60 million by year 2020 (CDC, 1994, 1998; Lawrence, Helmrick, & Arnett,

1998). Among these individuals at least 26% are partially disabled and about 10% are totally disabled. Arthritis and related diseases resulted in at least 45 million lost workdays yearly. These figures underscore the magnitude and the problems in diagnosis and management of these diseases. Furthermore, because most rheumatic diseases are chronic disabling conditions, these diseases as a group have significant social and economic ramifications. The rheumatic diseases detailed in this chapter, rheumatoid arthritis, spondyloarthropathies, and degenerative joint disease, are important because they are chronic disabling diseases that occur with relative frequency among individuals within the working population.

RHEUMATOID ARTHRITIS

THE PREVALENCE OF rheumatoid arthritis (RA) in most White populations approaches 1% among adults age 18 and older and increases with age, approaching 2% and 5% in men and women, respectively, by 65. The incidence also increases with age, peaking between the 4th and 6th decades. The annual incidence for all adults has been estimated at 67/100,000. Both prevalence and incidence are two and three times greater in women than in men (Hochberg, 1981).

Racial factors appear to be important in rheumatoid arthritis. American blacks, native Japanese, and Chinese may have a lower prevalence of rheumatoid arthritis than do whites, whereas several North American Indian tribes (the Yakima of central Washington State and the Mille-Lac Band of Chippewa in Minnesota) have a high prevalence of rheumatoid arthritis (Cunningham & Kelsey, 1984). Reasons for these differences are unknown but may relate to both genetic and environmental factors.

Genetic factors have an important role in the susceptibility to rheumatoid arthritis. The concordance among monozygotic twins is 25%–50%, whereas the concordance among dizygotic twins is only 10%. Studies have demonstrated a strong association between the major histocompatibility complex (MHC) Class II antigen HLA-DR4 and rheumatoid arthritis across several racial groups. Furthermore, a 5-amino-acid sequence on the beta-1 chain of the DR antigen appears to be shared among DR4 and non-DR4 individuals with rheumatoid arthritis, suggesting that the susceptibility to rheumatoid arthritis appears to be more specifically conferred by this 5-amino-acid sequence than by the entire DR4 molecule (Gregersen, Lee, Silver, & Winchester, 1987).

The role of environmental factors, particularly infectious agents, as a causal factor in rheumatoid arthritis remains under active investigation.

ETIOLOGY AND PATHOGENESIS

RHEUMATOID ARTHRITIS IS an autoimmune disease in which the normal immune response is directed against an individual's own tissue, including the joints, tendons, and bones, resulting in inflammation and destruction of these tissues. The cause of rheumatoid arthritis is not known, but current evidence suggests that the initiating event is an immune reaction to a foreign antigen such as a virus. In an individual with the genetic susceptibility for rheumatoid arthritis, this normal immune response is unchecked, perpetuating the inflammatory response. This theory is supported by the existence of an antibody called the rheumatoid factor, which is initially formed in the synovial fluid and can be found in the serum of about 80% of patients who have had rheumatoid arthritis for several months. This antibody is unique in that it interacts with normal immunoglobulin G, which is itself an antibody. An experimental arthritis in animals similar to rheumatoid arthritis can be induced following inoculation of protein substances similar to these antibodies, supporting this hypothesis in part (Holmdahl, Nordling, Rubin, Tarkowski, & Klareskog, 1986).

During this process of inflammation, cells of the immune system, including monocytes, T lymphocytes, B lymphocytes, and neutrophils, are activated to secrete a variety of chemical substances. These chemicals further stimulate proliferation of the synovial cells that normally line the joints, causing fluid accumulation in the joints (effusion), destruction of cartilage, and erosion of bone. The erosions in the bone can be observed radiographically and are characteristic of rheumatoid arthritis. Pathologically, the typical feature is the invasion of the cartilage and bone by the pannus, a vascular granulation tissue composed of various numbers of inflammatory cells, synovial cells, and new blood vessels. The tendons and ligaments can be similarly affected.

DESCRIPTION OF DISEASE

RHEUMATOID ARTHRITIS IS a systemic disease manifested primarily as polyarthritis. Although the diagnosis is made on clinical grounds, the most recent criteria, established by the ACR in 1987, afford a sensitivity of 91.2% and a specificity of 89.3% for diagnosing rheumatoid arthritis (Arnett et al., 1988). These include: (a) morning stiffness lasting at least 1 hour before maximal improvement; (b) arthritis of three or more joints or joint areas simultaneously for more than 6 weeks; (c) at least one of the joints involved should be the wrist, metacarpophalangeal joints (MCPs), or proximal interphalangeal joints (PIPs); (d) symmetrical pattern of joint involvement; (e) subcutaneous nodules over bony prominence, or extensor surfaces; (f) positive rheumatoid factor tested by any method that has been positive in less than 5% of normal control subjects; (g) radiographic changes that are typical of rheumatoid arthritis on posterioanterior (PA) views of the hands and wrists, including periarticular osteopenia or erosions.

Rheumatoid arthritis usually has an insidious, slow onset over weeks to months. About 15%–20% of individuals have a more rapid onset that develops over days to weeks. About 8%–15% actually have acute onset of symptoms that develop over days. The initial symptoms may be systemic or articular. In some patients, fatigue, malaise, low-grade fever, or diffuse musculoskeletal pain may be the first nonspecific complaints. Morning stiffness is frequently the first presenting symptom prior to onset of joint pain. Although symmetric pattern is common, asymmetric presentation is not unusual. The usual involvement is oligoarthritis progressing to polyarthritis in an additive but not migratory pattern. The most common joints involved in rheumatoid arthritis are MCPs (87%), PIPs (82%), and wrists (63%). Among larger joints, knees are most commonly involved (56%), followed by the shoulders (47%) and the hips. Medium-size joints are the least commonly involved, with the ankles (53%) affected more frequently than the elbows (21%) (Harris, 1997).

The natural history of rheumatoid arthritis is varied. In a minority of patients the intermittent course is marked by partial to complete remission without need for continuous therapy. This pattern of disease is usually mild. Initially, only a few joints are involved. Insidious return of the disease is often marked by progressive joint involvement. The majority of patients develop persistent disease requiring chronic therapy. At least 50% will develop erosive disease of cartilage in bone, which in a significant minority of patients is progressive and debilitating. Recent studies by Pincus and Callahan (1992) and others underscore the increased mortality and morbidity among patients with RA.

FUNCTIONAL PRESENTATION AND DISABILITY

IN THE INITIAL stages of each joint involvement, there is warmth, pain, and redness, with corresponding decrease of range of motion of the affected joint. In the hand, soft tissue swelling occurs as an early finding in rheumatoid arthritis and usually appears as fusiform enlargement of the PIPs. Patients describe difficulty in activity requiring motion of these joints, particularly in the morning. Progression of the disease results in reducible and later fixed deformities, including ulnar deviation, swan neck, or boutonniere deformities (Figures 23.1–23.3). The distal interphalangeal joints (DIPs) are seldom involved in rheumatoid arthritis. Many patients are able to continue performing activities of daily living as well as various nondexterous vocational tasks. The most severe form is arthritis mutilans, in which there is complete bone and

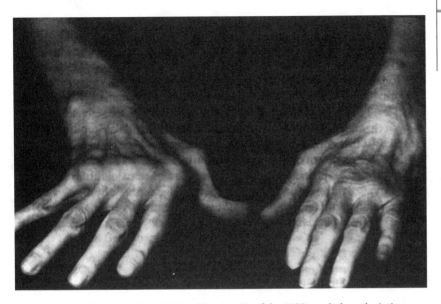

FIGURE 23.1   Rheumatoid arthritis with synovitis of the MCPs and ulnar deviation.
(Reproduced with permission from the American College of Rheumatology clinical slide
collection.)

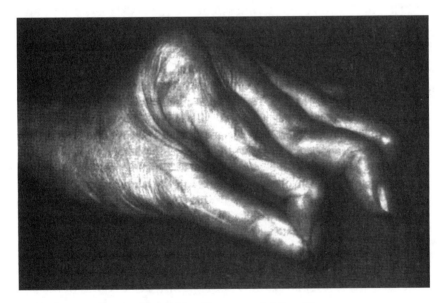

FIGURE 23.2   Rheumatoid arthritis with swan-neck deformity.

joint destruction and all movement is severely limited. At the wrist,
there is decreased ability to extend or flex, with progression toward
eventual fusion. An exaggerated flexion with near dislocation (subluxation) can occur in severe disease.

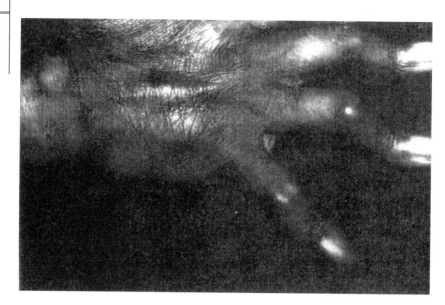

FIGURE 23.3 Rheumatoid arthritis with boutonnier deformity.

Deformities also occur at other joints. At the neck, there can be limitation in extension/flexion as well as rotation. The more serious deformities are those that result in neurological problems such as weakness and paralysis. The transverse ligaments that stabilize C-1 and C-2 vertebrae can become eroded. This results in C-1–C-2 (atlantoaxial) subluxation and can cause instability, with possible compression of the spinal cord or upward migration of the cervical spine and impingement of the medulla (brain). Such neurological involvement requires surgical intervention. The knees can decrease in flexion and can also develop flexion contracture. The hip may become limited in rotation or flexion extension. The ankle can be affected, with decreased ability to invert/overt or flex/extend. With inflammation or rupture of certain tendons, the foot can become flat. The toes mirror what occurs in the hands with involvement of the MTPs and PIPs. The most common deformities are hammer or cockup toes with metatarsal phalangeal joint (MTP) subluxation and callus formation of the planter surface.

Muscle weakness and atrophy develop early in the course of the disease in many patients. The exact cause of these problems is not clear. One observation is that perhaps the patients are unable to move because of pain, and this lack of movement can cause further muscle atrophy and weakness. The combination of pain and muscle atrophy further diminishes the patient's ability to perform activities requiring both strength and dexterity. Therefore, the vocational and functional skills of the patient may be impaired early by pain, inflammation, and weakness. If the inflammation clears after several weeks and no damage has been done to the bone or cartilage, there usually will be no residual impairment. If the inflammation persists, permanent deformities can develop such that the mechanics of the joint are altered and the joint cannot function well, even though pain and inflammation may subside eventually.

COMPLICATIONS

THERE ARE A number of complications in rheumatoid arthritis. These include carpal tunnel syndrome, Baker's cyst, vasculitis, subcutaneous nodules, Sjogren's syndrome, peripheral neuropathy, cardiac and pulmonary involvement, Felty's syndrome, and anemia (Hurd, 1984). With the exception of carpal tunnel syndrome and Baker's cyst, these complications usually occur in the presence of seropositive, progressive, and destructive disease.

Carpal tunnel syndrome occurs when the proliferating synovial tissue compresses on the median nerve as it travels through the narrow space in the flexor surface of the wrist. It is characterized by numbness, tingling, and eventual loss of feeling in the thumb, second, and third fingers. The small muscles of the thumb may weaken and atrophy when the compression is not relieved.

Baker's cyst occurs when the synovial fluid escapes from the knee and collects in the space behind the knee, with extension into the calf. Rupture of the Baker's cyst can occur abruptly and cause sudden pain and swelling in the calf. These symptoms must be distinguished from venous thrombophlebitis by ultrasound studies.

Vasculitis is the inflammation of blood vessel, affecting capillaries and small and medium-size blood vessels. It can lead to skin lesions such as ulcers and subcutaneous nodules and to more severe problems, such as mononeuritis multiplex.

Subcutaneous nodules may develop in approximately 20%–25% of patients. They typically occur in areas subject to pressure, such as the elbows, occiput, or sacrum. They may occasionally break down or become infected but generally are asymptomatic.

In Sjogren's syndrome, lymphocytes invade the glandular tissue of the mouth, nose, eyes, throat, and lungs, resulting in dry eyes (keratoconjunctivitis sicca) and dry mouth (xerostomia). The loss of glandular function may cause ulcers of the eye tissue, dental caries, and an inability to chew food normally. When dry eyes and dry mouth occur alone, the sicca syndrome is said to be present. When sicca syndrome is accompanied by rheumatoid arthritis, the condition is termed Sjogren's syndrome. The lymphocytes can also invade the kidneys, liver, lungs, and other internal organs, resulting in their dysfunction.

Many patients with rheumatoid arthritis can develop peripheral neuropathy and complain of mild numbness and tingling in their fingers and toes. Rarely, they can develop mononeuritis and lose complete function of a major nerve. This loss of nerve function is due to inflammation of the blood vessels that supply the nerve. When more than one nerve is involved, it is termed mononeuritis multiplex.

The most common cardiac involvement in rheumatoid arthritis is pericardial effusion, which is reported in about 40% of patients at autopsy but is usually clinically asymptomatic. When symptomatic pericarditis occurs, it will rarely proceed to pericardial tamponade. Sometimes a focal myocarditis may be recognized. Lesions similar to rheumatoid nodules may be found involving the myocardium and the valves. Valvular insufficiency, conduction abnormalities, and myocardial infarction secondary to these inflammatory lesions may occasionally be seen as clinical manifestations of rheumatoid heart disease.

Several forms of pulmonary disease can occur in patients with rheumatoid arthritis. Rheumatoid pleural disease, though frequently found at autopsy, is most commonly asymptomatic. Pleural effusions can develop, but rarely will they accumulate to significant size and cause respiratory distress. Multiple pulmonary nodules may occur bilaterally. Another, more serious pulmonary manifestation of rheumatoid arthritis is interstitial fibrosis with pneumonitis. This may progress to a honeycomb appearance on x-rays, with bronchiectasis, chronic cough, and progressive dyspnea. Lung biopsy can show chronic inflammatory cell infiltration accompanied by neutrophils and eosinophils. Laryngeal obstruction can also be caused by arthritis of the cricoarytenoid joint.

Felty's syndrome is characterized by splenomegaly, lymphadenopathy, anemia, thrombocytopenia, and neutropenia in association with chronic active rheumatoid arthritis. Systemic manifestations such as fever, fatigue, anorexia, and weight loss are common. Hyperpigmentation and leg ulcers may accompany Felty's syndrome.

The anemia of rheumatoid arthritis can be due either to chronic inflammation that primarily affects the production of red blood cells in the bone marrow or to iron deficiency secondary to occult blood loss among individuals treated with medications that can cause gastritis or peptic ulcer disease. Frequently, a combination of both factors can be present.

TREATMENT AND PROGNOSIS

A VARIETY OF medications are available in the treatment of rheumatoid arthritis (Harris, 1997). They can be divided into two broad categories: nonsteroidal antiinflammatory drugs (NSAIDs) and slow-acting, disease-modifying drugs (DMARDS). The specific drugs in each group are summarized in Table 23.1. The choice of therapeutic agents is individu-

TABLE 23.1 Agents Used to Treat Rheumatoid Arthritis

Agent	Dose*
A. Antiinflammatory agents	
1. Salicylates	1000–5000 mg/day (adjusted based on serum salicylate levels)
a. Aspirin	
b. Sodium salicylate	
c. Salicylic acid (Trilisate)	
d. Diflunisal (Dolobid)	
2. NSAIDs	
I. Non-selective NSAIDs	
a. Ibuprofen (Motrin)	400–800 mg t.i.d.–q.i.d.
b. Sulindac (Clinoril)	150–200 mg b.i.d.
c. Piroxicam (Feldene)	10–20 mg q.d.
d. Indomethacin (Indocin)	25–50 mg b.i.d.–q.i.d., 75 mg SR
e. Meclofenamate (Meclomen)	50–100 mg b.i.d.–q.i.d.
f. Naproxen (Naprosyn, Naprelene)	250–500 mg b.i.d.
g. Ketoprofen (Orudis, Oruvail)	50–75 mg b.i.d-q.i.d.
h. Phenylbutazone (Butazolidine)	50–100 mg b.i.d.–q.i.d.
i. Tolmetin (Tolectin)	200–400 mg b.i.d.–q.i.d.
j. Diclofenac (Voltaren, Cataflam)	25–75 mg b.i.d.
k. Flurbiprofen (Ansaid)	5–100 mg b.i.d.
l. Oxaprozin (Daypro)	1200 mg q.d.
m. Nemebutone (Relafen)	100–1500 mg q.d.
n. Meloxicam (Mobic)	7.5–15 mg q.d.
II. Selective COX-2 NSAIDS	
a. Rofecoxib (Vioxx)	25 mg q.d.
b. Celecoxib (Celebrex)	200–400 mg q.d.
c. Valdecoxib (Bextra)	10–20 mg q.d.
3. Corticosteroids	5.0–15 mg q.d. for arthritis
a. Oral prednisone	higher doses for extra-articular
b. Intra-articular	disease, varies with joint size
B. Disease-modifying agents (slow-acting agents)	
1. Gold	
a. Oral (Ridaura)	3 mg q.i.d.–b.i.d.
b. Parenteral (Solganol)	
2. D-penicillamine (Depen, Cupramine)	125–1000 mg q.d.
3. Hydroxychloroquine (Plaquenil)	200–400 mg q.d.
4. Sulfasalazine (Azulfidine)	1000–1500 mg b.i.d.
C. Immunosuppressive agents	
1. Methotrexate (PO, IM, IV)	5.0–30 mg per week
2. Azathioprine (Imuran)	25–150 mg q.d.
3. Leflunomide (Arava)	10–20 mg q.d.
4. Cyclosporin A (Neoral)	1–4 mg/kg/d
5. Cyclophosphamide (Cytoxan)	25–150 mg q.d.

(Continued)

TABLE 23.1 *(Continued)*

Agent	Dose*
D. Biological agents	
1. Anti-TNF agents	
a. Etanercept (Enbrel)	25–50 mg twice a week SQ
b. Infliximab (Remicaide)	3–10 mg/kg every 4–8 weeks IV
c. Adalimumab (Humira)	40 mg every week or every 2 weeks SQ
2. Anikinra (Kineret)	

*IV = intravenously; q.d. = once daily; b.i.d. = twice a day; t.i.d. = three times a day; q.i.d. = four times a day; SQ = subcutaneously; SR = slow release.

Adapted from "Inflammatory Arthritis" by G. Solomon (1991), in M. Jahss (Ed.), *Disorders of the foot and ankle* (2nd ed.), Vol. 2, New York: W. B. Saunders. Adapted with permission.

alized and dictated by a careful analysis of the severity of the patient's disease and rate of progression of the disease as well as an assessment of the patient's other comorbid conditions. Clinical assessment is supplemented by laboratory and radiographic assessment. Because articular cartilage or bone in humans cannot be replaced, the goal of the therapy must be to arrest the synovitis prior to any irreversible damage.

In early disease, symptoms can be relieved by NSAIDs, but these drugs do not arrest the disease process or prevent damage to the cartilage or bone. In individuals who have persistent disease, DMARDs should be initiated as soon as possible. Because all DMARDs are slow-acting agents, requiring 2–6 months to be effective, NSAIDs should be given simultaneously. The use of selective COX-2 inhibitors has decreased the risk of gastrointestinal adverse effects of NSAIDs in general. To date there are three COX-2 NSAIDs available: rofecoxib, celecoxib, and valdecoxib. In patients with extensive synovitis who do not obtain relief from NSAIDs, low-dose steroids can be given for temporary relief until DMARDs become effective. Once the disease is controlled or improved on DMARDs, steroid therapy should tapered and discontinued. Steroids alone should never be the mainstay of medical therapy because they do not prevent cartilage damage and because of their major side effects. Long-term steroid use can result in early cataract formation, osteoporosis, peptic ulcer disease, augmentation or initiation of hypertension and diabetes, increased skin and vascular fragility, delayed wound healing, muscle weakness, unsightly weight gain and fat accumulation on the face and the trunk, and poor resistance to bacterial and other opportunistic (e.g., fungal) infections.

There is now an increasing tendency to begin DMARDs earlier and more aggressively in the course of the patient's illness. This tendency resulted from the emerging view that there is a brief window of opportunity early in the patient's illness to halt the inflammatory process. Once articular damage occurs, the destructive process appears to self-perpetuate and cannot be reversed with medications. There is evidence that radiographic damage can occur within 2 years of onset of disease. Therefore, individuals who have evidence of disease activity as measured by swollen and tender joints, elevated C-reactive protein or sedimentation rate, constitutional symptoms including morning stiffness, fever, and weight loss should be aggressively treated with DMARDs so that remission is achieved as soon as possible. Methotrexate, Sulfasalazine, and hydroxychloroquine are the most frequently used medications. Parenteral gold and D-Penicillamine are less commonly used and have potential major side effects, including nephrosis (protein in the urine), anemia, leukopenia, thrombocytopenia, stomatitis, skin rash, and interstitial pulmonary fibrosis. Therefore, close laboratory and clinical monitoring is required while patients are on these medications. In order for the patient to accept these potentially toxic medications, the physician must adequately explain the necessity for their use. Oral gold and antimalarials have less toxic side effects but are also less likely to be effective. Because of the potential damage to the retina, regular ophthalmological examination is necessary while the patient is on antimalarials. Methotrexate has gained widespread use and is relatively easy to administer as it is given once a week. The drug is effective, but there are concerns about long-term toxicity, particularly pulmonary and hepatic fibrosis (Tugwell, Bennett, & Gent, 1987). Sulfasalazine has gained popularity in Europe as an effective DMARD (Pinals, Kaplan, Lawson, & Hepburn, 1986). The adverse effects associated with the use of this drug include blood dyscrasias, drug fever, hepatitis, allergic pneumonitis, drug-induced lupus, vasculitis, and significant cutaneous reaction including exfoliative dermatitis. Very few serious reactions have been reported in RA patients, and the adverse events appear to occur more commonly among slow acetylators. Leflunomide (Arava) is a reversible pyramidine inhibitor and appears similar to methotrexate and sulfalazine in efficacy; the major potential adverse effect is hepatotoxicity, and monitoring is required monthly. Other cytotoxic drugs (azathioprine, cyclophosphamide) appear effective but also have many potential side effects, particularly hepatic and hematologic toxicities, and require careful monitoring.

The newest class of DMARDs in the treatment of rheumatoid arthritis is the biological agents. These agents are unique in that they target a specific arm or subpopulation of cells within the immune system so that the inflammatory response in rheumatoid arthritis is abrogated. The majority of the approved agents target tumor necrosis factor (TNF). Etanercept (Enbrel) is an soluble TNF receptor antagonist and is a recombinant receptor fusion protein. Infliximab (Remicaide) is a chimeric anti-TNF monoclonal antibody (approximately 25% mouse protein) and approved for the treatment of RA in combination with methotrexate. Adalimumab (Humira) is a fully humanized anti-TNF monoclonal antibody. All the TNF agents have been found to be effective agents in preventing radiographic damage. Anikinra (Kineret) is an IL-1 receptor antagonist and the only approved IL-1 antagonist. Rituximab, a chimeric anti-CD20 monoclonal antibody which depletes B cells and was approved in 1997 for the treatment of B-cell lymphoma, is currently under active investigation in the treatment of rheumatoid arthritis. Preliminary data suggests one single course of treatment of rituximab for up to 48 weeks.

Another growing trend in the medical management of rheumatoid arthritis is the early use of combination drug therapy in aggressive disease. Smaller doses of multiple drugs with synergistic effects are used, in effect lowering the level of toxicity of individual drugs and enhancing the efficacy of treatment. Multiple studies have demonstrated that giving all the biologic agents in combination with methotrexate is more effective in preventing radiographic progression than when methotrexate or any of the biologic agents is given as monotherapy. The ultimate challenge for the future is to devise safe and effective therapies that can be administered in early stages of the disease.

Surgical treatment in rheumatoid arthritis should be used in combination with medical therapy. In patients with severe synovitis and in whom the slow-acting agents have not yet taken effect, early synovectomy (removal of the synovial tissue to as great a degree as possible) can be considered for the elbows and knees. When permanent deformities have developed despite medical therapy, surgery can be performed to correct these deformities to decrease pain and improve the patient's functional status. These procedures include joint fusions (e.g., wrist fusion to provide a stable and painless wrist), resections (e.g., resection of the distal ends of the metatarsal heads to reduce foot pain and improve comfort and walking), and joint prosthesis. The most successful total joint replacements are the hips and knees; joint replacement for the shoulder, elbow, and ankle are available but less successful.

Rehabilitation therapy is an integral part of treatment in rheumatoid arthritis. In early disease, the goal is to reduce pain and inflammation and to prevent deformities and muscle atrophy. As the disease progresses, it is an important modality to correct deformities and increase strength. The major goal at each stage is to improve functional skills in the patient. Modalities that are used to reduce pain and inflammation include moist heat, paraffin baths, and cold packs that allow more activities to be performed with less discomfort. The choice of treatment depends largely on patient's preference because there is little data upon which one can base the choice. The pain relief is temporary, lasting perhaps 2 hours. It is important, therefore, that the patient be taught how to perform these treatments at home. Placing a joint in plastic, fiberglass, or plaster splints will protect the joint and diminish the inflammation. There must be a balance between exercise and rest, however, to prevent deterioration of motion and muscle atrophy. Splints are most conveniently placed on the wrists or hands. For some, night use alone may be sufficient.

Exercise is important to help prevent contractures as well as preserve and improve muscle strength. Nonweight-bearing and isometric exercises will allow improvement in strength without joint inflammation. Passive range-of-motion exercises will help preserve motion without stress on the joints. Physical and occupational therapists should also evaluate the patient's functional limitations in activities of daily living and ambulation. Patients should be taught ambulation and transfer techniques. Devices such as reachers, hooks, and built-up utensil handles can be provided. The occupational therapist may also make energy- or labor-saving recommendations for the home, such as the raising or lowering of table tops or changing to more easily activated faucet handles. All of these measures aim to allow the patient to be more functional and independent.

The majority of patients with rheumatoid arthritis respond partially to some form of therapy, but few go into true remission, defined as absence of radiographic progression and clinical symptoms. The general course of rheumatoid arthritis, then, is gradual diminution of inflammation but progression of deformities (Pincus & Callahan, 1992). The speed with which the deformities occur varies from patient to patient. Factors associated with poor prognosis include persistent inflammation despite aggressive medical therapy of more than 1 year's duration; onset of disease below age 30; presence of extraarticular manifestation of rheumatoid arthritis, including subcutaneous nodules, vasculitis, Sjogren's syndrome, and neuropathy; and high-titer rheumatoid factor.

PSYCHOLOGICAL AND VOCATIONAL IMPLICATIONS

PATIENTS WITH RHEUMATOID arthritis undergo several stages of psychological adjustments. In the early stages of disease, it is common for patients with rheumatoid arthritis to be frightened because of the uncertainty of the prognosis of the disease and the degree of disability. Many patients also tend to blame themselves or a particular incident for the onset of the disease. Along with this feeling of guilt, there is also denial. Many patients do not give up hope that one day the disease and pain will miraculously vanish. This type of denial may lead to unrealistic expectations and resistance to medical treatment. As the disease progresses, the patient may express various degrees of anger, frustration, resentment, and depression. Some patients adapt to their disease and disability and function well with limited abilities, whereas other patients seem incapacitated by fairly minimal involvement. Adaptation to rheumatoid arthritis requires the patient to have self-confidence and willingness to adjust certain aspects of lifestyle without sacrificing independence. This adaptation is difficult and may be thwarted by pain denial, anger, and depression. Another reaction to the disease is hopelessness and increased dependency. Faced with the prospect of progressive deformities and apparent deterioration, the patient may give up trying to remain active by increasingly depending on others for care.

Not all individuals with rheumatoid arthritis progress unremittingly to disability. In the minority of patients with mild disease, fewer adjustments are required and vocational goals can be easily met. However, in individuals in whom the disease is an evolving and dynamic process, the vocational counselor should make frequent assessment of the patient's functional ability as the disease progresses and provide realistic goals and support through the more difficult periods so that employment can be sustained.

In general, motor coordination, finger and hand dexterity, and eye–hand–foot coordination are adversely affected by rheumatoid arthritis. Vocational goals dependent upon fine, dextrous, or coordinated movements of the hand are therefore not ideal for patients with rheumatoid arthritis. Loss of motion and pain on motion slow the patient's movements and diminish coordination. Therefore, the operation of machines requiring repetitive, dexterous, and rapid movements is also not a desirable choice. However, if the force required is quite low, dexterous tasks such as the use of an electric typewriter or computer are quite possible.

Most jobs requiring medium to heavy physical activity are also not desirable. Although most patients may be able to perform moderate manual labor (i.e., lift 25–30 lb), such level of activity will not be sustainable as the disease progresses. In addition, such a workload may be harmful to the joints. Activities such as climbing, balancing, stooping, kneeling, standing, or walking are all hampered by pain on weight bearing or with motion. Although these activities can be accomplished by most individuals with milder forms of rheumatoid arthritis, jobs requiring such activities repetitively and without periods of rest cannot be sustained and indeed may damage joints.

It is usual for patients with rheumatoid arthritis to detect changes in humidity, temperature, or barometric pressure. Therefore, extremes of weather or abrupt changes in temperature should be avoided, and an indoor climate in which the environment is relatively controlled is recommended. Excessive noise, vibration, fumes, gases, dust, and poor ventilation have no specific effects on patients with rheumatoid arthritis except for those individuals with appreciable pulmonary involvement.

Advanced or additional educational goals such as vocational training and/or college courses of 2 to 4 years should be strongly considered for individuals with recent-onset rheumatoid arthritis and those with long-standing disease despite increased mortality and morbidity among the latter. Educational goals should be guided by the patient's interest and aptitude. It is important to realize that the individual with rheumatoid arthritis does not have a permanent invariant disability but rather a changing disability with chronic pain (which can vary from day to day) that generally results in a progressive and unfavorable outcome. Such individuals require ongoing coordinated counseling that provides a combination of empathy, encouragement, and adequate evaluation and treatment.

SERONEGATIVE SPONDYLOARTHROPATHIES

THE SERONEGATIVE SPONDYLOARTHROPATHIES consist of a group of related disorders that include Reiter's syndrome, ankylosing spondylitis, psoriatic arthritis, and arthritis in association with inflammatory bowel disease. This group of diseases occurs more commonly among young men, with a mean age at diagnosis in the 3rd decade and a peak incidence between ages 25 and 34. The prevalence appears to be approximately 1%. The male-to-female ratio approaches 4 to 1 among adult Caucasians (Hochberg, 1992).

Genetic factors play an important role in the susceptibility to each disease. Among Caucasians, over 90% of patients with ankylosing spondylitis are HLA-B27, and approximately 20% of individuals with the HLA-B27 antigen will develop some form of spondyloarthritis. In addition, disease concordance for ankylosing spondylitis among monozygotic twins exceeds 50%. Linkage to other MHC Class I antigens that are cross-reactive with B27 (B7, B22, B40, B42) also has been observed, particularly among Blacks, in whom the association between ankylosing spondylitis and HLA-B27 (40%–50%) is not as striking as that in Caucasians (Arnett, 1984).

ETIOLOGY AND PATHOGENESIS

THE CAUSE OF spondyloarthritis is unclear, but there is strong evidence that the initial event involves interaction between genetic factors determined by Class I MHC genes and environmental factors, particularly bacterial infections. The onset of musculoskeletal symptoms following exposure to infections suggests an immunologically mediated process, as does the finding of lymphocytes at the sites of inflammation.

Reiter's syndrome may follow a wide range of gastrointestinal infections, including species of *Salmonella, Shigella, Yersinia, Campylobacter, and Escherichia coli* (Arnett, 1984). Recent work by Schumacher has identified chlamydial organisms in the synovial tissue. *Giardia, Brucella, and Streptococcus* organisms have also been implicated, as well as amoebas, and episodes of diarrhea in which no specific pathogen can be identified have been reported (Callin & Fries, 1976; Voltonen, Leirisalo, & Pentikainen, 1985). Arthritis also occurs in association with inflammatory bowel disease in patients who have undergone intestinal bypass operations for obesity and in Whipple's disease. Bowel inflammation has been implicated in the pathogenesis of endemic Reiter's syndrome, psoriatic arthritis, and ankylosing spondylitis. A putative link between these diverse conditions is the ability of enteric organisms to gain access to the systemic circulation and initiate an immune response in a genetically susceptible individual. The observation that some bacterial antigens share certain amino acid sequences with the HLA-B27 molecule suggests molecular mimicry as a plausible mechanism to explain the link between infection and arthritis in the presence of HLA-B27 (Inman, Chiu, Johnston, & Falk, 1992). This association, however, does not explain why only 20% of HLA-B27 individuals develop arthritis in the face of appropriate enteric infection. Whether there are fewer evident genetic differences between healthy and diseased HLA-B27-positive individuals remains under investigation.

DESCRIPTION OF DISEASE

THE SPONDYLOARTHROPATHIES SHARE certain common features, including the absence of serum rheumatoid factor, an oligoarthritis commonly involving large joints in the lower extremities, frequent involvement of the axial skeleton, familial clustering, and linkage to HLA-B27. Unlike rheumatoid arthritis, in which the predominant site of inflammation is the synovium, these disorders are characterized by inflammation at sites of attachment of ligament, tendon, fascia, or joint capsule to bone (enthesopathy).

Because the musculoskeletal presentation in each of the seronegative disorders is indistinguishable, current classification schemes are based on the presence of extraarticular features such as psoriasis, colitis, urethritis, aphthous stomatitis, inflammatory eye disease, nail changes, and keratoderma blenorrhagicum. Unfortunately, none of these features is unique to any particular disease. Psoriasis may occur in the setting of inflammatory bowel disease, aphthous stomatitis may occur in any of the seronegative disorders, keratoderma may be indistinguishable from pustularpsoriasis, and axial changes in psoriatic or colitic arthritis can be indistinguishable from primary ankylosing spondylitis. Overlap syn-

TABLE 23.2   Clinical Criteria for Ankylosing Spondylitis (AS) (New York, 1966)

Diagnosis
1. Limitation of the lumbar spine in all three planes—anterior flexion, lateral flexion, and extension
2. History of or presence of pain in the dorsolumbar junction or in the lumbar spine
3. Limitation of chest expansion to 1 inch (2.5 cm) or less measured at the level of the fourth intercostal space

Grading (requires radiographs of sacroiliac joints)
    Definite AS
        Grade 3–4 bilateral sacroiliitis with at least one clinical criterion
        Grade 3–4 unilateral or grade 2 bilateral sacroiliitis with clinical criterion 1 or with clinical criteria 2 and 3
    Probable AS
        Grade 3–4 bilateral sacroiliitis with no clinical criteria

From P. H. Bennett and T.A. Burch (1967), "New diagnostic criteria," *Bulletin on the Rheumatic Diseases,* 17, p. 453. Reprinted by permission.

dromes are common. Finally, there are patients with oligoarthritis and enthesopathy who lack sufficient extraarticular features to allow a specific diagnosis by existing criteria. HLA typing may provide a means of establishing that these patients have a disorder that falls within the spectrum of spondyloarthropathy. Given these pitfalls, the most accurate way of classifying a given patient may be to delineate fully the clinical features of the disease as well as the immunogenetic background in which it occurs.

Ankylosing spondylitis is the prototype disease among this group of disorders. The diagnosis is confirmed by clinical and radiographic findings. Existing criteria include the Rome and the New York criteria (Table 23.2) (Bennett & Burch, 1967). Ankylosing spondylitis is considered primary if no other rheumatological disorder is present and secondary if the patient has evidence of Reiter's syndrome, psoriasis, or colitis.

Reiter's syndrome was first described by Reiter in 1916 and consists of the triad of arthritis, urethritis, and conjunctivitis. Paronen (1948) subsequently pointed out the association of antecedent infectious urethritis or dysentery with the clinical triad. Arnett introduced the concept of incomplete Reiter's syndrome to describe those individuals who had only two of the features of the triad and underscored the association of the incomplete syndrome with HLA-B27 (Arnett, McClusky, & Schacter, 1976). The most current ACR criteria are much broader; they define Reiter's syndrome as a seronegative arthritis that follows urethritis, cervicitis, or dysentery. Possible associated features include balanitis, inflammatory eye disease, oral ulcers, and keratoderma. Callin

TABLE 23.3   Clinical Criteria for Reiter's Syndrome

Seronegative asymmetric arthropathy (predominately lower extremity)
Plus one or more of the following:
    Urethritis
    Cervicitis
    Inflammatory eye disease
    Mucocutaneous disease: balanitis, oral ulceration, or keratoderma

Exclusions
    Primary ankylosing spondylitis
    Psoriatic arthropathy
    Other rheumatic disease

From R. Fox, A. Callin, R. C. Gerber, & D. Gibson (1979), "The chronicity of symptoms and disability in Reiter's syndrome. An analysis of 131 consecutive patients." *Annals of Internal Medicine*, 91, p. 190. Reprinted by permission.

has proposed a broader definition (Table 23.3) that gives added weight to these extraarticular features (Fox, Callin, Gerber, & Gibson, 1979).

Psoriatic arthritis is not a single disease entity but consists of many different patterns of musculoskeletal disorders occurring in individuals with psoriasis. Patients may present with disease that is clinically indistinguishable from rheumatoid arthritis, ankylosing spondylitis, or Reiter's syndrome. The most widely used criteria are those of Moil and Wright (Table 23.4) (Bennett, 1967). Complicating this classification scheme is the observation that in up to 20% of patients the musculoskeletal disease antedates the onset of psoriasis. Therefore, an individual with dactylitis and radiographic evidence of pencil-in-cup deformities may be considered to have psoriatic arthritis even if the patient lacks skin disease. A family history of psoriasis or the presence of psoriasis-associated HLA alleles would further support this diagnosis (Mielants, Veys, & Cuvelier, 1985).

There are no distinct criteria for the enteropathic arthritis accompanying ulcerative colitis or Crohn's disease. A clinical spectrum of diseases similar to those seen in association with psoriasis may be observed. In an individual patient, axial disease, peripheral arthritis, or enthesopathy may predominate. Peripheral arthritis tends to parallel activity of bowel disease, whereas axial disease may progress independent of bowel activity. Complicating the concept of enteropathic arthritis as a distinct disease is the observation that low-grade bowel inflammation may be found on colonic or ileal biopsy in all of the seronegative disorders.

Patients with spondyloarthropathy may also develop inflammation of the aorta (aortitis) and the aortic valve, resulting in aortic insufficiency. Pulmonary fibrosis may also occur, resulting in diminished diffusion capacity and restrictive lung disease.

TABLE 23.4   Diagnosis of Psoriatic Arthritis

Criterion I	Psoriatic skin or nail involvement
Criterion II	Peripheral arthritis
Clinical	Pain and soft-tissue swelling with or without limitation of motion of the distal interphalangeal joints for over 4 weeks
	Pain and soft-tissue swelling with or without limitation of motion of the peripheral joints involved in an asymmetric peripheral pattern for over 4 weeks. This category includes diffuse swelling of an entire digit, known as the "sausage" digit
	Symmetric peripheral arthritis for over 4 weeks, in the absence of rheumatoid factor or subcutaneous nodules
Radiologic	"Pencil-in-cup" deformity, "whittling" of terminal phalanges, "fluffy periostitis," and "bony ankylosis"
Criterion III	Axial involvement
Clinical	Spinal pain and stiffness with restriction of motion present for over 4 weeks
Radiologic	Grade II symmetrical sacroiliitis according to the New York criteria or Grade II or IV unilateral sacroiliitis

Definite diagnosis of psoriatic arthritis requires Criterion I and any of the subheadings under Criteria II and III.

From "Psoriadic Arthritis" by R.M. Bennett (1979), in D.J. McCarthy (Ed.), *Arthritis and allied conditions: A textbook of rheumatology* (9th ed.), Philadelphia: Lea & Febiger. Reprinted by permission.

Functional Presentation and Disability

WHEN THE AXIAL skeleton is involved, the initial symptom is morning stiffness and lower-back pain. As the disease worsens, there is progressive diminution of motion of the spine. Eventually, the sacroiliac joints, lumbar, thoracic, and cervical spine become fused, although the process may skip over parts. At this stage, the spine is no longer painful, but the patient has lost all ability to flex or rotate the spine and generally develops a hunched-over posture with fused flexion of the cervical spine and flexion contracture of the hips to compensate for the loss of the lordosis curvature in the lumbar spine. The joints where the ribs attach to the vertebrae are also affected, and chest expansion and lung volume are decreased. Frequently, peripheral joints are involved, and the pattern is usually asymmetric oligoarthritis involving primarily the large or medium joints, including the hips, knees, and ankles. Rarely are smaller joints or the joints in the upper extremities involved. Enthesopathy can occur at multiple sites but more commonly presents as planter fasciitis, achilles tendonitis, and medial or lateral epicondylitis.

Loss of motion of the spine or pain in the spine with motion generally affects a patient's mobility, making certain chores difficult. Walking, however, remains unimpaired unless the hips and knees are affected. Frequent stooping and bending becomes impossible. Toilet activities and dressing may be difficult, but rarely does the patient become dependent. In fact, a patient with ankylosing spondylitis typically is able to continue vocational activity despite progressive stiffness, unless it requires significant back mobility or physical labor.

TREATMENT AND PROGNOSIS

NSAIDS ARE THE initial primary agents in the treatment of seronegative spondyloarthritis. Indomethacin is commonly regarded as being the most effective. Other NSAIDs, including naproxen, piroxicam, meclofenamate, and flurbiprofen, are also efficacious. Salicylates generally are not effective treatment. Corticosteroids, when given at significantly higher doses than that used in rheumatoid arthritis, can also be quite effective. If the inflammation does not completely resolve with NSAIDs alone or erosive disease is present at the initial evaluation, DMARDs should be given to prevent joint destruction and fusion. Just as in rheumatoid arthritis, the initiation of DMARDs in early disease is recommended to prevent progression of disease. The more common DMARDs used in the treatment of spondyloarthritis include sulfasalazine and methotrexate (Nissila, Lehtinen, & Leirisalo-Repo, 1988). Parenteral gold has been found to be effective therapy in patients with the form of psoriatic arthritis that mimics rheumatoid arthritis. Etanercept is the only biologic agent currently FDA approved in the treatment of psoriatic arthritis and ankylosing spondilitis, although the other two available anti-TNF agents have also been used. Surgical intervention includes either early synovectomy or total joint replacement in the later stages of disease. Physical therapy is also an integral part of treatment in this disease. Exercises should be done daily and should include those that enable the patient to maintain maximum chest expansion and erect posture as well as maximal axial flexibility.

Spondyloarthritis follows at least three different courses. The majority of the patients experience recurrent episodes of arthritis. A minority have only one self-limiting episode of the disease. A smaller minority of patients suffer a continuous and unremitting aggressive course. Although most patients can continue to work, most are affected and become disabled as the disease progresses (Fox et al., 1979).

VOCATIONAL IMPLICATIONS

THE PATIENT WITH spondylitis should be considered for vocational or professional education as resources and interests dictate. Although motor coordination, eye-hand coordination, and eye-hand-foot coordination will not be impaired among individuals with minimum peripheral arthritis, a stiff back will limit the patient's rotation and flexion so that overall dexterity may be affected. Tasks that require reaching or bending will be difficult. Work requiring lifting of over 10 to 15 lb may cause increased back pain. Climbing and balancing skills, stooping, and kneeling may be tolerated initially but become difficult as the disease worsens. Even with sedentary tasks, the patient must be allowed the opportunity to stretch the spine frequently. Although many individuals describe joint pain in relation to weather changes, patients with spondylitis should not necessarily require an indoor environment. Some noise, vibration, fumes, gas, dust, and poor ventilation should not be more intolerable than they are to an individual without spondyloarthritis unless significant pulmonary involvement is present. In general, patients with advanced education or clerical skills will frequently be able to continue meaningful employment, whereas those with only manual skills will become disabled.

DEGENERATIVE JOINT DISEASE

DEGENERATIVE JOINT DISEASE (osteoarthritis) is the most common rheumatic disease and is characterized by progressive loss of cartilage and reactive changes at the margins of the joint and in the subchondral bone. The disease usually begins in the 4th decade; prevalence increases with age, and the disease becomes almost universal in individuals aged 65 and older (Scott & Hochberg, 1984). It primarily affects weight-bearing joints such as the knees, hips, and lumbosacral spine. Frequently, the DIPs and PIPs are involved. Rarely, the shoulder can also be affected.

ETIOLOGY AND PATHOGENESIS

THE CAUSE OF degenerative arthritis is unclear. It is considered to be a "wear and tear" arthritis and is thought to occur as a consequence of some earlier damage or overuse of the joint. Obesity is frequently associated with degenerative joint disease in the weight-bearing joints (Hartz, Fischer, & Bril, 1986). Genetic factors play a role in the development of osteoarthritis of the PIPs and DIPs and appear to involve a single autosomal gene that is sex-influenced and dominant in females, resulting in an incidence 10 times greater than in men.

Degenerative changes begin as focal erosion of cartilage at various points of stress. There follows an increase in water content of the cartilage and quantitative and qualitative changes in the cartilage proteoglycans. Enzymes capable of degrading proteoglycans and collagen are increased in the osteoarthritis cartilage. As disease progresses, cartilage erosions become confluent and lead to large areas of denuded surface. The final outcome is full-thickness loss of cartilage down to bone. In contrast with this structural ulcerative breakdown, there is a proliferative cartilage and bone response leading to thickening of the subchondral bone and increased bony formation (osteophyte). Low-grade synovitis is common, particularly in advanced disease, and is due to release of inflammatory mediators or humoral and cell-mediated immune responses to damaged joint components (Pelletier, Martel-Pelletier, & Howell, 1985).

DESCRIPTION OF DISEASE

IN EARLY DISEASE, pain occurs only after joint use and is relieved by rest. As disease progresses, pain occurs with minimal motion or even at rest. Nocturnal pain is commonly associated with severe disease. Acute inflammatory flares may be precipitated by trauma or, in some patients, by crystal-induced synovitis in response to crystals of calcium pyrophosphate or apatite. Stiffness usually occurs only in affected joints. Local tenderness, pain on passive motion, and crepitus are prominent findings. Joint enlargement results from synovitis, synovial effusion, or proliferative changes in cartilage and bone (osteophyte formation). Clinical symptoms usually show positive correlation with radiological abnormalities. In a given patient, however, the lack of correlation between joint symptoms and radiographic findings may be striking.

Osteophytes formed at the DIPs are termed Heberden's nodes, and similar changes at the PIPs are called Bouchard's nodes. Flexor and lateral deviation of the DIPs are common. In most patients, Heberden's nodes develop slowly over months or years. These deformities are generally asymptomatic and primarily concern the patient for cosmetic reasons. In other patients, onset is rapid and associated with moderately severe inflammatory changes. This pattern of osteoarthritis is termed erosive osteoarthritis and frequently occurs during the 4th decade in women with a strong familial history. The first metacarpal (MP) joints are frequently involved, leading to tenderness at the base of the first MP bone and a squared appearance of the hand.

Osteoarthritis of the knee is characterized by localized tenderness over various components of the joint and pain on passive or active motion. Crepitans is usually present, and muscle atrophy is seen secondary to disuse. Disproportionate losses of cartilage localized to the medial or lateral compartments of the knee lead to secondary genu varum or valgum deformity. Chondromalacia patellae is commonly detected and is associated with softening and erosion of the patellar articular cartilage. Pain, localized around the patella, is aggravated by activity such as climbing stairs.

Osteoarthritic changes in the hip present with an insidious onset of pain. Pain is usually localized to the groin or along the inner aspect of the thigh, although patients often complain of pain in the buttocks, sciatic region, or the knee due to pain referral along contiguous nerves. Physical examination shows loss of hip motion, initially most marked on internal rotation or extension.

Osteoarthritis of the metatarsal phangeal joints (MTPs) can lead to MTP subluxation with corresponding hammer toe deformities. In the first MTP, the most common change is hallux valgus deformities. The severity of these deformities is usually aggravated by inappropriate footwear such as high heels and narrow, pointed, tight shoes.

Osteoarthritis of the spine results from involvement of the intervertebral disks, vertebral bodies, or posterior apophyseal articulations. Associated symptoms include local pain and stiffness and radicular pain due to compression of contiguous nerve roots. Lumbar stenosis is the term used when compression of the spinal cord occurs at multiple levels. The presenting symptom can be pain on walking and must be differentiated from claudication secondary to vascular incompetence. The presence of nocturnal pain can be a differentiating symptom for lumbar disease. In severe cases, myelopathy can develop, leading to muscle atrophy and disability. Surgical intervention is recommended when there are signs of neuropathy or myelopathy.

FUNCTIONAL DISABILITIES

OSTEOARTHRITIS AFFECTS THE patient's performance by impeding use of the involved joint. Because the hips, knees, and lower back are common sites of degenerative joint disease, walking and transfer activities may be impaired. At first the patient will be able to function well in a limited area, but as the disease progresses, the patient's functional capability decreases. Generally, however, activities of daily living, including dressing and eating, will not be significantly impaired.

TREATMENT AND PROGNOSIS

THE PRIMARY GOAL in the treatment of osteoarthritis is pain control and improvement of function in the affected joint. NSAIDs should be used in patients who show signs of inflammatory response in the affected joint. Analgesic agents such as acetaminophen may be used on a continuous basis, in combination with NSAIDs, to enhance pain control. Oral or parenteral therapy with corticosteroids is contraindicated in the treatment of osteoarthritis. Intraarticular injections of corticosteroids, however, may be beneficial when used judiciously in the management of acute flares, when inflammatory response appears to be a major component. Injections should be infrequent because joint deterioration may be accelerated by masking of pain and subsequent joint overuse or by a direct deleterious effect of these drugs on cartilage.

Newer therapies are in the horizon aimed at preserving the joint function and preventing further damage. These potential treatments can be divided into disease or structural modifying drugs and those which improve functional status only. The disease modifying agents include tetracyclines, gene therapy, and use of growth factors and cytokines (Howell & Altman, 1993). The mode of action is either through inhibition of collagenase activity, increase in the level of tissue inhibitor of metalloproteinases (TIMP), or manipulation of these factors via cytokines or gene therapy. Potential agents that are used only for symptomatic treatment of osteoarthritis include glucosamine sulfate, chondroitin sulfate, and intraarticular administration of hyaluronic acid derivatives. Glucosamine sulfate and chondroitin sulfate are available in the United States as nutritional supplements. Some evidence exists from Europe that these drugs may modify symptoms in selected patients, but no adequate controlled trial has been conducted to establish its effect in structural modification. Although hyaluronic acid derivatives are often mentioned as potential structure modifying drugs, these products are currently considered to be long-acting symptom-modifying drugs only (Peyron, 1993).

The goal in early physical therapy is to improve the functional status and prevent further deterioration of the affected joint. Patients should be instructed in daily non-weight-bearing exercise to strengthen muscles and thus protect joints from overuse. In addition, they should be taught weight-bearing techniques. Appliances such as canes are also beneficial.

Surgical procedures in the treatment of osteoarthritis include arthroplasty, osteotomy, and total prosthetic replacement. Hip and knee replacement procedures produce striking symptomatic relief and improved range of motion. Advances in arthroscopic techniques have led to increased surgical management such as debridement to remove loose bodies and abrasion chondroplasty earlier in the disease.

Osteoarthritis is a slowly progressive disease. Although medical and rehabilitative treatment can lead to improvement of function and diminution of pain in most patients, the effect is generally temporary. There is currently no established disease-modifying drug in the treatment of osteoarthritis. The eventual outcome is complete destruction of the joint, and ultimately surgical intervention is required.

Vocational Implications

Because osteoarthritis is not always a systemic disease, successful treatment of a single involved joint may result in continued employment in the patient's current job unless it requires dexterous or heavy use of the involved joint. Even if surgical or medical treatment results in an increased range of motion, diminished pain, and increased functional ability of the affected joint, the use of that joint should be limited. Heavy lifting, which repeatedly places stress on the hips, knees, or lumbosacral spine, should be avoided by those who have osteoarthritis in these areas. Light to medium work should be possible. Climbing, balancing skills, stooping, and kneeling will be impaired in many patients with osteoarthritis. The environment has no significant effect on patients with osteoarthritis even though changes in relative humidity and barometric pressures may cause transient joint discomfort.

Returning to work after undergoing successful surgery requires intensive postoperative rehabilitation and continued exercise to maintain muscle strength. As the patient's endurance and tolerance for activity normalize, work can be resumed. However, heavy manual work should be avoided, as the durability of the prosthetic implants is still limited. Stooping and kneeling may be accomplished without pain following surgery but should be limited. Certain motions involved with stooping and kneeling may cause dislocation of a prosthetic hip. Climbing and balancing can be accomplished, but such repetitive motions are hazardous and should also be limited. Most individuals with osteoarthritis are able to sustain gainful employment and a normal level of activity following successful medical and surgical therapy.

REFERENCES

American College of Rheumatology. Subcommittee on Rheumatoid Arthritis Guidelines. (2002). Guidelines for the management of rheumatoid arthritis. 2002 update. *Arthritis and Rheumatism, 46,* 328–346.

Arnett, F. C. (1984). HLA and the spondyloarthropathies. In A. Callin (Ed.), *Spondyloarthropathies* (pp. 297–321). Orlando, FL: Grune & Stratton.

Arnett, F. C., Edworthy, S. M., Bloch, D. A., McShane, D. J., Fries, J. F., Cooper, N. S., et al. (1988). The American Rheumatism Association 1987 revised criteria for the classification of rheumatoid arthritis. *Arthritis and Rheumatism, 31,* 315–324.

Arnett, F., McClusky, O. E., & Schacter, B. Z. (1976). Incomplete Reiter's syndrome:

Discriminating features and HLAB w27 in diagnosis. *Annals of Internal Medicine, 84*, 8–13.

Bathon, J. M., Martin, R. W., & Fleishmann R. M. (2000). A comparison of etanercept and methotrexate in patients with early rheumatoid arthritis. *New England Journal of Medicine, 343*, 1586–1593.

Bennett, P. H., & Burch, T. A. (1967). New York symposium on population studies in the rheumatic diseases: New diagnostic criteria. *Bulletin on the Rheumatic Diseases, 17*, 453–469.

Bennett, R. M. (1979). Psoriatic arthritis. In D. J. McCarty (Ed.), *Arthritis and allied conditions* (9th ed., pp. 453–466). Philadelphia: Lea & Febiger.

Bresnihan, B., Alvaro-Gracia, J. M., & Cobby, M. (1998). Treatment of rheumatoid arthritis with recombinant human interleukin-1 receptor antagonist. *Arthritis and Rheumatism, 41*, 2196–2204.

Callin, A., & Fries, J. F. (1976). An "experimental" epidemic of Reiter's syndrome, revisited: Follow-up evidence on genetic and environmental factors. *Annals of Internal Medicine, 84*, 564–574.

Centers for Disease Control. (1990). Prevalence of arthritic conditions in the United States. *Morbidity and Mortality Weekly Report, 39*(6), 99–102.

Centers for Disease Control and Prevention. (1994). Arthritis prevalence and activity limitations—United States, 1990. *Morbidity and Mortality Weekly Report, 43*, 433–438.

Centers for Disease Control and Prevention. (1998). Prevalence and impact of chronic joint symptoms—Seven states, 1996. *Morbidity and Mortality Weekly Report, 47*, 345–351.

Cunningham, L. S., & Kelsey, J. L. (1984). Epidemiology of musculoskeletal impairments and associated disability. *American Journal of Public Health, 74*, 574–579.

Dayer, J. M. (1990). Use of an IL-1 inhibitor in inflammation. In V. Strand (Ed.), *Proceedings: Early decisions in DMARD development: 2. Biologic agents in autoimmune disease* (pp. 44–46). Atlanta, GA: Arthritis Foundation.

Emery, P., Szczepaanski, L., & Szechinski, J. (2003). Sustained efficacy at 48 weeks after single treatment couse of reituximab in patients with rheumatoid arthritis [Abstract 1095]. *Arthritis and Rheumatism, 48*(Suppl.), S439.

Fox, R., Callin, A., Gerber, R. C., & Gibson, D. (1979). The chronicity of symptoms and disability in Reiter's syndrome: An analysis of 131 consecutive patients. *Annals of Internal Medicine, 91*, 190–207.

Gorman, J. D., Sack, K. E., & Davis, J. C., Jr. (2002). Treatment of ankylosing spondylitis by inhibition of tumor necrosis factor. *New England Journal of Medicine, 346*, 1349–1356.

Gregersen, P. K., Lee, S., Silver, J., & Winchester, R. (1987). The shared epitope hypothesis: An approach to understanding the molecular genetics of rheumatoid arthritis susceptibility. *Arthritis and Rheumatism, 30*, 1205–1213.

Harris, H. D., Jr. (1997). The clinical features of rheumatoid arthritis & treatment of rheumatoid arthritis. In W. N. Kelly, E. D. Harris, S. Ruddy, & C. Sledge (Eds.), *Textbook of rheumatology* (pp. 898–950). Philadelphia: W. B. Saunders.

Hartz, A. J., Fischer, M. E., & Bril, G. (1986). The association of obesity with joint pain and osteoarthritis. *Journal of Chronic Diseases, 39,* 311–319.

Hochberg, M. C. (1981). Adult and juvenile rheumatoid arthritis: Current epidemiologic concepts. *Epidemiology Review, 3,* 27–41.

Hochberg, M. C. (1992). Epidemiology. In A. Callin (Ed.), *Spondyloarthropathies.* Orlando, FL: Grune & Walton.

Holmdahl, R., Nordling, C., Rubin, K., Tarkowski, A., & Klareskog, L. (1986). Generation of monoclonal rheumatoid factors after immunization with collagen II-anti-collagen II immune complexes: An anti-idiotype antibody to anti-collagen II is also a rheumatoid factor. *Scandinavian Journal of Immunology, 24,* 197–212.

Howell, D. S., & Altman, R. D. (1993). Cartilage repair and conservaion in osteoarthritis. *Rheumatic Diseases Clinics of North America, 19,* 713–724.

Hurd, E. R. (1984). Extra-articular manifestations of rheumatoid arthritis. *Seminars in Rheumatic Diseases, 8,* 151–163.

Inman, R. D., Chiu, B., Johnston, M. E. A., & Falk, J. (1992). Molecular mimicry in Reiter's Syndrome: Cytotoxicity and ELISA studies of HLA-microbial relationships. *Immunology, 58,* 501–512.

Lawrence, R. C., Helmick, C. G., & Arnett, F. C. (1998). Estimates of the prevalence of arthritis and selected musculoskeletal disorders in the United States. *Arthritis and Rheumatism, 41,* 778–799.

Maini, R., St. Clair, E. W., & Breedveld, F. (1999). Infliximab versus placebo in rheumatoid arthritis patients receiving concomitant methotrexate, a randomized phase III trial. ATTRACT Study Group. *Lancet, 354,* 1932–1939.

Mielants, H., Veys, E. M., & Cuvelier, C. (1985). HLA B27 related arthritis and bowel inflammation: Part 2. Ileocolonoscopy and bowel histology in patients with HLA B27 related arthritis. *Journal of Rheumatology, 12,* 294–299.

Miller, B., Demerieux, P., & Srinivasan, R. (1980). Double-blind placebo-controlled crossover evaluation of levamisole in rheumatoid arthritis. *Arthritis and Rheumatism, 23,* 172–183.

Nissila, M., Lehtinen, K., & Leirisalo-Repo, M. (1988). Sulfasalazine in the treatment of ankylosing spondylitis: A 26-week placebo-controlled clinical trial. *Arthritis and Rheumatism, 31,* 1111–1117.

Paronen, A. (1948). Reiter's disease: A study of 344 cases observed in Finland. *Acta Medica Scandinavica, 131,* 1–143.

Pelletier, J. P., Martel-Pelletier, J., & Howell, D. S. (1985). Collagenase and nolytic activity in human osteoarthritic cartilage. *Arthritis and Rheumatism, 28,* 554–561.

Peyron, J. G. (1993). Intraarticular hyaluronan injection in the treatment of osteoarthritis: State-of-the-art review. *Journal of Rheumatology, 20*(39), 10–15.

Pinals, R. S., Kaplan, S. B., Lawson, J. G., & Hepburn, B. (1986). Sulfasalazine in rheumatoid arthritis. *Arthritis and Rheumatism, 29*(12), 1427–1434.

Pincus, T., & Callahan, L. F. (1992). Taking mortality in rheumatoid arthritis seriously: Predictive markers, socio-economic status and co-morbidity. *Journal of Rheumatology, 13,* 841–845.

Reiter, H. (1916). Über eine bisher unbekannte Spirochaeten Infektion (*Spirochaetosis arthritica*). *Deutsche Medicin Wochenschrift, 42,* 1535–1536.

Scott, J. C., & Hochberg, M. C. (1984). Osteoarthritis. *Maryland Medical Journal, 33,* 712–716.

Smolen, J. S., Kalden, J. R., & Scott, D. L. (1999). Efficacy and safety of leflunomide compared with placebo and sulphasalazine in active rheumatoid arthritis: A double-blind, randomized, multicentre trial. European Leflunomide Study Group. *Lancet, 353,* 259–266.

Solomon, G. (1991). Inflammatory arthritis. In M. Jahss (Ed.), *Disorders of the foot and ankle* (2nd ed., pp. 1681–1702). New York: W. B. Saunders.

Strand, V., Cohen, S., & Schiff, M. (1999). Treatment of active rheumatoid arthritis with leflunomide compared with placebo and methotrexate. European Leflunomide Study Group. *Archives of Internal Medicine, 159,* 2542–2550.

Tugwell, P., Bennett, K., & Gent, M. (1987). Methotrexate in rheumatoid arthritis: Indications, contraindications, efficacy, and safety. *Annals of Internal Medicine, 107,* 358–366.

Voltonen, V. V., Leirisalo, M., & Pentikainen, P. J. (1985). Triggering infections in reactive arthritis. *Annals of Rheumatic Diseases, 44,* 399–412.

Weinblatt, M. E., Keystone, E. C., & Furt, D. E. (2003). Adalimumab, a fully human anti-tumor necrosis factor a monoclonal antibody, for the treatment of rheumatoid arthritis in patients taking concomitant methotrexate: The ARMADA trial. *Arthritis and Rheumatism, 48,* 35–45.

Yocum, D. E., Klippel, J. H., & Wilder, R. L. (1988). Cyclosporin A treatment of refractory rheumatoid arthritis. *Annals of Internal Medicine, 1,* 863–873.

24

Spinal Cord Injury

ALLEN W. HEINEMANN, PhD, ABPP, AND
PURVA H. RAWAL, MA

S PINAL CORD INJURY resulting in permanent paralysis and loss of sensation would seem to be one of the most devastating experiences imaginable. Emptying one's bladder with a catheter, using a wheelchair, having difficulty entering one's home and public buildings, being unable to participate in enjoyed activities, and disrupted sexual expression may seem to the outsider like a life not worth living. The experience of celebrities such as Christopher Reeves captures media attention and focuses attention on paralysis, physical dependence, and loss, as well as research efforts to "cure" spinal injury. Yet the experience of most persons who live with spinal cord injury (SCI) is quite different. Advances in acute care and rehabilitation practices have reduced morbidity and mortality dramatically over the past 10 years (Brown, 1992; DeVivo, Stover, & Black, 1992). People who sustain SCI do live independent and fulfilling lives. The process by which they deal with disability-related limitations and attain a meaningful quality of life is the focus of this chapter.

This chapter summarizes recent advances in our understanding of the psychological and social aspects of spinal cord injury. In doing so, it reviews theoretical formulations of how spinal cord injury affects people, examines research evidence, and explores implications for psychological interventions. A context for integrating psychological and social theory is provided first by reviewing current data on quality of life and community reintegration following SCI.

QUALITY OF LIFE AND COMMUNITY REINTEGRATION

ALTHOUGH ENHANCED QUALITY of life as a goal of rehabilitation has emerged as an important topic (Anderson, 1982; Crewe, 1980), few studies have examined this subject explicitly. One source of information related to this topic is the National Spinal Cord Injury Statistical Center, which maintains a database on persons nationwide who have received care from the model SCI care system. DeVivo and Richards (1992) report information on residence, employment, and marital status from this database. They report that almost everyone (94%) who completes rehabilitation returns to a private residence; 10 years after rehabilitation, 98% reside in a private residence. As in the able-bodied population, nursing home residence is more likely as people age. While less than 2% of persons between 16 and 30 years of age reside in nursing homes, 22% of those over age 75 do so. Competitive employment for persons aged 16 to 59 years of age increases from 13% 2 years after injury to 38% 12 years after injury. Employment rates are associated with specific demographic factors. Employment is more likely for persons who are younger, male, white, have greater education, higher motivation, greater functional ability, and employment histories before injury. Disincentives to employment include Social Security Disability Income and Supplemental Security Income, and health insurance such as Medicare and Medicaid, which are available only to those who are not working.

Since DeVivo and Richards' (1992) work on demographic and injury trends, the Model Spinal Cord Injury Care Systems database of 25,054 individuals with SCI has continued to compile information (Nobunaga, Go, & Karunas, 1999). The average age at time of injury is rising, with people older than 60 years comprising over 10% of the SCI population, suggesting a greater number of falls and injuries in the elderly; the ratio of males to females with SCI remains 4:1, but the incidence of individuals with SCI has decreased significantly between 1994 and 1998 (Nobunaga et al.). The proportion of injuries related to violence from 1973–1977 to 1994–1998 increased from 13.9% to 21.8%, indicating an increase in injuries due to gunshot wounds, penetrating wounds, explosions, or person-to-person contact (Nobunaga et al.). Individuals involved in violent SCI tend to be younger, male, and African-American (Nobunaga et al.).

Krause (1992) reported similar results for patients receiving outpatient services at a urology clinic: employment is greater for persons with paraplegia who are younger, sustained injuries longer ago, and completed more years of education. A separate analysis of this sample (Krause, 1990) found that persons who were employed reported higher levels of overall adjustment compared with unemployed persons; those working in unpaid productive activities were at an intermediate level of satisfaction. Injury level was unrelated to level of productivity, though persons with quadriplegia spent fewer hours working per week. Time since injury was related to productivity such that employed persons had the longest average time since injury (15 years), followed by for unemployed individuals (14 years), and for productive but unemployed persons (12 years).

SCI affects the opportunity for marriage among single persons. Only 12% of never-married persons marry within 5 years of injury, whereas nearly three times that rate is expected for able-bodied peers. The impact of SCI on marriage is smaller. Five years after SCI, 81% of married persons were still married compared to a rate of 88% among able-bodied persons. Finally, 56% of postinjury marriages continued for 8 years compared to an expected rate of 77% in demographically similar, nondisabled adults. Divorce rates are higher for persons who are younger, female, African-American, have no children, are previously divorced, and are nonambulatory.

Quality of life is also reflected in the extent to which one is able to direct or independently carry out activities of daily living. Yarkony, Roth, Heinemann, Lovell, and Wu (1988) described the functional status of persons discharged from a model SCI care system over 3 years after rehabilitation. They reported that patients attain a relatively independent level of function in self-care and ambulation, which is maintained or improves in most cases. Level of injury (quadriplegia vs. paraplegia) and completeness of lesion (partial vs. total paralysis and sensory loss) are related to independent functioning in an expected manner: persons with incomplete lesions and those with paraplegia required less assistance.

A national survey of 719 community-dwelling veterans with SCI conducted by Saltz, Eisenberg, Fillenbaum, and George (1991) also provides information on quality of life. They collected information about impairment in five areas of functioning: social resources, economic resources, mental health, physical health, and activities of daily living. They concluded that the quality of life enjoyed by young and old veterans is relatively good, and for older veterans, better than for nondisabled men of a similar age. Disorders that limited activities of daily living included chronic pain, urinary tract disorders, and skin infections. The veterans' group was generally pleased with the quality of medical and other health services, which they primarily received from Veterans Administration hospitals.

Life satisfaction was the focus of a study reported by Krause and Dawis (1992), in which 286 urology clinic patients completed a questionnaire describing activities and satisfaction with specific life domains. The average age of the sample was 42 years; an average of 19 years elapsed from injury to study participation. Study participants also completed the Multidimensional Personality Questionnaire from which measures of positive and negative affect and constraint were derived. Greater life satisfaction was reported by people who experienced less emotional distress, lower levels of dependency (defined as lack of transportation, income and control, and family conflicts), fewer health problems, and greater positive affect. Current life satisfaction was also predicted with information gathered 4 years earlier. Persons who reported higher levels of adjustment and activity level, and fewer health problems and dependency at the initial assessment tended to report higher life satisfaction at the second time assessment. In contrast, dependency and employment were the best predictors of economic satisfaction both concurrently and from data collected 4 years earlier. Demographic characteristics were unrelated to satisfaction. The distinct nature of satisfaction in general life and economic-specific domains is illustrated by these results.

In contrast to studies investigating objective quality of life outcomes, qualitative research methods have been used to assess the subjective quality of life for individuals with spinal cord injury. Qualitative studies allow participants to relate their experiences in a less structured manner and give researchers the opportunity to gather novel information. A qualitative interview study of 40 participants described the subjective quality of life of individuals with SCI (Duggan & Dijkers, 2001). Individuals who rated themselves as having a high quality of life tended to be more financially secure, have more material assets, have more meaningful social roles, and had a longer time since injury pass. Individuals who rated themselves as having a medium level of quality of life were more likely to report positive social relationships, significant social support, and an overall positive change in their "values" (i.e., having a greater respect for life, existential issues). Individuals who rated themselves as having a low quality of life were more likely to have lower levels of educational attainment, financial security, and material resources. Overall, these studies suggest that quality of life has several components including physical, emotional, financial, and personality factors that contribute to overall life satisfaction.

Historically, a large component of community reintegration and rehabilitation outcomes has been employment for individuals with SCI. Krause (1992) examined whether people with SCI who reported better adjustment were likely to obtain employment or whether employment led to better adjustment in an effort to understand the directional nature of the relationship between adjustment and employment. In addition, Krause conducted one of the few longitudinal studies of individuals with SCI. He collected 11-year longitudinal data on 142 individuals (Krause, 1996). Results from both studies suggest that employment has a substantial impact on multiple facets of adjustment and that individuals with SCI who are better adjusted are not more likely to be employed. These results underscore the importance of vocational rehabilitation as being central to community reintegration. The most recently published follow-up of this sample extended to 20 years. Krause (1998) reported that years worked at a particular job increased linearly through the study period, that number of hours worked per week tended to increase over time, and that mean hours worked per week increased sharply in the first 11 years of the study and changed little afterwards. He concluded that the positive employment outcomes suggest that individuals with SCI show increasing adaptation and that employment opportunities have also increased over the study period (Krause, 1998).

In addition to research that has focused on community living and reintegration, other research has focused on psychological functioning and levels of distress after SCI. One study investigated the use of the Brief Symptom Inventory (BSI), a widely used psychological measure, in a sample of 225 people with SCI (Heinrich, Tate, & Buckelew, 1994). BSI scores were assessed at three time periods: at discharge from the hospital, from hospital discharge to 24 months, and over 24 months post-hospital discharge. The investigators sought to define BSI norms specific to individuals with SCI and also to assess levels of psychological distress in the sample. Individuals with SCI had significantly higher scores on all BSI subscales (somatization, obsessive-compulsive, interpersonal sensitivity, depression, anxiety, hostility, phobic anxiety, paranoid ideation, psychoticism) and global scales (total positive symptoms, average intensity of positive symptoms, and average item response) than did the normative group. When the investigators examined individuals' responses over time, they found a pattern suggesting a response to traumatic injury rather than an indication of general psychopathology. Scores were elevated from hospital discharge to 24 month post-discharge on the interpersonal sensitivity, depression, paranoia, and psychoticism scales; however, most scores decreased by 24 months post-discharge. The one exception was the paranoia scale, which remained elevated compared to levels at hospital discharge. Somatization, overall distress, and total number of positive symptoms were elevated for the first 24 months and then decreased. These results suggest improving physical and emotional stability over time following a difficult initial adjustment period that can last up to 24 months post-discharge. This early time period may be when mental health services are of greatest benefit.

With this functional and community living information providing a background, we are better able to ask what affects post-injury adjustment and identify the characteristics of persons who attain favorable outcomes.

THEORETICAL CONCEPTS IN
SPINAL CORD INJURY ADJUSTMENT

S CI IS A relatively low incidence impairment, with about 11,000 people sustaining injury resulting in permanent disability annually and
a prevalence of approximately 250,000 persons with SCI in the United
States (Stover & Fine, 1986; Spinal Cord Injury Information Network,
2001). Consequently, few unique theoretical approaches have been developed specifically related to spinal injury. Instead, psychologists have,
for the most part, borrowed theoretical models and approaches developed to explain health behaviors generally. Nonetheless, several recurring questions have focused specific concerns of rehabilitation
professionals in dealing with persons who sustain spinal cord injury.
Trieschmann (1992) identifies key clinical questions that emerge in light
of life expectancies that approach those of able-bodied peers and increasing opportunities for employment and community living. They include:
"How do we teach people to cope more effectively with this disability?"
"How can we facilitate better communication among professionals and
people with SCI to enhance independent functioning within the hospital and community environment?" "What are the best methods of promoting wellness in the SCI community?" "How do we teach coping skills
to [persons with] new SCI with a history of alcohol and drug abuse?"
Asking the right questions allows theory to relate usefully to the experience of persons with SCI.

Early theorists drew on their clinical experience and tended to focus
on patients' emotional responses immediately after injury and the life
disruption following SCI. Implicit in these models were several questions: How do people cope with SCI-related limitations? Are there predictable stages by which adjustment is attained? Is depression a necessary
reaction to injury? And, what kinds of people attain favorable adjustment? Early reports on post-injury adjustment often focused on describing emotional consequences and psychopathological reactions (Hohmann,
1975; Mueller & Thompson, 1950; Shontz, 1965; Siller, 1969; Stewart, 1978).
This focus reflected the fact that rehabilitation hospitalization could
extend up to a year, life expectancies were relatively short, and community accommodation of persons with disabilities was uncommon.

An early model of disability acceptance, which has influenced thinking about spinal injury reactions, was described by Dembo, Leviton,
and Wright (1956) and elaborated by Wright (1960, 1983). This model developed out of extensive interviews with veterans who sustained amputations. A model of value changes emerged by which the researchers
defined a concept they termed disability acceptance. Enlarging one's
scope of values, containing disability effects, emphasizing self-evaluation
with asset values rather than deriving one's self-worth by comparing

oneself with others, and subordinating the importance of physique and physical appearance were identified as the central value changes required to perceive oneself with a disability in nondevaluing terms. These concepts were based on Kurt Lewin's field-theoretic approach to personality (1935) and focus on intra-psychic processes. The process by which these value changes occur was not described.

An influential theoretical model of spinal injury adjustment was described by Trieschmann (1988). She bases her model on the assumption that disability adjustment is synonymous with balance in life, and that persons should be understood as integral mind-body systems. She describes a systems model in which behavior, health, and adjustment are determined by psychological resources, biological-organic state, and the environment. Within this model, she defines rehabilitation as "the process of teaching people to live with their disability in their own environment" (p. 26). Rehabilitation and life with SCI is regarded as a dynamic process; hence, no specific end-point of adjustment or rehabilitation is possible or desirable.

Shontz (1982) highlights the apparent paradox that exists when psychological adaptation to an unchangeable condition, such as disability, is successfully completed: the disability exists only while adaptation is in process. Yet, outsiders still react to visible signs of disability and often treat the person as having a handicap even when adaptation is complete. Extending Dembo's (1969) distinction between insiders (those with a condition) and outsiders, Shontz argues that from the perspective of the person who has successfully dealt with chronic illness or disability, one no longer adapts *to* illness or disability because the condition no longer exists. Instead,

> like everyone else, they adapt to the full array of possibilities and limitations that are afforded by the complete panorama of their biological states and their social and physical environments. . . . The question [for psychology] is how they come to satisfactory and satisfying terms with the same world in which everyone lives. (p. 155)

Like Trieschmann, he proposes that signs of psychological adjustment are no different for people with disabilities than for anyone else. Implicit in this perspective is that no special psychology of disability is needed. Satisfactory adaptation is, instead, evident when disability is no longer the dominant issue in a person's life space. The next section examines models that describe how this adaptive process occurs.

MODELS OF ADAPTATION

T HE BELIEF THAT persons sustaining SCI experience a more or less predictable sequence of reactions to loss accompanying injury has been described at length in the rehabilitation literature (Dunn, 1975; Gunther, 1969; Kerr, 1961). George Hohmann (1975) described his experiences dealing with SCI; to a large extent, his description of denial, withdrawal, hostility, and reactions against dependence parallel those of writers who describe reactions to other health crises and terminal illness (Kubler-Ross, 1969; Parkes, 1972). The possibility of sequential phases of adaptation has had an enduring allure for rehabilitation professionals. For example, intervention plans based on anticipated patient reactions have been described for nurses (French & Phillips, 1991).

One model with heuristic value was described by Fink (1967) and elaborated by Shontz (1965). It describes a disability such as spinal cord injury as a crisis-inducing event that is followed by four stages: shock, defensive retreat, acknowledgment, and adaptation. The consequences of progressing, or failing to progress, through these hypothesized stages have been the focus of several studies. One early study (Dinardo, 1971), found that persons who experienced depression after SCI attained poorer long-term adjustment, while denial was associated with greater better adjustment. The importance of socioeconomic factors was highlighted by Kalb (1971), who found that income was associated with greater depression, cooperation during hospitalization, and long-term adjustment. However, for middle-income men, cooperation with nurses was not a predictor of rehabilitation success and depression was unrelated to outcome. For low-income men, denial of depression appeared to be the best course. Neither of these early studies found evidence to support a process model of adaptation.

Stage models of adjustment have been criticized for a lack of empirical evidence (Trieschmann, 1988) and for failing to account for variability in individuals' response to life disruption (Silver & Wortman, 1980). One would expect that time since injury would be a crude marker of an adjustment process. Krause and Crewe (1991) examined the effect of age, time since injury, and time of measurement on post-SCI adjustment. Two groups of subjects, recruited in 1974 and 1985 from patients seeking services at a renal clinic, were assigned to one of five cohorts based on age and time since injury. The group originally recruited in 1974 was reassessed in 1985; both groups were an average of nearly 10 years post-injury. Indices of activity, medical stability, adjustment, interpersonal satisfaction, and economic satisfaction were derived from a Life Satisfaction Questionnaire. They found that the nature of SCI-related changes depended on the nature of adjustment considered. Activities were more strongly related to chronological age, while medical problems were more strongly related to time since injury. Both age and time since injury were related to psychological indices of adjustment, such as life satisfaction and self-rated adjustment. Older persons reported less activity, as measured by sitting tolerance and frequency of leaving one's home, and less rewarding lives, as measured by number of weekly visitors, satisfaction with sex life, and self-rated adjustment. However, older persons were more satisfied with their living arrangements, worked more hours per week, and were more satisfied with their employment. Time since injury was associated with enhanced psychological functioning as measured by satisfaction with living arrangements and employment, self-rated adjustment, number of hours working per week, and medical adjustment. These findings suggest that age and time since injury may work in opposing directions. Persons injured at younger ages not only have greater opportunity to deal with consequences of their injury, but may be dealing with different developmental issues in their lives. These results illustrate the outcomes of a developmental process, the phases or turning points of which are not clear.

A 20-year follow-up of the same study provides more information on a developmental process in adjusting to SCI. The most recent cohort was comprised of 112 participants with a mean age of 49.9 years and a mean of 28.7 years since injury (Krause, 1998). Overall, Krause found that outcomes related to activity levels, health, and employment were positive. Specifically, sitting tolerance increased over the 20 years, number of hospitalizations and number of days hospitalized decreased overall, years of education increased by 1.6 years over the study period, and the number of years worked at a job increased linearly. The mean number of hours worked per week increased sharply from 1974 to 1985 and then remained stable. Despite objective improvements, subjective assessments of satisfaction (i.e., social life, sex life) did not improve over the 20-year period; only employment satisfaction improved linearly. He also reports evidence to suggest that individuals who were more active and better adjusted in 1974 continued to be more active and better adjusted in 1994, highlighting the importance of individual differences and personality in adaptation. Present adjustment showed a quadratic trend with scores increasing in the 1st decade and decreasing in the 2nd decade; future adjustment demonstrated a negative linear trend over the 20 years. This series of reports suggests that adjustment following SCI is not a linear process; rather, individuals are faced with different challenges through their development.

Antonak and Livneh (1991) also approach the issue of disability adaptation from a developmental perspective in which gradual acceptance of changes to body, self, and social interactions occur. They report evidence for a hierarchy of reactions to disability using an ordering-theoretic data analysis procedure. Support for a nonlinear, multi-dimensional process was found with a sample of 118 adults who sustained disabilities an average of 8 years earlier; in addition to SCI, the impairments sustained by the sample included stroke, myocardial infarction, amputation, sensory impairment, and degenerative conditions. They used their Reactions to Impairment and Disability Inventory to assess eight emotional states: shock, anxiety, denial, depression, internalized anger, externalized hostility, acknowledgment, and adjustment. A pattern of nonlinear, empirical contingencies was found among this set of reactions in which five of the six nonadapted responses were found to be prerequisites for the two adapted responses (acknowledgment and adjustment). Anxiety, depression, internalized anger, and externalized hostility were found to be prerequisite to adaptation. However, considerable variability in the sequence of these reactions was found. These results are consistent with the observation that people sometimes regress to earlier phases or bypass phases because of their life situation or capacity to cope effectively. The experience of shock was observed to be a prerequisite of depression and internalized anger which, in turn, are prerequisites of acknowledgment and adaptation. Only denial was found to be independent of the two sets of reactions. This result is consistent with Wright's position (1983) that years may pass before a person is able to realize fully the implications of a disability. This model allows for persons to acknowledge a disability but not attain full adjustment. The statistical method used in this study is noteworthy in that it allows contingent relationships to be examined in a cross-sectional design.

Another approach to understanding adaptation is illustrated by Heinemann and Shontz' (1984, 1985) personological investigation of emotional and cognitive experiences following SCI. They studied two carefully selected persons as a means of evaluating a process model of adaptation. The goal of this representative case study was to determine the extent to which adjustment proceeds in a sequential fashion, and the extent to which adjustment follows patterns that are characteristic of the person before injury. Both persons were 24 years old and had sustained quadriplegia as the result of traumatic injury more than 2 years earlier. They were similar in socioeconomic (middle income), religious (Roman Catholic), and educational (post-baccalaureate) backgrounds. They differed in terms of gender, the extent to which they were the perpetrator (hang-gliding crash) or victim (passenger in an auto crash), and previously established coping style (emotionally expressive vs. reserved). They completed a number of nomothetic measures of intelligence, depression, disability acceptance, and to personality. Idiographic measures included Kelly's (1955) Role Repertory Technique to identify personal constructs related to disability acceptance, and a Q-sort designed to tap stages of reaction to crisis described by Fink (1967). A modification of Flanagan's (1954) Critical Incident Technique was used to obtain course-of-life landmarks before and after injury.

The two participants provided strikingly different data. One participant, Deirdre, provided data that supported a model of sequential emotional reactions and value changes, while the other participant, Craig, did not. Deirdre reported experiencing a period of depression prior to adjustment, though the sequence of stages was not in the expected order. Instead, her reactions were strongly related to external events in her family and to rehabilitation. In contrast Craig, who had attempted suicide earlier as a means, he said, of restoring control over his life, never consciously mourned his loss, but instead quickly assumed a position of doing the best he could. Congruence with preinjury coping styles was apparent in both cases, as one (Deirdre) used intellectualizing, fantasy, and obsessive patterns of thinking as mechanisms to cope with stress, and the other (Craig) avoided introspection and attempted to master his body and physical environment. Both achieved academic success despite their different pattern of adjustment, disability-related value changes, and coping styles.

Deirdre's readiness to mourn her lost abilities provides a notable contrast with Craig's tendency to focus on physical values and tackle rehabilitation tasks without attending to his emotional reactions. No single, common underlying process of adjustment was illustrated by these two cases. Instead, they illustrate two different solutions to life problems that seem similar because of the similar impairment. These results show that symbolic integration of loss was more complete in the person who experienced a sequence of reactions than in the person who did not. Emotional and behavioral reactions are then affected by who it is that experiences injury, the meaning each person attributes to the loss, the person's already established means of dealing with life disruption, and the context within which the person undergoes rehabilitation and community re-entry.

Adopting a developmental perspective that considers the life course before SCI, identity established before injury, and commitments made allows us to understand how SCI affects psychological well-being. More recently, reports have focused on effective problem-solving and coping strategies, the role of social support in enhancing adjustment, the value of caregiver roles and peer support, substance abuse as a maladaptive coping strategy, and quality of life more generally. These topics are considered next.

APPLICATIONS OF STRESS AND COPING MODELS

THE COGNITIVE-PHENOMENOLOGICAL PERSPECTIVE of Lazarus and Folkman (1984), which explains stress resulting from disability-related life changes and coping efforts to manage these changes, has been used by several clinicians to describe the experiences of persons undergoing rehabilitation. Stress and coping theory allows us to view adverse life events as experiences that tax adaptive resources, threaten well-being, and place individuals at risk for stress-related dysfunction and psychopathology.

One often-cited study applied social psychological theory to understanding the adjustment of persons with SCI. Bulman and Wortman (1977) examined the short-term adjustment of 29 persons with SCI during initial rehabilitation hospitalization. They found that persons who blamed themselves for causing their injury and who perceived the injury as unavoidable coped better with disability as rated by rehabilitation staff. All had questioned why the injury occurred, and all but one developed answers to explain why. A need for meaning was implicit in this process. While criticized for its small sample size, the use of staff-rated coping, and an outsiders' perspective of problem-selection and interpretation (Shontz, 1982), this study illuminates what may well be a universal process when misfortune occurs: Efforts to ascribe meaning to the event. This study did not find better outcomes to be associated with specific types of meaning. Instead, quite different meanings were provided by those who were rated as coping effectively.

A longer term relationship between self-blame and adjustment was reported by Nielson and MacDonald (1988). In a sample of community residents, they found results quite different from those of Bulman and Wortman (1977): self-blame was negatively associated with adjustment, sociability, pessimism, hostility, and dysphoria. Further, they found that perceiving injury as avoidable was positively related with coping and adjustment. They concluded that self-blame is maladaptive after community re-entry.

A replication and extension of these studies was conducted by Heinemann, Bulka, and Smetak (1988) with a sample of 52 community residents with quadriplegia. While similar in terms of age at injury, gender, and injury etiology to Bulman and Wortman's (1977) sample, this group completed more years of education and employment. Similarly, this group reported equivalent levels of self-blame, perceived avoidability, and present happiness, though they rated SCI as a life event in significantly more positive terms. Greater disability acceptance was associated with younger age, greater time since injury, and the absence of maladaptive coping efforts such as drinking. Like Bulman and Wortman's sample, nearly all (94%) had asked themselves why their injury occurred; in contrast, 65% of those asking the question reported no specific answer. Neither specific attributions for injury nor satisfaction with the answer were associated with greater disability acceptance. However, perceiving some good as coming from injury was positively related to disability acceptance. Support for adaptation as a developmental process is apparent in the relationship between time since injury and disability acceptance: the value changes described by Wright (1983) were more strongly endorsed with greater time since injury.

However, a study with a sample of 31 found nonsignificant results in the relationship between self-blame and coping (Sholomskas, Steil, & Plummer, 1990). No positive or negative relationship between participant attributions of self-blame and ratings of coping were detected; however, investigators did find that alcohol use prior to injury, and endorsing the belief that the accident was avoidable were related to self-blame post-injury. However, the strongest predictor of self-blame was alcohol use prior to the injury. Interestingly, blaming others for injuries was also related to poorer coping; in fact, the authors suggested that blaming others might be a stronger predictor of poorer coping than self-blame. Blaming others was significantly predicted by a belief that the other person could have avoided the accident, having a longer period of time elapse since the accident, not having used alcohol prior to the accident, and believing that the accident could have been avoided. Attributions regarding negative life events probably play differential roles in various individuals, and questions regarding what roles they play in coping with negative life-events remain.

While there is some evidence that self-blame and specific attributions for injury may be adaptive shortly after injury, they do not appear to serve this function with greater time. The passage of time appears to allow people to reframe their experience of injury and disability in ways that promote greater self-valuation. While the question "why me?" is compelling shortly after injury and some reasonably satisfactory answer appears to be important, it is the resolution of the question that allows psychological energy to be re-directed to the external world, relationships, and important goals.

The effect that individual differences in coping styles have on psychological distress and depression has also been explored to clarify the process by which adaptation occurs. Frank, Umlauf, and associates (1987) used cluster analysis, on scores from the Ways of Coping Checklist and the Millon Health Locus of Control Scale, to identify two subgroups of persons with recent SCI. One group more strongly endorsed all coping factors and relied less on internal attributions of beliefs than did the second group. The two groups also differed on measures of depression, negative life events, and general distress: the first group experienced higher (though not clinically significant) depression, experienced more negative life stress, and more negative life events in the previous year. Persons in the two groups did not differ in terms of level of injury, age, and time since injury, or in positive life stressors during the past year. While the cross-sectional nature of the study does not allow causal relationships to be identified, the authors speculate that the coping efforts of persons in the first group were less effective. They interpret their results to suggest that an external health locus of control is associated with greater distress and depression, and that external events may be important in affecting mood and attributional styles. Consistent with Wright's emphasis on value changes that allow positive self-valuation, they support the clinical practice of helping people with SCI come to value their internal resources.

The same group of investigators also examined the relationship between coping styles and psychological distress in 57 inpatients with SCI who were undergoing rehabilitation a median of 3.6 months after injury (Buckelew, Baumstark, Frank, & Hewett, 1990). In this cross-sectional study, only 26% of the sample reported high levels of distress as measured by the Symptom Checklist (SCL) (*T*-score greater than 70). When divided into three equal-sized groups defined by distress level, persons experiencing high distress also reported being more likely to use coping strategies that included self-blame, wish-fulfilling fantasy, emotional expression, and threat minimization compared to persons with moderate and low levels of distress. Groups of patients defined by SCL scores did not differ by age, time since injury, gender, level of injury, or marital status. However, self-blame was strongly correlated with distress, suggesting that this coping strategy is maladaptive. Evidence for a developmental process of adaptation was not supported by a correlation with time since injury. These results build on a related study (Frank & Elliott, 1987) in which psychological distress as measured by the SCL was related to life events independent of time since injury. They demonstrate that external events can disrupt one's well-being both for people whose injuries are recent or older. The authors note that frequent use of coping strategies is not necessarily a successful means of managing psychological distress and may instead reflect characteristic (and ineffective) efforts to deal with stress.

These authors extended their 1990 study to examine the role of coping strategies in adjustment following SCI (Hanson, Buckelew, Hewett, & O'Neal, 1993). They reported that active coping strategies (e.g., cognitive restructuring) are more positive than passive coping strategies (e.g., wish fulfilling fantasy). However, coping is a long-term process and strategies used immediately after injury do not always predict adjustment outcomes. Thus, family members and clinicians must recognize the long-term nature of coping and that coping strategies change over time as individuals with SCI face new and varying developmental challenges.

Social problem-solving abilities also play a role in adjustment to SCI. One study examined the relationships between social problem-solving abilities and psychological and physical adjustment in people with recent-onset SCI (Elliott, 1999). At admission, higher levels of depressive behaviors were associated with lower levels of disability acceptance at discharge (Elliott, 1999). Impulsive and careless problem solving and negative problem orientation were associated with lower disability acceptance at discharge, whereas rational problem-solving skills were associated with better disability acceptance at discharge. These traits had consequences for career decisional and informational needs in that depressive symptoms and lower acceptance of disability were associated with greater decisional needs at discharge. Thus, cognitive factors such as social problem-solving abilities may play important roles in disability acceptance, psychological adjustment, and subsequent coping.

It is clear that external factors, such as rehabilitation practices, can affect well-being above and beyond the effect of cognitive and affective processes. The effects of developmental factors and changes in rehabilitation practices on psychological well-being were explored in a study reported by Buckelew, Frank, Elliott, Chaney, and Hewett (1991). They compared two samples of 53 persons who sustained SCI between 1981 and 1982 or between 1984 and 1986, and who were an average of 3.6 and 1.7 years post-injury, respectively, on measures of health locus of control and psychological distress. Age and time since injury were unrelated to health beliefs and to psychological distress. However, the group with more recent injuries reported more anxiety, phobic anxiety, psychoticism, and hostility than did the first group. Shorter lengths of stay and earlier transfers to rehabilitation distinguished the groups. This study suggests that changes in rehabilitation practices that reflect recent efforts to contain health care costs may affect psychosocial outcomes. In such an economic climate, the questions of who experiences greater levels of well-being, how adaptation proceeds, and how adaptation can be supported attain even more importance.

SOCIAL SUPPORT AND ADJUSTMENT

RESEARCH AND CLINICAL interest in the effects of social support on adjustment after SCI have increased in parallel with theoretical developments in this field. Overlapping and unclear definitions of social support have limited understanding in this area of inquiry, beginning with Cobb's (1976) landmark article that described the benefits of social support. Barrera (1986) contributed to conceptual clarity by distinguishing among social embeddedness, perceived social support, and enacted support as three major categories of social support. Sarason, Shearin, Pierce, and Sarason (1987) concluded that, despite distinctions between support concepts, most measures of social support assess a sense of being accepted, loved, and involved in relationships where open communication exists.

Cohen and Wills (1985) reviewed studies which evaluated two hypothesized processes by which social support benefits health: (1) global benefits of support and (2) social support as a buffer against the impact of stressful life events. They concluded that empirical evidence supports both models. Heller, Swindle, and Dusenbury (1986) note that the way in which social ties provide health protective effects are unclear, even though many studies demonstrate a correlation between social support and physical and psychological outcomes. Broadhead and associates (1983) summarized social support and health relationships. They noted 11 characteristics of social support, including temporal, strength, consistency, and dynamics of social support. They reviewed evidence that poor social support precedes adverse psychological outcomes, is consistently related to outcomes across various groups defined by age, sex, racial, ethnic, and illness characteristics, and is dependent on life events.

The effects of social support on long-term adjustment of persons with SCI were examined by Schulz and Decker (1985) in a cross-sectional study. They studied a group of 100 middle-aged and older community residents an average of 20 years postinjury. They found a level of self-reported well-being that was only slightly lower than that of peers without disabilities. High levels of social support, satisfaction with social contacts, and perceived control over one's well-being were associated with higher levels of well-being after controlling statistically for health and income. In contrast to Bulman and Wortman's (1977) results in which self-blame and staff-rated coping were strongly correlated, Schulz and Decker found only a modest correlation between self-blame and life satisfaction. They interpret their results by emphasizing that participants appeared to attain favorable self-perceptions by selectively focusing on attributes in which they had an advantage, ascribing meaning to injury, and by defining standards of adjustment in which they could excel. This coping process illustrates how Wright's (1983) value changes, which define disability acceptance, can proceed. In Wright's terms, favorable coping was achieved by subordination of physique and employing asset values.

Rintala, Young, Hart, and associates (1992) replicated and extended the work of Schulz and Decker by selecting a more representative community sample in which women were over-sampled, and objectively measuring health status and secondary medical complications (e.g., urinary tract infections, pressure ulcers), which might affect well-being.

The sample of 140 persons was an average of 10.6 years post-injury. Using Schulz and Decker's (1985) questionnaire, they found that greater levels of social support were associated with greater life satisfaction, better self-assessed physical health and the absence of urinary tract infections. Greater satisfaction with one's social support was associated with lower levels of depression and greater life satisfaction; however, the secondary medical complications were unrelated to satisfaction with support. The association between social support and life satisfaction was about twice as strong for men as it was for women. The authors speculate about the mechanisms that underlie the correlation between physical health and social support; these mechanisms may include others influencing health maintenance activities, social support acting to reduce stress, or others providing goods or services that enhance health. Alternately, healthy persons may attract the support of others or be more likely to seek out support from others.

Further evidence for a relationship between social support and long-term adjustment was reported by Coca (1991) in a sample of 80 men who sustained injury an average of 17 years earlier and who received outpatient services at a Veterans Administration hospital. Perceived social support from family and friends was strongly associated with disability acceptance and psychological distress, such that persons perceiving greater support from family and friends reported greater disability acceptance and lower levels of psychological distress. Income and social support from friends were the best predictors of disability acceptance. Friends' support was positively correlated with coping efforts, which involved planful problem solving and seeking social support, while it was negatively correlated with self-controlling coping efforts and escape-avoidance. In addition, marital status and spousal support specifically are associated with higher perceived life satisfaction and quality of life (Holicky & Charlifue).

A study of 120 individuals with SCI investigated the patterns of social support and coping over time, and the direction of the effects of coping on social support (McColl, Lei, & Skinner, 1995). Data were collected at 1 month (time 1), 4 months (time 2), and 12 months (time 3) after rehabilitation discharge. Social support had a significant direct effect on coping at future data points, but not vice versa; both social support and coping were predictive of future social support and coping, respectively. The effects of social support on coping were not linear at three evaluation points; in fact, at time 1, social support had a positive effect on coping at time 2, but time 2 social support had a negative effect on time 3 coping. This pattern of associations suggests that high levels of social support decrease the likelihood of flexible and effective coping on the part of the individual with SCI. Types of social support also changed from informational support through the 1st month to emotional support from 4 to 12 months. Overall, the results indicate that the relationship between social support and coping is dynamic and changes as individuals with SCI move through phases of adjustment.

Another line of research explored relationships between social support, assertiveness, and psychological adjustment in which assertiveness was hypothesized to be a mediator resulting in positive or negative effects of social support (Elliott et al., 1991). Elliot and colleagues examined the hypothesis that higher levels of assertiveness in individuals with SCI would be associated with greater social support and may positively impact depression and psychological adjustment (Elliott et al.). Assertive patients reported lower levels of depression; higher levels of social integration and reassurance of self-worth were associated with lower depression scores; and higher levels of nurturance by social supports were associated with higher levels of depression. An interaction between assertiveness and guidance by social supports suggested that assertive patients were more depressed when they received high levels of guidance and less depressed when they received low levels of guidance. Similarly, assertiveness was also inversely related to guidance in examining level of impairment. Thus, individual levels of assertiveness appeared to moderate the relationships between social support and depression and adjustment.

Elliott's research team also examined problem-solving abilities in individuals with SCI. They reported that better problem-solving abilities were associated with levels of depressive symptoms and lower impairment scores, and moderated the effects of social support (Elliott, Herrick, & Witty, 1992). Effective problem solving was associated with lower levels of depression and psychosocial impairment. Effective problem solving was also associated with lower levels of impairment when guidance from social supports was low; however, it was associated with less impairment when reliable alliance (material support) was high. If health care professionals are able to address problem-solving abilities in individuals with SCI, it may promote more effective use of social supports. These findings have important implications for professionals working with people with SCI; the relationships between social support and adjustment and depression are complex. Individual differences mediate the effects of social support and subsequent adjustment and coping.

The relationship between social support and depression was investigated further by Elliott, Herrick, Witty, Godshall, and Spruell (1992). Their sample of 182 patients was interviewed an average of 8 years after injury. People who reported lower levels of depressive symptomatology also reported stronger support in the form of relationships that reassured self-worth and a sense of social integration. Time since injury was related modestly to depression such that people with more recent injuries tended to report higher levels of depression. Time since injury was unrelated to any of the social-support measures. Although a longitudinal design is needed to clarify causal relationships, these results suggest that people who are able to solicit social support may experience better mental health.

One context in which some people socialize and experience social support involves drinking alcohol. The relationship between alcohol and other drug use and SCI is the focus of the next section.

SUBSTANCE ABUSE AND SPINAL CORD INJURY

PROBLEMS RESULTING FROM alcohol and other drug abuse provide another example of how issues in the mainstream of health psychology have been extended to persons with spinal injuries. The prevalence of substance abuse problems in persons who incur traumatic SCI has emerged as an important issue for psychologists in rehabilitation settings. Alcohol and other drug abuse can contribute to onset of disability when a person is intoxicated, limit rehabilitation gains by impairing learning, and hamper rehabilitation outcomes by contributing to increased morbidity and mortality. This section describes our knowledge about (a) the prevalence of alcohol and other drug use by persons with SCI, (b) the rate at which treatment for substance use problems is received, (c) the effects of substance use on rehabilitation, and (d) the effects of alcohol and other drug use on rehabilitation outcome.

PREVALENCE OF ALCOHOL AND OTHER DRUG USE

INTOXICATION AS A frequent contributor to SCI onset has been recognized by several investigators. O'Donnell, Cooper, Gessner, Shehan, and Ashley (1981–2) reported a 68% rate of self-reported use at SCI onset, with 68% resuming drinking during hospitalization. Depending on the site and sample, the rate of intoxication for persons incurring traumatic injury has been estimated to vary between 17% and 49% (Frisbie & Tun, 1984; Fullerton, Harvey, Klein, & Howell, 1981; Galbraith, Murray, Patel, & Knitt-Jones, 1976; Gale, Dikmen, Wyler, Temkin, & McClean, 1983; Heinemann, Goranson, Ginsburg, & Schnoll, 1989).

One recent study used toxicology screens with 87 consecutively admitted rehabilitation patients with acute spinal cord injuries and found that 47% of patients were intoxicated at the time of injury, while 53% had positive toxicology screens (McKinley, Kolakowsky, & Kreutzer, 1999). Young, unmarried males had the highest likelihood of positive toxicology screens. Patients incurring violent SCI were more likely to have positive screens than patients involved in non-violent SCI, suggesting an increased risk for violence-related injuries when substances were involved. Intoxication resulting in impaired judgment appears to be responsible for increased risk-taking that results in many injuries.

Several studies have reported the prevalence of alcohol use and abuse following initial care for traumatic disability. Johnson (1985) reported a rate of moderate and heavy drinking by vocational rehabilitation and independent living center clients with SCI that was nearly twice the rate reported in the general population (46% vs. 25%), while the rate of alcoholic symptoms has been observed to vary from 49% of persons with recent SCI (Heinemann, Donohue, Keen, & Schnoll, 1988) to 62% of vocational rehabilitation facility clients (Rasmussen & DeBoer, 1980). However, age-related differences in drinking problems were highlighted in a study of primarily older veterans with SCI (Kirubakaran, Kumar, Powell, Tyler, & Armatas, 1986). These investigators found that alcohol and drug use was less than the rate reported in the National Institute on Drug Abuse's National Household Survey (NIDA, 1988). These findings support the conclusion that age-related differences in the rate of alcohol and other drug abuse in the able-bodied population also exist in persons with SCI.

The prevalence of intoxication at time of injury onset was examined in a sample of 88 cases at admission to a regional SCI rehabilitation center (Heinemann, Schnoll, Brandt, Maltz, & Keen, 1988). Serum ethanol greater than 50 mg/dl was observed in 40% of the cases, followed by urine analysis evidence of cocaine (14%), cannabinoids (8%), benzodiazepines (5%), and opiates (4%). Overall, 35% of the sample had evidence of substances with abuse potential in their urine. A total of 62% had either serum ethanol greater than 50 mg/dl or a positive urine analysis. These results cannot be regarded as compelling evidence of chemical dependence since false-positive results may reflect occasional or low-dose use of substances with abuse potential, which was detected by toxicology screens.

Chronicity of substance use was addressed by assessing histories of 103 persons with recent SCI (Heinemann, Donohue, Keen, & Schnoll, 1988), including those described above for whom toxicology screens were obtained. Inclusion criteria included age between 13 and 65 years at injury; absence of cognitive impairment, which would limit self-report; injury within the past year; and English-speaking. The mean age of the sample was 28 years; 75% were men. Lifetime exposure to and recent use of several substances with abuse potential were greater in this sample than for a like-age national sample. Compared with a national sample collected by the National Institute on Drug Abuse (1988), the SCI sample of 18 to 25 year olds reported significantly greater exposure to amphetamines, marijuana, cocaine, and hallucinogens. This age group also reported recent use of alcohol, amphetamines, marijuana, cocaine, and hallucinogens which was significantly greater than for a like-aged national sample. The SCI group of 26 years of age and older reported significantly greater exposure to narcotic analgesics and tranquilizers than did the national sample. They also reported recent use of tobacco, alcohol, amphetamines, and marijuana which was at least ten percentage points greater than the national sample. Finally, greater proportions of the SCI sample in the 18 to 25 year old and the 26-year and older groups reported greater recent use of nine of ten substance categories compared to the national sample. Within the SCI sample, young adults (18 to 25 year olds) reported greater recent use of marijuana before injury and greater cocaine exposure than did the 26 years of age and older group. However, the 26 years of age and older group reported greater tobacco exposure. Intoxication at time of injury was an important marker for prior substance use, as the 39% who reported being intoxicated at injury also reported greater exposure to tobacco, amphetamines, marijuana, hallucinogens, tranquilizers, and sedatives, and recent use of tobacco, alcohol, amphetamines, cocaine, and hallucinogens.

These results suggest that persons with SCI are more likely to use and abuse alcohol and other drugs than are persons in the general population. However, before classifying persons that incur SCI as probable drug abusers and further enhance their stigma, several methodological considerations must be considered when interpreting these comparisons. Although the methodologies in the SCI samples and the National Household Survey (NHS) are essentially the same, minor differences in definitions of recent use require mention. For instance, NIDA's recent use criterion of one or more times during the past month vs. the NHS's criterion of three or more times during the past 6 months may not assess substance use in a comparable manner. Despite the complication in interpreting the results, these findings highlight a previously undocumented fact: substance use and abuse occurs frequently, may complicate the rehabilitation process, and limit long-term outcomes and the capacity for independent living.

The first epidemiological study of substance abuse problems in individuals with disabilities using a nonreferred national sample found distinct patterns of substance use (Gilson, Chilcoat, & Stapleton, 1996). Individuals with disabilities were defined as those who responded that they were unable to work due to a disability. Thus, only unemployed individuals with a disability were included. Disability was defined broadly and included those with substance abuse problems. Despite the limitation of not defining specific disabilities, the authors assert that the study provides a useful marker for the extent of substance abuse in individuals who self-identify as having a disability. The National Household Survey on Drug Abuse found that 18 to 24 year olds with disabilities were more likely to report heroin or crack cocaine use than non-disabled individuals, disabled individuals from 24 to 35 years were more likely to report use of marijuana than nondisabled individuals, and those over 35 years were more likely to report using non-medically prescribed sedatives and tranquilizers than nondisabled individuals (Gilson et al., 1996). Interestingly, there were no significant differences in odds of alcohol use among any of the age groups. One of the conclusions of this study was that persons with severe disabilities at an early age have a higher likelihood of being associated with high-risk drug use, thereby identifying a point of potential intervention.

Moore and Li (1998) examined patterns of illicit drug use in a sample of 1,876 individuals receiving vocational rehabilitation services. Prevalence of most illicit and nonmedical drugs was higher in the disability sample than in the general population. For example, the rates of crack cocaine use both in the past month and year were more than three times the rate of use in the general population. Factors associated with substance use included: being younger, male gender, low income, family and/or friends using illicit drugs, greater feelings of hostility and risk-taking, lower self-esteem, and believing that having a disability entitles one to use substances.

Intoxication at SCI onset appears to be a marker of pre-injury substance use, and thus it is important to screen for substance abuse in persons who incur traumatic injury. Implications for clinicians are apparent since the lifetime exposure to and recent use of substances reported by this sample indicate that many persons with SCI are at risk for substance abuse. This risk is underscored by studies that report a relationship between previous substance use and subsequent use of other drugs (Dembo, Blount, Schmeidler, & Burgos, 1985). Substance use is not necessarily substance abuse or dependence. Nor does use necessarily result in specific problems. However, it is important to understand the context, expectancies, and motives for use. For example, substance use may be a means of re-establishing social relationships, of managing stress, or an escalating pattern of addiction. Clinicians should take note of substance use and observe if it is related to other problems. These results highlight the importance of assessing alcohol and drug-abuse-related problems so that a potential dual disability is identified and treated in a timely fashion.

Other investigators have examined the possibility that intoxication at injury may be related to individual differences such as sensation seeking. Mawson, Jacobs, Winchester, and Biundo (1988) reported that persons who scored high on a measure of sensation seeking were younger and more likely to be using substances at the time of injury. In contrast, Rohe and Basford (1990) found that only the MacAndrew Alcoholism Scale of the Minnesota Multiphasic Personality Inventory scale distinguished patients with positive blood alcohol concentrations from patients with negative blood alcohol concentrations and a normative sample. Further research is needed to clarify this issue.

TREATMENT FOR SUBSTANCE USE PROBLEMS

THE RATE OF self-reported alcohol problems, perceived need for treatment, and receipt of treatment by persons with recent SCI has also been the focus of research (Heinemann, Doll, & Schnoll, 1989). Participants reported alcohol use information across three time periods: 6 months before injury, the first 6 months after injury, and the next 12 months after injury. Drinking on three or more occasions was reported by 93% of the participants at one or more of the assessment periods; 71% reported experiencing one or more drinking problems. Of the entire sample, only 15% reported perceiving a need for treatment of alcohol abuse, and 11% actually received treatment. Post-injury alcohol abuse in persons who did not experience pre-injury abuse appears to occur infrequently, as 65% reported drinking problems before injury while only 6% reported drinking problems for the first time after injury. Longer-term follow-up is needed to verify this impression since participants were followed for only 18 months. Even though the incidence of self-recognized alcohol problems may be low, the total number of persons affected by alcohol problems may be substantial. Routine assessment of substance abuse and provision of treatment services to persons with traumatic SCI are indicated to prevent a potential dual disability.

There is also an increasing emphasis on preventing substance abuse problems in rehabilitation populations. There are a growing number of examples signifying this change. First, interdisciplinary models for rehabilitation and substance abuse prevention have been created under grants from the National Institute on Disability and Rehabilitation Research (NIDRR) and the J.M. Foundation at the Rehabilitation Institute of Chicago (RIC). RIC has developed a model approach for substance-abuse prevention as an essential aspect of rehabilitation. The model accomplishes this by recognizing the potential role of all rehabilitation professionals; thus, it is interdisciplinary in its structure and approach. Second, the Rehabilitation Services Administration (RSA) of the Department of Education awarded a contract to provide training to vocational rehabilitation counselors on substance abuse issues, thereby addressing the needs of vocational rehabilitation clients with comorbid conditions. Third, the Institute on Alcohol, Drugs, and Disability brought together leaders in these fields to create action plans for implementing policies to improve access to substance abuse prevention services for individuals with disabilities (Cherry, 1991). Lastly, the second National Conference on Substance Abuse and Coexisting Disabilities, held in 1992, convened leaders in the fields of substance abuse treatment, policy, research, and consumer advocacy to progress toward a consensus on issues that could potentially improve recovery and vocational services for individuals with multiple disabilities (Substance Abuse

Resources and Disability Issues [SARDI], 1992). The conference participants made several recommendations, including (a) ensuring that the disability community receive an equitable share of available resources, (b) establishing a vision of employment as integral to recovery and as an outcome goal, (c) providing education to consumers, service providers, employers and others that reduces stigma and discrimination, (d) implementing integrated service delivery systems that include vocational rehabilitation and substance-abuse treatment services, and (e) ensuring the integration of substance abuse, mental health, and vocational rehabilitation services.

EFFECTS OF ALCOHOL AND OTHER DRUG USE ON THE REHABILITATION PROCESS

THE RELATIONSHIP BETWEEN substance use and lifestyle activities after SCI was the focus of a study completed by Heinemann, Goranson, Ginsburg, and Schnoll (1989). A sample with recent injuries described their activity patterns during their inpatient rehabilitation stay using the Activity Pattern Indicators timeline format during a structured interview. More drinking before injury and more family drinking problems predicted a greater number of drinking problems after injury. In turn, those who reported more drinking problems reported spending less time in quiet activities such as sleeping and resting during rehabilitation, but spent more time in quiet recreation activities such as watching television and reading. Of greatest concern, persons who drank more before injury spent less time in productive activities such as rehabilitation therapies. These relationships are of concern because the often fast pace and increasingly short rehabilitation stays may limit rehabilitation outcomes.

Readiness-to-change concepts have been adopted by rehabilitation researchers to improve substance abuse treatment design and implementation for individuals with SCI. Alcohol use and readiness-to-change patterns were assessed in 58 individuals with recent SCI onset (Bombardier & Rimmele, 1998). Investigators found that 35% of the sample were alcohol dependent and 50% were at risk for developing alcohol dependence. Approximately 45% of the sample was in the contemplation phase of changing their drinking behavior and 34% were in the action phase, indicating they were ready for treatment. A substantial number of individuals with recent onset SCI were at least considering changing their drinking behaviors, suggesting that assessing stages of change during inpatient rehabilitation hospitalization might be an opportune time to implement change in alcohol use behaviors.

Although further study is needed to determine the consequences of drinking on long-term rehabilitation outcome, these results suggest that heavy pre-injury drinking may be associated with a constellation of psychological factors which impact adversely on rehabilitation. In addition, assessing an individual's readiness to change their substance use behaviors, especially early in the rehabilitation process, may improve outcomes for individuals with SCI.

EFFECTS OF SUBSTANCE USE ON REHABILITATION OUTCOME

THE WAYS IN which changes in employment, substance use, depression, and disability acceptance may be related were studied in a sample of community residents following SCI (Heinemann, Kiley, Schnoll, & Yarkony, 1989). Beck's Depression Inventory and Linkowski's Acceptance of Disability Scale were completed, and Hollingshead and Redlich's Social Position Index (SPI; 1958) was used to code social status. Pre- to post-SCI employment status was unchanged in 21%; 16% were employed and had increased their job status; 23% became employed; 18% became unemployed; and 22% remained unemployed. Use of diazepam (Valium), alcohol, marijuana, and cocaine was lower among employed individuals. Persons who were unemployed at injury and became employed reported greater disability acceptance, as did persons who increased in SPI score between injury and interview. Finally, persons who used prescription medications either as prescribed or in a nonprescribed manner were more depressed and less accepting of their disability than were persons who did not use prescription medications.

Heinemann and Hawkins (1995; Hawkins & Heinemann, 1998) examined the relationship between medical complications, including pressure ulcers and urinary tract infections (UTIs), and substance abuse in a series of studies based on a sample of 71 inpatient subjects. Their 1995 study examined outcomes related to medical complications across three time intervals: 6 months prior to injury (time 1), 6 months following injury (time 2), and 7–18 months after injury (time 3). They found that individuals reporting alcohol use from time 1 to time 2 decreased from 90% to 58%, then increased to 66% by time 3. Moderate and heavy drinkers were the most likely to develop UTIs at time 1 (Heinemann & Hawkins). However, post-injury abstainers with a history of problem drinking had the highest likelihood of developing pressure sores and UTIs through the study period. Illicit drug use and prescription medication misuse post-injury were related to medical complications. Their 1998 study focused on medical complications resulting in hospital stays and the relationship of alcohol and illicit substance use to hospitalization (Hawkins & Heinemann). Individuals with long histories of alcohol abuse prior to injury onset but abstained after injury were at an increased risk for developing UTIs 7 to 12 months post-injury and for incurring longer inpatient lengths of stay; these results suggest that newly abstinent patients may not have acquired sufficient self-care and coping mechanisms. Illicit substance use 12 to 18 months post-injury was related to an increased incidence of pressure ulcers 19 to 30 months following SCI onset. Older individuals were at greater risk for pressure ulcers 1–6 and 19–30 months after SCI; younger individuals were at greater risk 12 months after injury; level and completeness of SCI were risk factors for pressure ulcers only during the 1st year after injury. It may be important to distinguish subtypes of drinkers in order to understand the complex relationship between alcohol and drug use and medical complications in SCI patients. Adherence to self-care regimes becomes critical following SCI. The critical issues appear to be the individual's willingness and ability to assume responsibility for self-care, and factors such as substance abuse that create barriers to self-care.

A study by Elliott and colleagues examined medical and psychological adjustment in individuals with SCI and alcohol abuse problems (Elliott, Kurylo, Chen, & Hicken, 2002). Alcohol abuse was significantly associated with medical complications, specifically pressure sore occurrence, in individuals with SCI. Their results are consistent with findings reported by Hawkins and Heinemann (1998), indicating a relationship between alcohol abuse and medical complications following SCI. However, Elliott and colleagues did not find a relationship between alcohol abuse and depression or disability acceptance immediately after injury for SCI patients. The psychological effects of SCI on individuals abusing substances may become more apparent during community reintegration.

These results reveal how long-term psychological and medical rehabilitation outcomes can be affected by substance use, even when sanctioned medically. The reasons underlying prescription use, whether for management of spasticity, chronic pain, or other problems, should be examined psychologically. These are issues that rehabilitation and health psychologists can address as members of a multidisciplinary team.

IMPLICATIONS FOR CLINICAL INTERVENTIONS

REHABILITATION AND HEALTH psychologists are coming to realize that the expectation that persons with SCI will either experience predictable emotional reactions in a specific sequence or develop clinical depression is unsupported by the literature and potentially harmful (Frank, Elliott, Corcoran, & Wonderlich, 1987). Suicide is a leading cause of death in individuals with SCI, and is especially a problem within the first 5 years of injury (DeVivo, Black, & Stover, 1993). Even though the rate of suicide may be two to six times greater in persons with SCI than in their able-bodied peers (Charlifue & Gerhart, 1991), specific characteristics appear to place people at risk. These characteristics include pre- and post-injury despondency; a sense of shame, apathy and hopelessness; family disruption before injury; alcohol abuse; active involvement in SCI etiology; and antisocial behavior. Based on a review of case histories, Judd and Brown (1992) add to this list schizoid, depressive, and narcissistic personality characteristics; post-injury depression; and important others viewing death as a preferred option to living with SCI. Depression, particularly severe depression where suicide is considered, may be an understandable but maladaptive reaction to crisis. The psychological structure and life experiences of some individuals may well place them at risk for negative reactions. Understanding these personal characteristics and the meaning individuals ascribe to the experience of injury is necessary before an intervention is made. The importance of this approach is illustrated by the observation that rehabilitation staff frequently overestimate the level of depression experienced by patients (Cushman & Dijkers (1990).

This appreciation for individual differences in adaptation following SCI is reflected in Hammell's statement (1992) that

> the rehabilitation team will need to become more flexible in recognizing the heterogeneity of the life values of the individual. . . . The lifelong process of adjustment to disability and to interacting with society and the environment is not complete at discharge from an inpatient facility. Rather, this is when true adjustment and adaptation begins. (p. 324)

Intervention strategies that reflect a sensitivity to individuals' experience of coping with crisis are described by Livneh (1986). He proposes that the timing of psychotherapeutic strategies—supportive, insight-oriented, cognitive, and behavioral—consider the experience and needs of clients.

In addition to psychological and social needs, substance abuse issues are often important during rehabilitation. Unfortunately, these issues have often been overlooked in rehabilitation settings. This oversight results from staff who do not know how to recognize substance abuse problems and consequently are unlikely to intervene in a timely and effective manner, and from rehabilitation programs which have not recognized substance abuse treatment as part of their mission. However, it is clear that early identification of persons with SCI who abuse or are addicted to substances should minimize the incidence of secondary complications, decrease the cost of rehabilitation, and improve rehabilitation outcome. Specific suggestions regarding assessment and management of substance abuse also emerge from this literature review. Assessment of alcohol use and alcoholism should be a routine part of inpatient screenings in acute care and rehabilitation programs for persons incurring SCI. Responsibility for this screening could be assumed by a variety of team members, though rehabilitation and health psychologists are in a unique position to appreciate the interplay of medical, functional, psychological, and social forces in a developmental context. Continuing education to recognize alcohol abuse may be required in order to allow these professionals to provide this assessment. Professionals involved with alcoholism and other drug abuse treatment program can be consulted to acquire this knowledge. Relationships with substance abuse treatment providers are also necessary in order to address problems before a dual disability is established. Establishing these links is likely to require education for substance abuse treatment counselors about the special needs of persons with SCI. Not only are disability-related issues such as architectural accessibility and functional abilities important to address, but so are attitudes toward persons with disabling conditions that may limit program access. In larger communities, chemical dependence treatment programs designed specifically for persons with physical disabilities are another treatment alternative (Anderson, 1980–1; Lowenthal & Anderson, 1980–1; Sweeney & Foote, 1982).

FUNDING AND POLICY ISSUES

HEALTH CARE FUNDING is an important issue for people with long-term disabilities such as SCI. Issues related to private insurance, Medicaid, managed care, and access to health care have an impact on many of the topics covered in this chapter, from adjustment and coping to interventions. One example of research on this topic was reported by Shigaki and associates. They focused on individuals with disabilities in central Missouri in order to assess their access to health care under a Medicaid fee-for-service reimbursement model (Shigaki, Hagglund, Clark, & Conforti, 2002). Over 85% of individuals with SCI in the sample reported difficulty accessing services, with dental care, personal care services, medical supplies, eyeglasses, durable medical equipment, physical therapy, specialist care, occupational therapy, in-home therapy, speech therapy, care for minor health problems, and prescriptions being noted as problem areas in order of decreasing difficulty. In addition to physical health services, psychological services were difficult to access for over 25% of the sample that believed these services were needed. Given the breadth of psychological issues faced by individuals with SCI, limited access to mental health services creates major problems. The authors found an association between poorer health status and difficulty accessing services in Missouri; the most frequently reported reason for not having access to services was providers not accepting

Medicaid or Medicaid not paying for specific services. This study illustrates how individuals with disabilities, including SCI, are faced with numerous health access problems that may exacerbate physical and psychological problems.

Another struggle that confronts many individuals with SCI is choosing which health care option best serves their needs. There is a growing body of research investigating how well managed care—HMOs or Medicaid—meets the needs of people with SCI. A study investigating differences between individuals with SCI enrolled in a managed care program in Massachusetts found few differences (Meyers, Bisbee, & Winter, 1999). The authors concluded that prepayment managed care programs may not be harmful to providing satisfactory care; however, the study was based on a single managed care program tailored for people with disabilities and was cross-sectional in its design, limiting its generalizability. Studies such as these highlight the increasing need to adequately finance health care for people with disabilities.

An evolving perspective on disability and the growing need to address the needs of people with disabilities is being addressed on a national level. NIDRR published a Long Range Plan for research outlining goals to integrate disability research into national economic and health care policy. NIDRR has described a New Paradigm that is holistic in its approach to understanding the needs of people with disabilities. Much like the influential perspective of seminal rehabilitation psychologists (e.g., Wright, 1983), it focuses on the transactional nature of persons and their environments as a framework for conducting research, influencing policy, and delivering services and supports for people with disabilities (National Center for the Dissemination of Disability Research, 2003). The Plan addresses a range of diverse objectives, including (a) knowledge and information needs that enable people with disabilities to achieve greater self-direction, independence, inclusion, and functional competence; (b) information needs of providers for new techniques and technologies that will enable them to assist in rehabilitation; (c) researchers' needs to advance the body of scientific knowledge; (d) societal needs for strategies to facilitate the contributions of all citizens; and (e) translational research needs from basic to applied research. Congressional support for legislation such as the Rehabilitation Act and funding for disability and rehabilitation research through agencies such as NIDRR help assure that these objectives can be achieved.

Several private organizations also recognize the urgent need to understand better the health care needs of persons with SCI. Several SCI-specific organizations advocate for improved health services, including the Paralyzed Veterans of America (http://www.pva.org/) and its research affiliate, the Spinal Cord Research Foundation (http://www.pva.org/res/scrf/scrf.htm), the Eastern Paralyzed Veterans of America (http://

www.unitedspinal.org/), and the National Spinal Cord Injury Association (http://users.erols.com/nscia/index.html). Federal government efforts to improve the quality of life of persons with disabilities is coordinated by the Interagency Committee on Disability Research. This committee was authorized by the Rehabilitation Act of 1973, as amended, and is mandated "to promote coordination and cooperation among Federal departments and agencies conducting rehabilitation research programs." The committee provides valuable links to various disability and health policy sites (http://www.icdr.us/links.htmlp). Its subcommittees focus on disability statistics, medical rehabilitation, the New Freedom Initiative, technology, and technology transfer. The World Institute on Disability (http://www.wid.org/) is a nonprofit research, training, and public policy center promoting the civil rights and full societal inclusion of people with disabilities. The Disability Research Institute (DRI) at the University of Illinois at Urbana–Champaign (http://www.als. uiuc.edu/dri/) is funded by the Social Security Administration and serves as SSA's disability research partner. Its research and education activities seek to address the needs of the more than 8 million Supplemental Security Income and Disability Income applicants and recipients. The DRI's activities focus on research, information dissemination, training and education, and facilitation of data usage. Finally, NIDRR sponsored a Rehabilitation Research and Training Center on Managed Health Care and Disability at National Rehabilitation Hospital (http://www.ilru.org/ mgdcare/rtcinfo.html) that addresses health care access and outcome issues for persons with disabilities.

SUMMARY

THE PROCESS BY which people make sense of a major life disruption, such as SCI, emerges as a critical concern for psychologists working in rehabilitation settings. This issue was described originally in terms of a series of stages of emotional reactions. Theorists and clinicians differed in how they described the order and rigidity of this process. More recently, a stress and coping model has been applied, and the importance of social support in achieving successful outcomes has been studied. Making sense of injury is an early task in rehabilitation. "Why did this happen to me?" is a question many people ask themselves during and shortly after rehabilitation. Finding an answer appears to be important, though the particular attribution made does not appear to be critical. In dealing with disability, it is helpful to regard the adaptive task as involving not just the specific functional and behavioral limitations resulting from impairment, but rather the full array of life options, some of which may seem to be abridged by disability. No best route to adaptation is evident in our current understanding of this process. In fact, respect for and sensitivity to individual differences has emerged as a key principle in helping people make sense of their experience. Barriers to long-term adjustment, such as handicapping attitudes, employment biases, lack of social support, and alcohol and other drug abuse, have been identified. Research investigating means of enhancing the process by which favorable long-term adjustment is achieved is needed in order to assist this population effectively.

REFERENCES

Anderson, P. (1980–1). Alcoholism and the spinal cord disabled: A model program. *Alcohol Health and Research World, 5,* 37–41.

Anderson, T. P. (1982). Quality of life of the individual with a disability. *Archives of Physical Medicine and Rehabilitation, 63,* 65.

Antonak, R. F., & Livneh, H. (1991). A hierarchy of reactions to disability. *International Journal of Rehabilitation Research, 14,* 13–24.

Barrera, M. (1986). Distinctions between social support concepts, measures and models. *American Journal of Community Psychology, 14,* 413–445.

Bombardier, C., & Rimmele, C. (1998). Alcohol use and readiness to change after spinal cord injury. *Archives of Physical Medicine & Rehabilitation, 79,* 1110–1115.

Broadhead, W. E., Kaplan, B. H., James, S. A., Wagner, E. H., Schoenbach, V. J., Grimson, R., et al. (1983). The epidemiologic evidence for a relationship between social support and health. *American Journal of Epidemiology, 117,* 521–537.

Brown, D. J. (1992). Spinal cord injuries: The last decade and the next. *Paraplegia, 30,* 77–82.

Buckelew, S. P., Baumstark, K. E., Frank, R. G., & Hewett, J. E. (1990). Adjustment following spinal cord injury. *Rehabilitation Psychology, 35,* 101–109.

Buckelew, S. P., Frank, R. G., Elliott, T. R., Chaney, M. A., & Hewett, J. (1991). Adjustment to spinal cord injury: Stage theory revisited. *Paraplegia, 29,* 125–130.

Buckelew, S. P., Hanson, S., & Frank, R. G. (1991). Psychological factors and adjustment to spinal cord injury. *NeuroRehabilitation, 4,* 36–45.

Bulman, R., & Wortman, C. (1977). Attributions of blame and coping in the "real world:" Severe accident victims react to their lot. *Journal of Personality and Social Psychology, 35,* 351–363.

Charlifue, S. W., & Gerhart, K. A. (1991). Behavioral and demographic predictors of suicide after traumatic spinal cord injury. *Archives of Physical Medicine and Rehabilitation, 72,* 488–492.

Cherry, L. (1991). *Summary report, alcohol, drugs, disability*. National Policy and Leadership Development Symposium, Institute on Alcohol, Drugs, and Disability, San Mateo, CA.

Cobb, S. (1976). Social support as a moderator of life stress. *Psychosomatic Medicine, 38*, 300–314.

Coca, B. (1991). *Coping, social support and acceptance of disability among persons with SCI*. Paper presented at the 99th annual convention of the American Psychological Association, San Francisco, CA.

Cohen, S., & Wills, T. A. (1985). Stress, social support, and the buffering hypothesis. *Psychological Bulletin, 98*, 310–357.

Crewe, N. (1980). Quality of life: The ultimate goal in rehabilitation. *Minerva Medica, 63*, 586–589.

Cushman, L. A., & Dijkers, M. P. (1990). Depressed mood in spinal cord injured patients: Staff perceptions and patient realities. *Archives of Physical Medicine and Rehabilitation, 71*, 191–196.

Dembo, R., Blount, W., Schmeidler, J., & Burgos, W. (1985). Methodological and substantive issues involved in using the concept of risk in research into the etiology of drug use among adolescents. *Journal of Drug Issues, 4*, 537–553.

Dembo, T. (1969). Rehabilitation psychology and its immediate future: A problem of utilization of psychological knowledge. *Rehabilitation Psychology (Psychological Aspects of Disability), 16*, 63–72.

Dembo, T., Leviton, G., & Wright, B. A. (1956). Adjustment to misfortune: A problem in social-psychological rehabilitation. *Artificial Limbs, 3*, 4–62.

DeVivo, M. J., & Richards, J. S. (1992). Community reintegration and quality of life following spinal cord injury. *Paraplegia, 30*, 108–112.

DeVivo, M. J., Stover, S. L., & Black, K. J. (1992). Prognostic factors for 12-year survival after spinal cord injury. *Archives of Physical Medicine and Rehabilitation, 73*, 156–162.

DeVivo, M. J., Black, K. J., & Stover, S. L. (1993). Causes of death during the first 12 years after spinal cord injury. *Archives of Physical Medicine and Rehabilitation, 74*, 248–254.

Dinardo, G. (1971). Psychological adjustment to spinal cord injury (Doctoral dissertation, University of Houston, 1971). *Dissertation Abstracts International, 32*, 4206B–4207B.

Duggan, C. H., & Dijkers, M. (2001). Quality of life after spinal cord injury: A qualitative study. *Rehabilitation Psychology, 46*, 3–27.

Dunn, M. (1975). Psychological intervention in a spinal cord injury center: An introduction. *Rehabilitation Psychology, 22*, 165–178.

Elliott, T. R. (1999). Social problem-solving abilities and adjustment to recent-onset spinal cord injury. *Rehabilitation Psychology, 44*, 315–332.

Elliott, T. R., Herrick, S. M., Patti, A. M., Witty, T. E., Godshall, F., & Spruell, M. (1991). Assertiveness, social support, and psychological adjustment following spinal cord injury. *Behaviour Research & Therapy, 29*, 485–493.

Elliott, T. R., Herrick, S. M., & Witty, T. E. (1992). Problem-solving appraisal and the effects of social support among college students and persons with physical disabilities. *Journal of Counseling Psychology, 39,* 219–226.

Elliott, T. R., Herrick, S. M., Witty, T. E., Godshall, F., & Spruell, M. (1992). Social support and depression following spinal cord injury. *Rehabilitation Psychology, 37,* 37–48.

Elliott, T. R., Kurylo, M., Chen, Y., & Hicken, B. (2002). Alcohol abuse history and adjustment following spinal cord injury. *Rehabilitation Psychology, 47,* 278–290.

Fink, S. (1967). Crisis and motivation: A theoretical model. *Archives of Physical Medicine and Rehabilitation, 48,* 592–597.

Flanagan, J. (1954). The critical incident technique. *Psychological Bulletin, 51,* 327–358.

Frank, R. G., & Elliott, T. R. (1987). Life stress and psychologic adjustment following spinal cord injury. *Archives of Physical Medicine and Rehabilitation, 68,* 344–347.

Frank, R. G., Elliott, T. R., Corcoran, J. R., & Wonderlich, S. A. (1987). Depression after spinal cord injury: Is it necessary? *Clinical Psychology Review, 7,* 611–630.

Frank, R. G., Umlauf, R. L., Wonderlich, S. A., Askanazi, G. S., Buckelew, S. P., & Elliott, T. R. (1987). Differences in coping styles among persons with spinal cord injury: A cluster-analytic approach. *Journal of Consulting and Clinical Psychology, 55,* 727–731.

French, J. K., & Phillips, J. A. (1991). Shattered images: Recovery for the SCI client. *Rehabilitation Nursing, 16,* 134–136.

Frisbie, J. H., & Tun, C. G. (1984). Drinking and spinal cord injury. *Journal of the American Paraplegia Society, 7,* 71–73.

Fullerton, D. T., Harvey, R. F., Klein, M. H., & Howell, T. (1981). Psychiatric disorders in patients with spinal cord injuries. *Archives of General Psychiatry, 38,* 1369–1371.

Galbraith, S., Murray, W. R., Patel, A. R., & Knitt-Jones, R. (1976). The relationship between alcohol and head injury and its effects on the conscious level. *British Journal of Surgery, 63,* 128–130.

Gale, J. L., Dikmen, S., Wyler, A., Temkin, N., & McClean, A. (1983). Head injury in the Pacific Northwest. *Neurosurgery, 12,* 487–491.

Gilson, S. F., Chilcoat H., & Stapleton, J. M. (1996). Illicit drug use by persons with disabilities: Insights from the National Household Survey on Drug Abuse. *American Journal of Public Health, 86,* 1613–1615.

Gunther, M. (1969). Emotional aspects. In D. Ruge (Ed.), *Spinal cord injuries* (pp. 93–108). Springfield, IL: Thomas.

Hammell, K. R. W. (1992). Psychological and sociological theories concerning adjustment to traumatic spinal cord injury: The implications for rehabilitation. *Paraplegia, 30,* 317–326.

Hanson, D., Buckelew, S. P., Hewett, J., & O'Neal, G. (1993). The relationship between coping and adjustment after spinal cord injury: A 5-year follow-up study. *Rehabilitation Psychology, 38,* 41–52.

Hawkins, D., & Heinemann, A. (1998). Substance abuse and medical complications following spinal cord injury. *Rehabilitation Psychology, 43,* 219–231.

Heinemann, A. W., Bulka, M., & Smetak, S. (1988). Attributions and disability acceptance following traumatic injury: A replication and extension. *Rehabilitation Psychology, 33,* 195–206.

Heinemann, A. W., Doll, M., & Schnoll, S. (1989). Treatment of alcohol abuse in persons with recent spinal cord injuries. *Alcohol Health and Research World, 13,* 110–117.

Heinemann, A. W., Donohue, R., Keen, M., & Schnoll, S. (1988). Alcohol use by persons with recent spinal cord injuries. *Archives of Physical Medicine and Rehabilitation, 69,* 619–624.

Heinemann, A. W., Goranson, N., Ginsburg, K., & Schnoll, S. (1989). Alcohol use and activity patterns following spinal cord injury. *Rehabilitation Psychology, 34,* 191–206.

Heinemann, A., & Hawkins, D. (1995). Substance abuse and medical complications following spinal cord injury. *Rehabilitation Psychology, 40,* 125–140.

Heinemann, A. W., Kiley, D., Schnoll, S., & Yarkony, G. (1989, November). *Effects of substance use on vocational outcome following spinal cord injury.* American Congress of Rehabilitation Medicine, San Antonio, Texas.

Heinemann, A. W., Schnoll, S., Brandt, M., Maltz, R., & Keen, M. (1988). Toxicology screening in acute spinal cord injury. *Alcoholism: Clinical and Experimental Research, 12,* 815–819.

Heinemann, A. W., & Shontz, F. C. (1984). Adjustment following disability: Representative case studies. *Rehabilitation Counseling Bulletin, 28,* 3–14.

Heinemann, A. W., & Shontz, F. C. (1985). Methods of studying persons. *Counseling Psychologist, 13,* 111–125.

Heinrich, R. K., Tate, D. C., & Buckelew, S. P. (1994). Brief symptom inventory norms for spinal cord injury. *Rehabilitation Psychology, 39,* 49–56.

Heller, K., Swindle, R. W., & Dusenbury, L. (1986). Component social support processes: Comments and integration. *Journal of Consulting and Clinical Psychology, 54,* 466–470.

Hohmann, G. (1975). Psychological aspects of treatment and rehabilitation of the spinal injured person. *Clinical Orthopedics, 112,* 81–88.

Holicky, R., & Charlifue, S. (1999) Ageing with spinal cord injury: The impact of spousal support. *Disability and Rehabilitation, 21,* 250–257.

Hollingshead, A., de Belmontand, A., & Redlich, F. (1958). *Social class and mental illness.* New York: John Wiley and Sons.

Johnson, D. C. (1985). *Alcohol use by persons with disabilities.* Wisconsin Department of Health and Social Services, Madison, WI.

Judd, F. K., & Brown, D. J. (1992). Suicide following acute traumatic spinal cord injury. *Paraplegia, 30,* 173–177.

Kalb, M. (1971). An examination of the relationship between hospital ward behaviors and post-discharge behaviors in spinal cord injury patients (Doctoral dissertation, University of Houston, 1971). *Dissertation Abstracts International, 32,* 3005B–3006B.

Kelly, G. (1955). *A theory of personality: The psychology of personal constructs.* New York: Norton.

Kerr, N. (1961). Understanding the process of adjustment in disability. *Journal of Rehabilitation, 27,* 16–18.

Kirubakaran, V. R., Kumar, V. N., Powell, B. J., Tyler, A. J., & Armatas, P. J. (1986). Survey of alcohol and drug misuse in spinal cord injured veterans. *Journal of Studies on Alcohol, 47,* 223–227.

Krause, J. S. (1990). The relationship between productivity and adjustment following spinal cord injury. *Rehabilitation Counseling Bulletin, 33,* 188–199.

Krause, J. S. (1992). Employment after spinal cord injury. *Archives of Physical Medicine and Rehabilitation, 73,* 163–169.

Krause, J. S. (1996). Employment after spinal cord injury: Transition and life adjustment. *Rehabilitation Counseling Bulletin, 39,* 244–256.

Krause, J. S. (1998). Changes in adjustment after spinal cord injury: A 20-year longitudinal study. *Rehabilitation Psychology, 43,* 41–55.

Krause, J. S., & Crewe, N. M. (1991). Chronologic age, time since injury, and time of measurement: Effect on adjustment after spinal cord injury. *Archives of Physical Medicine and Rehabilitation, 72,* 91–100.

Krause, J. S., & Dawis, R. V. (1992). Prediction of life satisfaction after spinal cord injury. *Rehabilitation Psychology, 37,* 49–60.

Kubler-Ross, E. (1969). *On death and dying.* New York: Macmillan.

Lazarus, R., & Folkman, S. (1984). *Stress, appraisal and coping.* New York: Springer.

Lewin, K. (1935). *A dynamic theory of personality.* New York: McGraw-Hill.

Livneh, H. (1986). A unified approach to existing models of adaptation to disability: Part II—Intervention strategies. *Journal of Applied Rehabilitation Counseling, 17,* 6–10.

Lowenthal, A., & Anderson, P. (1980–1). Network development: Linking the disabled community to alcoholism and drug abuse programs. *Alcohol Health and Research World, 5,* 16–19.

Mawson, A. R., Jacobs, K. W., Winchester, Y., & Biundo, J. J. (1988). Sensation-seeking and traumatic spinal cord injury: Case-control study. *Archives of Physical Medicine and Rehabilitation, 69,* 1039–1043.

McColl, M. A., Lei, H., & Skinner, H. (1995). Structural relationships between social support and coping. *Social Science in Medicine, 41,* 395–407.

McKinley, W., Kolakowsky, S., & Kreutzer, J. (1999). Substance abuse, violence, and outcome after traumatic spinal cord injury. *Archives of Physical Medicine and Rehabilitation, 78,* 306–312.

Meyers, A. R., Bisbee, A., & Winter, M. (1999). The "Boston Model" of managed care and spinal cord injury: A cross-sectional study of the outcomes of risk-based, pre-paid, managed care. *Archives of Physical Medicine and Rehabilitation, 80,* 1450–1456.

Moore, D., & Li, L. (1998). Prevalence and risk factors of illicit drug use by people with disabilities. *American Journal on Addictions, 7*, 93–102.

Mueller, A. (1950). Personality problems of the spinal cord injured. *Journal of Consulting Psychology, 4*, 189–192.

National Center for the Dissemination of Disability Research. (2003). Overview of NIDRR's long-range plan. Retrieved September 15, 2003, from http://www.ncddr.org/rpp/lrp_ov.html

National Institute on Drug Abuse. (1988). *National Household Survey on Drug Abuse: Main findings.* Rockville, MD: Author.

Nielson, W. R., & MacDonald, M. R. (1988). Attributions of blame and coping following spinal cord injury: Is self-blame adaptive? *Journal of Social and Clinical Psychology, 4*, 163–175.

Nobunaga, A. I., Go, B. K., & Karunas, R. B. (1999). Recent demographic and injury trends in people served by the model spinal cord injury care systems. *Archives of Physical Medicine and Rehabilitation, 80*, 1372–1382.

O'Donnell, J. J., Cooper, J. E., Gessner, J. E., Shehan, I., & Ashley, J. (1981–2). Alcohol, drugs and spinal cord injury. *Alcohol Health & Research World, 6*, 27–29.

Parkes, C. (1972). *Bereavement: Studies in grief in adult life.* New York: International University Press.

Rasmussen, G. A., & DeBoer, R. P. (1980). Alcohol and drug use among clients at a residential vocational rehabilitation facility. *Alcohol Health and Research World, 5*, 48–56.

Rehabilitation Act of 1973, Pub. L. No. 93-112, 87 Stat. 355 (codified as amended in scattered sections of 15 U.S.C., 20 U.S.C., 29 U.S.C., 36 U.S.C., 41 U.S.C., and 42 U.S.C.

Rintala, D. H., Young, M. E., Hart, K. A., Clearman, R. R., & Fuhrer, M. J. (1992). Social support and the well-being of persons with spinal cord injury living in the community. *Rehabilitation Psychology, 37*, 155–164.

Rohe, D. E., & Basford, J. R. (1990). Traumatic spinal cord injury, alcohol, and the Minnesota Multiphasic Personality Inventory. *Rehabilitation Psychology, 34*, 25–32.

Saltz, C. C., Eisenberg, M. G., Fillenbaum, G., & George, L. K. (1991). Functional status and service use among community-based spinal cord injured male veterans. *NeuroBehavior, 4*, 25–35.

Sarason, B. R., Shearin, E. N., Pierce, G. R., & Sarason, I. G. (1987). Interrelations of social support measures: Theoretical and practical implications. *Journal of Personality and Social Support, 52*, 813–832.

Schulz, R., & Decker, S. (1985). Long-term adjustment to physical disability: The role of social support, perceived control and self-blame. *Journal of Personality and Social Psychology, 48*, 1162–1172.

Shigaki, C. L., Hagglund, K. J., Clark, M., & Conforti, K. (2002). Access to health care services among people with rehabilitation needs receiving Medicaid. *Rehabilitation Psychology, 47*, 204–218.

Sholomskas, D. E., Steil, J. M., & Plummer, J. K. (1990). The spinal cord injured revisited: The relationship between self-blame, other-blame, and coping. *Journal of Applied Social Psychology, 20*, 548–574.

Shontz, F. C. (1965). Reactions to crisis. *Volta Review, 67*, 364–370.

Shontz, F. C. (1982). Adaptation to chronic illness and disability. In T. Millon, C. Green, & R. Meagher (Eds.), *Handbook of clinical health psychology* (pp. 153–172). New York: Plenum.

Siller, J. (1969). Psychological situation of the disabled with spinal cord injuries. *Rehabilitation Literature, 30*, 290–296.

Silver, R., & Wortman, C. (1980). Coping with undesirable life events. In J. Garber & N. Seligman (Eds.), *Human helplessness: Theory and applications.* New York: Academic Press.

Spinal Cord Injury Information Network. (2001). Facts and figures at a glance. Retrieved from http://www.spinalcord.uab.edu/show.asp?durki=21466

Stewart, T. D. (1978). Coping behavior and the moratorium following spinal cord injury. *Paraplegia, 15*, 338–342.

Stover, S. L., & Fine, P. R. (1986). *Spinal cord injury: The facts and figures.* Birmingham: University of Alabama at Birmingham.

Substance Abuse Resources and Disability Issues (SARDI). (1992). Retrieved accessed September 15, 2003, from http://www.med.wright.edu/citar/sardi/rrtc_conference.html

Sweeney, T. T., & Foote, J. E. (1982). Treatment of drug and alcohol abuse in spinal cord injury veterans. *International Journal of the Addictions, 17*, 897–904.

Trieschmann, R. B. (1988). *Spinal cord injuries: Psychological, social, and vocational rehabilitation* (2nd ed.). New York: Demos Publications.

Trieschmann, R. B. (1992). Psychosocial research in spinal cord injury: The state of the art. *Paraplegia, 15*, 58–60.

Wright, B. A. (1960). *Physical disability: A psychological approach.* New York: Harper and Row.

Wright, B. A. (1983). *Physical disability: A psychosocial approach.* New York: Harper and Row.

Yarkony, G., Roth, E., Heinemann, A. W., Lovell, L., & Wu, Y. (1988). Functional skills after spinal cord injury rehabilitation: Three year longitudinal follow-up. *Archives of Physical Medicine and Rehabilitation, 69*, 111–114.

25

Hemiplegia

LEONARD DILLER, PhD, AND ALEX MOROZ, MD

MEDICAL BACKGROUND

STROKE IS THE third leading cause of death in the USA and the leading cause of disability. Approximately 550,000 people suffer strokes
each year and nearly one third die from them, while three million people are alive following stroke with various residual neurologic impairments. Stroke is the leading cause of focal neuropsychologic impairment.

Ancient writers of history, science, and poetry used the word
apoplexy, meaning a sudden strike of paralysis, dumbness, or fainting
from which the victim often failed to recover. Such a stroke of illness,
whether delivered by the gods or disease, was a spontaneous event of the
same character as a "stroke of genius," a "stroke of luck," or, more aptly,
a "stroke of misfortune" (Roth & Harvey, 1996). Today the term stroke
connotes the sudden and surprising nature of symptomatic cerebrovascular disease and is preferred over the more scientific sounding
phrase "cerebrovascular accident" since the event may not be cerebrovascular nor accidental (Wiebe-Velasquez & Hachinski, 1991).

Stroke is a clinical syndrome characterised by rapidly developing
clinical signs of focal (or global) disturbance lasting 24 hours or longer
or leading to death with no apparent cause other than of vascular origin (Aho et al., 1980). The definition of stroke incorporates haemorrhagic
and ischemic lesions, with additional subtypes in both categories.
Approximately three quarters of strokes are caused by cerebral infarct.
Intracerebral or subarachnoid hemorrhages account for 15%.

The epidemiology of stroke reflects well-established risk factors for
vascular disease. Risk factors for stroke can be divided into two groups.
Modifiable risk factors include transient ischemic attack, diabetes mel-

litus, hypertension, atrial fibrillation, substance abuse, obesity, and smoking. Hypertension remains the most important modifiable risk factor. Among non-modifiable risk factors, the most prominent is age. Strokes increase dramatically with age and tend to double with each decade at age 55. First ever strokes account for 75%, while recurrent strokes account for 25% of the incidence. However, gender, race, and family history can contribute as etiologic factors. Strokes occur more often in males than females and more often in Afro Americans than in Caucasians. In Western countries there appears to be a decline in stroke, perhaps because of public education with regard to the modifiable risk factors (Gresham, Duncan, Stason, et al., 1995).

Of those who survive the initial onset, the most frequent presenting problem is hemiplegia or hemiparesis, which occurs in about 75%–88% of survivors at 30 days with an equal number of right and left hemiparetics. Generally the paralysis occurs on the side of the body opposite the brain damage so that an individual with right brain damage (RBD) will sustain a paralysis or weakness on the left side of the body. An individual with left brain damage (LBD) will sustain a paralysis or weakness on the right side of the body. During the acute period there is a high incidence of associated neurologic deficits ranging from 12% to 56%. The deficits include ataxia (20%), hemianopsia (26%), visual perceptual defects (32%), aphasia (30%), dysarthria (48%), sensory deficits (56%), cognitive deficits (36%), depression, bladder control(29%), and dysphagia (12%) (Gresham et al., 1995). The deficits often coexist so that management is complicated. On long-term follow-up 6 to 12 months later, there is a lower incidence of deficits in bladder control, dysarthria, aphasia, and dysphagia. The long-term cognitive and emotional sequelae will be discussed below. One important medical concern is the incidence of comorbidities which might affect management and rehabilitation potential (Moroz, Bogey, Bryant, Geiss, & O'Neill, 2004). Among these comorbidities are hypertensive heart disease, obesity, coronary heart disease, arthritis, diabetes mellitus, and congestive heart failure.

Tracking the course of recovery over time is an important consideration. Most recovery takes place within the first 1–3 months. Although recovery may continue particularly with regard to language and visual perception, the pace of recovery slows. Since rehabilitation, particularly at the inpatient level, usually takes place during the first 3 months, it is often difficult to tell whether gains are due to natural recovery or rehabilitation. Recent studies suggest that for patients undergoing rehabilitation, functional recovery of motoric independence can continue beyond 3 months despite the lack of gain in neurologic markers. Furthermore, while rehabilitation in stroke may result in reduction of neurologic impairment as well as disability, disability is reduced even in those in those patients who show no change in impairment. This suggests that gains in disability are not due to recovery alone, but may be the result of interventions in rehabilitation (Roth et al., 1998). A study conducted in Japan, where insurance requirements differ from those in most Western countries, comparing patients who entered rehabilitation within 30 days of onset, vs. 91 to 180 days, vs. 180+ days, showed that all three groups improved in ambulation, with most improvement in the first two groups (Yagura, Miyai, Seike, Suzuki, & Yanangihara, 2003), suggesting that improvement occurs when rehabilitation is applied after 6 months although gains will be less.

FUNCTIONAL LIMITATIONS

TRADITIONAL MEDICINE HAS been concerned with disease management and cure. Rehabilitation has moved beyond these concerns to issues in living with the effects of disease and trauma. Although neurologic deficits are generally associated with impairments, rehabilitation is concerned with functional limitations and handicap. Functional limitations involve the quality of daily activities which are commonly expressed by the degree of dependence in the physical, cognitive, social, emotional, and vocational domains of daily living. Instruments to assess functional limitations permit quantifiable observation which can be used to track outcomes, recovery, and individual and program differences. An indication of the rapid development in the field can be seen by examining the most common method of assessing functional limitations—Functional Independence Measure (FIM). The FIM has been adopted by 1,300 participating facilities and 70,000 trained clinical raters. By the end of 1997, data have been collected on more than 3,000,000 patients (Granger, 1998).

Studies in community based samples of hemiparetics who have not undertaken formal rehabilitation indicate that while only 27% of survivors were independent in walking during the 1st week after stroke, 85% were independent at 6 months. In activities of daily living, help was needed for bowel and bladder incontinence, grooming, toileting, feeding, dressing, bathing, or transfers in 77–88% of the cases at 3 weeks after onset (Wade & Hewer, 1987; Dombovy, 1993). On follow-up 6 months to 5 years later, help was needed in 24–53% of the cases. In patients who have completed inpatient rehabilitation, FIM scores on motor activities improved by 38% and cognitive scores improved by 11% at discharge. The benefits of these improvements have been translated into a reduction of person hours in caretaker burden (Roth et al., 1998).

Eighteen percent of stroke survivors participate in rehabilitation. The most prominent reason for rehabilitation in stroke is hemiplegia or hemiparesis. Of those patients who do not enter rehabilitation, the majority are discharged home with or without outpatient services, or they are discharged to nursing homes (10%–29%). Discharge destination depends in large part on the person's clinical status as well as social factors. For example, there is a higher incidence of discharge to nursing homes or sheltered dwellings among persons living alone at the time of stroke than those coming from intact families (Powell, Diller, & Grynbaum, 1976).

PSYCHOLOGICAL PROBLEMS

A PSYCHOLOGICAL PROBLEM may be defined as a difficulty in meeting the task demands in rehabilitation and/or in assuming the premorbid or normative role expectations following discharge, due to a problem in the person and/or the environment. In this chapter we are largely concerned with the difficulties in the person, hence we focus on the psychological problems. Psychological problems may be related to cultural or environmental circumstances and may be referred to as psychosocial problems. Psychological difficulties attributable to the environment during rehabilitation may require an examination of the attitudes of the rehabilitation team or significant others.

Psychological problems may be expressed as difficulties in learning, attitudes, and/or behaviors which interfere with maximum utilization of the program, increasing length of stay, accidents, disturbance in well-being of the patient, problems in management by the rehabilitation staff, or difficulties in family relationships. The psychologist generally translates presenting problems into difficulties in cognition, emotion, and/or motivation as they interact with current circumstances. The translation also factors in premorbid personality which might influence the response to the current situation (Langer, 1992). In a retrospective chart survey of 200 inpatients, approximately 13% had evidence of prior psychiatric histories (Padrone, 1995).

Clinically, it might be useful to describe mental life in terms of cognition, affect, and motivation. This categorization permits the organization of a large body of psychological studies in a framework which is meaningful for rehabilitation. One can indicate the incidence of impairments, the relationship to rehabilitation, some common methods which are used in their assessment, and finally treatment methods. It encompasses the historical emphasis of different professional approaches. While psychologists have emphasized information processing and affective responses, other therapists in rehabilitation tend to use the label "lack of motivation" in describing a difficult patient.

Cognition is "the mental process or faculty by which knowledge is acquired, or that which comes to be known through perception, reasoning, or intuition" (*Webster's New College Dictionary*, 1995). Cognitive changes may be end points of processes involving language, attention, perception, and memory. A diffuse or global decline in cognitive functioning yields the clinical picture of dementia.

Complex and specific patterns of cognitive dysfunction have been identified. Among the most prominent are apraxia, aphasia, and visual perceptual deficits. Apraxia is a neurologically based difficulty in following a motor command that is not due to a primary motor deficit or a language impairment in strength, coordination, sensation, or lack of comprehension. Apraxias have been observed on both clinical testing and activities of daily living (ADLs). Aphasia is a disturbance in communication in language-related events generally resulting from damage to the dominant hemisphere and occurs more often in individuals with right hemiparesis than left hemiparesis. Aphasia is manifested by problems in comprehension, speech, verbal comprehension, reading, and writing. It is distinguished from the neuromotor components of language such as dysarthria, where the difficulty may lie in executing a sequence of voluntary movements. Perceptual difficulties may appear in several ways, including visual field defects, color recognition, diplopia, visual gaze, and defect in depth perception which may impact rehabilitation. The most prominent problem is that of visual neglect or hemi-inattention. It occurs more often in right brain damage (RBD) with left hemiparesis than in left brain damage (LBD) with right hemiparesis. Hemi-inattention is a complex disorder with a diminished awareness of space on the side opposite to the damaged hemisphere. The diminished attention is manifested by errors of omission. It occurs with regard to location on the body (body image) as well as external to the body (extrapersonal space). It can involve visual and tactile modalities and to a lesser extent auditory modalities. Hemi-inattention can be observed in clinical testing as well as in activities of daily living (Gordon & Diller, 1983).

Emotional reactions are generally divided into depression, anxiety, and hostility. Post-stroke depression has been cited as the most common untreated disability secondary to stroke (Gordon & Hibbard, 1997). Although reported in the stroke literature since the turn of the last century, it was not regarded as a serious problem in rehabilitation settings until the 1980s. Earlier observers focused on denial of affective reactions in stroke patients. Depression has several features including attitudes reflecting hopelessness and pessimism, non-verbal demeanor, and vegetative disturbances in eating and sleeping. While earlier observers attributed depression to a grieving response or a catastrophic response to frustrations and losses associated with stroke, recent observers have implicated biologic factors via locus of brain damage (Starkstein & Robinson, 1994) and social factors via the social isolation following stroke. Depression in stroke has a high frequency of characteristics of anxiety. Other psychiatric disturbances such as hallucinations, mania, delusions, personality alterations, and obsessive-compulsive disorders occur less often.

Motivation is an individual's response to a rehabilitation program in terms of participation or compliance with its task demands (Hyman, 1972; Thompson, 1991). Although poor motivation can be attributed to many factors, two stand out. First, there maybe a lack of congruence between the patient's goals and the goals of the rehabilitation team. For example, if the patient wants only a cure for his/her condition, anything less is viewed as a failure in treatment. The goals may be influenced by a number of circumstances including retention of a premorbid self-concept; emotional flooding by anger or depression; cognitive incompetence which is related to neurologically based unawareness, pain, or cultural factors which influence the meaning of the occurrence of a stroke. Second, apathy or hypoarousal which might be a direct consequence of the stroke. The patient's passivity may be misconstrued as a lack of interest or depression rather than a neurologically based problem (Diller, Goodgold, & Kay, 1988).

The cognitive, emotional, and motivational domains interact and influence each other. While the domains may exist separately, in practice a cognitive problem is likely to occur along with an emotional and/or motivational problem and vice versa (Diller et al., 1988).

There are no formal data on actual psychological problems since their manifestations are diverse. An informal survey of the time spent by occupational and physical therapists indicates that in one large rehabilitation facility, more than 40 hours of therapist time in a given week was taken up with the management of behavioral problems (Padrone, 1995). Despite the absence of documentation on the incidence of psychological problems, there is a great deal of information on cognitive, emotional, and motivational factors which play a role in rehabilitation. This information can be used to understand and help management of psychological problems.

Stroke patients perform more poorly on standard cognitive tests than normals (Egelko et al., 1989) and orthopedic patients (Osmon, Smet, Winegarden, & Ghandavadi, 1992). Cognitive performance is lower in patients after a stroke at 6 month follow-up in comparison with actual pre-stroke scores (Kase et al., 1987). While cognitive disturbances are most acute at the time of onset they may persist for longer periods (Egelko et al.). For example at 3 months, problems in memory still remained for 29% of a group which returned to the community (Wade, Parker, & Langton-Hewer, 1986). In another study using a more functional test of memory, 49% were found to be below the lowest scores of non-brain-damaged persons at 7 months after onset. Hemi-inattention is present in 72% of right brain damaged (RBD) and 62% of left brain damaged (LBD) patients at 3 days after stroke. At 3 months it is still present in 75% of rbds who originally showed neglect and 33% of lbds who originally showed neglect (Stone et al., 1991). Wide variation in estimates occur, in part because of the variation in tests which are used. However, it appears that the more extensive and inclusive the test battery the higher the reported incidence (Schenkenberg, Bradford, & Ajax, 1980; Wilson et al., 1986).

Affective disturbance places patients at risk and is clearly a problem. In comparison with a pre-stroke indicator of depression, at 6 months after stroke patients are significantly depressed. However, it is difficult to draw firm conclusions regarding major issues. For example, estimates of depression vary from 11%–68% (Gordon & Hibbard, 1997), depending on the hemispheric and anatomic location, but even more importantly on methods of assessment. Assessment of depression in hemiparetic patients is difficult because instruments to assess depression involve self-report which may be influenced by the presence of aphasia, lack of awareness, cognitive confusion, or somatic manifestations. These manifestations might be attributed to organic conditions such as lability, or to being in a hospital which might influence eating and sleeping patterns (Gordon & Hibbard). Time of assessment may also play a role (Schubert, Burns, Paras, & Sioson, 1992a). Depression is underreported in self-report or medical intake interview and is likely to decrease during a rehabilitation program (Schubert et al., 1992a, 1992b). Data are ambiguous with regard to long-term status (Gordon & Hibbard; Thompson, 1991). It is apparent that some with earlier major depression still remain in this state at 2 years and even longer, and that minor depression may get worse (Parikh et al., 1990).

With regard to motivation, a substantial number of stroke patients are unaware of various aspects of stroke. Unawareness tends to be greater in the acute phase (Hier, Mondlock, & Caplan, 1983). However, after the acute phase unawareness is unrelated to time since onset (Hibbard et al., 1992). Unawareness is not a unitary phenomenon. More people are aware of physical impairments than of affective and cognitive impairments (Anderson & Tranel, 1989; Hibbard, Gordon, Stein, Grober, & Sliwinski, 1992). Although half of stroke patients are aware of memory and mood disorders, patients tend to exaggerate memory problems and minimize self-report of perceptual problems (Diller & Weinberg, 1993) and depression (Hibbard et al.). Patients may misattribute their problems. For example, an individual with a perceptual problem who denies the presence of a problem, when pressed may state that a problem exists but it is a memory problem (Diller & Weinberg). From a management standpoint, there are differences between individuals who overtly deny the presence of a problem and those who passively acknowledge a problem but remain unresponsive otherwise. The level of denial is related to cognitive competence (Diller & Weinberg).

While motivation may be affected by the neurobiology of stroke, cultural factors play a role. Stroke patients in a public vs a private university medical rehabilitation program with similar neurologic impairments differed in attitudes to authority and feelings about controlling their health-related activities (Powell et al., 1976).

Another aspect of lack of motivation is that of hypoarousal. RBD stroke patients make fewer movements than lbd patients in performing a block design task (Ben Yishay, Diller, Mandleberg, Gordon, & Gerstman, 1984), even when solving a problem correctly. Right and left hemiplegics are slower in reaction time tasks than normals and their response rate is slower (Egelko et al., 1989). Although some find that reaction time improves during a rehabilitation program, others report that even with improvement it is a most persistent impairment at 1 year follow-up (Egelko et al.). Prigitano and Wong (1997) note that speed of finger tapping, but not grip strength, is impaired in the hand which is ipsilateral to the side of brain damage in unilateral stroke patients. Theoretically, speed should be affected only on the side contralateral to the brain damage. They argue that the degree of impairment is an indicator of the degree of bilateral damage and that the task activates bilateral cerebral hemispheres.

PSYCHOLOGICAL PROBLEMS AND PROGRAM PARTICIPATION

MANY ASPECTS OF ADL are related to perceptual and cognitive problems. Patients with spatial constructional problems perform poorly in dressing, eating, walking, and grooming (Warren, 1990). Patients with visual neglect have difficulty (Gordon & Diller, 1983) in academic tasks (reading, writing, written arithmetic), grooming (shaving in men, makeup in women), instrumental activities (reading a menu, using a telephone, household activities), driving, telling time from a clock (Titus, Gall, Yerxa, Robertson, & Mack, 1991). Since a given ADL task may depend on the integration of several abilities, failure may occur for different reasons by patients with different patterns of cognitive deficits. Thus in learning to transfer to and from a wheelchair, overall gain is related to cognitive competency. In individuals with left hemiparesis, mastery is associated with fewer errors on spatial tasks. In individuals with right hemiparesis mastery is associated with speed in processing information (Diller, Buxbaum, & Chiotelis, 1972). Similarly, with regard to the occurrence of accidents on a rehabilitation program, left hemiparetics with neglect on a visual cancellation test are more likely to have multiple accidents. Right hemiparetics who are too slow on the same test are more likely to have accidents (Diller & Weinberg, 1970). A further example of a common path of difficulty due to different sources of dysfunction may be found in the observation that problems in recognizing affective dimensions of verbal expression (aprosodia) occur equally in right and left brain damaged stroke patients. The groups, however, show different patterns of impairment in their response to auditory frequencies, arguing for the fact that aprosodia may be related to different patterns of deficit in auditory frequency.

Poor performance on cognitive tasks predicts outcome in inpatient rehabilitation (Ben Yishay, Gerstman, Diller, & Haas, 1970) and on long-term follow-up (Wade et al., 1986). Although different combinations of tests have been used, motor impersistence and logical memory have contributed to predictions (Ben Yishay, Gerstman, Diller, & Haas, 1968). Visual neglect in rehabilitation predicts poorer ADLs on long-term follow-up (Denes, Semenza, Stoppa, & Lis, 1982; Kinsella & Ford, 1980). Prigitano and Wong (1997) found that speed of reaction time using the hand ipsilateral to the brain damage predicts goal attainment in rehabilitation. They suggest that this is a behavioral marker of the integrity of the intact hemisphere which could be used to predict rehabilitation outcome.

Depression has been shown to be related to increased length of stay in inpatient programs (Schubert, Burns, et al., 1992b), lower ADL scores (Schubert, Taylor, Lee, Mentari, & Tamaklo, 1992a), discharge to a facility rather than to home (Cushman, 1988), and cognitive impairment (Starkstein & Robinson, 1994). While falling behaviors among stroke victims living in the community are typically associated with balance and gait problems, they are also associated with depression (Hyndman, Ashburn, & Stack, 2002). Depression is associated with decline in social (Parikh et al., 1990) and sexual activities (Monga, Lawson, & Inglis, 1986). While depression is not originally associated with severity of impairment, with time depression becomes increasingly related to severity of impairment (Robinson, Bolduc, & Price, 1987; Thompson, 1991). In an outpatient sample, depression was associated with a lack of meaning in life and overprotection (Thompson). In a follow-up of patients 10 years post-onset, Morris, Robinson, Andrzejwski, Samuels, and Price (1993) found that patients diagnosed as depressed on examination 1 to 3 weeks after a stroke had a mortality rate 3.4 times higher than non-depressed patients. Depression and other mental health diagnoses were found to have a higher mortality rate (Williams, Ghose, & Swindle, 2004).

Motivation in outpatient treatment has been related to overprotection, lower cognitive functioning, lower sense of meaning, and less hope (Thompson, 1991). Those who hold themselves responsible for the stroke had a poorer adjustment (Thompson).

IDENTIFYING PSYCHOLOGICAL PROBLEMS

SPECIFIC PROBLEMS MIGHT be detected in initial clinical impression, the medical chart, report by the family or the staff, or self-report. Since the incidence of cognitive and/or emotional impairments is high, routine screening is recommended to identify stroke patients at risk of not benefiting from a program or posing management problems. In initial medical screenings, chart reviews suggest that depression (Schubert, Taylor, Lee, Mentari, & Tamaklo, 1992b) and visual perceptual problems (Weinberg & Diller, 1966) may be overlooked.

Although brief screening for psychosocial problems may be part of an initial medical examination, further levels of screening by a psychologist should be considered. An informal survey of consecutive admissions to an inpatient service of 200 patients, of whom 30% were stroke patients, found the presence of depression/anxiety in 63% (Padrone, 1995). With the scarcity of available time and the increasing trend towards curtailing lengths of stay in inpatient rehabilitation, psychologists are in the position of having to choose between concentrating their efforts on a few problem patients who may require extensive in depth evaluations vs. many patients with different degrees of psychological problems. The former approach may involve a few patients who might consume more team resources, while the latter approach may involve less in-depth contact and permits the psychologist to participate more actively in case management by the rehabilitation team. The psychologist in this approach samples in a more limited way domains of language, attention, perception, memory, and psychomotor proficiency as well as patient goals, concerns, and affective state. The psychologist is in a position to be more effective with a larger number of patients, although the diagnostic judgements are based on less fine-grained analysis of impairments. The former approach pursues the development of more refined test batteries to parse deficits, while the latter approach seeks shorter batteries to deal with the logistics of decision making and management. Hajek, Gagnon, and Ruderman (1997) found that measures of disability which are designed to detect cognitive factors such as FIM are often insensitive to cognitive impairments. For example, stroke patients who perform well on the cognitive sections of the FIM may not do well on neuropsychologic tests. A brief test which maybe useful for screening purposes is the Neurobehavioral Cognitive Status Examination (Osmon et al., 1992). A more complete description of instruments which might be used for screening can be found in Caplan and Schechter (1995) and in Wagner, Nayak, and Fink (1995).

To permit quantified measures of cognitive disability rather than impairments, functionally based measures of cognitive tasks which are useful for stroke patients have been introduced. The basic idea is to sample an area of cognitive function by using tasks from daily life, such as following a series of directions and then recalling the directions, or reading a menu, rather than items derived from psychometric tasks with no intrinsic use in daily life. Such tasks are useful to assess visual neglect—Rivermead Behavioural Inattention Test (Wilson, Cockburn, & Halligan, 1987) and memory—Rivermead Behavioural Memory Test (Wilson,

Cockburn, & Baddley, 1989). Subjective ratings of memory impairment by patients and by their relatives are more related to the Rivermead Behavioural Memory Test than they are to conventional memory tests.

The assessment of emotional state utilizes information from history, clinical interview, and external observers. Methods include symptom check lists as well as formalized scales. Although formal scales such as Zung, Beck Depression Inventory, and Geriatric Depression Scale have been used in epidemiologic and community-based studies, for clinical purposes they may not be useful. Toedter and colleagues (1995) found that stroke patients were unreliable reporters of their mood states. Changes in depression may not be detected by formal instruments but may be reported by observers (Diller, 1992; Schubert et al., 1992b). Biochemical markers such as the Dexamethasone Suppression Test (DST) have yielded questionable results in detecting poststroke depression (Grober et al., 1991).

In the absence of standardized tests, assessment of motivational problems generally is based on history, interview, and clinical observation. Review of medical chart records in a population of spinal cord injured patients suggests that motivational problems are the most frequently cited complaint (Bleiberg & Merhitz, 1985). While a patient whose goals deviate from those of the team might be at risk for poor cooperation, a modest degree of denial expressed as an optimistic outlook is a useful prognostic sign (Powell et al., 1976). Patients typically rate their progress greater than therapists do and attribute their success to factors different from those that their therapists cite. Caregivers typically rate satisfaction greater than the patients do (Heinemann, Cichowski, & Kan, 1997).

TREATMENT

THE PATIENT WHO refuses to go to classes, the patient who is depressed or angry, or the patient who is apathetic may have disturbances in perception, affect, and/or motivation. It is useful to consider a treatment plan which addresses all of the elements (Heinemann et al., 1997). For example, cognitive perceptual remediation is not effective if it is seen as a series of straightforward exercises without taking into account the fact the patient may be unaware of a problem or too upset to participate. Anger may be internally derived but its management must take into account the staff's response.

TREATMENT OF PERCEPTUAL COGNITIVE DISORDERS

HEMI-INATTENTION MAY BE a simple phenomenon to illustrate. For example, the patient may omit drawings on the left side of the page.

When one breaks down the responses for treatment purposes, there is a nest of behaviors which can be used as key points in therapy. Typically, one begins to scan the visual environment by starting from the left and directing the gaze to the right. Patients with hemi-inattention will have difficulty in finding a reference point or a starting point to anchor the beginning of a search for the stimulus; once anchored, some patients will respond impulsively and skip important features of their environment. Patients may have problems in two-dimensional space, such as reading, as well as in three-dimensional space, such as locating the body in space and may bump into objects or misreach objects set on a table. Patients may have difficulty in benefitting from feedback; patients may be unaware of specific difficulties and, out of a fear that they are losing their minds, they may try to cover up problems by denying their existence, or they may misattribute their errors to a memory problem. Each of these points can be incorporated into a strategy which combines arranging tasks with graded degrees of difficulty and relating them to problems in the environment outside of the test room. For example, a patient in early stages of rehabilitation with major difficulties in neglect can be given simple bedside exercises to track pictures on the wall or squares on the hospital ceiling. Patients may be taught to slow impulsive responses by pacing, that is, by pointing and reciting targets aloud. A therapeutic concern is to maintain awareness of the problem and show strategies to resolve it while demonstrating its relevance for important features of daily living.

These points have been translated into specific techniques (Diller & Riley, 1993) in a series of controlled studies. Improvements were noted in academic skills such as reading and written arithmetic; appreciation of space on and off the body; and perceptual organization. While the experimental group maintained the level of gain at follow-up at 5 months after discharge, the controls improved to the same level as the treated group, except for the fact that the treated patients spent more free time in reading (Gordon et al., 1985). In a study comparing the effectiveness of concentrated practice on a narrow range of tasks, a "depth" approach versus practice over a wide range of tasks, a "broad" approach, both performed better than a control group. This suggested that a narrow focus involving repetitive practice with the same materials is more helpful for severely impaired patients, while less intense exercise with a broader range of materials is more useful for milder patients. In addition, exercises to stimulate arousal made the program more effective (Diller, Goodgold, & Kay, 1988). The basic strategy has also been applied to patients with mild neglect, which was presented as a problem in memory and losing track of conversations (Diller & Weinberg, 1986); to patients with severe neglect and underarousal (Diller & Weinberg, 1993); and to patients who had difficulty in recognizing faces (Weinberg & Diller,

2000). Strategies have been elaborated to translate or modify the principles for use by a whole team to be incorporated into ADL training (Hanlon et al., 1992), improving training in transfer activities (Calvanio, Levine, & Petrone, 1993), improving table reaching behavior (Zoccolotti & Judica, 1991), and avoiding obstacles in wheelchair maneuvers (Webster et al., 1995). In all of these applications, there is recognition of the difficulties in generalizing the effectiveness of the training into functional activities.

Alternative behavioral approaches with somewhat different emphases have been suggested. Activation of movement on the impaired side of space to increase awareness has been shown to be effective. Thus activation of the impaired limb yields improvement in personal space (hair combing), locomotor space (circuit walking), and reaching space behavior (placing buns in a tray), although only the gains in reaching space behavior were maintained on follow-up (Robertson, Hogg, & McMillan, 1998). The theory behind this approach is that stimuli from the intact hemisphere overwhelm stimuli from the impaired hemisphere to dampen activation in the impaired hemisphere. Attention to stimuli in the space opposite to the impaired hemisphere is impoverished. Activating the impaired hemisphere by movement of the opposite side of the body will offset the dominance of the intact hemisphere. From a somewhat different vantage point it might be argued that a major feature of the syndrome is the displacement of the normal body axis which served as a referent for egocentric or personal body space. This can easily be demonstrated by touching an RBD patient on the back along the shoulder blades and asking to indicate when the "backbone" or midpoint is reached. RBD patients displace the midline to the right, while left brain damaged patients and normals are accurate in locating the midline. Wiart and others (1997) have been able to train patients to improve in egocentric space by using trunk rotation to track a target. A summary and critical review of the different approaches, their benefits and limitations, may be found in Pearce and Buxbaum (2002). The different approaches suggest that neglect may be a heterogeneous phenomenon with treatments targeting arousal events, deficient visual attention, and spatial representation deficits.

The results of these studies indicate that psychologists can play a useful role with regard to the perceptual problems presented by RBDs either by direct intervention programs or by serving as consultants to occupational and physical therapists.

MANAGEMENT OF EMOTIONAL PROBLEMS

As with emotional problems in individuals who have not suffered a stroke, both psychopharmaceutical as well as psychotherapeutic methods are used. The pharmaceutical approach uses antidepression medication such as nortryptoline (Lipsey, Robinson, Pearlson, Rao, & Price, 1984), or psychostimulants such as methylphenidate. There are few controlled studies, with small numbers of patients, so that results must be interpreted cautiously. Electroconvulsive therapy has also been used, but despite some reports of favorable outcomes, there are noticeable side effects in a significant number of cases so that it should only be considered as a last resort (Gordon & Hibbard, 1997). A complication with all of the biologic approaches may be a patient's unwillingness to consent to the treatments. In addition, pharmaceutical approaches require sophistication in managing polypharmacological reactions.

With regard to the psychotherapeutic treatment of depression in stroke, a variety of therapies is available. Perhaps the most common is supportive therapy. Psychodynamic (Langer, 1992) and cognitive behavioral approaches are clinically useful (Hibbard, Grober, et al., 1990). Some modifications have to be made to take into account language and perceptual problems (Langer). Psychotherapists must also take into account cognitive limitations resulting from brain damage. In addition to limitations in processing information, there is a possibility of the patient perseverating affective states as well as ideas and language. Thus, in response to the question "Why are you crying?" the patient responded "Because my sister died two years ago."

There is only one formal clinical trial on the efficacy of psychotherapy up to this point. When depressed stroke patients were placed into groups which offered differing combinations of psychotherapeutic and pharmacologic therapy and a no-therapy control, 74% of psychotherapy patients showed an elevation in mood while only 36% of controls showed an elevation (Gordon, 1992). While results did not differ by hemispheric locus, different-sided hemispheric-lesioned patients showed different correlates with improvement. One of the by-product findings was the refusal of patients to enlist in a psychopharmacological study. There are useful clinical case descriptions of psychodynamic (Langer, 1992; Langer & Padrone, 1992) as well as cognitive behavioral approaches (Hibbard, Grober, Gordon, Aletta, & Freeman, 1990).

In a novel approach, a paraprofessional coach, working under supervision, combined methods of perceptual remediation and applications of solution-focused therapy to family systems (DeShazer, 1988). An experimental group (n = 10) of outpatient hemiparetics, when compared with a control group (n = 12), showed an increase in instrumental ADLs (dressing/bathing), increased out-of-home visits, better caregiver mood, less likely to report worsening of mood, and increased time in reading. The approach is promising because it is a service which can be delivered at home by a graduate student working under close supervision (Diller, 1992).

Group therapy approaches are very useful, with modifications to take account of cognitive limitations. A variant of group therapy includes psychoeducational groups where information is presented in a psychotherapeutic context. In inpatient settings, the logistics can pose a problem because of the wide range of impairments and shortened lengths of stay. Sherr and Langenbahn (1992) describe an outpatient program which places great emphasis on group approaches. They have developed a hierarchic model for teaching problem solving which provides a methodology for dealing with cognitive as well as emotional factors before training in logical thinking.

VOCATIONAL REHABILITATION

WHILE STROKE IS usually associated with old age, it has been estimated that 30% of strokes occur in people under 65 years of age. In a sample of more than 400 cases of hemiplegia due to stroke in which patients engaged in inpatient rehabilitation over a 1-year period, 10% were between the ages of 45–54 (Diller, 1992). Thus, many of the survivors of stroke are of working age. Unfortunately the public at large, physicians, families, and even professionals who work with such patients have little hope of stroke patients' successful return to work. The stigma associated with stroke carries over to the patients, who lose confidence in their abilities and give up hope. The estimates of return to work vary widely; however, in the largest follow-up study of patients 21–65 years of age, Black-Schaffer and Osberg (1990) found that of 79 patients who were working at the time of stroke, 49% had returned to work 6 months after rehabilitation. The mean time to return to work was 3.1 months. Ninety percent returned to their old jobs, but only 23% were working the same number of hours. Other follow-up studies report lower figures (Zuger & Boehm, 1993).

It is apparent that physical factors play a role. The presence of aphasia adds complications in vocational planning, so that even those aphasics who return to work take much longer to do so (Weissberg, Esibell, & Zuger, 1971). Socioeconomic and family support play important parts. As might be expected, individuals with more education and greater pre-stroke job skills were more successful. Individuals without families and members of minority groups are less likely to return to work. Support from families and employers is very important. Clinically the problem of too much support becomes an issue. The popular notion that stroke may be caused by stress contributes to this idea (Zuger & Boehm, 1993).

It is important to have a proper vocational evaluation and access to a full range of vocational services including a rehabilitation counselor, proper work sampling methods, counseling, and supportive employment in which support is rendered by a job coach who conducts in situ evaluations with action plans for all parties relevant to the employment process. All of these activities should occur only after a careful analysis of the patient's premorbid life style (Zuger & Boehm, 1993). In general, vocational rehabilitation must be rendered on a case-by-case basis.

TREATMENTS UNDER INVESTIGATION

BODY WEIGHT SUPPORT (BWS) consists of walking the patient on a treadmill at their maximum comfortable speed while a percentage of their body weight is supported centrally at the trunk by an overhead harness. The percentage of body weight supported typically ranges from 0 to 40%. Unloading of the lower extremities appears to be an important factor in unmasking the potential for recovery of gait, and the degree of support is typically decreased as the patient advances in therapy. Gait improvements during supported locomotion can be sustained and transferred to full-weight-bearing over-ground walking after a training regimen. The net result is more functional gait, with improved balance, motor control, walking velocity, and distance. The advantages of partial body weight support are that it allows upright posture, minimizes fall risk, facilitates a reciprocal stepping pattern, and is task-specific, with the potential for multiple repetitions (Bogey, Geis, Bryant, Moroz, & O'Neill, 2004).

Virtual reality (VR) has many advantages in the rehabilitation setting. Compared to more commonly used therapies, VR simulates "real-life." This may allow users to "forget" that they are in a testing environment, and allows presentation of valid testing and training scenarios and/or cognitive challenges. VR allows the rehabilitation specialist to control stimuli presentation. As a function of this control, the clinician allows presentation of repetitive stimuli which can be varied from simple to complex contingent upon success. It gives immediate performance feedback in a variety of forms and the capacity for complete performance recording. Many activities of daily living may be hazardous to persons after stroke (e.g., driving). VR simulates potentially hazardous situations without the risk. It provides a safe learning environment and allows the user to experience mistakes to promote learning and self-awareness. The VR approach may lead to the design of individualized training environments, with modification of sensory presentation and response requirements based on the user's impairments (e.g., movement, hearing, and visual disorders). It permits an individual to train at their own pace.

Virtual reality can be viewed as an advanced form of human-computer interface that allows the user to interact with and become immersed in a computer-generated environment. Much like an aircraft simulator, which serves to test and train piloting ability, computer-generated virtual environments (VEs) can be created to assess and rehabilitate cognitive and functional abilities, providing interactive scenarios designed to target simulated "real-world" tasks.

Interaction in three dimensions (3D) is a key characteristic that distinguishes a VR experience from watching a movie. The realistic virtual experience is fostered by employing such specialized technology as head-mounted displays (HMDs), tracking systems, earphones, and gesture-sensing gloves. An HMD is an image display system worn on the head, which remains optically-coupled to the user's eyes as he/she turns and moves. A tracking system senses the position and orientation of the user's head (and HMD) and reports that information to a computer that updates (in real time) the images for display in the HMD. In most cases, full-color stereo image-pairs are produced and earphones may also deliver relevant 3D sound. The combination of a HMD and tracking system allows the computer to generate images and sounds in any computer-modeled virtual scene that corresponds to what the user would see and hear from their current position if the scene were real. The user may walk and turn around to survey a virtual landscape, or inspect a virtual object by moving towards it and peering around its sides or back. While HMDs are most commonly associated with VR, other methods incorporating 3D projection walls and rooms, as well as basic flat-screen computer systems, have been used to create interactive scenarios for rehabilitative purposes. Methods for navigation and interaction such as data gloves, joysticks, and some high-end feedback mechanisms which can provide tactile feedback can be used to further enhance realism. Application of this innovative technology in rehabilitation is promising (Bogey et al., 2004).

OUTCOME PREDICTION

P REDICTING FUNCTION AFTER a stroke has been difficult because of the number of variables involved (Jongbloed, 1986). Age, sex, presence of comorbidities, history of prior stroke, pre-stroke level of function, presence of support in the form of a caregiver and available financial resources, time since onset, cognitive status, presence of visual field or perceptual deficits, degree of motor impairment, sensory loss, balance and postural control, presence of bladder or bowel incontinence, functional status on admission, laboratory abnormalities during the acute stage, and size, location and type of the stroke are all considered important predictors of function after a stroke. However, few factors are agreed upon as universally predictive.

There have been several attempts to use predictions by rehabilitation practitioners as a measure of functional outcome. While physical and occupational therapists were able to predict some measures of hand impairment and mobility, they were not able to prognosticate activities of daily living status, need for assistance, or discharge destination (Kwakkel, van Dijk, & Wagenaar, 2000). A study intended to support the ability of physical therapists to predict the discharge functional status actually showed that function on discharge is related to admission function rather than age or side of lesion (Korner-Bitensky, Mayo, Cabot, Becker, & Coopersmith, 1989). Stroke patients were able to predict their function at 12 weeks essentially as well as the physiotherapists (Jones, 1998). Despite solid scientific basis for stroke pathophysiology and treatment, prediction of outcome after a stroke remains a clinical art.

FUTURE RESEARCH

I T IS OF interest to note that in the *Clinical Practice Guidelines on Post Stroke Rehabilitation* (Gersham et al., 1995) published by the Department of Health and Human Services, of the 57 recommended practices pertaining to stroke, 13 refer to practices in the acute hospital phase, 15 to screening procedures during admission to rehabilitation programs, 24 to management practices in the rehabilitation setting, and 5 to community transition. Of all the recommendations, only 4 are based on scientific evidence, that is 2 random controlled trials, 10 are based on fewer than 2 randomly controlled trials, whereas the remaining 45 are based on clinical consensus. Eight of the scientifically based recommendations are for rehabilitation practices during the acute care period.

While the major focus of rehabilitation programs has been on reduction of disability as measured by observation of outcomes, more recent approaches have incorporated subjective components of experience. Typically this approach utilizes indicators of quality of life and measures of satisfaction (Tulski & Rosenthal, 2002). Doyle (2002) has proposed a patient-reported measure of functioning and well being to address the limitations of current approaches, the Burden of Stroke Scale (BOSS), in which a single concept, burden of care, is partitioned among three domains: physical, cognitive, and emotional. The domains incorporate activity limitations as well as experienced difficulty.

REFERENCES

Aho, K., Harmsen, P., Hatano, S., Marquardsen, J., Smirnov, V. E., & Strasser, T. (1980). Cerebrovascular disease in the community: Results of a WHO collaborative study. *Bulletin World Health Organization, 58,* 113–130.

Anderson, S., & Tranel, D. (1989). Awareness of disease states following cerebral infarction, dementia, and head trauma: Standardised assessment. *Clinical Neuropsychology, 3,* 327–339.

Antonucci, G., Guariglia, C., Judica, A., Magnotti, L., Paolucci, S., Pizzamiglio, L., et al. (1995). Effectiveness of neglect rehabilitation in a randomized group study. *Journal of Clinical Experimental Neuropsychology,* 383–389.

Ben-Yishay, Y., Diller, L., Mandleberg, I., Gordon, W. A., & Gerstman, L. (1972). Similarities and differences in block design performance between older normal and brain-injured persons: A task analysis. *Journal of Abnormal Psychology, 78,* 17–25.

Ben Yishay, Y. B., Diller, L., Mandleberg, I., Gordon, W. A., & Gerstman, L. J. (1974). Differences in matching persistence behavior during block design performance between older normal and brain damaged persons *Cortex, 6.*

Ben Yishay, Y., Gerstman, L. J., Diller, L., & Haas, A. (1968). The relationship between impersistence, intellectual function, and outcome of rehabilitation in patients with left hemiplegia. *Neurology, 18,* 852–861.

Ben Yishay, Y., Gerstman, L. J., Diller, L., & Haas, A. (1970). Prediction of rehabilitation outcomes from psychometric parameter in left hemiplegia. *Journal of Consulting and Clinical Psychology, 34,* 36–41.

Black-Schaffer, R. M., & Osberg, J. S. (1990). Return to work after stroke: Development of a predictive model. *Archives of Physical Medicine and Rehabilitation, 71,* 285–290.

Bogey, R. A., Geis, C. C., Bryant, P. R., Moroz, A., & O'Neill, B. J. (2004). Stroke and neurodegenerative disorders. 3. Stroke: Rehabilitation management. *Archives of Physical Medicine and Rehabilitation, 85*(3 Suppl. 1), S15–20.

Calvanio, R., Levine, D., & Petrone, P. (1993). Elements of Cognitive Rehabilitation after right hemisphere stroke. *Neurology Clinics, 3,* 25–57.

Campodonico, J. R., & McGlynn, S. M. (1995). Assessing awareness of deficits: Recent research and applications. In L. A. Cushman & M. J. Sherer (Eds.), *Psychological assessment in medical rehabilitation.* Washington, DC: American Psychological Association.

Caplan, B., & Shecter, J. (1995). The role of nonstandard neuropsychological assessment in rehabilitation: History, rationale, and examples. In L. A. Cushman & M. J. Sherer (Eds.), *Psychological assessment in medical rehabilitation.* Washington, DC: American Psychological Association.

Cushman, L. A. (1988). Secondary neuropsychiatric complications in stroke; Implications for acute care. *Archives of Physical Medicine and Rehabilitation, 69,* 877–879.

Denes, G., Semenza, C., Stoppa, E., & Lis, A. (1982). Unilateral spatial neglect and recovery from hemiplegia. A follow-up study. *Brain, 105,* 543–552.

DeShazer, S. (1988). *Clues: Investigating solutions in brief therapy.* New York: Norton.

Diller, L. (1992). *Psychological and social adjustment after stroke. Final report.* NIDRR Rehabilitation Research and Demonstration Grant #H133A 80057-88, Department of Rehabilitation Medicine, NYU School of Medicine.

Diller, L., Buxbaum, J., & Chiotelis, S. (1972). Relearning motor skills in hemiplegia: Error analysis. *Genetic Psychology Monographs, 85,* 249–286.

Diller, L., Goodgold, J. G., & Kay, T. (1988). *Rehabilitation of traumatic brain injury and stroke; Final report.* New York: Research & Training Center, Department of Rehabilitation Medicine, NYU School of Medicine.

Diller, L., & Riley, E. (1993). The behavioral management of neglect. In I. H. Robertson & J. C. Marshall (Eds.), *Unilateral neglect: Clinical and experimental studies.*

Diller, L., & Weinberg, J. (1970). Evidence for accident-prone behavior in hemiplegic patients. *Archives of Physical Medicine and Rehabilitation, 51,* 358.

Diller, L., & Weinberg, J. (1986). Learning from failures in perceptual cognitive retraining in stroke. In B. Uzzell & Y. Gross (Eds.), *Clinical neuropsychology of intervention.* Boston: Martinus Nijhoff.

Diller, L., & Weinberg, J. (1993). Styles of response in perceptual retraining. In W. A. Gordon (Ed.), *Advances in stroke rehabilitation.* Andover, MA: Andover Medical Publishers.

Dombovy, M. L. (1993). Rehabilitation and the course of recovery after stroke. In J. P. Wishnant (Ed.), *Stroke: Populations, cohorts, clinical trials.* Oxford, MA: Butterworth-Heineman.

Doyle, P. (2002). Health outcomes in stroke survivors. *Archives of Physical Medicine and Rehabilitation, 83*(Suppl. 2), S39–S43.

Egelko, S., Simon, D., Riley, E., Gordon, W., Ruckdeschel-Hibbard, & Diller, L. (1989). First year after stroke: Tracking cognitive and affective deficits. *Archives of Physical Medicine and Rehabilitation, 70,* 297–302.

Gordon, W. A. (1992). *The treatment of affective deficits in a stroke population. Final report.* NIH; NS24608, New York: Department of Rehabilitation Medicine, Mt. Sinai Hospital.

Gordon, W. A., & Diller, L. (1983). Stroke; Coping with a cognitive deficit. In T. G. Burish & L. A. Bradley (Eds.), *Coping with chronic disease.* New York: Academic Press.

Gordon, W. A., & Hibbard, M. R. (1997). Poststroke depression: An examination of the literature. *Archives of Physical Medicine and Rehabilitation, 78,* 658–663.

Gordon, W. A., Hibbard, M., Egelko, S., Diller, L., Shaver, M. S., Lieberman, A., et al. (1985). Perceptual remediation in patients with right brain damage: A comprehensive program. *Archives of Physical Medicine and Rehabilitation, 66,* 353–364.

Gordon, W. A., Hibbard, M. R., Egelko, S., Riley, E., Simon, D., Diller, L., et al. (1991). Issues in the diagnosis of post-stroke depression. *Rehabilitation Psychology, 36,* 142–160.

Granger, C. V. (1998). The emerging science of functional assessment: Our tool for outcome analysis. *Archives of Physical Medicine and Rehabilitation, 79,* 235–242.

Gresham, G. E., Duncan, P. W., Stason, W. B., Adams, H. P., Jr., Adelman, A. M., Alexander, D. N., et al. (1995). *Post Stroke Rehabilitation.* Clinical Practice

Guideline, no. 16. Rockville, MD: Agency for Health Care Policy and Research, U.S. Public Health Service.

Grober, S. E., Gordon, W. A., Silwinski, M., Hibbard, M. R., Aletta, E. G., & Paddison, P. L. (1991). Utility of the Dexamethasone Test in the diagnosis of post-stroke depression. *Archives of Physical Medicine and Rehabilitation, 72,* 1076–1079.

Hajek, V. E., Gagnon, S., & Ruderman, J. A. (1997). Cognitive and functional assessments of stroke patients: An analysis of their relation. *Archives of Physical Medicine and Rehabilitation, 78,* 1327–1331.

Heinemamm, A. W., Cichowski, K., & Kan, E. (1997). Mapping differences in patient satisfaction. *Archives of Physical Medicine and Rehabilitation, 78,* 900.

Hibbard, M. R., Gordon, W. A., Stein, P., Grober, S., & Sliwinski, M. A. (1992). Awareness of disability following stroke. *Rehabilitation Psychology, 37,* 103–119.

Hibbard, M. R., Grober, S. E., Gordon, W. A., Aletta, E. A., & Freeman, A. (1990). Cognitive therapy and the treatment of poststroke depression. *Topics Geriatric Rehabilitation, 5,* 43–55.

Hier, D. B., Mondlock, J., & Caplan, L. (1983). Behavioral abnormalities after right hemisphere stroke. *Neurology, 33,* 337–344.

Hyman, D. M. (1972). The stigma of stroke. *Geriatrics,* 132–141.

Hyndman, D., Ashburn, A., & Stack, E. (2002). Fall events among people with stroke living in the community: Circumstances of falls and characteristics of fallers. *Archives of Physical Medicine and Rehabilitation, 83,* 165–170.

Jones, F. (1998). The accuracy of predicting functional recovery in patients following a stroke, by physiotherapists and patients. *Physiotherapy Research, 3*(4), 244–256.

Jongbloed, L. (1986). Prediction of function after stroke: A critical review. *Stroke, 17*(4), 765–776.

Kase, C., Wolf, P. A., Kelly-Hayes, M., Kannel, W. B., Bachman, D. L., & Linn, R. T. (1987). Intellectual decline following stroke: The Framingham study. *Neurology, 37*(Suppl. I), 119.

Kinsella, G., & Ford, B. (1980). Acute recovery patterns in stroke patients: Neuropsychological factors. *Medical Journal of Australia, 2,* 663–666.

Korner-Bitensky, N., Mayo, N., Cabot, R., Becker, R., & Coopersmith, H. (1989). Motor and functional recovery after stroke: Accuracy of physical therapists' predictions. *Archives of Physical Medicine and Rehabilitation, 70*(2), 95–99.

Kwakkel, G., van Dijk, G. M., & Wagenaar, R. C. (2000). Accuracy of physical and occupational therapists' early predictions of recovery after severe middle cerebral artery stroke. *Clinical Rehabilitation, 14*(1), 28–41.

Langer, K. G. (1992). Psychotherapy with the neurologically impaired adult. *American Journal of Psychotherapy, 46.*

Langer, K. G., & Padrone, F. J. (1992). Psychotherapeutic treatment of awareness in acute rehabilitation in traumatic brain injury. *Neuropsychological Rehabilitation, 2,* 59–71.

Levine, D. (1990). Unawareness of visual motor and sensory defects: An hypothesis. *Brain, 13,* 233.

Lipsey, R., Robinson, R. G., Pearlson, G. D., Rao, K., & Price, T. (1984). Norotriptine treatment of post stroke depression: A double blind study. *Lancet, 11,* 297–300.

Monga, T. N., Lawson, J. S., & Inglis, J. (1986). Sexual dysfunction in stroke patients. *Archives of Physical Medicine and Rehabilitation, 67,* 19–22.

Moroz, A., Bogey, R. A., Bryant, P. R., Geis, C. C., & O'Neill, B. J. (2004). Stroke and neurodegenerative disorders. 2. Stroke: Comorbidities and complications. *Archives of Physical Medicine and Rehabilitation, 85*(3 Suppl. 1), S11–S14.

Morris, P. L. P., Robinson, R. G., Andrzejwski, P., Samuels, J., & Price, T. R. (1993). Association of depression with 10 year mortality in stroke. *American Journal of Psychiatry, 150,* 124–129.

Osmon, D. C., Smet, I. C., Winegarden, B., & Ghandavadi, B. (1992). Neurobehavioral Cognitive Status Examination: Its use with unilateral stroke patients in a rehabilitation setting. *Archives of Physical Medicine and Rehabilitation, 73,* 414–418.

Padrone, F. (1995). *Review of adjustment of stroke in patients in rehabilitation.* New York: Ruck Institute of Rehabilitation Medicine.

Parikh, R. M., Robinson, R. G., Lipsey, J. R., Starkstein, S. E., Federoff, J. P., & Price, T. E. (1990). The impact of post stroke depression on recovery of activities of daily living over a two year follow-up. *Archives of Neurology, 47,* 785–790.

Pearce, R. P., & Buxbaum, L. J. (2002). Treatments of unilateral neglect: A review. *Archives of Physical Medicine and Rehabilitation, 83,* 256–268.

Powell, B., Diller, L., & Grynbaum, B. (1976). Rehabilitation performance and adjustment in stroke patients: A study of social class factors. *Genetic Psychology Monographs, 93,* 287–352.

Prigitano, G. P., & Wong, J. L. (1997). Speed of finger tapping and goal attainment after unilateral cerebral accident. *Archives of Physical Medicine and Rehabilitation, 78,* 847–852.

Rapport, L. J., Webster, J. S., Fleming, K. L., Lindberg, J. W., Godlewski, M. C., Brhee, J. E., et al. (1993). Predictors of falls among right hemisphere stroke patients in the rehabilitation setting. *Archives of Physical Medicine and Rehabilitation, 74,* 621–626.

Reynolds, E. H., & Wilson, J. V. K. (2004). Stroke in Babylonia. *Archives of Neurology, 61,* 597–601.

Robertson, I. H., Hogg, K., & McMillan, T. M. (1998). Rehabilitation of unilateral neglect; Improving function by contralateral limb activation. *Neuropsychological Rehabilitation, 8,* 19–30.

Robinson, R. G., Bolduc, P. L., & Price, T. R. (1987). A two year longitudinal study of post stroke mood disorders; Diagnosis and outcome at two years. *Stroke, 18*, 837–845.

Roth, E. J., & Harvey, R. L. (1996). Rehabilitation of stroke syndromes. In R. L. Braddom (Ed.), *Physical medicine and rehabilitation*. Philadelphia: W. B. Saunders.

Roth, E. J., Heinemann, A. W., Lovell, L., Harvey, R. L., McGuir, J. R., & Diaz, S. (1998). Impairment and disability: Their relation during stroke rehabilitation. *Archives of Physical Medicine and Rehabilitation, 79*, 329–341.

Schenkenberg, T., Bradford, D. C., & Ajax, E. T. (1980). Line bisection and unilateral visual neglect in patients with visual impairment. *Neurology, 30*, 509–517.

Schubert, D. S., Burns, R., Paras, W., & Sioson, E. (1992a). Decrease of depression during stroke and amputation rehabilitation. *General Hospital Psychiatry, 14*, 135–141.

Schubert, D. S., Burns, R., Paras, W., & Sioson, E. (1992b). Increase of medical hospital length of stay by depression in stroke and amputation patients; A pilot study. *Psychotherapy Psychosomatics, 52*, 61–66.

Schubert, D. S., Taylor, C., Lee, S., Mentari, A., & Tamaklo, W. (1992a). Physical consequences of depression in the stroke patient. *General Hospital Psychiatry, 14*, 69–76.

Schubert, D. S., Taylor, C., Lee, S., Mentari, A., & Tamaklo, W. (1992b). Detection of depression in the stroke patient. *Psychosomatics, 33*, 290–294.

Starkstein, S. E., & Robinson, R. G. (1994). Neuropsychiatric aspects of stroke. In H. Coffey & J. L. Cummings (Eds.), *Textbook of geriatric psychiatry*. Washington, DC: American Psychiatric Association.

Stone, S. P., Wilson, B., Wroot, A., Halligan, P. W., Lange, S. L., Marshal, J. C., et al. (1991). The assessment of visual spatial neglect after acute stroke. *Journal of Neurology Neurosurgery and Psychiatry, 54*, 345–350.

Thompson, S. C. (1991). The search for meaning following stroke. *Basic & Applied Social Psychology, 12*, 81–86.

Titus, M. N., Gall, N. G., Yerxa, E. J., Robertson, T. A., & Mack, W. (1991). Correlation of perceptual performance and activities of daily living in stroke patients. *American Journal of Occupational Therapy, 45*, 510–518.

Toedter, L. J., Schall, R., Reese, C. A. S., Hyland, D. T., Berk, S. N., & Dunn, D. S. (1995). Psychological measures: Reliability in the assessment of stroke patients. *Archives of Physical Medicine and Rehabilitation, 76*, 719–725.

Tulski, D., & Rosenthal, M. (2002). Quality of life measurement in rehabilitation. *Archives of Physical Medicine and Rehabilitation, 83*(Suppl. 2), S1–S3.

Wade, D. T., Parker, V., & Langton-Hewer, R. L. (1986). Memory losses after stroke: Frequency and associated losses. *International Rehabilitation Medicine, 8*, 68–74.

Wagner, M. T., Nayak, M., & Fink, C. (1995). Bedside screening of neurocognitive function. In L. A. Cushman & M. J. Scherer (Eds.), *Psychological assessment in medical rehabilitation*. Washington, DC: Amer Psychol Assoc.

Warren, M. (1990). Identification of visual scanning deficits in adults after cerebrovascular accidents. *American Journal of Occupational Therapy, 44,* 391–399.

Webster, J. S., Jones, S., Blanton, P., Gross, R., Beissel, G., & Wofford, J. (1984). Visual training with stroke patients. *Behavior Therapy, 15,* 129–143.

Webster, J. S., Roades, L. A., Morrill, B., Rapport, L. J., Abadee, P. S., Sowa, M. V., et al. (1995). Rightward orienting bias, wheelchair maneuvering, and fall risk. *Archives of Physical Medicine and Rehabilitation, 76,* 924–928

Webster's New College Dictionary. (1995). New York: Houghton-Mifflin.

Weinberg, J., & Diller, L. (1966). Denial of a reading disability. *American Psychology, 74.*

Weinberg, J., & Diller, L. (1968). On reading newspapers by hemiplegics—Denial of visual disability. *Proceedings of the 76th Annual Convention of the American Psychological Association,* pp. 655–656.

Weinberg, J., & Diller, L. (2000). Dealing with rationalization and unawareness in the treatment of visual inattention. In K. E. Langer, L. Laatsch, & L. Lewis (Eds.), *Psychotherapy in individuals with acquired brain injury.* New Haven, CT: International University Press.

Weinberg, J., Diller, L., Gordon, W. A., Gerstman, L., Lieberman, A., Lakin, P., et al. (1977). Visual scanning training effect on reading-related tasks in acquired right brain damage. *Archives of Physical Medicine and Rehabilitation, 58,* 479–486.

Weinberg, J., Diller, L., Gordon, W. A., Gerstman, L., Lieberman, A., Lakin, P., et al. (1979). Training sensory awareness and spatial organization in people with right brain damage. *Archives of Physical Medicine and Rehabilitation, 60,* 491–496.

Weinberg, J., Piasetsky, E., Diller, L., & Gordon, W. A. (1982). Treating perceptual organization deficits in non-neglecting RBD stroke patients. *Journal of Clinical Neuropsychology, 4,* 59–75.

Weissberg, S., Esibell, N., & Zuger, R. R. (1971). Factors in the vocational success of hemiplegic patients. *Archives of Physical Medicine and Rehabilitation, 52,* 441–447.

Wiart, L., Saint Come, A. B., Debelleix, X., Petit, H., Joseph, P. A., Mazaux, J. M., et al. (1997). Unilateral neglect syndrome rehabilitation by trunk rotation and scanning training. *Archives of Physical Medicine and Rehabilitation, 78,* 424–436.

Wiebe-Valesquez, S., & Hachinski, V. (1991). Overview of clinical issues in stroke. In R. A. Bornstein & G. Brown (Eds.), *Neurobehavioral aspects of cerebrovascular disease* (pp. 111–130). New York: Oxford University Press.

Wilson, B. A., Cockburn, J., & Baddley, A. (1989). *The Rivermead Behavioural Memory Test—II.* Bury St. Edmunds, UK: Thames Valley Test.

Wilson, B. A., Cockburn, J., & Halligan, P. (1987a). *The Rivermead Behavioural Inattention Test.* Bury St. Edmunds, UK: Thames Valley Test.

Wilson, B. A., Cockburn, J., & Halligan, P. C. (1987b). Development of a behavioral test of visuospatial neglect. *Archives of Physical Medicine and Rehabilitation, 68,* 98–102.

Williams, L. S., Ghose, S. S., & Swindle, R. W. (2004). Depression and other mental health diagnoses decrease mortality after ischemic stroke. *American Journal of Psychiatry, 6,* 1090–1095.

Yagura, H., Miyai, I., Seiki, I., Suzuki, T., & Yanangihara, T. (2003). Benefit of inpatient multidisciplinary rehabilitation up to 1 year after stroke. *Archives of Physical Medicine and Rehabilitation, 84,* 1687–1692.

Zoccolotti, P., & Judica, A. (1991). Functional evaluation of hemineglect by means of a semistructures scale: Personal extrapersonal differentiation. *Neuropsychological Rehabilitation, 1,* 29–44.

Zuger, R. R., & Boehm, M. (1993). Stroke: A new challenge for vocational rehabilitation. In W. A. Gordon (Ed.), *Advances in stroke rehabilitation* (pp. 258–268). Boston: Andover Medical Publishers.

26

Substance Use Disorders in Rehabilitation

CONSTANCE SALTZ CORLEY, MSW, PhD,

MARCIA J. LAWTON, PhD, AND MURIEL GRAY, PhD

THE ABUSE OF and dependence on recreational, medicinal, and otherwise harmful substances have been noted historically for centuries, accompanied by a wide range of explanations of causality. Although a discussion of etiology is beyond the scope of this chapter, awareness of the impact of harmful substances on persons presenting in health care settings (whether due to the consequences of one episode of using crack or a long-term addiction to tobacco) is essential for practitioners. The thrust of this chapter is to help those in a gatekeeper role to identify addiction and to know how to refer the client to an appropriate component of the continuum of care.

The chapter begins with an overview of the prevalence, cost, and consequences of chemical abuse and dependency, with a brief presentation of definitions and terminology. The chapter then focuses on addiction, using the substance of alcohol to explore the addiction process, screening, intervention, treatment, and recovery. Relevant considerations pertaining to several other major addictions (especially cocaine and nicotine) are addressed, and the growing importance of substance use and abuse by older persons is also noted (Corley, Gray, & Yakimo, in press). Implications for treatment on both the practice and policy levels are discussed in the concluding section of the chapter.

PREVALENCE

THE MOST RECENT national survey on drug abuse (Substance Abuse
and Mental Health Services Administration [SAMHSA], 2003) found
that overall drug use has leveled off since 1995. However, a substantial
number of persons in the United States continue to abuse one or more
of the following substances: alcohol, tobacco, marijuana, cocaine/crack,
heroin, hallucinogens, inhalants, and psychotherapeutic drugs used for
nonmedical purposes (e.g., sedatives, tranquilizers, stimulants, analgesics, and anabolic steroids).

According to the National Survey on Drug Use and Health (formerly
known as the National Household Survey on Drug Abuse) (SAMHSA,
2003), legal drugs are the most used and abused. The per capita alcohol
consumption has increased, so alcohol continues to be the most commonly used and abused substance. It is used by about half of the U.S.
population age 12 years and older. Of those users, about 22.9% engaged
in binge drinking, and 6.7% were heavy drinkers. An estimated 7% of
adults have an alcohol use disorder (either abuse or dependence)
(National Institute on Alcohol Abuse and Alcoholism [NIAAA], 2003)
and 30.5% of the traffic crash deaths in the United States are attributed
to alcohol consumption (NIAAA, 2003). Alcohol in combination with
other drugs was mentioned in 39% of deaths reported in medical examiner cases (SAMHSA, 1995). The prevalence of substance use disorders
in general and alcohol disorders in particular is difficult to determine.
Data gathered from the National Hospital Discharge Surveys concluded
that hospital discharge records may underrepresent the extent of disorders related to alcohol use. It found that, whereas 7.4% of hospital patients
had an alcohol-related diagnosis, when screened specifically for alcohol
problems, 22% screened positive (NIAAA, 1997). Substance use disorders
also lead to a myriad of social, legal, and job-related problems.

Tobacco, like alcohol, is a highly addictive legal substance. It is used
regularly by 30.4% of the U.S. population age 12 years and older. According
to the Monitoring the Future study (National Institute on Drug Abuse
[NIDA], 1996), cigarette smoking among youth continues to decline.
However, it has been noted that cigarette smokers are more likely to use
alcohol and illicit drugs than nonsmokers (NIDA, 1996).

Approximately 8.3% of the U.S. population 12 years of age and older
reported current use of an illicit substance in the 2002 (SAMHSA, 2003).
Marijuana is the most commonly used illicit substance. Of current illicit
drug users, 75% reported marijuana use (SAMHSA, 1997). According to
the 2002 NSDUH, the rate of marijuana initiation has been approximately the same since 1995 but the initiation age is estimated to be
between 10 and 11 years of age (SAMHSA, 2003).

The proportion of the population age 12 years and older who are current cocaine users remains stable at approximately 0.9% (SAMHSA, 2003). However, cocaine was the most frequently reported substance in drug abuse deaths. According to data from the Drug Abuse Warning Network (SAMHSA, 2004), it was reported in nearly half of drug-related deaths.

According to 1995 medical examiner data, heroin is the second most often mentioned substance in drug abuse deaths (SAMHSA, 1997). Results from the 1996 National Household Survey on Drug Abuse show decreasing overall heroin use but an increased number of new users between the ages of 12 and 17 years. They also show that most new heroin users are under the age of 26 years (SAMHSA).

The Drug Abuse Warning Network (SAMHSA, 2003) reports concern about abuse of prescription painkillers—especially narcotic analgesics—and notes a 117% increase in related emergency department visits. While most emergency department mentions of narcotic analgesics did not increase from 2000 to 2001, mentions of OxyCodone increased 70%. In 2001, the average age of patients visiting the emergency department because of narcotic analgesic abuse was 37 years.

Consequences and Costs

Regular use of harmful drugs (some sometimes even a single incident of use of a drug such as crack) can have major adverse medical, psychological, psychiatric, economic, and social consequences. The medical complications resulting from alcoholism (Kinney & Leaton, 1991), especially among older adults (Cummings, Bride, & Rawlins-Shaw, in press), perhaps best illustrate how one widely available substance can affect almost every body system: the cardiovascular, gastrointestinal, genitourinary, endocrine, nervous, musculoskeletal, and immune systems. Major nutritional deficits as well as changes in the skin and hair can result from chronic alcoholism (Kinney & Leaton). Hematological disorders are more common in alcoholics than in the population at large, and at least 10% of all cancers occur in sites affected by heavy drinking (Kinney & Leaton).

In terms of psychological/psychiatric consequences of misuse of alcohol and/or most other harmful substances, the following may result: intoxication, craving, depression/mood swings, anxiety, paranoia, hallucinations/delusions, organic brain syndromes (both acute and chronic), and flashbacks (Kinney & Leaton, 1991). Suicide is a major risk among alcoholics: an estimated 7% to 21% of alcoholics commit suicide (Kinney & Leaton).

Although calculating the economic costs of substance abuse and dependence is more difficult than for other illnesses, the costs of abuse of alcohol, tobacco, and other drugs are estimated as close to or in excess of $400 billion (Center on Addiction and Substance Abuse [CASA], 1993).

Although the primary costs are those of health care expenditures, such figures also take into account lost productivity from employee substance abuse and social losses from premature deaths, substance-induced psychiatric disorders, and family disruption. The impact of substance use disorders on the family will be discussed below.

DEFINITIONS AND TERMINOLOGY

SEVERAL CONCEPTS ARE important in defining and identifying maladaptive effects of harmful substances. These include abuse, dependence, tolerance, withdrawal, addiction, and denial.

Two diagnostic categories that broadly cover chemical misuse are included in the Diagnostic and Statistical Manual Disorders (4th edition, herein referred to as DSM-IV): psychoactive substance abuse and psychoactive substance dependence (American Psychiatric Association [APA], 1995).

CRITERIA FOR SUBSTANCE DEPENDENCE

A MALADAPTIVE PATTERN of substance use, leading to clinically significant impairment of distress, as manifested by three (or more) of the following occurring at any time in the same 12-month period:

1. tolerance, as defined by either of the following:

   a. a need for markedly increased amount of the substance to achieve intoxication or desired effect
   b. markedly diminished effect with continued use of the same amount of the substance

2. withdrawal, as manifested by either of the following:

   a. the characteristic withdrawal syndrome for the substance (refer to Criteria A and B of the criteria sets for withdrawal from the specific substances)
   b. the same (or a closely related) substance is taken to relieve or avoid withdrawal symptoms

3. the substance is often taken in larger amounts or over a longer period than was intended
4. there is a persistent desire or unsuccessful efforts to cut down or control substance use
5. a great deal of time is spend in activities necessary to obtain the substance (e.g., chain-smoking, or recovering from its effects)

6. important social, occupational, or recreational activities are given up or reduced because of substance use
7. the substance use is continued despite knowledge of having a persistent or recurrent physical or psychological problem that is likely to have been caused or exacerbated by the substance (e.g., current cocaine use despite recognition of cocaine-induced depression, or continued drinking despite recognition that an ulcer was caused by alcohol consumption) (p. 181).

CRITERIA FOR SUBSTANCE ABUSE

A. A maladaptive pattern of substance use, leading to clinically significant impairment of distress, as manifested by one (or more) of the following occurring within a 12-month period:

1. recurrent substance use resulting in a failure to fulfill major role obligations at work, school, or home (e.g., repeated absences or poor work performance related to substance use; substance related absences, suspensions or expulsions from school; neglect of children or household)
2. recurrent substance use in situations in which it is physically hazardous (e.g., driving an automobile or operating a machine when impaired by substance use)
3. recurrent substance-related legal problems (e.g., arrests for substance-related disorderly conduct)
4. continued substance use despite having persistent or recurrent social or interpersonal problems caused or exacerbated by the effects of the substance (e.g., arguments with spouse about consequences of intoxication, physical fights)

B. The symptoms have never met the criteria for Substance Dependence for this class of substance (pp. 182–183).

Tolerance occurs with the regular consumption of a substance over an extended period and is one of the defining characteristics of alcohol addiction (Kinney & Leaton, 1995). *Withdrawal* results in the development of adverse physical symptoms when the use of a substance is stopped (Beasley, 1990).

Addiction, the primary emphasis of this chapter, is a physiological process in which the person with an addiction craves one or more substances, uses the substance(s) compulsively (daily and/or in binges), and continues using the substance(s) despite a range of adverse consequences (Beasley, 1990). Tolerance and withdrawal occur with many forms of addiction (e.g., alcohol).*Denial* of addiction itself is usually also a hallmark of addiction.

Given the multifactorial nature of addiction, the following factors must be taken into account during assessment, intervention, treatment, and recovery: biological, psychological, social/economic, and spiritual. This will be referred to as the biopsychosocial-spiritual approach. The process of addiction to alcohol through the steps to recovery is now presented to exemplify this approach.

ALCOHOLISM AS AN EXAMPLE OF ADDICTION

THE NATURE OF the addiction process has been most extensively studied and is best understood with alcoholism. Therefore, alcoholism is used here to demonstrate the highlights of the addiction process: screening, recovery, intervention, and treatment.

ADDICTION PROCESS

ALCOHOLISM HAS GENERALLY been accepted, since the American Medical Association (AMA) declaration in 1956, as a primary, chronic, progressive, family disease. The most notable aspect of alcoholism (or any addiction) is the development of the denial system. This is not simply a psychological defense used to cope with anxiety but a complex system composed of multiple mechanisms (blaming, minimizing, rationalizing, intellectualization, humor, and others, depending on the individual), which becomes an unconscious way to protect a lifestyle focused on alcohol. One of the best practical resources on understanding denial, from Hazelden (1975), describes it as follows:

> The development of a denial system is a cardinal and integral feature of chemical dependency. It is one of the major symptoms of this disease and develops along with the more visible symptoms, that is, harmful consequences. To a greater or lesser extent, it can be found in all chemically dependent persons. Denial is the fatal aspect of alcoholism and other drug dependencies. It impairs the judgment of affected individuals and results in self-delusion which keeps them locked into an increasingly destructive pattern. It is the denial system which, for example, permits a chemically dependent person [sic] to ignore a physician's advice of "stop or you will die." (p. 9)

In addition to the denial system, alcoholism is characterized by certain predictable signs and symptoms that manifest themselves as the illness progresses. There are some discrepancies as to what constitutes alcoholism or at what point one crosses the imaginary line. There does appear to be a fairly wide acceptance that once a person reaches a stage where there are physical consequences (tremors, liver damage, etc.) and loss of ordinary willpower, alcoholism is in the picture. Other consequences may occur earlier in the process: psychological (e.g., guilt), mental (e.g., preoccupation with alcohol), and spiritual (e.g., moral deterioration) signs; these deserve as much attention as do the physical consequences.

A very important aspect of this chronic illness is relapse; it is addressed later in more detail. What triggers this relapse or resumption of use varies. Gorski (Miller, Gorski, & Miller, 1982) and Marlatt (Marlatt & Gordon, 1985), coming from different philosophical orientations (the former from a disease orientation, and the latter from a learned-behavior one), both stress the significance of relapse. Indicators that the addiction is being activated even before the person with an alcohol addiction resumes drinking include recurrence of the denial system, tendencies toward loneliness, a feeling that nothing can be solved, progressive loss of daily structure, thoughts of social drinking, and unreasonable resentments.

The role of the family in maintaining or returning to addiction to alcohol has been increasingly studied (Wegschneider, 1981). Alcoholism has been described as a hanging mobile; as one member changes, the others have to make adjustments to acquire an equilibrium. Jackson (1954) spells out the seven adjustment stages through which family members go as a person with an alcohol addiction progresses in his or her disease: attempts to deny the problem, social isolation, disorganization of family structure, efforts to reorganize in spite of the problem, attempts to escape the problem, reorganization of part of the family, and, finally, recovery and reorganization of the whole family.

In understanding the significance of the family, it is important to address two concepts: enabling and codependency. Enabling is any behavior on the part of anyone that protects the denial system of a person with an alcohol addiction. Codependency is a term full of confusion in the addiction field today. It currently has a variety of meanings, many of which focus on it as an addiction in its own right, whereby the person with codependent behavior is addicted to having someone else provide emotional support and in fact defines his or her own identity by that relationship. Probably the best and most useful definition of codependency is the following: "Codependency is a pattern of painful dependency upon compulsive behaviors and on approval from others in search for safety, self-worth and identity. Recovery is possible" (Lawton, 1990, p. 1).

SCREENING FOR ALCOHOLISM

AN OVERALL RECOMMENDATION is that the practitioner begins work with an individual to examine at a conscious level the client's relationship with alcohol. If the client is comfortable in that relationship and does not let alcohol control his or her behavior and the ability to deal effectively with life stresses and problems, then he or she probably is not a person with an alcohol addiction. To assist further in the decision about drinking behavior, Alcoholics Anonymous (AA) has prepared a brief pamphlet that includes 12 questions such as "do you wish people would mind their own business about your drinking—stop telling you what to do?" (Alcoholics Anonymous, 1973). As a guideline, if the client answers yes to 4 or more of the 12 questions, then there is probably trouble with alcohol. The counselor can review this material with the client along with information on the progressive signs of alcoholism (e.g., using the chart developed by Glatt in 1957, based on Jellinek's research published in 1954). Additional tools are available in the form of the Trauma Scale (Skinner, Holt, Schuller, Roy, & Israel, 1984), the CAGE (Ewing, 1984), the Michigan Alcoholism Screening Test (MAST) (Selzer, 1971), and formalized interviews such as the Addictions Severity Index (ASI) McLellan, Luborsky, Woody, & O'Brien, 1980).

The CAGE is composed of four simple questions:

1. Have you ever tried to Cut down on your drinking?
2. Do you get Annoyed when drinking is criticized?
3. Do you feel Guilty about your drinking?
4. Do you use alcohol as an "Eye-opener"?

The MAST is a self-report test with 25 items regarding the consequences of problem drinking; a positive answer of 12 or 13 deserves taking some action. The ASI is a structured clinical interview suitable for use with persons with either an alcohol or drug addiction. It can be administered by a technician in about 20 to 30 minutes and provides a problem severity profile reflecting six areas: medical, psychological, legal, family/social, employment/support, and chemical abuse. Each area is measured independently, and the severity is derived from two kinds of information: the client's subjective judgment and objective data (e.g., lab reports).

There are some clinical lab tests available (serum gamma-glutamyltransferase and aspartate amniotransferase) that can indicate an alcohol problem, but unfortunately they lack diagnostic specificity and are not positive until later stages of addiction when denial is strongest (NIAAA, 1990). Sometimes, particularly negative consequences of alcoholism (e.g., citations for driving under the influence) can be indicators of alcoholism; the helpful role these can play in presenting the reality of the illness will be discussed in the intervention section.

RECOVERY FROM ALCOHOL

ON THE JELLINEK chart referred to earlier (Glatt, 1957), recovery is pictured as a mirror-image representation of the addiction process. However, more research done by Brown (1985) on a dynamic, developmental model of recovery belies this description. Brown discovered a process whereby the individual undergoes a second-order change regarding the ability to control drinking. The stages are (a) drinking: "I can control my drinking." "I am not an alcoholic [sic]."; (b) transition: "I cannot control my drinking." "I am an alcoholic [sic]."; (c) early recovery: same as transition but with a beginning awareness of the environment and a slight interpersonal focus; (d) ongoing recovery: same as transition but with increased awareness of environment and relationship between self and others.

Brown (1985) acknowledges the role of AA in accomplishing these changes. Since its inception in 1935, AA has been beneficial to many persons with an alcohol addiction as a support system that recognizes the internal healing that occurs in recovery. This self-help movement emphasizes self-responsibility and surrender to a higher power. The focus is on spirituality, the energy force within each person, rather than on religion as an institution with a set of rules created by people (Lawton, 1991a). This is the spiritual component mentioned in the biopsychosocial-spiritual approach discussed in the introduction and in Kuhn's (1988) article, which provides a spiritual inventory for the person with a medical illness. It should be noted that recovery is an internal healing process with its own developmental stages and is distinct from the external treatment given to an individual.

INTERVENTION WITH THE ALCOHOLIC

BECAUSE THE DENIAL system is the most crucial aspect of addiction, it is essential that it be addressed to stop the cycle and promote recovery. Johnson (1980) found that, by involving significant others (or concerned persons) in the planning part of the intervention and helping break through their denial, there was increased likelihood of reaching the person with an alcohol addiction. A trained professional teaches the concerned persons about alcoholism as a disease, helps them collect factual data about the consequences of the drinking of an individual with an alcohol addiction, and works through the concerned person's anger and judgmental attitudes through attendance at counseling meetings and AA support groups. The group then formalizes a concrete plan with clear alternatives, such as "go to treatment" or "accept my having to leave the family."

Following a real crisis (such as arrest for driving under the influence), when the guilt of the individual with an alcohol addiction is the highest and defenses are the weakest, the group meets with the individual with an addiction and presents the prepared choices. When done in a factual, nonjudgmental, caring manner that taps into the core being of the person with an alcohol addiction, it is most likely to achieve changes.

TREATMENT FOR ALCOHOLISM

SINCE ITS INCEPTION in 1949, the Minnesota Model developed at Hazelden (www.hazelden.org) has gained widespread recognition as the treatment of choice for the person with an alcohol addiction and his/her family. It focuses on the holistic nature of alcoholism:

1. Philosophy of treatment: assumption that alcoholism/chemical dependency exists; it is a multiphasic illness; focus on the phenomenon of addiction as the major presenting problem; denial is part of the illness.
2. Goals of treatment: improved mental and physical health achieved through total abstinence.
3. Content of treatment: help people take better care of themselves by understanding chemical dependency as well as the strategies that will help maintain sobriety.
4. Quality of interdisciplinary staff: trained people who meet professional standards to address the physical, social, family, spiritual, and psychological areas; important that recovering chemically dependent people are part of the staff.
5. Duration of treatment: length of stay based on the average time it takes a typical patient to complete primary care; treatment duration must remain individualized.
6. Intensity of treatment: living in a therapeutic community that includes lectures, group meetings, individual meetings with professionals as needed, aftercare planning.
7. Context of treatment: atmosphere conducive to self-evaluation; environment in which people are treated with dignity and respect by staff who are caring and concerned—a caring community.
8. Quality assurance measures: process and outcome quality measurements (Engleman, 1989).

Although the Minnesota Model focuses on a therapeutic community to provide services, earlier detection of alcoholism and limited insurance coverage for treatment have led to a broader and more varied choice of options, with emphasis on utilizing outpatient services initially, if not exclusively in some instances. A diagram of the current continuum of care in the addiction field (adapted from Jans, 1991) is depicted in Figure 26.1.

Although this picture appears somewhat confusing to the uninitiated, efforts are under way to help clarify placement criteria. In particular, the American Society of Addictive Medicine (ASAM) and the National Association of Alcohol Treatment Programs (NAATP) cooperated in developing a set of guidelines that has been well accepted by the field (Lawton, 1991b). Four different levels of care are highlighted: out-

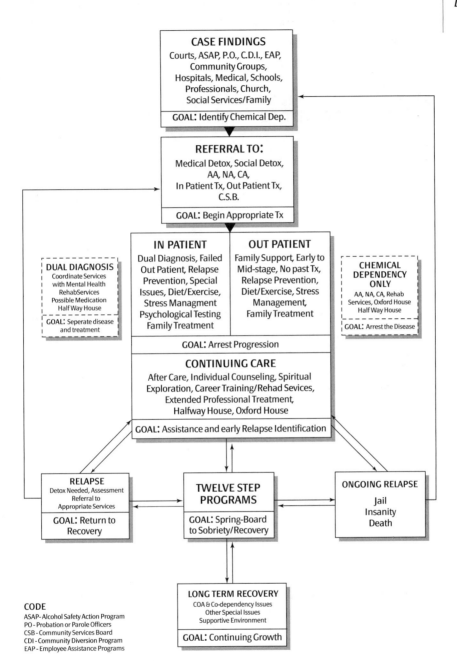

FIGURE 26.1 Continuum of care.

patient, outpatient with partial hospitalization, medically monitored intensive inpatient, and medically managed intensive inpatient. The assignments are not limited to "medical necessity" but include biopsychosocial considerations.

SPECIAL CONSIDERATIONS WITH OTHER ADDICTIONS

COCAINE

ALTHOUGH COCAINE IS a stimulant rather than a depressant, the person with a cocaine addiction (like the person with an alcohol addiction) nevertheless manifests the characteristics common to addiction, such as the denial system, preoccupation, and loss of control. "Coke" addiction has its own distinctive signs and symptoms (e.g., weight loss, chronic runny nose, frequent upper respiratory infections, loss of interests, auditory hallucinations, and repetitive compulsive acts such as tapping fingers or playing with hair). They occur in a sequence of three phases: crash, withdrawal, and extinction.

The fatal nature of cocaine may more likely be played out in heart failure than in liver or pancreatic diseases as seen in alcoholism (Nuckols, 1989). One substantial difference encountered in cocaine addiction is the problem of intense cravings, which serve to perpetuate the use of cocaine. This appears to be the result of the vivid euphoric memories associated with cocaine binges. Also, with cocaine addiction there is the issue of illegality, which can intensify the isolation because of the perceived need to keep the use secret for fear of the legal consequences. Finally, a further complication resulting from cocaine addiction is the situation in which intravenous needles are used, leading to an increased possibility of acquired immune deficiency syndrome (AIDS).

In treating cocaine addiction it appears that simply using the standard addiction approach of breaking denial is not sufficient. Additionally, pharmacological nonaddictive antidepressants (e.g., imipramine) are being tried, along with psychotherapeutic treatment focusing on the systematic desensitization of the person with an addiction to craving-loaded cues like razor blades or syringes (Gawin, 1990).

NICOTINE

ALTHOUGH NICOTINE FOLLOWS the benchmarks for addiction in its own right, it is mentioned here because of another interesting aspect: it can be a gateway and/or trigger to another addiction, especially alcohol. Evidence is mounting to suggest that it plays a part in preventing quality sobriety or in fact even abstinence from other substance. Treatment is increasingly moving way from dealing with one addiction at a time and including trigger addictions as part of the initial treatment. For example, hospital units use decaffeinated coffee and have "no smoking" rules (Henningfield, Clayton, & Pollin, 1990; Pletcher, Lysaght, & Human, 1990).

OTHER ADDICTIONS

SO FAR, EXCEPT for codependency, which appears to be in a class of its own, the discussion has been on drug addictions (primarily alcohol, cocaine, and nicotine). It is also possible to demonstrate the same major characteristics of addiction (denial system, loss of control, preoccupation, and moral deterioration) with other compulsive behaviors such as over-eating and gambling. It is not within the scope of this chapter to address the many details associated with a specific addiction. Two general resources that cover the substance addictions in more depth are *Concepts of Chemical Dependency* (Doweiko, 1996) and *Visions of Addiction* (Peele, 1988).

Misuse and abuse of prescription and over-the-counter medications also are receiving increased attention. Older persons "are at a particularly high risk for addiction due to their more frequent use of medications to treat a variety of acute and chronic medical conditions . . . and to a high prevalence of depression and anxiety disorders" (Lowinson, Ruiz, Millman, & Langrod, 1992, p. 849). Polyaddiction among persons who are older may be masked by the greater prevalence of multiple medical conditions.

SUBSTANCE USE AND OLDER ADULTS

THERE IS GROWING interest in addressing the impact of substance use disorders among older adults, who are the highest utilizers of both prescription and over-the-counter drugs. While not traditionally viewed as a population with high utilization of alcohol and illicit substances, older adults are more vulnerable to the adverse effects of alcohol (Cummings et al., in press), particularly in combination with medications.

Services targeted to this population are limited, yet there is a pressing need to address new cohorts of older adults whose patterns of substance use and abuse are more intense than in previous generations (e.g., the Baby Boomers who are turning 65 in 2011). In addition, differentiating early-onset alcoholism and late-onset alcoholism and its impact (McInnis-Dittrich, 2002) is critical (e.g., late-onset alcoholics are less likely to see their alcohol use as a problem). Additionally, defining what constitutes "problem drinking" is controversial, since older adults may not demonstrate the more prominent impairments seen in younger populations (e.g., financial or occupational). Instead, health impacts such as increased falls, high blood pressure, and/or memory loss may mask an addiction and only be treated symptomatically (McInniss-Dittrich). Issues of assessment, diagnostic validity, and treatment modalities tailored to older adults are increasingly being addressed (Corley et al., in press).

RELAPSE PREVENTION

R EGARDLESS OF THE substance, primary intensive treatment alone is not sufficient for these disorders. Relapse prevention as a biopsychosocial strategy to maintain abstinence and a healthy lifestyle is critical (Gray, 2004).

Although relapse prevention is individualized to address client needs (e.g., older adults), most such treatment plans include social support approaches, lifestyle change approaches, cognitive-behavioral approaches, and pharmacological approaches (USDHHS, 1995; Wormer, 1995).

Research studies (NIAAA, 1997) cite the fact that the availability of social resources following primary intensive inpatient treatment increased the rate of abstinence among patients. Special resources may include psychosocial therapy, relationship enhancement, aftercare groups, family networks, and many types of support groups. The most prevalent type of support groups associated with abstinence from substance use and the prevention of relapse are 12-step programs such as AA and Narcotics Anonymous. Rational Recovery, a support group utilizing the Addictive Voice Recognition Technique (AVRT) (Trimpey, 1996), and SMART (Self Management and Recovery Training) Recovery, a support group using a cognitive-behavioral approach based on Rational Emotive Behavior Therapy (REBT) (Knaus, 1995), are relatively new support groups offering alternatives to the spiritually-based 12-step programs. Other support groups, like Women for Sobriety, are population-specific, and still other approaches (e.g., One Church One Addict) are religion- and church-based.

Approaches addressing lifestyle changes focus on breaking ties with people who use drugs and teaching ways of coping with negative behaviors while acquiring a new social identity as a person who does not use drug substances. Many of these approaches utilize the cognitive-behavioral approach to teach self-efficacy and avoidance skills, using such instrument as the Situational Confidence Questionnaire (Annis & Graham, 1988) and workbooks such as the *Staying Sober Workbook* (Gorski, 1989) to identify warning signs and internal and external cues associated with cravings.

According to *Effectiveness of Substance Abuse Treatment* (USDHHS, 1995), many pharmacotherapies are now available for the treatment of substance use disorders and the prevention of relapse. For opiate addiction, such drugs as buprenorphine, clonidine, methadone, naltrexone, and LAAM (levo-alpha-acetyl methanol) are approved as opiate-craving blockers. Some of these also have been found effective in the treatment of alcohol use disorders, specifically, disulfiram (Antabuse), an alcohol-sentizing agent for avoidance of alcohol consumption, and naltrexone for alcohol craving and opiate addiction. Some antidepressant medication trials have found mixed results in reducing cocaine abuse. The efficacy of these therapies continues to be studied.

IMPLICATIONS

GREATER SOCIETAL AWARENESS of the multidimensional impact of chemical abuse and dependency has led to increased prevention efforts as well as awareness of the need for early recognition and treatment. Health care professionals are in a critical position (as gatekeepers to a range of services and programs) to provide and/or refer those at risk to educational, diagnostic, intervention, and treatment options.

Addiction per se must be considered a primary illness in health care settings. If overlooked or inadequately treated, it will continue to take its toll on individuals, their families, and society at large. Identifying and managing triggers (e.g., caffeine and nicotine) for other chemical use and addiction, especially among younger persons and those who are compromised by health problems or otherwise vulnerable because of changes in social status (such as unemployment or homelessness), are essential. It is increasingly important to increase awareness of the needs of diverse populations (including older adults) and to increase the number of culturally sensitive prevention and intervention programs (Cummings et al., in press; Grant et al., 2004).

Building support for persons at risk may require community-based treatment and referral, with long-term follow-up and services to pertinent family members and significant others. Although they are beyond the scope of this chapter, there are additional considerations in working with persons who abuse or are addicted to multiple substances and in addressing those persons who may also have a psychiatric history (i.e., dual diagnosis). Access to care and follow-up for those with multiple treatment needs is often inadequate and sometimes inappropriately provided.

Addiction, like other chronic disorders, is a lifelong illness requiring a comprehensive approach. Given the rapid and confusing changes in the organization and financing of health care services, treatment for persons with addictions and/or their families may be compromised.

This is particularly evident with the introduction of managed care and cost-containment approaches intended to control cost in the traditional medical acute-care setting, where treatment is based on medical necessity and physician's orders. The same criteria are not always applicable to the rehabilitation model needed for addiction, a chronic, multidimensional illness for which family support and aftercare services are critical (Spicer, 1991). Managed care will undoubtedly have an impact on the current role of employee assistance programs (EAPs), which serve as an identification/referral arm for industry in the area of chemical abuse and dependency. EAPs could be considered as duplication of, replacement for, and/or supplements to managed care programs. In some instances, the company providing the EAP services may also have a separate contract to administer and manage mental health and substance abuse related treatment needs. In any event, the trend is toward reduced reimbursement of fewer services, which will profoundly affect access to essential treatment and follow-up for addicted persons and their families.

In spite of the negative aspects of addiction, with its stigma and pervasive prevalence, there is a very positive aspect to be considered. Since the beginning of AA in 1935 there has emerged increasing hope for converting the crisis of addiction into an opportunity to improve the overall quality of one's life. With the advent of the Hughes Act in 1970 (Comprehensive Alcohol Abuse and Alcoholism Prevention, Treatment, and Rehabilitation Act), the chances to capitalize on these opportunities were enhanced as the stigma was decreased and appropriate resources were developed. Although currently there seems to be a loss in momentum and a shift backward toward an emphasis on controlling drug use through restricting supply and/or punishment of users, the progress and gains of the past several decades are still available for those with the motivation and access to services. Using the biopsychosocial-spiritual approach, it is the role of those with professional credentials to identify the addiction, challenge the denial system of the person, and work with the person and his or her family to find the resources necessary for treatment and recovery. With appropriate and adequate care, persons who abuse or are addicted to harmful substances can return to and/or maintain healthy and productive lives.

REFERENCES

Alcoholics Anonymous. (1973). *Is AA enough?* New York: Alcoholics Anonymous World Services.

American Psychiatric Association. (1995). *Diagnostic and statistical manual of mental disorders* (4th ed., revised). Washington, DC: Author.

Annis, H., & Graham, J. (1988). *Situational Confidence Questionnaire (SCQ-39) user's guide*. Toronto, Canada: Addiction Research Foundation.

Beasley, J. (1990). *Diagnosing and managing chemical dependency*. Durant, OK: Essential Medical Information Systems.

Brown, S. (1985). *Treating the alcoholic: A developmental model of recovery*. New York: John Wiley.

Center on Addiction and Substance Abuse. (1993). *The cost of substance abuse to America's health care system: Report 1: Medicaid hospital costs*. New York: Columbia University Press.

Corley, C. S., Gray, M., & Yakimo, R. (in press). Substance abuse service networks and aging. In B. Berkman & S. D'Ambruoso (Eds.), *Handbook of social work and aging*. New York: Oxford University Press.

Cummings, S. M., Bride, B., & Rawlins-Shaw, A. M. (in press). Alcohol abuse treatment for older adults: A review of recent empirical research. *Journal of Evidence-Based Social Work Practice*.

Doweiko, H. (1996). *Concepts of chemical dependency*. Pacific Grove, CA: Brooks/Cole.

Ewing, J. A. (1984). Detecting alcoholism: The CAGE questionnaire. *Journal of the American Medical Association, 252*, 1905–1907.

Gawin, F. (1990). Cocaine addiction: Psychology and neurophysiology. *Science, 251*, 1580–1585.

Glatt, M. M. (1957). Group therapy in alcoholism. *British Journal of Addiction, 54*, 21–28.

Gorski, T. (1989). *The staying sober workbook*. Independence, MO: Harold House Press.

Grant, B., Dawson, D., Stinson, F., Chou, S., Dufour, M., & Pickering, R. (2004). The 12-month prevalence and trends in DSM-IV alcohol abuse and dependence: United States, 1991–1992 and 2001–2002. *Drug and Alcohol Dependence, 74*, 223–234.

Gray, M. (2004). Relapse prevention. In L. Straussner (Ed.), *Clinical work with substance abusing clients*. New York: Guilford Press.

Hazelden Foundation. (1975). *Dealing with denial*. Caring Community Series. Center City, MN: Hazelden.

Henningfield, J., Clayton, R., & Pollin, W. (1990). Involvement of tobacco in alcoholism and illicit drug use. *British Journal of Addiction, 85*, 279–292.

Jackson, J. K. (1954). The adjustment of the family to the crisis of alcoholism. *Quarterly Journal of Studies on Alcoholism, 15*, 562–586.

Jans, P. (1991). *Delivery of services: Continuum of care*. Unpublished manuscript, Virginia Commonwealth University, Richmond.

Jellinek, J. K. (1954). *The disease concept of alcoholism*. New Haven, CT: College and University Press.

Johnson, V. E. (1980). *I'll quit tomorrow*. New York: Harper & Row.

Kinney, J., & Leaton, G. (1991). *Loosening the grip: A handbook of alcohol information*. St. Louis, MO: Mosby-Year Book.

Knaus, W. (1995). *S.M.A.R.T. Recovery: A sensible primer.* Longmeadow, MA: Author.

Kuhn, C. C. (1988). A spiritual inventory of the medically ill patient. *Psychiatric Medicine, 6*(2), 87–100.

Lawton, M. J. (Ed.). (1990). Codependency: The search for definition. *Addiction Letter, 6*(8), 1.

Lawton, M. J. (Ed.). (1991a). A thread in the tapestry of life. *Addiction Letter, 7* (11), 8.

Lawton, M. J. (Ed.). (1991b). Two provider groups propose patient placement criteria. *Addiction Letter, 7*(2), 3.

Lowinsin, J., Ruiz, P., Millman, R., & Langrod, J. (1992). *Substance abuse: A comprehensive textbook* (2nd ed.). Baltimore: Williams and Wilkins.

Marlatt, G., & Gordon, J. (1985). *Relapse prevention.* New York: Guilford Press.

McLellan, A. T., Luborsky, L., Woody, G., & O'Brien, C. (1980). An improved diagnostic evaluation instrument for substance abuse patients: The Addiction Severity Index. *Journal of Nervous and Mental Diseases, 168,* 26–33.

McInnis-Dittrich, K. (2002). *Social work with elders: A biopsychosocial approach to assessment and intervention.* Boston: Allyn & Bacon.

Miller, M., Gorski, T., & Miller, D. (1982). *Learning to live again.* Independence, MO: Independence Press.

National Institute on Alcohol Abuse and Alcoholism. (1990). *Alcohol and health.* Washington, DC: U.S. Government Printing Office.

National Institute on Alcohol Abuse and Alcoholism. (1997). *Alcohol and health.* Washington, DC: U.S. Government Printing Office.

National Institute on Alcohol Abuse and Alcoholism. (2000). *10th Special Report to the U.S. Congress on Alcohol and Health.* Available: http://www.niaa. nih.gov/publications//10report/intro.pdf

National Institute on Drug Abuse. (1991). *Drug abuse and drug abuse research.* Washington, DC: U.S. Government Printing Office.

National Institute on Drug Abuse. (1996). *The Monitoring the Future Study, 1975–1995.* Washington, DC: U.S. Government Printing Office.

National Institute on Drug Abuse. (1997). *Epidemiologic trends in drug abuse* (Volume 1: NIH Publication No. 97-4204). Rockville, MD: National Institutes of Health.

Nuckols, C. C. (1989). *Cocaine: From dependency to recovery.* Blue Ridge Summit, PA: TAB Books.

Peele, S. (Ed.). (1988). *Visions of addiction: Major contemporary perspectives on addiction and alcoholism.* Lexington, KY: Lexington Press.

Pletcher, V., Lysaght, L., & Human, V. (1990). *Treating nicotine addiction.* Center City, MN: Hazelden.

Selzer, M. L. (1971). The Michigan Alcoholism Screening Test: The quest for a new diagnostic instrument. *American Journal of Psychiatry, 127*(12), 89–94.

Skinner, H., Holt, S., Schuller, R., Roy, J., & Israel, Y. (1984). Identification of alcohol abuse using laboratory tests and history of trauma. *Annals of Internal Medicine, 101,* 847–851.

Spicer, J. (1991, May). The rehabilitation concept in managed care: Uneasy partners. *Professional Update*, p. 3.

Substance Abuse and Mental Health Services Administration. (1995). *Drug Abuse Warning Network annual medical examiner data 1995*. Washington, DC: U.S. Government Printing Office.

Substance Abuse and Mental Health Services Administration. (1997). *Preliminary results from the 1996 national household survey on drug abuse*. Washington, DC: U.S. Government Printing Office.

Substance Abuse and Mental Health Services Administration, Office of Applied Studies. (2002). *National Survey on Drug Use and Health (NSDUH), The Monitoring the Future, 2001 and 2002*. Ann Arbor: University of Michigan.

Substance Abuse and Mental Health Services Administration. (2003). *Results from the 2002 National Survey on Drug Use and Health: National Findings*. (OAS, NHSDA Series H-22, DHHS, Publication number SMA 03-3836). Rockville, MD: U.S. Government Printing Office.

Substance Abuse and Mental Health Services Administration, Office of Applied Studies (OAS). (2004). *Mortality data from the Drug Abuse Warning Network (DAWN), 2002*. DAWN Series D-25, DHHS Publication number (SMA) 04-3875. Rockville, MD: U.S. Government Printing Office.

Trimpey, J. (1996). *Rational recovery: The new cure for substance addiction*. New York: Simon & Schuster.

U.S. Department of Health and Human Services. (1995). *Effectiveness of substance abuse treatment* (DHHS Publication No. SMA95-3067). Washington, DC: U.S. Government Printing Office.

Wegschneider, S. (1981). *Another chance: Hope and health for the alcoholic family*. Palo Alto, CA: Science and Behavior Books.

Wormer, K. (1995). *Alcoholism treatment: A social work perspective*. Chicago: Nelson-Hall Publishers.

27

Visual Impairments

BRUCE P. ROSENTHAL, OD, FAAO, AND
ROY GORDON COLE, OD, FAAO

VISION IMPAIRMENT, WHICH can be defined as a visual acuity of 20/50 or worse vision in the better eye even with eyeglasses, affects a significant proportion of middle-aged and older Americans. Vision impairment also has a significant affect on the national economy and is estimated to cost $4 billion in benefits and lost taxable income (Vision Problems in the U.S., 2002).

The estimated prevalence rates at age 75 years is 2% in the white population and 4% in the Hispanic and black population, according to the National Eye Institute. By age 80 years the prevalence dramatically increases to 14% in the Hispanic population, 9% in Blacks, and 8% in Whites. In another study, one in six adults (17%) age 45 years and older, representing 13.5 million Americans, reports some form of vision impairment even when wearing glasses or contact lenses (The Lighthouse, National Survey on Vision Loss, 1995). The prevalence of visual impairment increases with age and is estimated as follows (Robinson, Acorn, Miller, & Lyle, 1997; The Lighthouse, National Survey on Vision Loss):

1. 15% of Americans age 45–64 years, representing 7.2 million persons.
2. 17% of Americans age 65–74 years, representing 3.1 million persons.
3. 26% of Americans age 75 years and older, representing 3.5 million persons.

According to a Gallup poll, blindness is "the worst thing that can happen" to 42% of the Americans polled (Research to Prevent Blindness, 1989). It has also been reported that 71% of Americans age 45 years and older fear being blind more than being deaf, and 76% fear being blind more than having to use a wheelchair (The Lighthouse, 1995). Fortunately, the blindness that people often think of (cannot see light, needs a guide dog, has to learn braille) rarely occurs. It is not uncommon, however, to have a loss of vision to the point that one has a significant problem in maintaining a satisfactory quality of life. What this means can vary from individual to individual, so a careful evaluation of the patient's abilities and needs is required before attempting to implement a rehabilitation program.

WHERE WE'VE COME FROM AND WHERE WE ARE

VISION REHABILITATION REALLY got its start after World War II (as did medical rehabilitation), when the blinded veterans who came back from the war recovered from their wounds but were still blind (or otherwise handicapped). Attention was paid more to psychosocial and vocational issues, and care was provided by an interdisciplinary team. Unfortunately, these two rehabilitation programs (vision and medical) split apart, and the first civilian Low Vision Rehabilitation Center was opened at the VA Hospital in Hines, Illinois, in 1948. Initially this system (vision rehabilitation) worked mainly with healthy blind veterans, but in 1978 there was an amendment to the Rehabilitation Act of 1973 designating funds for independent living skills training for older adults. Since older adults develop many other health problems, it would make sense for these two system to come back together, and that is what seems to now be happening (Wainapel, 2001).

There are currently two parallel systems in the U.S. that provide services to older adults, but they have not really collaborated: the Blindness System (sometimes referred to as an educational model), and the Health Care System (sometimes referred to as a medical model). There is also a third system, the Aging System, that works with aging and sick adults, but not really with the visually impaired or blind. Aging visually impaired people sometimes fall through the cracks, each group (vision and aging) feeling that the other should be taking care of this person. Again, this seems to be being addressed somewhat at present (Warren, 2000).

Besides the fact that occupational therapists have been getting more involved in providing vision rehabilitation care, thus bringing together the health and vision issues of the patient, there have been changes in Medicare, and also legislative attempts, to provide more care and coverage for these visually impaired or blind adults.

MEDICARE, THIRD PARTY COVERAGE, AND LEGISLATION

THE PROBLEM WITH Medicare coverage in the past was that there was no distinct national policy. Local medical review policies were inconsistent and/or non-existent. Vision-impaired patients were denied full and consistent access to rehabilitation services. This started to change with statements in two appropriations bills in 2 consecutive years:

> The Committee is concerned that although one in six people over the age of 65 has a vision impairment, the Medicare program has not been responsive to the needs of visually impaired older adults, and coverage of low vision services is inconsistent and inadequate. *The Committee urges HCFA to study the impact of vision loss on beneficiary health status and health care costs.* (Appropriations Bill, 2001) (emphasis by author)

> Medicare beneficiaries who are blind or visually impaired are eligible for physician-prescribed rehabilitation services from approved health care professionals on the same basis as beneficiaries with other medical conditions that result in reduced physical functioning. *The Committee urges CMS to direct its carriers to inform physicians and other providers about the availability of medically necessary rehabilitation services for these beneficiaries.* (Appropriations Bill, 2002) (emphasis by author)

These statements resulted in the issuing of a Program Memorandum by Medicare (AB-02-78) on May 29, 2002. It clarified equal access and coverage of necessary rehabilitation services, and it directed the local carriers to publish the Memorandum in provider newsletters/bulletins. Without going into detail, it stated that Medicare-covered therapeutic services could include mobility, activities of daily living, and other rehabilitation goals that are medically necessary. It discusses coverage and limitations, lists the applicable HCPCS Therapeutic Procedures and the ICD-9 Codes for Vision Impairment that support medical necessity. One major change that this Memorandum brought was the fact that visually impaired people who are NOT legally blind can get coverage. It raised the acuity level requirement from 20/200 (severely impaired—legally blind) to 20/70 (moderately impaired), and added a number of visual field conditions that could also now be covered (Program Memorandum accessed 4/24/04 at http://www.empiremedicare.com/news/njarchives02/053002med.htm).

In 2003, Congress encouraged CMS to recognize the additional component of in-home care:

> The committee commends CMS for issuing a program memorandum to clarify that Medicare [benefits] . . . and believes that vision rehabilitation

services provided in a clinical setting may be enhanced by a brief course of additional vision rehabilitation in the home. *The committee encourages CMS to direct carriers and intermediaries to recognize the delivery of additional vision rehabilitation in the home that are included in a clinical care plan.* (Appropriations Bill, 2003) (emphasis by author)

There have been legislative attempts at coverage since 1999, but none have passed either House as of early 2004. The latest language coming out of Congress (as of early 2004) was in the Medicare Drug Bill, Section 645. When the compromise bill finally came out, it directed the Secretary to study the feasibility and advisability of Medicare payment for services of vision rehabilitation professionals:

SEC. 645. STUDIES RELATING TO VISION IMPAIRMENTS

(a) COVERAGE OF OUTPATIENT VISION SERVICES FURNISHED BY VISION REHABILITATION PROFESSIONALS UNDER PART B.—

(1) STUDY.—The Secretary shall conduct a study to determine the feasibility and advisability of providing for payment for vision rehabilitation services furnished by vision rehabilitation professionals.

(2) REPORT.—Not later than January 1, 2005, the Secretary shall submit to Congress a report on the study conducted under paragraph (1) together with recommendations for such legislation or administrative action as the Secretary determines to be appropriate.

(3) VISION REHABILITATION PROFESSIONAL DEFINED.—In this subsection, the term "vision rehabilitation professional" means an orientation and mobility specialist, a rehabilitation teacher, or a low vision therapist. (accessed 4/22/04 at http://www.apha.org/legislative/legislative/hr1-conflegtext.pdf)

Two other provider proposals came out in 2003 in the CONFERENCE REPORT ON H.R. 2673, CONSOLIDATED APPROPRIATIONS ACT, 2004—(House of Representatives—November 25, 2003):

H12580: Directs the Secretary to report on the provision of services by vision rehabilitation professionals (including in the home) under "general" supervision:

By January 1, 2005, the Secretary shall develop policy recommendations and issue a report to Congress by which vision rehabilitation services would be provided by vision rehabilitation professionals in an appropriate setting, including the patient's home environs, acting under a qualified physician's general supervision. The report may include adopting a national credentialing measure, or other steps deemed necessary by the

Secretary, that would ensure patient quality of care. In developing the recommendations, the Secretary should consult with the National Vision Rehabilitation Cooperative, the Association for Education and Rehabilitation of the Blind, the Academy for Certification of Vision Rehabilitation and Education Professionals, the American Academy of Ophthalmology, and the American Optometric Association and other interested organizations. (accessed 4/22/04 at http://www.congress.gov-/cgi-bin/query/F?r108:1:./temp/~r108sXo5gC:e2549639:)

H12745: Requests a demonstration to examine the impact of "standardized" national vision rehabilitation provided in the home by physicians, occupational therapists and vision rehabilitation teachers:

VISION REHABILITATION

The Secretary of the Department of Health and Human Services is directed to carry out a nationwide outpatient vision rehabilitation services demonstration project. The purpose of this demonstration project is to examine the impact of standardized national coverage for vision rehabilitation services provided in the home by physicians, occupational therapists and certified vision rehabilitation teachers.

This demonstration project should be conducted over a period of five years beginning July 1, 2004. The Secretary shall expend from available funds appropriated to him in FY 2004, including transfers authorized under existing authorities from the Federal Supplementary Insurance Trust Fund, an amount not to exceed $2 million for FY 2004 to carry out this demonstration project. (accessed 4/22/04 at http://www.congress.gov-/cgi-bin/query/F?r108:1:./temp/~r108DPNrgO:e3813204:)

Because other third-party coverage generally follows Medicare, it is expected that other policies will soon cover vision rehabilitation, if they are not already doing so. It should be noted that Medicare does not cover the low vision examination done by optometrists and ophthalmologists. The medical part of the exam would be covered, but there is generally a charge to the patient for the non-covered part ("refractive" or "optical"). Medicare also does not currently cover the provision of low vision devices that are so beneficial to most of these patients. The American Academy of Ophthalmology and the American Optometric Association are currently trying to address these issues. In the current climate of downsizing and budget limitations, this will not be an easy task.

NOTE: Physicians (MDs) can contact the American Academy of Ophthalmology (Vision Rehabilitation Committee), and optometrists (ODs) can contact the American Optometric Association (Low Vision Rehabilitation Section) to find out the latest status of coverage.

FACTORS AFFECTING VISUAL FUNCTION AND THEIR TREATMENT

THE MAIN IMPAIRMENTS affecting visual function are reduced visual acuity, visual field loss, poor contrast sensitivity, and lighting and glare problems. These factors and their treatment are discussed below. Other impairments generally of less importance include color vision problems and binocular vision problems.

VISUAL ACUITY

BASED ON 1990 estimates, approximately 2.3 million Americans aged 40 years and older have a best corrected visual acuity of worse than 20/40 but better than 20/200 in the better eye, and 912,000 individuals are legally blind (Prevent Blindness America, 1994).

Measured visual acuity gives us an indication of the patient's ability to resolve detail. "Normal" acuity (i.e., 20/20) is based on the assumption that an individual should be able to separate objects that are 1 minute apart in visual angle. People can have better vision (20/15 and even 20/10). The limitation on acuity level is generally determined by the spacing of the cones. Cone spacing predicts that the smallest features of the acuity target should be about half a minute apart, corresponding to a Snellen acuity of 20/10 (Arditi, 1997). Visual acuity is generally written as a fraction, the numerator of which represents the test distance and the denominator of which represents the letter size.

$$\text{Visual Acuity} \ = \ \frac{\text{testing distance}}{\text{letter size}}$$

The letter size is actually a distance measurement: the distance at which the letter must be held to subtend a visual angle of 5 minutes at the eye. When test distances in feet are used, we see acuities such as 20/20 or 20/200. When metric distances are used, these acuities become 6/6 and 6/60. All acuities can be represented as decimal acuities, and this is done by "dividing out the fraction"; that is, 20/20 becomes 1.0; 20/200 becomes 0.1. Another way that visual acuity can be defined is as follows:

$$\text{Visual Acuity} \ = \ \frac{\text{distance at which letter was read}}{\text{distance at which letter subtends 5' of arc}}$$

When working with people whose vision is significantly reduced, the acuity can still be measured accurately. One technique simply involves walking the patient up to the test chart, thus reducing the test distance and increasing the sensitivity of the chart. Another technique is to use a test chart with larger letters or numbers and a larger selection of intermediate sizes. In this case, very low levels of vision can still be measured, even worse than 20/2000.

A patient with reduced visual acuity is unable to resolve detail. In some cases, all that is needed is an up-to-date refraction, resulting in a new pair of glasses for general wear. When glasses by themselves are not adequate, additional interventions must be initiated. This is generally accomplished by making the image on the retina larger, that is, using some form of magnification. Magnification can be provided in one of three ways: making the object larger (e.g., large-print books), moving the object closer (e.g., sitting closer to the television or bringing the reading material closer to the eyes when using stronger reading glasses), or using some optical device to make the object look bigger (e.g., a telescope to see distant objects better or a magnifier for reading). One of the goals of the low-vision examination (discussed below) is to determine and prescribe the appropriate level and type of magnification.

VISUAL FIELD

WHEREAS VISUAL ACUITY gives us an indication of the patient's ability to resolve detail, the visual field gives us information regarding the patency of the whole retina (the central and peripheral areas of the retina). When we test the visual field, we are generally, but not exclusively, evaluating "peripheral vision." This is important for the patient to be able to detect objects around him. Once the individual detects an object, he/she can look at it and identify it (using visual acuity). The visual field becomes an especially important factor when discussing and considering training for mobility problems.

Perimetry, which is the technique of measuring the visual field, employs a variety of techniques. These may include manual as well as automated evaluation of the entire visual field with kinetic or static stimuli. The automated perimeter has paved the way for more standardized and accurate visual field testing in all types of patients, including those with low vision (Bass & Sherman, 1996).

There are different ways that the visual field can be affected. A loss of vision in a specific area is referred to as a scotoma. It should be noted that scotomas in the visual field can have almost any size and shape, and the number of scotomas a patient has can also vary significantly. Scotomas can be located in the center of the macula (referred to as a central scotoma), affecting straight-ahead vision with a concurrent reduction in visual acuity. The magnification principles discussed above would apply. Scotomas also can be located adjacent to the central area (paracentral scotoma). In this case, acuity is usually not affected; interference comes from the scotoma's closeness to what is being viewed.

An overall peripheral field defect can interfere with mobility. This is the situation when only a small central part of the visual field remains. Mobility problems generally occur when the overall remaining central field subtends an angle of about 5° or less, but some patients are bothered even earlier. Scotomas also can be limited to one side of the visual field (hemianopia). These can be very detrimental to patient function because the patient cannot see objects to that side. This can interfere significantly with general mobility, as well as with near tasks like reading and writing.

In some cases, scotomas are caused by the treatment the patient receives. The multiple small scotomas that occur following laser photocoagulation for conditions such as macular degeneration and diabetic retinopathy are examples of this.

The treatment of a visual field defect will vary, depending on the size, location, number, and severity of the scotomas. Generally, there is no good optical treatment available, although in some cases either prisms or mirrors can be of help. Generally, the patient must learn to live with and compensate for the defect. Orientation and mobility training (especially cane travel), and also visual scanning training will often be helpful.

CONTRAST

VISUAL ACUITY CHARTS measure high-contrast vision (very black letters on very light backgrounds). Most of the world, however, is not high contrast, and this can explain some situations in which patients feel their vision has worsened although the measured acuity is the same. If tested on a contrast sensitivity chart, the doctor might find that the contrast sensitivity of the patient has changed; this would then account for the subjective change in perceived vision.

The benefit of contrast sensitivity testing is that it often gives us an indication of who will respond poorly to standard magnification levels or who will need higher levels of lighting to perform their desired tasks. It is not unusual, in fact, to see patients function with significantly weaker lenses when very bright light (e.g., using a halogen bulb) is incorporated into the task (along with appropriate glare-control techniques).

LIGHTING AND GLARE

IT IS OFTEN impossible to predict how much light a patient needs. Too much can be as detrimental as not enough. The best way to test for lighting level is to see how the patient responds to different light levels and note the effect of the light levels on patient performance. Patients also complain about glare. One broad definition of glare is "light that does not contribute to retinal imagery but has an adverse effect on visual efficiency, visual comfort, or resolution" (Waiss & Cohen, 1991, p. 436). Intraocular glare problems can sometimes be solved by removing the source of the glare (e.g., cataracts). If the glare source is external, one can either modify the environment or filter out the distracting wavelengths causing the glare problem by using special filters, such as yellow or amber lenses, or visors.

DEFINITIONS AND STATISTICS

LEGAL BLINDNESS

PROBABLY THE MOST common definition of blindness states that an individual is legally blind if either the best corrected visual acuity (with standard lenses) is 20/200 (6/60) or worse in the better eye or if the remaining central visual field is restricted to 20° or less in the widest meridian of the better eye.

The leading causes of new cases of legal blindness, according to the National Eye Institute, are macular degeneration, glaucoma, and diabetic retinopathy.

The acuity part of this definition dates back to 1935, when the Social Security Act, with its benefits to the blind, was passed. The visual field part was added as an amendment the following year (Simons, 1991). This definition has been adopted widely by federal, state, and local agencies throughout the United States. It is even used by the Internal Revenue Service to determine tax benefits.

The problem with this definition of legal blindness is that it has little or no validated experimental basis. Anyone working in the field has had patients with relatively poor visual acuity or visual field (considered legally blind) who functioned very well and other patients with relatively good visual acuity and fields (not legally blind) who could barely do anything for themselves. Thus, from a rehabilitation point of view, it makes more sense to talk in terms of visual disability.

DISORDER, IMPAIRMENT, DISABILITY, AND HANDICAP

THERE HAVE BEEN many attempts at defining visual impairment. The World Health Organization (WHO, 1993) devised a classification of impairments, disabilities, and handicaps that has been applied to vision. This *International Classification of Impairments, Disabilities, and Handicaps* (ICIDH) is a classification system that distinguishes between the consequences of diseases, accidents, and disorders on these three different levels (Visio, 1993).

A visual impairment can be defined generally as any loss or abnormality of an anatomical structure or of a physiological or psychological function. Some examples of visual impairments would be reduced visual acuity, visual field loss, and loss of contrast. The visual impairment may be categorized as normal, near-normal, moderate, severe, profound, near-total, or total vision loss, depending on the degree of loss of visual acuity or visual field.

There is a continuum in the classification of visual performance. Individuals classified with low vision may have visual acuity ranging between 20/30 and 20/40 to 20/1000, with the term *blindness* applied to all categories with performance worse than this (hand motion, light perception, no light perception) (WHO, 1977).

Another classification system, developed by August Colenbrander (1977), shows how *impairment* relates to *disorder* and *disability*. A disorder may be defined as "any deviation from normal structure and or function of the body or parts thereof" (e.g., a cataract). A disorder can lead to an impairment, which is "a disorder interfering with an organ function" (e.g., reduced visual acuity, reduced visual field, reduced contrast sensitivity). An impairment can lead to a disability, which is "the lack, loss, or reduction of an individual's ability to perform certain tasks" (e.g., cannot read a newspaper). It should be noted that *impairment* refers to the basic functions performed by a part of the body, whereas *disability* refers to tasks performed by a person.

A handicap is "a disadvantage for a given individual, resulting from an impairment or a disability, that limits or prevents the fulfillment of a role that is normal (depending on age, sex, and social-cultural factors) for that individual" (Visio, 1993). A patient could be considered *handicapped* if reading the newspaper is an activity that is important in this person's life and he cannot do it. Individuals who do not need to read the newspaper and do not want to should not be considered handicapped by this disability.

It is interesting to note that the World Health Organization has adopted new terms for "disability" and "handicap," namely, "activity" and "participation," respectively. Thus, an impairment leads to an inability to do an activity (the disability), which can lead to an inability of participation in society (the handicap) (accessed 12/28/04 http://www3.who.int/ief/beginners/bg.pdf).

Arditi and Rosenthal (1996) defined visual impairment as a significant limitation of visual capability resulting from disease, trauma, or congenital condition that cannot be fully ameliorated by standard refractive correction, medication, or surgery. An impairment is manifested by one or more of the following:

1. Insufficient visual resolution (worse than 20/60 in the better eye with best correction of ametropia).
2. Inadequate field of vision (worse than 20° along the widest meridian in the eye, with the more intact central field, or homonymous hemianopia).
3. Reduced peak contrast sensitivity (< 1.7 log CS binocularly).

OVERVIEW OF TOTAL VISION REHABILITATION

BEFORE A NY type of visual rehabilitation is considered, the patient must have a thorough medical eye evaluation, along with the initiation of any medical and or surgical interventions. The ultimate goal in the rehabilitation of a visually impaired person is to maximize the use of any residual vision and compensate for vision loss.

MAXIMIZING THE USE OF RESIDUAL VISION WITH CLINICAL LOW-VISION CARE

BEFORE ANY TYPE of vision rehabilitation services are recommended and implemented, it is important that a low vision examination be done. The low-vision examination will identify the patient's functional goals (visual), assess the patient's current level of visual functioning, and determine whether any modifications can be made to attain these goals. As mentioned, the objective of the low-vision examination is to maximize the use of the residual vision. Based on the results of this examination, the patient will be categorized as either "sighted" or "blind" and will be guided into the appropriate rehabilitation model. Thus, the low-vision examination is the key component tying together the medical model and the rehabilitation model and making certain that patients are channeled into the correct programs.

In January 1990, a conference was held at which 14 vision rehabilitation agencies from around the country collaborated on the growing problem of age-related vision loss (Lighthouse, 1990a). During this conference, there was discussion of low vision as the core service. The low-vision examination provides older persons their first opportunity to work with a low-vision clinician who will assess their residual vision, detail how the vision loss has personally affected their functional abilities, and explore in a receptive environment ways in which that vision may be enhanced or maximized. This is a unique service that is only carried out by either a low-vision practitioner, a free-standing low-vision service, or a vision rehabilitation agency. The expertise that exists among low-vision specialists and vision rehabilitation agencies should be developed and marketed because it is this service that most responds to the chief complaint of older persons with vision loss (Lighthouse, 1990b, p. 3). The chief complaint of a majority of older persons was previously identified (in this same reference) as "I want to see better."

COMPENSATING FOR VISION LOSS WITH VISION REHABILITATION

ONCE THE CLINICAL low-vision care has been completed or at least initiated to the point that current functional levels and desired goals have been determined, the general vision rehabilitation of the patient can be initiated. (It should be noted that there are occasions when the entry point for the patient into rehabilitation services occurs in the agencies providing general vision rehabilitation care. However, a low-vision examination must be an essential, and early, component of any of the rehabilitation services described in the text that follows.) The rehabilitation can include but is not necessarily limited to the following:

Activities of daily living training, to enable the patient to perform satisfactorily those activities that are commonly needed in one's day-to-day living style. These include such things as food preparation and consumption ("seeing" the food on the plate), personal grooming techniques (applying makeup, shaving, etc.), selecting the appropriate clothing (coordination of colors, etc.), and general house maintenance and cleaning.

Communications skills training, to develop the ability of the patient to handle common interactions with other individuals. This includes both direct verbal communication between individuals, writing techniques, and use of the telephone, special hearing amplifying devices, and the like.

Orientation and mobility training, to enable the patient to navigate safely both indoors and outside. Travel training stresses safe travel and teaches techniques that can be used when traveling alone or with someone else (sighted-guide technique), including detecting obstacles ahead, crossing the street, locating the destination, and using public transportation.

Educational and vocational training, to provide the patient with an educational background (possibly including college and graduate school) for a specific goal. At a minimum, this would be the educational experience needed to attain a basic level of competency. Then, with vocational training, the patient can learn the work skills necessary to be employed and to maintain a certain degree of independence. Included in this is the provision of any special optical devices needed for the specific task being performed, as well as any special equipment (e.g., special computer systems) needed by the patient.

Psychological and social counseling, to help the patient deal with problems in acknowledging and accepting the loss of vision and interacting with other people. Support groups may also provide help for adjusting to vision loss.

Family and peer counseling, to help family and friends understand and deal with the problems the patient is having.

Other needed services: Some patients have very specific and unusual needs. It is important that the patient be carefully questioned as to the problems and needs to be addressed and that the patient be referred to the appropriate individual or agency to receive the necessary services.

Note that these descriptions and definitions can vary from one agency or organization to another and should be taken only as guidelines. It is important to contact the local agencies in your area to find out the specific programs that are offered, how to refer patients, and other information.

THE ROLE OF PATHOLOGY IN VISUAL IMPAIRMENT

ONE OF THE ways to understand the various pathologies that cause a visual impairment is to understand how light travels through the eye.

The cornea and the lens, which are the primary refracting structures of the eye, are the main systems that focus images onto the retina, which is located at the back of the eye. After passing through the lens, the light must travel through the vitreous, which is a clear, jellylike material that fills the interior of the eye. Problems such as cataracts and corneal disease affect these systems and generally result in the patient experiencing an overall blurred image (reduced visual acuity), decreased contrast, and glare.

Eventually, the light will fall on the retina, a structure that is, in effect, a dual image-processing system. The central portion of the retina (macular area) is associated with straight-ahead vision, including detail discrimination and color. The macular area plays a major role in such functions as reading, facial discrimination, and object identification. Problems in the macular area can cause a reduction in visual acuity or a loss of central visual field (a central scotoma, or blind spot). Some of the common conditions in which the macular region is affected include macular degeneration, diabetic retinopathy, and albinism.

The second portion of the retina, the peripheral retina, is associated with object awareness and motion detection. Its function is to allow one to become aware of objects to the side (peripherally, i.e., up, down, right, left, etc.), and it plays a major role in mobility (one's ability to navigate around objects and people without bumping into them). Conditions that affect the peripheral retina result in a loss of side vision, with or without a concurrent reduction in visual acuity. Some of these conditions are glaucoma, retinitis pigmentosa, strokes, and tumors.

The retina changes light into electrical impulses, which leave the eye through the optic nerve and travel a route through the brain (the visual pathways) to the occipital region, in particular, areas 17, 18, and 19, where the interpretation and interaction with other body systems take place.

CATARACT

Description of Medical Condition. The lens is composed of three layers: the nucleus (center), the cortex, and the capsule. It is clear at birth, but throughout life the lens continues to produce cells that become increasingly yellow with age. A cataract (opacity or clouding of the lens) may develop as a result of aging, trauma, hereditary factors, birth defects, or a systemic condition such as diabetes.

Cataracts are a normal part of aging. Approximately 50% of Americans between 65 and 74 years of age and 70% over age 75 years have cataracts (Faye, Rosenthal, & Sussman-Skalka, 1995). Caucasians are three times as likely as Blacks to develop cataracts, smokers are 60% more likely, and those taking medication for gout are twice as likely to develop cataracts.

Functional Presentation of Medical Condition. The greater the progression of the cataract, the greater the visual impairment from the effects of decreased visual acuity, loss of contrast, and glare.

Treatment and Prognosis. Normally, cataracts can be treated very simply: surgical excision and replacement of the cataract with an intraocular lens (IOL). Cataract extraction, which is generally done on an outpatient basis, is considered one of the safest surgical procedures. Assuming a healthy retina, the prognosis for functional cure of any patient problems is high. There is a problem, however, when an underlying ocular pathology such as macular degeneration has been difficult to detect because the opaqueness of the cataract prevents a good look at the inside of the eye. If another condition exists, it must be dealt with in its own regard.

Cataract surgery is indicated when (a) visual function is impaired and it becomes difficult to pursue normal activities such as reading or independent travel or (b) there are medical complications occurring from very advanced cataracts.

Two types of cataract surgery are generally performed. Extracapsular extraction involves the removal of the lens nucleus in one piece from the capsular bag. An IOL is then inserted in the posterior chamber of the eye (behind the iris) during surgery to replace the lens that has been removed.

A second procedure, more commonly implemented in developing countries, is an intracapsular extraction, in which the entire contents (lens and capsule) are removed during surgery. The surgical removal of the lens is then followed by an optical correction with an aphakic spectacle correction or contact lenses.

In some cases, the capsule that is left in the eye can become opaque some time after the initial surgery is done. This is referred to as a secondary cataract or secondary membrane. This can usually be simply treated in the office with a YAG (yttrium aluminum garnet) laser, which opens a hole in the membrane. Patients go in with poor vision, and generally leave with very good vision (assuming there are no problems elsewhere in the eye).

If cataract surgery cannot be done or complications occur, the patient should be referred for a low-vision examination. Although magnification itself might not be as successful as in other eye conditions, approaches using lighting, glare control, and contrast enhancement can often go a long way in helping the patient.

Psychological and Vocational Implications. Assuming no complications, there should be no psychological or vocational implications following cataract surgery. In fact, many individuals are amazed that the visual acuity and color vision is so improved with surgery and that the glare disability has disappeared.

CORNEAL DISEASE

Description of Medical Condition. It has been reported that diseases of the cornea are the leading cause of visits to physicians for medical eye care in the United States (Leonard, 1996; National Eye Institute, 1993). Composed of three layers and two membranes, the cornea is normally clear, but changes in any of the corneal layers or membranes can cause the retinal image to be blurred. The cornea is a structure that is prone to dystrophies, deposition, non-inflammatory progressive thinning (keratoconus), infection, viral diseases, and trauma. It can sometimes be restored with medical treatment but may require either laser treatment or a corneal transplant.

Functional Presentation of Medical Condition. Interference with corneal integrity can result in a blurred or distorted image on the retina. A totally opaque cornea can prevent light from reaching the retina altogether. Patients with corneal disease may experience severe glare, cloudy vision, and also problems with reduced visual acuity.

Treatment and Prognosis. Keratoplasty is the primary method of restoring vision for an individual with a diseased, irregular, or scarred cornea. The procedure involves transplanting a healthy cornea from a compatible donor. It is done to improve the visual acuity as well as preserve the anatomy and physiology of the cornea, remove active disease tissue, and improve the cosmetic appearance of the cornea. The four leading indications for corneal transplantation in the United States are keratoconus, corneal edema after cataract surgery, corneal scarring, and Fuch's dystrophy (Krachmer & Palay, 1991; Lindquist, McGlothan, Rotkis, & Chandler, 1991). Recently, lasers have been used to treat some corneal problems. Where surgery is contraindicated, a scarred or disfigured cornea can be cosmetically "corrected" with a contact lens to match the fellow eye.

If the treatment is not totally successful in restoring vision, the patient should be referred for a low-vision examination. Although magnification itself might not be as successful as in other eye conditions, approaches using lighting, glare control, and contrast enhancement can often go a long way in helping the patient.

Psychological and Vocational Implications. In addition to improving visual function with corneal surgery, a cosmetic contact lens or prosthetic shell should be considered when the cosmetic appearance will enhance professional or personal goals. Consultations with a prosthetic specialist should be considered as early as possible. Vocational goals will be dependent on the degree to which the retinal image is compromised.

MACULAR DEGENERATION

Description of Medical Condition. Macular degeneration is considered one of the leading causes of visual impairment in older adults. There were an estimated 1,651,335 people over the age of 50 with an age-related macular degeneration according to the National Eye Institute (Vision Problems in the U.S., 2002).

As previously noted, the light-sensitive tissue of the eye, the retina, is composed of a central and a peripheral area of receptors, and is analogous to the film in a camera. The macula is centrally located in the retina, and is the area where most of the color photoreceptors (the cones) are concentrated and tightly packed. The central retina specializes in object identification (acuity/resolution tasks such as facial recognition, letter reading, etc.), daylight vision, and color perception. The peripheral retina contains the majority of the rods, which are specialized for night vision as well as object detection and motion detection.

The macula is composed of the fovea (the area having the highest resolution and best visual acuity), the parafovea, and the perifoveal areas. Most frequently associated with the aging process, age-related maculopathy is categorized as either the "dry" or "wet" (exudative) type. It is caused by degenerative changes that can result in atrophy, hemorrhage, exudates, fibrovascular scars, or cyst formation of the macular and paramacular areas.

Risk factors associated with macular degeneration include White race, family history, high blood pressure or a history of hypertension, and light iris color (Maguire, 1997). Another risk factor associated with macular degeneration is smoking. There appears to be an incidence of macular degeneration in smokers that is two to four times the rate in nonsmokers. It is still too early to state whether supplementing the diet with antioxidant vitamins, such as C and E, and selenium, along with the beta carotenoids, such as lutein and zeaxanthin, will have any effect on the reduction of macular disease, but clinical studies are starting to show a positive correlation.

Functional Presentation of Medical Condition. The effect of structural changes in the macula may be visually manifested as distortions, a decrease in visual acuity, a decrease in color recognition, a loss of contrast, or an absolute or relative area of no vision (scotoma). Reading may become progressively more difficult as the disease progresses, driving may have to be discontinued, and employment may be impossible without special low-vision intervention. In addition, macular degeneration has been linked with depression.

Treatment and Prognosis. Fluorescein angiography and indocyanine green (ICG; Yannuzzi, Slakter, Sorensen, et al., 1992) are two of the diagnostic procedures that are used to evaluate the proliferative angiogenic processes of macular degeneration and determine whether treatment might be indicated to slow the progression of the disease. Laser photocoagulation may be indicated to slow down the exudative or hemorrhagic (wet) type of macular disease if detected in the early stages. Patients are also able to monitor the course of the disease with the Amsler grid to determine whether there is a change in the macular area. Any sudden change of the grid (such as waviness or distortion) may be indicative of a leaking retina that might be amenable to laser treatment, especially if done very early. Additional treatments that have been investigated for macular degeneration include the use of radiation therapy, laser treatment of drusen, photodynamic therapy, submacular surgery, retinal cell transplantation, and the use of vascular endothelial growth factor (VEGF). The effectiveness of these treatments has not yet been established.

Fortunately, patients with macular degeneration can often be helped with low-vision interventions. A low-vision examination is recommended to determine which lenses are of value for distant, intermediate, and near tasks. The power and type of magnification is determined by the extent of the visual loss. Except in a minority of cases, functional ability is generally retained to the end, with the use of low-vision devices such as microscopic and telescopic lens systems and absorptive lenses. Talking books are available, free of charge, from the local library system through the federal government. Bold felt-tip pens, talking clocks, and checkbook stencils are some other nonoptical devices that are available for the person with macular disease and low vision. Through the use of low-vision devices, individuals are often able to function with visual acuity as low as 20/1000. Other types of rehabilitation, as discussed in this chapter, are also generally beneficial to the patient.

Psychological and Vocational Implications. As with most visual losses, individuals are most concerned that the condition will progress to complete blindness. Where possible, the eye-care provider and low-vision specialist must reassure the patient that low-vision devices will generally permit the patient to return to normal activities of daily living, such as reading, maintaining a checkbook, or going to museums and the theater. If necessary, other rehabilitation services, such as training in orientation and mobility and activities of daily living, should be advised.

DIABETIC RETINOPATHY

Description of Medical Condition. It is estimated that 16 million people in the United States have diabetes, of whom more than half are not aware that they have the disease (American Diabetes Association, 1995; Leonard, 1996). Late-onset diabetes is the most common form and accounts for 90% of all persons with diabetes (American Diabetes Association, 1988; Flom, 1992). In this country, diabetes accounts for about 5,000 new cases of blindness each year, and diabetic individuals have a 25 times greater risk for blindness than the general population (Flom). Approximately 40% of persons with diabetes have diabetic retinopathy, one of the most devastating conditions affecting the eye. The early, or background, stage manifests itself with small hemorrhages in the eye. This eventually may lead to the more serious proliferative type, which can cause retinal scarring, hemorrhaging into the vitreous, and even retinal detachment.

Functional Presentation of Medical Condition. Diabetic individuals often experience fluctuating or severely decreased visual acuity, which in turn may cause difficulty in reading and seeing the markings on a syringe. They also may experience problems due to glare, reduced contrast sensitivity, and various types of visual field problems. In addition, diabetic individuals can even have transient episodes of diplopia.

Treatment and Prognosis. The Diabetes Control and Complications Trial (DCCT) study showed that strict control of blood sugar is required to reduce the incidence of complications once considered an inevitable result of diabetes (DCCT Research Group, 1995; Fuchs, 1996). Despite regulation of the condition with diet, oral medication, or insulin, however, many individuals still continue to have progressive visual loss. Photocoagulation may be indicated when there is leaking of the blood vessels. In addition, panretinal photocoagulation of the peripheral retina may be indicated to preserve remaining vision, and a cataract may have to be removed.

Despite continued vision loss, low-vision devices will often be of value in enabling an individual to maintain everyday activities. Prisms also have been used to correct for the transitory diplopia. Prognosis, however, must remain guarded.

Psychological and Vocational Implications. Individuals are often depressed and should be directed to a social worker, psychiatrist, psychologist, or discussion group for support. Rehabilitation considerations must include not only vision but also the effect of this debilitating disease on other systems.

GLAUCOMA

Description of Medical Condition. Glaucoma is a disease that, if left untreated, results in the destruction of the peripheral retina. The causes of glaucoma are varied and may be congenital, hereditary, systemic, traumatic, secondary, drug-induced, neoplastic, or surgically induced.

The philosophy of the etiology of glaucoma has been changing. There are basically three types of glaucoma that affect the eye: (1) chronic (open-angle) glaucoma, in which elevated pressure over time eventually affects the optic nerve and visual field; (2) acute (closed-angle) glaucoma, in which there is a rapid increase or spiking of the intraocular pressure that may be accompanied by intense pain and even nausea or vomiting; and (3) low-tension glaucoma, which may be caused by a decrease in blood flow to the optic nerve.

Functional Presentation of Medical Condition. Over a period of time, especially if left untreated, irreversible optic nerve and visual field damage will take place, impairing night vision, visual acuity, mobility, and even the reading skills of the patient. In addition, glare and light sensitivity are also prevalent in individuals with glaucoma.

Treatment and Prognosis. Medications that decrease production of aqueous humor or facilitate outflow of fluid through the trabecular meshwork are generally the first treatments instituted with the glaucoma patient. Some of the drugs used to reduce the IOP (intraocular pressure) are the anticholinergic drugs, beta-blocking agents, carbachol, carbonic anhydrase inhibitors, epinephrine, and pilocarpine. Argon laser trabeculoplasty (ALT), in use since 1979, relieves buildup of pressure by creating drainage holes. Another procedure is a trabeculectomy, which is designed to lower pressure by cutting out a small section of the drainage system (Harrison, 1996).

Low-vision devices, including spectacles, hand and stand magnifiers, closed circuit television (CCTV), lighting, and nonoptical devices are used to return an individual with glaucoma to normal, or at least improved, visual function. Absorptive lenses, especially those that transmit in the yellow visible portion of the spectrum, seem to be especially beneficial for outdoor as well as indoor wear. These lenses enhance the apparent brightness of the scene and often aid in mobility.

Psychological and Vocational Implications. Progressive loss of vision, even with the most rigid compliance, may result in difficulty in performing one's job or pursuing normal activities. Modifications in the work space may be required, with high technology including voice-output devices. Intervention and support groups also should be considered, along with orientation and mobility training for independent travel.

ALBINISM

Description of Medical Condition/Disability Condition. Albinism is a trait that is inherited through autosomal recessive or sex-linked transmission and results in characteristics that affect the pigmentation of the skin and hair as well as the iris and retina. In addition, nystagmus and a significant refractive error are also generally associated with albinism. There is a lack of the pigment in the body and the eye in the tyrosinase-negative (ty-neg oculocutaneous) form of albinism. This "typical" person with albinism has white or platinum hair and irises that appear to be pink. In the tyrosinase-positive (ty-positive oculocutaneous) type of albinism there is some degree of pigmentation in the eye and skin. The ocular albino, however, is distinctive in that the lack of pigmentation is restricted to the eyes only. This person has a normal (and often dark) skin and hair coloring.

Functional Presentation of Medical Condition/Disability Condition. Photophobia varies with the type of albinism. For example, the ty-negative albino is characteristically more sensitive to light than the ty-positive or ocular albino. Nystagmus is also more noticeable in the ty-neg albino than in the ocular albino.

Persons with albinism have a decrease in visual acuity due to macular aplasia, but, as mentioned, the severity of the loss of vision varies with the type of albinism. With regard to visual acuity, the ty-neg albino has the severest visual impairment, and the ocular albino has the least.

Treatment and Prognosis. Because refractive errors are generally significant, the albino should be evaluated for corrective spectacle lenses as early as possible, as well as for absorptive lenses to reduce light sensitivity. The individual with albinism also responds favorably to low-vision devices, including strong microscopic reading lenses, magnifiers, absorptive lenses, and telescopic lenses and should be referred to a specialist in low vision prior to entry into school. The presence of nystagmus is in no way a contraindication to the use of low-vision devices, and people with albinism are often our best low-vision patients.

Psychological and Vocational Implications. The individual with albinism is generally singled out early in life by her or his peers as being different because of physical appearance. Parents and children should have family counseling by an individual familiar with visual disabilities. Vocational implications have changed dramatically, with the acceptance of persons having albinism into most occupations, including medicine.

RETINITIS PIGMENTOSA

Description of Medical Condition/Disability Condition. Retinitis pigmentosa (RP), which is a progressive eye disease that affects the pigmentary layer of the retina, is the most common cause of inherited blindness (National Eye Institute, 1993). In addition, approximately 30% of people with RP report some degree of hearing loss (National RP Foundation, 1995). Though there are many variants of RP, it most commonly affects the periphery or midperiphery of the retina. The speed of the progression of visual field loss varies with each individual; some progress to a significant loss of functional visual field.

The electroretinogram (ERG) is essential in differential diagnosis of RP. The ERG will typically reveal a decreased or absent scotopic response and a reduction in the photopic response as the condition progresses. The visual field is also diagnostically significant in recording the progression of the visual field loss. It is impossible, however, to predict whether an individual diagnosed in the early stages will rapidly progress to a loss of functional vision.

Functional Presentation of Medical Condition/Disability. Night vision and peripheral vision loss go hand in hand. The more advanced the RP, the greater the loss of peripheral vision and the more difficult it is to travel. Legal blindness, as previously noted, is a field restricted to 20° or less in the better eye. Mobility, however, does not generally become a significant problem until the remaining visual field is 5° or less. Reading also becomes progressively more difficult as the visual field becomes small.

Glare or light sensitivity is frequently associated with RP, especially when a small posterior subcapsular cataract is associated with the condition. The need for good lighting, however, is a very important factor in providing optimal visual function.

Treatment and Prognosis. At present no medical or surgical treatments are known to stop or decrease the progression of RP. Periodic eye examinations are essential in monitoring the progression of the condition. Refractive corrections are necessary, along with absorptive lenses to cut down on glare or light sensitivity. In addition, contrast-enhancing lenses such as the NOIR or Corning CPF series may be very beneficial in enhancing performance and reducing adaptation times between outdoors and indoors.

The closed-circuit television (CCTV) is also indicated when reading becomes too difficult with optical devices. The CCTV provides the ability to reverse polarity so that white letters can be seen on a black background, and it enables one to regulate the brightness and contrast of

TABLE 27.1   Summary of Eye Disease Prevalence Data

Prevalence of Cataract, Age-Related Macular Degeneration (AMD), and Open-Angle Glaucoma Among Adults 40 Years and Older in the United States

Age	Cataract		Advanced AMD		Intermediate AMD		Glaucoma	
Years	Persons	(%)	Persons	(%)	Persons	(%)	Persons	(%)
40–49	1,046,000	2.5	20,000	0.1	851,000	2.0	290,000	0.7
50–59	2,123,000	6.8	113,000	0.4	1,053,000	3.4	318,000	1.0
60–69	4,061,000	20.0	147,000	0.7	1,294,000	6.4	369,000	1.8
70–79	6,973,000	42.8	388,000	2.4	1,949,000	12.0	530,000	3.9
≥ 80	6,272,000	68.3	1,081,000	11.8	2,164,000	23.6	711,000	7.7
Total	20,475,000	17.2	1,749,000	1.5	7,311,000	6.1	2,218,000	1.9

Prevalence of Diabetic Retinopathy Among Adults

Age	Type 1 Diabetes		All Diabetes—40 Years and Older	
Years	Persons	(%)	Persons	(%)
18–39	278,000	0.3	NA	NA
40–49	172,000	0.4	589,000	1.4
50–64			1,582,000	3.8
65–74	317,000	0.4	1,068,000	5.8
≥ 75			824,000	5.0
Total	767,000	0.4	4,063,000	3.4

Prevalence of Blindness and Low Vision Among Adults 40 Years and Older in the United States

Age Years	Blindness* Persons	(%)	Low Vision* Persons	(%)	All Vision Impaired Persons	(%)
50–59	45,000	0.1	102,000	0.3	147,000	0.4
60–69	59,000	0.3	176,000	0.9	235,000	1.2
70–79	134,000	0.8	471,000	3.0	605,000	3.8
≥80	648,000	7.0	1,532,000	16.7	2,180,000	23.7
Total	937,000	0.8	2,361,000	2.0	3,298,000	2.7

Estimated Prevalence of Myopia and Hyperopia Among Adults 40 Years and Older in the United States

Age Years	Myopia (Nearsightedness) Persons	(%)	Hyperopia (Farsightedness) Persons	(%)
40–49	15,460,000	36.4	1,534,000	3.1
50–59	7,355,000	23.3	2,325,000	7.7
60–69	3,459,000	17.0	2,538,000	13.2
70–79	2,481,000	15.2	3,112,000	19.3
≥80	1,603,000	17.5	2,168,000	23.6
Total	30,358,000	25.4	11,677,000	9.9

From: Blindness and Visual Impairment (2002).
*Blindness is defined in the U.S. as the best-corrected visual acuity of 6/60 (20/200) or worse in the better-seeing eye; low vision is defined as the best-corrected visual acuity less than 6/12 (20/40) in the better-seeing eye (excluding those who were categorized as being blind by the U.S. definition).
We thank the National Eye Institute for use of their statistics.

the image viewed. Special prism lenses have been used in the later stages of RP to increase the awareness of the periphery. The Nightscope, which was intended to be used for mobility under dim illumination by individuals with RP, has been found to have very limited use.

As the progression continues, so will the loss in mobility. A traveling cane, special laser cane, sensory device, or seeing-eye dog may be indicated to assist in independent travel.

Psychological and Vocational Implications. The fear of total blindness and loss of independence is uppermost in the minds of most individuals with RP. Psychological and family counseling are indicated, as well as genetic counseling for persons contemplating having children.

In accordance with motor vehicle laws, individuals with serious progressive visual field loss should not contemplate occupations that will necessitate driving. They also might have trouble driving because of the field loss even though their acuity it still relatively good.

PERIPHERAL VISUAL FIELD LOSS FROM STROKES OR TUMORS

Description of Medical Condition. Peripheral visual field loss can be the result of inflammatory, vascular, congenital, toxic, or degenerative changes which can occur anywhere in the visual pathway as well as the eye itself. A person who has a stroke or tumor can be left with a resultant visual field loss that may be partial, bilateral, unilateral, homonymous, eccentric, bitemporal, superior, inferior, or nasal. This problem may be compounded by the cognitive, motor, and language disorders that may result from stroke or head trauma (Cohen & Waiss, 1994). In addition there are more complex aspects of the visual process that can be affected. These include perception of visual form, color, object meaning, recognition, and attention. There also may be disorders of the visual system such as hallucinations (Brown & Murphy, 1992).

Functional Presentation of Medical Condition. A complete bilateral loss of the left or right side of vision (homonymous hemianopia) is often the result of a vascular accident in the head. Reading disability is greater when the defect falls in the right visual field. The strategy behind the treatment of hemianopia is to take the visual information present in the nonseeing portion of the field and transfer it for processing into the functioning area of the field (Cohen & Waiss, 1996). Optical treatment generally involves the use of prisms and mirrors. Mobility and night vision may be impaired, and losing one's place while reading is often the result if there is a loss in the either the left visual field (finding the beginning of the next line to be read) or the right visual field (reading to the end of the line being read).

Treatment and Prognosis. Generally, visual field loss is accompanied by "spatial neglect" in the area of the field loss. Prisms have been used to enhance rather than expand spatial awareness when there is a loss in the peripheral visual field. Also, mirrors have been placed on glasses, with less success than prisms, to facilitate peripheral field awareness. Low-vision devices, including the CCTV, have also been of value in reading and vocational pursuits.

Psychological and Vocational Implications. Individuals with peripheral field loss may need counseling to understand the extent of the loss. Driving, though legal, may be dangerous when there is a significant peripheral loss, especially to one side. Individuals with this condition should therefore be discouraged from driving.

REFERENCES

American Diabetes Association. (1988). *Physician's guide to non-insulin dependent (Type II) diabetes: Diagnosis and treatment* (2nd ed.). Alexandria, VA: Author.

American Diabetes Association. (1995). *Diabetes facts and figures* [On-line]. Available from http://www.diabetes.org/ada/c2of.html

Arditi, A. (1997). The macula's role in the acuities. *Aging and Vision News, 9*(2), 3.

Arditi, A., & Rosenthal, B. (1996, July). *Developing an objective definition of visual impairment.* Paper presented at the VISION 96 International Conference on Low-Vision Proceedings, Book 1, Madrid, Spain.

Bass, S. J., & Sherman, J. (1996). Visual field testing in the low vision patient. In B. P. Rosenthal & R. G. Cole (Eds.), *Functional assessment of low vision.* St. Louis, MO: C. V. Mosby.

Blindness and visual impairment: A public health issue for the future as well as today. *Archives of Ophthalmology, 122,* 451–452.

Brown, G. C., & Murphy, R. P. (1992). Visual symptoms associated with choroidal neovascularization: Photopsias and the Charles Bonnet Syndrome. *Archives of Ophthalmology, 110,* 1251.

Cataract Management Guideline Paper. (1993). *Cataract in adults: Management of functional impairment. Clinical Practice Guideline, number 4.* Rockville, MD: U.S. Department of Health and Human Services, Public Health Service, Agency for Health Care Policy and Research (AHCPR Pub. No. 93-0542).

Cohen, J. M., & Waiss, B. M. (1994). An overview of visual rehabilitation for stroke and head trauma patients. *Aging and Vision News, 6,* 3, 11.

Cohen, J. M., & Waiss, B. M. (1996). Visual field remediation. In R. G. Cole & B. P. Rosenthal (Eds.), *Remediation and management of low vision* (pp. 1–126). St. Louis, MO: C. V. Mosby.

Colenbrander, A. (1977). Dimensions of visual performance. *Transactions of the American Academy of Ophthalmology and Otolaryngology, 83,* 322.

Diabetes Control and Complications Trial Research Group. (1995). *Ophthalmology, 102,* 647–661.

Faye, E. E., Rosenthal, B. P., & Sussman-Skalka, C. J. (1995). *Cataract and the aging eye*. New York: The Lighthouse.

Flom, R. (1992). Low vision management of the diabetic patient. *Problems in Optometry, 4*, 2–3.

Fuchs, W. (1996). Preventing diabetic vision loss. *Aging and Vision News, 8*(1), 6–7.

Guyer, D. R., Yannuzzi, L. A., Slakter, J. S., Sorenson, J. S., & Freund, B. (1994). Digital indocyanine green videoangiography of central serous chorioretiopathy. *Archives of Ophthalmology, 112*, 1057–1062.

Harrison, R. (1996). Glaucoma: New concepts, new treatments. *Aging and Vision News, 8*(1).

Krachmer, J., & Palay, D. (1991). Corneal disease. *New England Journal of Medicine, 325*, 1805–1806.

Leonard, R. (1996). *Statistics on vision impairment: A resource manual*. New York: The Lighthouse, Arlene R. Gordon Research Institute.

The Lighthouse. (1990a). *Proceedings of the Lighthouse National Center for Vision and Aging, Miami Conference, January 13–14, 1990*. New York: Author.

The Lighthouse. (1990b). *Statistics on blindness and vision impairment: A resource manual*. New York: Author.

The Lighthouse. (1995). *The Lighthouse National Survey on Vision Loss: The experience, attitudes, and knowledge of middle-aged and older Americans*. New York: Author.

Lindquist, T. D., McGlothan, J. S., Rotkis, W. M., & Chandler, J. W. (1991). Indications for penetrating keratoplasty 1980–1988. *Cornea, 110*, 210–216.

Maguire, M. (1997). Who is at risk? *Aging and Vision News, 9*(2), 5.

National Eye Institute. (1993). *Vision research: A national plan 1994–1998* (NIH Publication No. 95-3186). Bethesda, MD: Author.

National Eye Institute. (2004). Statistics. (Available: http://www.nei.nih.gov/eyedata/tables.asp)

National RP Foundation. (1995). *Fact sheets: Information about retinitis pigmentosa*.

Prevent Blindness America. (2002). *Vision problems in the U.S. Prevalence of adult eye disease and vision impairment in America*. (Available: http://www.preventblindness.org/resources/vision_data.html

Robinson, B., Acorn, C. J. M., Millar, C. C., & Lyle, W. M. (1977). The prevalence of selected ocular diseases and conditions. *Optometry and Vision Science, 74*(2), 79–91.

Simons, K. (1991). Visual acuity and the functional definition of blindness. In W. Tasman & E. A. Jaeger (Eds.), *Duane's clinical ophthalmology* (Vol. 5, rev. ed., pp. 1–21). Philadelphia: J. B. Lippincott.

Visio. (1993). *Interdisciplinary model for the rehabilitation of visual impaired and blind people* (Report No 93-2, English version). Huizen, Netherlands.

Vision Problems in the U.S. (2002). Prevalence of Adult Eye Disease and Vision Impairment in America, Prevent Blindness America. (Available: http://www.preventblindness.org/resources/vision_data.html)

Wainapel, S. F. (2001). Low vision rehabilitation and rehabilitation medicine: A parable of parallels. In R. W. Massof & L. Lidoff (Eds.), *Issues in low vision rehabilitation—Service delivery, policy, and funding* (pp. 55–59). New York: AFB Press.

Waiss, B., & Cohen, J. (1991). Glare and contrast sensitivity for low vision practitioners. *Problems in Optometry, 3,* 433–448.

Warren, M. (2000). An overview of low vision rehabilitation and the role of occupational therapy. In M. Warren (Ed.), *Low vision: Occupational therapy with the older adult* (pp. 11–14). MD: American Occupational Therapy Association.

World Health Organization. (1977). *International classification of diseases* (ICD-9; 9th revision). Geneva, Switzerland: Author.

World Health Organization. (1993). *International classification of impairments, disabilities, and handicaps. A manual of classification relating to the consequences of disease* (new ed.). Geneva, Switzerland: Author.

Yannuzzi, L. A., Slakter, J. S., Sorenson, J. A., et al. (1992). Digital indocyanine green videoangiography and choroidal neovascularization. *Retina, 12,* 191–223.

Part III

Special Topics

28

Alternative Medicine and Its Relationship to Rehabilitation

MARY F. BEZKOR, MD, AND

MATHEW H. M. LEE, MD

HEALTH OR WELLNESS is a dynamic and constantly evolving process. It can be encompassed in the ancient symbol of yin-yang (see Figure 28.1). The symbol contains two equal forces in perpetual motion. Each contains an element of the other and exists in an interrelated fashion. Yang is often depicted as day, brightness, heaven, sun, and male. Yin is often depicted as night, darkness, earth, moon, and female. Their harmonious balance is used to represent the cosmos.

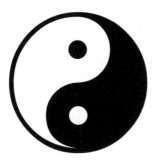

FIGURE 28.1   Yin–yang symbol.

It is an excellent symbol to represent the body in balance, or home-ostasis, free of turmoil or dis-ease (disease). Many alternative therapies are based on flow of vital energy (chi) and homeostasis, holistic (whole body) balance. This symbol of beautiful simplicity may be used to understand the process of feeling well by attaining equilibrium.

Practitioners of conventional Western medicine are familiar with the techniques of specialization, exacting precision, and detail. Preservation of a whole picture or a holistic quality may often be lost. Whole-body issues deal with function, a subjective sense of wellness, and interrelation of coexisting body states. Often the healer and sufferer may be at odds in attaining a "cure." By aligning what the two are seeking, a more effective combined result is often achieved. Open communication between practitioner and patient is a key element in the healing process. It may account for an expanding role and demand for alternative healing therapies.

Alternative routes may sometimes surprise the traditional practitioner. Often old remedies, consisting of plant life (belladonna/atropine) or practical manual application (compression/massage), have later led to traditional technical-medical practice. Sometimes ancient remedies are looked at with fresh eyes and new applications (e.g., acupuncture) are found. The modern person, who is looking at a longer lifespan but possibly facing risks of associated disability, pain, or dysfunction, may feel that traditional avenues have not completely answered his or her needs. A natural tendency is to explore alternative solutions. This process will begin with or without the knowledge or consent of the practitioner. If an open line of communication is preserved, a more harmonious balance can be expected.

The practitioner can assist in educating, screening, and interrelating alternative and traditional selections. The traditional practitioner need not necessarily advocate nor practice alternative arts. By simply being aware of the risks and potential benefits involved in alternative practices, the traditional practitioner can better integrate these therapies to assist the patient. An important role would be to warn the patient of hazardous interactions. If the practitioner is open to new ideas, patients are more likely to maintain an open dialogue about alternative therapies they are participating in. Therefore, any treatment interactions can be more successfully anticipated. Alternative therapies can be easily and effectively used as an adjuvant to traditional care. Often they are a needed source of hopefulness when traditional methods have been exhausted.

Alternative therapies are often based on the five senses (vision, hearing, touch, smell, taste). Some visual therapies are art therapy and certain hypnotic techniques. Music therapy involves the auditory system;

changing, singing, primal scream, and vocalization also involve auditory responses. Reiki, touch therapy, pet therapy, and massage all use tactile qualities. Aroma therapy uses the sense of smell. Taste is very important in the successful incorporation of diet and herbal therapy to seek harmonious balance. The five senses are, in fact, the basis of the traditional review of systems for health maintenance. The addition of movement and mechanical principles, such as active exercise, postural exercise, movement therapy, kinesiology, yoga, tai chi, dance therapy, and many other disciplines, is the very basis of rehabilitation.

Health is a dynamic and flowing energy system. The therapeutic environment is another essential feature in alternative healing. Older arts, such as *feng shui* (wind and water), focus on the arrangement of the home and work environment to create a peaceful and harmonious atmosphere. This is said to be achieved through the use of texture, color, sound, and light, as well as other qualities, to allow free energy flow within a specific environment. Horticultural therapy makes use of plants and a quiet healing atmosphere to help promote feelings of wellness, productivity, and self-esteem. It is often the description or definition of these techniques that makes traditional practitioners either comfortable or uneasy with the solution. Proper lighting, noise level, and visual stimulation in work and home environments have often been studied in industry and architecture to shape productivity and task performance. They are also used to enhance tranquility, relaxation, and healing in hospital environments.

Alternative solutions often call for an environment free of the hospital structure, and this has long been a source of conflict between patient and practitioner. Now, as patients are facing shorter and shorter periods of hospitalization, healing environments outside the traditional hospital setting are not only necessary but much sought after. More of the recuperative process occurs outside the traditional structure. The sufferer or recovering person is also allowed a more active and more effective role in his or her health recovery, becoming a more dynamic element in the solution.

CRITIQUING AND ASSESSMENT OF ALTERNATIVE TREATMENTS

IT IS DIFFICULT for the practitioner to assess the wide range of alternative therapies available. The absence of regulation, double-blind studies, and other traditional avenues of exploration or scientific method makes the situation more confusing. Again the need for openness and communication is stressed. If a method is reliable, it should therefore be reproducible. A safe, effective, and beneficial treatment should not crumble in the light of examination.

The following may help the clinician to evaluate some of the proposed methods and therapies: a number of therapies that differ widely in acceptance, efficacy, and traditional foundation. They may stimulate the reader to further knowledge, exploration, and examination of the roots of so-called traditional methods.

ACUPUNCTURE

ACUPUNCTURE IS AN ancient Chinese healing art that has been available and growing in increased acceptance in the United States since the 1970s. Thin, sterile, stainless steel needles are inserted into the body in precisely mapped acupuncture points. There is minimal skin penetration, and no chemicals are injected. There is usually no bleeding. Pain relief can be variable. There are reports of pain reduction, relaxation, a sense of drowsiness, or even euphoria. One hypothetical model for acupuncture efficacy is the release of endorphins, the natural morphine-like substance that occurs in the body.

The principles of acupuncture are often extended into such techniques as acupressure, Shiatsu, acupoint massage, and trigger points. The ancient art describes the enhancement or flow of chi (life energy). Precise mapping of acupuncture points encompasses almost all bodily functions. However, in Western adaptations the most reliable applications seem to be in pain relief and analgesia. Precautions include strict observation of sterile technique and universal precautions for care of needles.

BIOFEEDBACK

BIOFEEDBACK UTILIZES THE electrical and other natural signals generated by the body to promote the retraining of functions that may elude traditional voluntary training methods. Electromyography (EMG), electroencephalography (EEG), and electrocardiography (ECG) may all be used. Self-regulation of biological functions can be used for relaxation, pain reduction, and anxiety relief. A training effect often requires several sessions. Sometimes follow-up sessions are required to attain a sustained effect.

HYPNOSIS AND OTHER TECHNIQUES

THE USE OF hypnosis, guided imagery, and other such techniques can be effective in controlling an individual's reaction to life events and can aid in pain reduction and relief of anxiety. Often, positive images are used to alleviate otherwise stressful situations and circumstances. The subject is engaged in a number of treatment and training sessions and is then encouraged to use the process in an independent setting. This is a more self-directed solution, and there is better control of one's symptoms because the treatment can be done in an independent setting.

MUSIC THERAPY

MUSIC THERAPY CAN involve the production of or the appreciation of music. Playing an instrument or singing requires the subject to take part in an active process and also creates vibratory and auditory feedback. Production of music on a performance level can integrate the subject into a communal surrounding and deal with issues of self-esteem and self-actualization.

The appreciation of or listening to music can produce relaxation and pain reduction, as well as enhance knowledge and information. Communal participation is again involved when music appreciation occurs in a group setting. Music therapy is often involved in reducing the pain and anxiety involved in medical testing, stressful situations, and ongoing chronic pain and disability.

HORTICULTURAL THERAPY

HORTICULTURAL THERAPY ADVOCATES the concept of the healing environment and active participation in the growth process. Live plants, in a quiet and serene environment that incorporates the principles of planting, growing, and ultimately healing, aid in producing a therapeutic effect. Horticultural therapy may be used to deal with healing, renewing, and coping with loss. When done in a therapeutic setting, communal interaction may be another beneficial element.

PET THERAPY

IN PET THERAPY live animals are used to encourage contact, positive expression, and companionship. This therapy is often practiced in therapeutic settings and geriatric centers, and reporting of results has been generally positive. Proper supervision, with attention to the health and care of both people and animals, is most important. Screening for health-related issues is always essential. Some positive aspects may be the opportunity to express closeness, friendship, and love in settings where these important elements of life have been severely diminished. Reports of lowered blood pressure, increased energy, relaxation, and possible longevity in people who have positive interactions with animals may be upheld by further study.

ART THERAPY

ART THERAPY MAY be used for the production or appreciation of various forms of art. Materials such as paint, pencils, and clay can enhance manual dexterity. The active process of creation encourages expression. A subject too difficult or complex to verbalize may be portrayed in an artistic form. Art encompasses painting, sculpture, pottery, drawing, and other creative forms. It offers an outlet for visual and tactile expression.

DANCE THERAPY

DANCE THERAPY INCORPORATES movement, contact, and auditory appreciation and may be used as a source of nonverbal personal expression. The capacity for individualization and personal styling is infinite, and dance is often more engaging than repetitive routine exercise. Music appreciation is an incorporated feature.

AROMA THERAPY

OLFACTORY SENSATION IS used to promote a therapeutic effect through the use of sprays, scents, or essential oils. Aromatic substances are used on the body, fabric, or in a soothing bath to promote various responses such as relaxation, sleep enhancement, energy promotion, revitalization, or stress relief. This is one of the few therapies to center on the importance of olfactory input. The sense of smell is often intimately linked to taste. It may have key emotional triggers and associations. It is interesting that this area is now attaining some renewed interest.

FENG SHUI

THIS ANCIENT EASTERN art that translates as "wind and water" stresses the importance of a suitable home and work environment for proper energy flow, or *chi* (life flow). Although the importance of mirrors, water, furniture, color, or fabric within the home or work environment is stressed, there are other things to be considered. The patient/sufferer may spend many hours in a home or therapeutic setting. The amount of light, noise, temperature, and stimulation may be an essential factor in promoting or detracting from a healing environment. The traditional practitioner may wish to consider this ancient Chinese art as a tool in understanding the effect of environment.

CRYSTAL HEALING

THE USE OF precious and semiprecious stones and crystals to promote a therapeutic effect involves holding and applying these objects to the body. A stone may have certain attributes associated with it, for example, amethyst (healing powers) and rose quartz (attraction for universal love). These claims have yet to be proved, but there is something to be said for the association of an object and a positive wish or image for an individual. The simple use of quartz in an ultrasound or Doppler machine makes us traditionally comfortable.

DIET

THE USE OF diet and nutrition is sometimes viewed as an alternative practice. A good nutritional state is the very basis of sound medical practice. Often the patient requires guidance from the practitioner to make sound assessments. Hypertension and diabetes are often managed by the patient's nutritional state. Proper balance of food groups, essential amino acids, vitamins, and minerals is necessary. Many times a person must be cautioned of health risks associated with extreme dietary plans. This particularly applies to diets that incorporate periods of fasting. Proper intake of water also should be stressed. It is beneficial for the practitioner to participate in the educational process associated with sound nutritional health.

YOGA

YOGA AS A form of exercise and movement therapy may be beneficial in some conditions (pain, muscle stiffness, stress). The practitioner should be aware of certain positions that may stress underlying lumbar conditions. Persons inexperienced in yoga may experience peroneal nerve stress during lotus positioning. Yoga provides an additional element of relaxation that may be of some benefit for chronic pain sufferers.

TAI CHI

TAI CHI IS an Eastern martial art that may also serve as a form of movement therapy. In fact it is practiced by the elderly in China as a type of maintenance exercise. The art involves various positions or forms and is often compared to shadow boxing. Combining the effect of movement and posturing, tai chi translates as "supreme ultimate."

WATER THERAPY AND MASSAGE THERAPY

WATER AND MASSAGE therapies are traditional mainstays of rehabilitation practice and may be seen in various interpretations among alternative treatments. The use of a soothing bath in aroma therapy may have positive therapeutic qualities. Sometimes it is our explanation of the mechanism of benefit that differs. Massage may be practiced by a traditional physical therapist as well as by one who is aware of the arts of shiatsu and acupoint. It is of interest that many aspects of the effects of water and massage and the resultant systemic response can still benefit from further exploration. At times nontraditional therapies may have a very similar treatment or practice but their beneficial effects are attributed to different mechanisms.

REIKI

REIKI IS A system of touch therapy that promotes balance and harmony of the body energy flow; it has both Tibetan and Japanese origins. The translation is "universal life force." Light touch of the hands is applied to the body of the subject to promote the free flow of life energy. The energy fields of both the subject and the healer are important. Physical contact, stress relief, and interpersonal relatedness may be some of the essential features of this therapy. It is good to consider one of the five spiritual principles of *reiki*: "Just for today I shall not worry."

HOMEOPATHIC AND HERBAL THERAPY

HOMEOPATHY IS THE use of small amounts of a substance that would normally produce a symptom in order to potentiate a systemic effect and allow the body to combat the symptom or disease state. Essentially, this means stimulating the body response or immune system. Although many traditional practitioners may be uncomfortable with the term *homeopathy*, there is complete ease with the principle of immunology.

Homeopathy is based on the principle of Hahnemann's law of similars, which states that "like cures like," and the law of infinitesimals, which notes that the lower the dose of the remedy, the greater the potential for efficacy. Those suffering from cancer, HIV-associated disease, and chronic pain, as well as the severely disabled, are often interested in the possibilities offered by homeopathic solutions. Homeopathy is often classified as a New Age solution.

Efficacy or failure of homeopathic remedies may lie in the proposed amounts or purity of the product used to produce the so-called immune effects. Another argument in efficacy may be the chosen routes of administration. Many of the remedies are orally delivered.

The National Center for Homeopathy states that practitioners include physicians, osteopaths, naturopaths, nurse practitioners, physician assistants, dentists, and others. The practitioner is advised to be aware of the effects, claimed benefits, and potential risks of homeopathic and herbal products, as noted in the following:

Ginseng claims are for vitalization, energy boost, sexual stamina, and stimulation of the immune system. There is a potential risk of increasing hypertension and a caution for pregnant women and nursing mothers. Some extracts may contain significant levels of alcohol.

Ginkgo biloba is claimed to lessen the effects of memory loss, of interest to persons affected by Alzheimer's disease. To date its efficacy is not proven but may merit further research.

DHEA (dehydroepiandrosterone) is claimed to boost energy and immune qualities as a "fountain of youth," but its effects have yet to be proven. It is a naturally occurring substance in the body produced by the adrenal gland.

Ma huang is claimed to enhance energy and sport performance, as well as aiding in weight loss. It contains ephedrine and has been associated with heart attack, stroke, seizure, dizziness, and arrhythmias.

Echinacea is essentially an extract from the sunflower, reportedly enhancing immune qualities and often used as a cold remedy. Definitive proof of its efficacy is still pending, but it may merit further investigation.

Ionic zinc is claimed to reduce the duration and symptoms associated with the common cold. Double-blind study results have been reported.

St. John's wort is claimed to alleviate symptoms of depression. In considering possible side effects of this substance, of note are the many associated side effects reported in standard antidepressant medications.

OTHER THERAPIES

IT MAY BE difficult for the practitioner to review and critique the entire range of alternative approaches. The following are examples:

Iridology: mapping of the iris as a gauge of physical wellness.

Electromagnetic therapy: magnet application (often worn within garments) to enhance energy flow.

Reflexology: stimulation and mapping of the points of the feet to reflect total body health.

If the practitioner is unfamiliar with what the patient may be engaged in it is best to simply listen to a technique as described. It may not be possible to comment on efficacy, but it may be very simple to caution regarding hazards and conflicting health risks.

REGULATION, LICENSING, CERTIFICATION

SOME ALTERNATIVE THERAPIES offer their own process of credentialing. It is possible for a *reiki* healer to be certified and ultimately become a *reiki* master. There are two fully accredited naturopathic medical schools in Seattle, Washington, and Portland, Oregon. A Washington law required insurers to cover services from licensed providers of the state, including alternative therapies such as massage, acupuncture, and naturopath; however, the law was invalidated at a federal judicial level.

Levels of credentialing, training, testing, regulation, double-blind experimentation, and research may vary widely among the alternative therapies. Reimbursement is often not available for such therapies, necessitating a significant personal expenditure on the part of the patient. Alternative therapies are demanding acceptance and availability. One positive aspect of this movement is the open assessment and disclosure of alternative practices. Perhaps an improved system of supervision and investigation may provide a safer and higher quality product for the general public. If the practices are sound and safe, further disclosure and inquiry should uphold their potential for efficacy.

Trust is an important factor in the choice of nontraditional solutions. The simple distrust of the traditional approach does not guarantee the safety or efficacy of a nontraditional route. Lack of traditional recognition does not invalidate a particular approach; for example, acupuncture is gaining greater acceptance and availability. This result was furthered by expansion of knowledge and investigation. Communication and cultural exchange may contribute to harmony and life flow.

SUGGESTED READINGS

Bezkor, M. F., & Lee, M. H. M. (1997). Noninvasive techniques for managing pain. In *Expert pain management* (p. 179). Springhouse, PA: Springhouse Corp.

Dossey, B. M., Keegan, L., Guzzetta, C. E., & Kolkmeier, L. G. (1995). *Holistic nursing: A handbook for practice* (2nd ed.). Gaithersburg, MD: Aspen.

Henig, R. M. (1997, April–May). Medicine's new age. *Civilization*, p. 42.

Holman, J. R. (1997, July). Can these pills make you live longer? *Reader's Digest*, pp. 81–86.

It's magic! The Alzheimer's dog. (1997, Winter). *Vim and Vigor*, p. 4.

Lee, M. H. M. (1989). *Rehabilitation, music and human well-being.* St. Louis, MO: MMB Music.

Liao, S. J., Lee, M. H. M., & Ng, L. K. (1994). *Principles and practice of contemporary acupuncture.* New York: Marcel Dekker.

Page, L. (1997). Demand for alternative care not quashed by Washington ruling. *American Medical News, 40*(22), 3.

Rand, W. L. (1995). *Reiki, the healing touch: First and second degree manual.* Southfield, MI: Vision Publications.

Stewart, J. C. (1993). *The reiki touch.* Houston, TX: The Reiki Touch.

Wolf, S. L., Coogler, C., & Tingsem, Y. (1997). Exploring the basis for tai chi chuan as a therapeutic exercise approach. *Archives of Physical Medicine and Rehabilitation, 78*, 886–892.

29

Rehabilitation Nursing: Educating Patients Toward Independence

Jeanne Dzurenko, RN, MPH

PROSPECTIVE PAYMENT AND managed care have changed the face of traditional rehabilitative services, with many implications for patient education as a result. Patients now transfer to rehabilitation facilities with their acute medical processes still in need of attention. The rehabilitation unit must learn to incorporate these sicker patients and begin restoration to optimal functioning in less time. Six-day-a-week therapy services have been added to meet the needs of patients in shortened lengths of stay. Home care and outpatient rehabilitative services have expanded in an effort to continue patient therapies in lower-cost environments. Thus, patients are required to learn without the round-the-clock presence of professionals. The family becomes an essential member of the rehabilitative team, to support and reinforce those self-care techniques taught by the professional staff.

The goals of any rehabilitation program are to maximize independence and minimize the effects of a chronic illness or acute traumatic injury. In addition to treating the physical disability, the therapeutic philosophy of rehabilitation addresses the emotional, social, and psychological problems of patients. Existing rehabilitation programs are based on the pioneering efforts of Dr. Howard A. Rusk, which were developed in 1942 to assist injured World War II personnel.

Rehabilitation nurses continue to provide support in the form of patient and family education and empower these individuals when they go home or return to work or school (Association of Rehabilitation Nurses [ARN], 2003). They care for a variety of disabled persons. The case mix may be composed of individuals who have had amputations, joint replacements, strokes, spinal cord injuries, and cardiac events that require rehabilitation. Whether adult or pediatric, inpatient or outpatient, education is a key component of any comprehensive rehabilitation program. Following traumatic injury or chronic illness, restorative therapy teaches patients to bathe, dress, and feed themselves. The ultimate goal is to enable the individual to perform activities of daily living (ADL) independently. Measuring functional ability after setting realistic, attainable goals will foster success (Williams, 1994).

The approach to rehabilitation should be interdisciplinary as well as multidisciplinary. Physical therapy, occupational therapy, speech, vocational rehabilitation, therapeutic recreation, psychology, social services, and nursing are the disciplines involved. This approach allows each specialty to focus on the individual's affected function that its department aims to maximize. Depending upon the person's age, the goals of the rehabilitation program may vary. In the elderly, vocational training may not be relevant, as retirement may have occurred prior to the onset of disability; therefore, functional independence is the highest achievable goal. On the other hand, a young individual may require functional retraining as well as educational and vocational programs because both goals are important.

As part of an interdisciplinary model, the ability of the nurse to understand the other professionals' techniques and focus on a common goal allows for a comprehensive integrated program. The education component is at the core of every rehabilitation program. The sections that follow describe prevalent diagnoses found in dedicated rehabilitation hospitals and the roles of the nurse in educating individuals with these disabilities.

WHAT IS A STROKE?

STROKE IS THE third leading cause of death in the United States (American Heart Association, 2004). Although the majority of stroke victims are elderly, stroke can affect middle-aged individuals as well. Some patients may recover from this event with little residual dysfunction; however, many patients demonstrate physical and behavioral changes. An educational program about stroke should include the following:

* Definition of stroke
* Risk factors
* Functional changes
* Behavioral changes
* Visual changes
* Cognitive changes
* Communication deficits
* Sensory changes
* Complications of stroke

Because of the varying levels of injury, the nursing care should include both group and individual teaching. Group sessions can be utilized to cover the definition of stroke, associated risk factors, and prevention; individual sessions will help patients and their caregivers to better understand specifically what has happened to them. Combining both methods with frequent reinforcement and clear, concise audiovisual aids and handouts will improve the patient's ability to cope with the changes associated with stroke. Weinhardt and Parker (1999) demonstrated increased knowledge about the warning signs and what to do to seek treatment early with the use of a stroke education video. The following discussion highlights key points recommended for inclusion in a stroke program.

A stroke results from a blockage (cerebral thrombosis) or a ruptured blood vessel (cerebral hemorrhage). The severity of this event, which occurs in the brain, determines how bodily functions are affected. Depending on which side of the brain the stroke occurs in, stroke patients will present with different disabilities. Audiovisual aids describing blood flow to the brain and pictorials demonstrating a thrombosis versus a hemorrhage should be available. Risk factors can be grouped into two categories, those that can be controlled and those that cannot. Discussing risk factors according to these categories is essential for patients and families to better understand why strokes occur. High blood pressure, heart disease, and transient ischemic attacks are medical problems that increase a person's risk for a stroke. Cigarette smoking also has been demonstrated to be a cause of stroke. Medical management of the first three and abstinence from the fourth risk factor should be reinforced.

The non-controllable risk factors include age (older people are at greater risk), being male, being of African-American heritage, having a history of a prior stroke, and having a family history of stroke.

THE EFFECTS OF STROKE

A LEFT CEREBRO-VASCULAR accident (CVA) results in right hemi-paresis. Nursing care objectives for patients in this group are an understanding of right-sided paralysis, speech-language deficits such as aphasia and dysarthria, behavioral changes manifested by slow, disorganized movements, and memory deficits associated with a left CVA. For a right CVA, paralysis on the left side of the body, spatial-perceptual deficits, impulsive behavior, and memory deficits should be the topics of learning. Descriptive examples of behavioral changes and expected responses will assist patients and families to adjust to the cognitive changes associated with stroke.

After the general explanation of the two types of strokes, the nurse's focus must be centered on routine care and management. Prevention of blood clots and pressure ulcers due to immobility are important aspects of care.

Safe transfers and mobility to prevent falls and related injuries should be addressed. Toileting routines can be difficult and frustrating for both patient and family. Incontinence, although usually temporary in stroke patients, must be controlled to maintain personal hygiene and the dignity of the patient. Teaching the family to use external or indwelling catheters, incontinence briefs, and enemas routinely facilitates coping with these sequelae. To achieve a return to self-management, stroke rehabilitation often involves repetitive therapy. Because the patient may present with cognitive and perceptual deficits, this retraining may seem non-purposeful. Assisting patients and family members to understand the meaning of repetition and how it relates to their personal goals can restore confidence and reduce anxiety (Folden, 1994).

In addition to psychological support, the interdisciplinary team must be sensitive to role changes that occur as a result of chronic illness. Entenlante and Kern (1995) found that wives' roles are altered significantly following their husbands' stroke. Assessment of the wife's ability to act as economic provider, financier, and homemaker must be completed during the inpatient hospitalization. Adults are able to identify their own learning needs; therefore, it is crucial to include them in the educational plan of care. A study that compared the educational wants of male and female family members assessed the importance of four categories: assisting disabled adults, maintaining their own well-being, maintaining family well-being, and learning about health and human resources (Vanetzian & Corregun, 1995). According to the results, male family members rated learning to assist disabled adults highest, whereas female family members prioritized learning about health and human resources. This study reinforces the need for careful assessment and planning of any educational program.

SPINAL CORD

S PINAL CORD INJURIES (SCI) occur from falls, sports, or motor-vehicle-related trauma. Impairments result in varying degrees of disability, depending on the location of the injury. SCI rehabilitation can be grouped into five general categories which can be addressed by nursing care:

* Effects of SCI on mobility.
* Effects of SCI on bladder function.
* Effects of SCI on bowel function.
* Sexuality.
* Discharge planning.

In order for patients to better understand the nature of their disability, a discussion about the anatomy and physiology of the nervous system, types of injuries, and levels of impairments should be the introductory phase of the program. Paraplegia versus quadriplegia, complete versus incomplete injuries, and functional levels will demonstrate to patients the variation within spinal cord impairment.

Utilization of audiovisual aids to define the central nervous system function and differentiate between the types of injuries is essential. Reinforcement of learning through pictorials will foster a better understanding of what has happened. There are various videos currently available that will assist the nurse in explaining spinal cord function and the effects of injuries. Nursing education often focuses on the bladder and bowel management. In addition, sexual function is a major concern of the individual and should be addressed.

BLADDER MANAGEMENT

BLADDER MANAGEMENT IS an important focus of SCI care. The use of indwelling catheters and their care should be discussed. Patients must have an understanding of catheter care, whether suprapubic or urethral. If the patient requires intermittent catheterization, the procedure and care of the catheters (cleaning, storage) must be taught. A study survey of 175 rehabilitation facilities found that, although health care professionals use sterile catheters and gloves in the hospital setting, patients are taught to cleanse and reuse catheters in the home setting (Rainville, 1994). Soap and water are the most popular cleansing agents for home use. Bladder management should focus on preventing urinary tract infections; therefore, catheter care is an integral part of the program.

Patients should be taught signs and symptoms of infection. Complications related to altered bladder function, such as reflux, bladder or kidney stones, infections, and signs and symptoms of these complications, also should be reviewed.

BOWEL MANAGEMENT

BOWEL MANAGEMENT IS another area that requires attention in SCI patients. A successful bowel routine should be completed within 45 minutes to minimize complications and avoid accidents. Components of a bowel management education program may vary depending on whether the bowel is spastic or flaccid. Medications for the neurogenic bowl include laxatives, stool softeners, and suppositories. Proper dosing and scheduling enhance the development of a routine.

Potential problems associated with a neurogenic bowel include constipation and impaction, diarrhea, and autonomic dysreflexia. Maximizing independence with bowel routine is achieved through detection of these complications and early intervention. Coping with bowel incontinence is attainable through education.

A spastic bowel results from upper motor neuron disease. It is demonstrated by the presence of anal tone on examination. Diet, stool softeners, laxatives, and a suppository will regulate a spastic bowel. A bowel routine might include medications, digital stimulation, and the Valsalva maneuver. In patients with autonomic hyperreflexia, stimulation should be minimized with the use of a topical anesthetic jelly. In a flaccid bowel with absent anal tone, bulk formation rather than stool softening is indicated.

The nurse should facilitate an understanding of the need for a bowel routine and hopefully foster compliance. Individuals with SCI may take weeks or even months to establish a routine. In any case, the combination of one-to-one instruction and attendance at SCI group sessions should be encouraged. While individual instruction addresses each person's own situation, group instruction for SCI has the advantages of motivation, sharing of experience, and peer support. Research has demonstrated that SCI patients respond positively to group instruction (Payne, 1993).

SEXUALITY

SEXUALITY IS A topic that should be raised with all SCI patients and their partners. Whether they are young or old, this population requires assistance in expressing their fears about sexuality as well as in learning alternatives to genital intercourse.

Depending on the level of SCI, a patient may experience altered physical sensation. The SCI patient should be made to realize that sexuality is not merely physical but rather part of the emotional being of the individual.

Sex education has two elements: cognitive and personal application (Leyson, 1991). The first element includes watching videos and reading; the personal application is more individualized.

In both cases, the nurse must have competence about the topic and feel comfortable discussing issues of sex and sexuality. Leyson (1991) describes competence as including knowledge about sexual responses of males and females, dysfunctions and their treatment, and the ability of the counselor to encourage experimentation while minimizing feelings of embarrassment. Comfort with the topic is equally important. Many health care professionals have difficulty discussing sexuality issues because of the sensitivity of the content. As with any other education program, repetition will increase comfort because each session will build on previous knowledge and experience.

Sexuality covers a broad range of issues. The concerns of women are different from those of men. The focus of sex education programs should be on addressing sexual behavior, desire, orgasms, erection, and infertility. Volumes have been written on these topics. Whatever an individual's education need, it is essential that the learning process preserve his or her dignity.

Sexual behavior in our society usually is associated with the act of sexual intercourse. Our emotions and the center of the brain control sexuality. Pleasure results from all forms of intimacy, and SCI individuals must be allowed to explore "de-genitalized" sexual behavior to meet their needs and desires (Stien, 1992).

Personal expectations must be a focus of education. For example, the nurse should not minimize a man's need to experience an erection if that is what is important to him. For that person, therapeutic rehabilitation may include review of technical and pharmacological aids or penile implants.

In any case, SCI patients should have the opportunity to discuss and learn about options. Focusing on receiving pleasure as well as giving it will boost confidence. Adapting to SCI will include taking responsibility for one's own sexual pleasure. Often the focus lies in pleasing the partner, or "performing." Effective education in this area will redirect the individual to explore his or her own sexuality and discover that the only difference between SCI patients and others is the interrupted connection between the higher centers of the brain and the lower body. As our ability to experience sexual pleasure is located in the brain, SCI individuals are no different from the rest of us (Stien, 1992).

CARDIAC REHABILITATION

CARDIAC REHABILITATION EMPLOYS the utilization of a multidisciplinary program to maximize activity tolerance following an acute cardiac event. Since 1980, cardiac rehabilitation has been a standard impatient therapy, having evolved from progressive ambulation following an acute myocardial infarction in the early 1900s. Currently, various models are utilized in both inpatient and outpatient settings. Overall, research has demonstrated that the implementation of cardiac rehabilitation programs has brought about a 20% reduction in cardiovascular deaths and a 37% reduction in sudden death within the 1st year following an acute myocardial infarction (Pashkow, 1993).

This secondary prevention will minimize the risk for further injury through a combined program of education and therapy. Medication compliance to control hypertension, weight management, and dietary modification can decrease the complications associated with coronary artery disease (Mullinax, 1995). Regardless of the treatment arena, nursing care is a key component in the cardiac rehabilitation plan of care. The following components should be considered.

Medication compliance during the recovery phase of an acute cardiac episode provides patients with the pharmacotherapeutical support necessary to stabilize heart function. Reinjury to the heart is potentiated by noncompliance; therefore, instruction on dosing, drug actions, side effects, and how to manage missed doses is of paramount importance. Daily reinforcement by the nursing staff complements any formalized medication instruction. In addition, patient involvement in a self-administered medication program is encouraged. Because the goal of any rehabilitation program is to foster independence, self-medicating while still in a hospital setting reassures the patient and caregiver. The support offered by members of the interdisciplinary team can lead to confident self-management of the medication regimen. The self-medication concept and program implementation have been discussed at length in a previous chapter.

Management of hypertension, dietary modification, and weight control are additional topics that should be incorporated into the overall cardiac rehabilitation program. Minimizing risk through education about salt intake, dietary cholesterol, and obesity and its effect on heart function can increase both patient and caregiver knowledge. Written materials about these topics should be utilized to reinforce teaching post-discharge. Organizations such as the American Heart Association (2004) produce comprehensive "Patient Management Tools" that are informational and easy to understand. As with any educational tool, be sure that the content fits your institutional philosophy, serves as a supplement to your educational process, and is appropriate for the intended audience.

The age of your patient should be considered when planning an individualized program. An acute cardiovascular event may change your patient's lifestyle, role, or disposition. Psychosocial support should be offered to all cardiac rehabilitation patients. When activity tolerance and endurance is altered, the patient's life can dramatically change. Addressing these issues with patients as individuals or in groups will promote healing. For the elderly, psychosocial functioning was demonstrated to be significantly better in patients who participated in self-management education following the onset of cardiovascular disease (Clark et al., 1992).

Involving all members of the rehabilitation team can improve the overall health status of this patient population. While therapists focus on ADL and endurance, nutritionists help promote proper dietary modification. Social workers and psychologists help patients to cope with altered lifestyles and family roles. Nurses assess progress and reinforce the goals of the program. With physician guidance, the team ultimately maximizes the patient's functional ability post-injury.

AMPUTEES

AMPUTEES REQUIRE A comprehensive rehabilitation program. The loss of a limb is devastating to both patient and family. In addition to being disabled, the patient has to cope with an altered body image. The nursing care plan should include psychological support and education focusing on stump care, phantom pain, prostheses, and mobility as key components.

Having identified the need for a national movement to address amputation rehabilitation, the Veterans Administration has developed the Special Team for Amputation, Mobility and Prosthetics/Orthotics (STAMP). The multidisciplinary approach includes guidelines for care of the residual limb, limb wrapping, phantom pain, transfer techniques, and prosthetic care (Heafy, Golden-Baker, & Mahoney, 1994).

Nursing care will include skin care of the residual limb, such as assessment of the suture line for signs of infection and methods to prevent skin breakdown. Limb wrapping is generally taught early in the postoperative phase to minimize edema and prepare the stump for prosthesis. Safe transfer training and mobility must be taught. Adaptive equipment needs also should be assessed and education about safe use should be implemented.

Advanced prosthetics technology has allowed for lighter and more comfortably fitting artificial limbs. Care and maintenance of the prosthetic socket and knowledge about proper donning and doffing will help the patient to manage independently (Yetzer, Kauffman, Sopp, & Talley, 1994).

Finally, the need for psychological support should not go unnoticed. The grieving process should be encouraged as a normal reaction for both patient and family members. Learning to verbalize the feelings associated with a loss may be difficult; therefore, nurses must teach the involved parties what to expect and how to cope. Depending on the existing coping skills, support groups or individualized psychotherapy may be appropriate. The involvement of a social worker and psychologist will help the patient to adjust to the anticipated lifestyle changes.

OTHER NURSING EDUCATION ISSUES

ALTHOUGH NURSING EDUCATION can be disability-focused, general plans of care are common to all rehabilitation patients. Pressure ulcer prevention for any patient with limited mobility should be incorporated into the nursing care plans. Frequent position change, skin care, and adequate nutritional intake should be addressed. The AHCPR has developed clinical practice guidelines for pressure ulcer prevention. Proper wheelchair positioning to minimize pressure over bony prominences through the use of cushions and other devices can be beneficial to any rehabilitation candidate with limited mobility. Keeping skin clean and dry and the inclusion of moisturizers and barrier creams for patients with incontinence may be added to this daily routine. Finally, adequate nutrition intake, particularly for a patient susceptible to skin breakdown, will minimize the adverse effects to the skin.

Foot care is another focus of education for rehabilitation candidates. Self-assessment of toes and feet, cleansing, and gentle care will minimize the complications that can develop.

Discharge planning can never be discussed too much, although patients are interviewed about the discharge plan early in the hospitalization and the discussion continues until the actual discharge. Common topics included in the program are equipment and its uses, community referrals, follow-up visits, and medication regimens.

This type of program also allows family members who may have missed some of the one-to-one meetings with the social workers or discharge planner to seek answers and reassurance from the rehabilitative staff.

PATIENT EDUCATION METHODS

PATIENT EDUCATION CLASSES have been replaced by other methods. Computer-based learning offers access to extensive information on various topics. Patients and family can access this information at their convenience, thus increasing participation. It is essential for nurses to assist them in accessing reliable sources that provide evidence-based information that is accurate (Lewis, 2003).

Videotapes also provide learning on demand. Patients may access the tape at any time. Many rehabilitation facilities provide this method on closed circuit televisions. This allows patients to watch the info at their choosing, supporting learning on demand. One example is the production of a discharge video. Since the lengths of stay have dropped significantly, the classroom methodology doesn't capture enough patients. A video reaches a larger population of patients and allows the flexibility of 24-hour availability.

After the individual disciplines have completed their therapeutic regimens, patients may participate in self-care days accompanied by a family member. With the assistance of the interdisciplinary team, the patient progresses toward a higher level of independence, and family members observe the patient as he or she completes the tasks of self-care. The interdisciplinary team also evaluates the patient's readiness for an independent living experience (ILE). Once the patient has mastered self-care, the ILE is arranged.

The ILE is the final step in the rehabilitation continuum prior to discharge. Its objectives are fourfold:

1. to promote a realistic experience,
2. to provide an opportunity to apply newly learned ADL skills,
3. to develop confidence, and
4. to develop abilities to manage community living.

The patient and caregiver are invited to this "day at home" simulation in an apartment-like setting. A nurse will observe and supervise the patient through all of the activities learned during the hospitalization. Proper transfer techniques, bathing, showering, dressing, and meal preparation will be performed. This program facilitates the experience of a post-discharge routine for patient and caregiver while they are still in the supportive environment of the hospital. Patients and their families are offered this "trial and error day" to experience their anticipated challenges of living at home and to allay their fears.

Often, patients are able to perform ADLs in the rehabilitation setting, but the techniques learned are forgotten because of the stress of being home alone or because of the changed environment. For example, a patient may have mastered bathing independently in the roll-in shower at the rehabilitation facility; however, once home, showering requires the additional step of transferring to a tub chair. Because of the extra energy and step involved, the patient may become discouraged and never attempt to shower. The ILE will occur in a environment similar to the home and permit the patient to practice the activity. This process can be individualized to mimic the barriers of the permanent home. Through a thorough home assessment, the nurse or therapist can recreate the setting and foster independence within the home constraints.

Families are encouraged to participate, share their concerns, discuss fears, and ask questions. Their involvement in the ILE will offer insight to the future patient living at home. The goal and plan that have been set for admission can demonstrated with confidence. Depending on individual needs, patient and family may grocery-shop, prepare a meal, or launder clothes. The choice of activities is left to patient and family, but patients are encouraged to select the tasks they feel most unsure performing. Ultimately, the ILE will restore the patient's ability to function within the community.

COMMUNITY REFERRALS

THE TRANSITION FROM hospital to home requires additional support to patients and their families. An efficient discharge plan from a rehabilitation setting includes referrals to community agencies. Various disease-related organizations offer comprehensive services to their members. Support groups for both patients and family members can be found for diseases such as stroke, SCI, and multiple sclerosis. The Center for Independent Living of the Disabled in New York (CIDNY) offers counseling, equipment loan, entitlement advice, and housing information. Other agencies may offer transportation, recreational activities, and respite care. Early assessment of individual patients' communities will enable the interdisciplinary team to incorporate the services of community agencies into the discharge plan.

SUMMARY

AS THE HEALTH care industry moves toward managed care, the ways in which rehabilitative services are provided will change. As lengths of stay shorten, it will become even more imperative that health care professionals perform accurate evaluation and begin therapy immediately.

Patient and family education is the backbone of every rehabilitation plan of care and helps to facilitate a smooth transition from hospital to home. Individual and group classes reinforce the accomplishments achieved in physical, occupational, and speech therapy. Motivation and progress are fostered through an interdisciplinary approach that includes the patient and family as integral participants in the process. To do this effectively, goals must be individualized, mutual, and realistic. No matter how small the gains may seem to others, it is these small achievements that produce the larger and ultimate goals of independence. The nurse plays a key role in delivering care that ultimately enhances the quality of life for those affected by disability or chronic illness (Association of Rehabilitation Nurses, 1995).

REFERENCES

American Heart Association. (1994). *Recovering from a stroke*. Dallas, TX: Author.

American Heart Association. (2004). Impact of stroke. Dallas, TX: Author.

Association of Rehabilitation Nurses. (1995). *ARN purpose*. Glenview, IL: Author.

Clark, N. M., Janz, N. K., Becker, M.H., Schork, M. A., Wheeler, J., Liang, J., et al. (1992). Impact of self-management education on the functional health status of older adults with heart disease. *Gerontologist, 32*, 438–443.

Entenlante, T., & Kern. J. (1995). Wives' report role changes following a husband's stroke: A pilot study. *Rehabilitation Nursing, 20*, 155–160.

Folden, S. (1994). Effect of a supportive educative nursing intervention on older adults' perceptions of self-care after a stroke. *Rehabilitation Nursing, 19*, 163–168.

Heafy, M., Golden-Baker, S., & Mahoney, D. (1994). Using nursing diagnoses and interventions in an inpatient amputee program. *Rehabilitation Nursing, 19*, 163–168.

Lewis, D. (2003). Computers in patient education. *Computers, Informatics, Nursing, 21*, 88–96.

Leyson, J. (Ed.). (1991). *Sexual rehabilitation of the spinal cord injured*. Clifton, NJ: Human Press.

Mullinax, C. (1995). Cardiac rehabilitation programs and the problem of patient dropout. *Rehabilitation Nursing, 20*(2), 90–92.

Pashkow, F. (1993). Issues in contemporary rehabilitation: A historical perspective. *Journal of the American College of Cardiology, 21*, 822–834.

Payne, J. (1993). The contribution of group learning to the rehabilitation of spinal cord injured adults. *Rehabilitation Nursing, 18*, 375–379.

Rainville, N. C. (1994). The current nursing procedure for intermittent urinary catheterization in rehabilitation facilities. *Rehabilitation Nursing, 19*, 330–333.

Stien, R. (1992). Sexual dysfunctions in the spinal cord injured. *Paraplegia, 30*(1), 54–57.

Vanetzian, E., & Corregun, B. (1995). A comparison of the educational wants of family caregivers of patients with stroke. *Rehabilitation Nursing, 20*, 149–154.

Weinhardt, J., & Parker, C. (1999). Developing a patient education video as a tool to case manage patients who have had strokes. *Nursing Case Management 4*, 198.

Williams, J. (1994). The rehabilitation process for older people and their careers. *Nursing Times, 90*(15), 32–34.

Yetzer, E. A., Kauffman, G., Sopp, F., & Talley, L. (1994). Development of a patient education program for new amputees. *Rehabilitation Nursing, 19,* 163–168.

30

Social Work and Rehabilitation

ESTHER CHACHKES, DSW

HISTORY OF MEDICAL SOCIAL WORK

SOCIAL WORK IN a rehabilitation setting extends the role of the social worker in a medical setting. Medical social work is a professional discipline with skills and knowledge that facilitate realistic treatment planning and patient management of illness and disability.

Medical social work has a long history beginning at the turn of the last century. At the end of the 19th century, concerns were being raised about the living conditions of the medically ill and the connection between social conditions and the delivery of medical care. Dr. Richard Cabot, a physician at the Massachusetts General Hospital in Boston, has been credited with founding the first department of hospital-based social work in 1905, influenced by a program developed by Johns Hopkins College in which medical students made home visits to learn about the social and family problems of patients. Dr. Cabot believed that the root causes of illness were found in social conditions as well as in physiological ones and thus saw collaboration with social services as essential. He advocated an approach that supported social, educational, and preventative activities. Working from a public health perspective, he understood the role of community organization and patient advocacy and identified functions of the social worker, including those of teacher, interpreter, referee, and investigator. Cabot knew the difference between neighborliness, charity, and professional intervention (Cabot, 1915).

Cabot's view of social work profoundly influenced the development of the profession in medical care. The specialization grew and in 1918 the American Association of Hospital Social Workers was founded (Sites, 1955). During the depression era, social work in public hospitals expanded and a social work component was introduced to public relief agencies. From the 1950s through the 1970s, hospitals expanded. This was the result of the shift from a chronic care focus to an acute care focus, the result of new treatments, including antibiotics, and new technologies which were developed after World War II that made major strides in the rehabilitation of patients and in survival rates of acutely ill patients. Departments of Social Work grew, as well, in response to increases in the numbers of beds and of patients served, and to the subsequent demands for increased support services.

In the 1960s and 1970s, hospitals as medical centers incorporated a community perspective which emphasized the importance of social work, with its knowledge of social welfare issues and community resources, and fostered its growth. The social work role expanded to include advocacy, outreach, case finding, and information and referral (Bartlett, 1961; Bracht, 1978; Carlton, 1984; Rehr, 1985; Chachkes, 1994).

In more recent years, with changes in the direction of hospital organization and administration, the profession has maintained several important functions, primarily discharge planning and psychosocial counseling to facilitate coping and adaptation to illness and disability. Currently, social work has joined in the efforts to reduce length of hospital stay and minimize unnecessary patient use of hospital resources.

When rehabilitation centers were developed, social work was incorporated into the multidisciplinary approach to care that is the hallmark of the rehabilitation setting. Social work training in providing assistance to patients and families who must make quick decisions and problem-solve around the life-changing crises that characterize disability is consistent with rehabilitation goals. In addition, social workers mobilize community resources, help patients and families identify inner strengths and utilize the resources of the family support system— critical aspects in enhancing adaptation and managing the disability post discharge.

SOCIAL WORK IN REHABILITATION

ILLNESS AND DISABILITY can result in intense psychosocial and emotional turmoil as the patient and family try to cope with often drastic changes in their lives. For the patient and the patient's family, many elements of a supportive plan of care must be put into place for the patient to organize his/her life to manage the impact of the disability and to restore as much functioning and quality of life as is possible. The patient is called upon to tolerate the limitations of the disability, to adapt to these limitations by acceptance, to develop compensatory defenses, and to organize his/her psychosocial environment in order to facilitate adjustment. This includes rethinking aspirations, goals, and expectations and accepting changes in interpersonal relationships as well as in managing the physical environment. Coping, adaptation, and adjustment are the major emotional strategies that must be employed (Russell, 1988).

In the rehabilitation setting, social work focuses on the patient and family understanding of the nature and level of disability, adjustment to the disability, assessment of motivation, expectations and goals for rehabilitation, and plans for discharge and community reintegration. The social worker is a member of the rehabilitation team and is the link between the inpatient setting and community resources, providing for the patient's safe transition back into the community. The National Association of Social Workers (NASW) states that no other profession or occupational group has this focus on the utilization of resources on behalf of people (NASW, 1996).

Because the team is a critical aspect of treatment planning in rehabilitation, team skills such as the ability to collaborate and to advocate for the patient are important to how effective the social worker will be. Russell emphasizes that the rehabilitation team provides the diagnosis, treatment, and follow-up care for the patient who is disabled or handicapped. He adds that the social worker must approach the team with an understanding of his/her own competency. The competence and special skills of each profession contributes to the overall competency of the group (Russell, 1988).

As part of the team, the social worker brings information gathered from a psychosocial assessment to the treatment planning discussion. A psychosocial assessment includes information about the total social and emotional environment of the patient from the physical layout of the home to the nature of the patient's informal support system, the patient's ego strengths, past history of the patient and family that is pertinent to the current plan of care, and other factors. Basically, a psychosocial assessment identifies strengths and resources that can be mobilized to assist the patient in the process of coping, adaptation, adjustment, and barriers to this process, whether they are psychological, environmental, or interpersonal (Carlton, 1984; Compton & Galaway, 1989).

One of the challenges for social workers in rehabilitation is helping the patient and the family come to terms with the permanence of the disability and the expectations that may be held regarding outcome and future functioning. Helping people to deal with this information about prognosis demands that the social worker establish a trusting and supportive relationship and assess the strengths, capacities, and vulnerabilities of the patient/family. The intervention most needed is helping the patient/family to obtain the information about the disability, the anticipated treatment plan, and the prognosis and to help them process and integrate this information so that they can make appropriate decisions and problem-solve in an effective manner. As family needs compete, decisions must be made as to which needs will hold priority and in what time frame. This involves thought and discussion which leads to negotiation, compromise, and planning. Honest communication between family members is essential. These situations are not short-term and they will not generally resolve quickly or easily. Therefore problem-solving is an on-going effort and the family must learn to view this as a constant element in their lives.

The major processes for accomplishing social work goals and the scope of practice in the rehabilitation setting are: discharge planning, psychosocial counseling, psychosocial health education, and case management. The focus of practice includes the patient and the patient's family and significant others who will carry caregiving responsibilities.

DISCHARGE PLANNING

DISCHARGE PLANNING IS a major social work function in the rehabilitation setting. Although discharge planning is a multidisciplinary effort, the social worker generally takes the lead in developing and coordinating the plan. The discharge plan provides for the transition from the acute rehabilitation setting to the community or to an alternative level of care. Most disabled patients, however, are not institutionalized and can go home. Increased availability of transportation, assistive devices, and outpatient services provide previously homebound patients with access to the community and allow them to participate in community and work more easily. Linkage to appropriate resources in the community is essential to ensure a safe discharge plan and to promote the patient's reentry into community life.

Discharge planning is a complex process. The plan must match individual and family needs. The plan must include resources that are both available and affordable. Many discharge plans are relatively easy to arrange, particularly when informal support systems are available and finances are not a problem. However, in many cases planning is more complicated. Home care needs which require the services of professionals in the home or custodial care for patients who cannot be left alone, assistive devices and equipment not covered by insurance policies, and specialized programs for ongoing care may be difficult to arrange. Even more difficult may be the organization of a caregiving system that will be available to the patient. The social worker often must help families negotiate the availability of family members for caregiving tasks and the sharing of caregiving burdens. Issues of dependency and emotional reactions such as anger, anxiety, and depression must be identified, explored, and dealt with in order for the discharge plan to be appropriate and realistic (Volland, 1988; Kadushin & Kulys, 1993; Brashler, 1994; Young, 1994).

Discharge planning then demands a combination of skills, from psychosocial counseling and advocacy to knowledge of community resources and the ability to negotiate bureaucratic systems to obtain them. Currently this extends to dealing with managed care companies and the structures developed to manage cost and utilization of medical resources and the shift in reimbursement policies that have shortened the length of stay in acute rehabilitation facilities or decreased the number of outpatient sessions available to individual patients (Byrne & Sauselein, 1994).

Young warns that managed care and capitation may drive patients through the system faster, with subacute and step-down care offered in another setting. The demand for reduced acute care stays impacts on the consistent caregiving that a longer stay and stable environment provide. Discharge planning must help patients and families to understand these quicker transitions and the discharge planner must be the guide to helping them prepare for and anticipate the impact of changing venues of care (Young,1994).

Brashler believes that decreasing lengths of stay leave some patients and families unprepared to leave the hospital and that their anger is displaced onto the social worker as the discharge planner. Families have less time to participate in community reentry activities or practice new skills at home on therapeutic passes. Their confidence level is lower and their anxiety levels are higher. They are often less sure of their abilities to manage what is needed (Brashler, 1994).

It is essential, therefore, that the rehabilitation team help patients and families to understand what and how care will continue to be provided and to assess the appropriateness of care in the home, in outpatient programs, or in residential placements. This is a considerable challenge for the discharge planner. If resources appear to be inadequate for the family, the social worker is often called upon to advocate with the managed-care case manager and other third-party payers to expand on limited benefits and resources. Success in obtaining these expansions of services is often not possible. Social workers acting as advocates have become more skilled in establishing justification for extra days or extra sessions when this is clinically appropriate in collaboration with physiatrists, physical therapists, and other staff, and they have also become more aware of the role patients and families can play, encouraging and assisting them to advocate for the patient with insurers and employers.

However, for many patients, increased time in the rehabilitation facility is not possible. Referrals to subacute facilities often housed in nursing homes or continued treatment in the home are necessary for the patient to continue to receive needed services. Patients and their families need to understand the limits of what can be offered when services are not covered by their insurance policies. Social workers are called upon to help when the patient and/or family is concerned about the amount of treatment that will be received and resists the referrals to alternative treatment sites because the setting does not appear to be optimal, or when the patient has a strong emotional reaction to discharge from the acute setting. Although dealing with these types of concerns is traditionally a part of the discharge planning process it becomes more significant when expectations for care by the patient and family are not met because of the realities of reimbursement policies. The role for social work in helping to prepare patients and families for these financial and service-related realities and to evaluate all sources of potential payment has expanded as length of stay in rehabilitation facilities has decreased.

While the linkage with community resources after discharge is a basic focus of the discharge plan, counseling is an essential aspect and core of the process. Engaging patients and families who are experiencing crises and helping them identify needs and resources in order to make dramatic and critical life decisions is a challenge to even the most skilled professional. Patients and families need to have real control over their lives and the decision-making process. They must understand the full range of choices that are realistic and available to them and they must be able to deal with the limitations that the disability imposes. The involvement of the patient and family in the discharge planning process can provide an opportunity for education and support that is significant in facilitating control, understanding, and coping (Lawrence, 1988). In the following situation, the difficult decision about planning for discharge is illustrated:

> Dr. Jones, a 75-year-old married physician, sustained a severe stroke, resulting in hemiplegia and aphasia. He was wheelchair bound and incontinent of urine. The patient and his wife had been married for 40 years and his wife was the office manager for the patient's medical practice. She was accustomed to spending all her time with him. After the stroke, she felt helpless, unable to care for his physical needs, and extremely distressed over the aphasia. The patient was always the strong figure in the family and now was extremely physically dependent and depressed. Experiencing his impairments as a loss, his wife had difficulty accepting

his limitations and pushed him to do more than he could. The social worker met with her and her children to help them understand the patient's ongoing care needs and facilitate a decision-making process. The process entailed weighing realistic options and mourning the loss of the husband and father that they knew and of future retirement plans together. It was very difficult for the wife to admit that she could not manage him at home and she saw herself as a failure and disloyal. With the social worker's help, she was able to define a new role for herself and deal with her feelings about being unable to care for her husband. This allowed the family to speak more openly with the patient and to pursue a more realistic discharge plan. The patient was discharged to a skilled nursing facility.

PSYCHOSOCIAL COUNSELING

SOCIAL WORK COUNSELING is centered on the identification of individual and environmental strengths. Social work values are based on the belief that therapeutic interventions should focus on releasing individual capacities and enhancing the environment in which these can be best mobilized and put to use (Compton & Galaway, 1989; Loewenberg & Dolgoff, 1992). These values are also congruent with recent changes in the view of disabled individuals, as a result of the disability movement and the Americans with Disabilities Act of 1990. The view of disability as "sickness" and of disabled people as unable to work or participate in a range of social activities has changed. As such, interventions that help to identify and capture the capacity for adaptation, change, and growth and involve the patient as an active and responsible partner in care have gained prominence (Mackelprang & Salsgiver, 1996). Social work values fit easily with the goals of rehabilitation, which are to facilitate maximum functioning and quality of life, encouraging independence and patient involvement.

Social work counseling techniques rely more on interventions that characterize shorter-term treatments and crisis intervention than those associated with longer-term psychotherapeutic techniques. These are by necessity time-limited and solution-focused, encouraging problem-solving around concrete goals and active dynamic involvement of the patient and family (Steinglass & Horan, 1988; Steinglass, 1992; Reiss, Steinglass, & Howe, 1993).

The social work perspective is a person-in-environment one that focuses on the individual in his/her social and interpersonal world. This involves assessments that extend from a review of the physical arrangement of living quarters to strategies that strengthen family cohesiveness and support. A critical element in the process is helping the individual focus on ego strengths, enhance decision-making capacities, self-image, and skills to maximize independence and self-sufficiency. A major aspect of this approach is the focus on the caregiving and support network that will surround the patient in the community (Gitterman & Germain, 1980; Lawrence,1988). Because the family usually provides most of the caregiving to the patient, the family is a primary focus for social work intervention.

FOCUS ON FAMILIES

MOST FAMILIES DO not abandon their loved ones and, historically, the sick have been cared for within the locus of family. Only in the past 2 centuries or so has health care been professionalized, and even during most of this period, family members have continued to take a leading role in caring for the sick. Today's changing health care delivery system has imposed renewed responsibilities on the family to augment care provided by professionals. In particular, the trend towards managed care and concomitant pressures to lower costs have resulted in a shift of the service site from inpatient to ambulatory care settings or the home and a reduced length of hospital stay. If the family is well prepared and able to support the patient during the hospital stay and after discharge, the result may be more efficient use of medical resources and more effective caregiving. In order to do so, however, many families will need the education, psychosocial counseling, and support that take into account the unique complexities of each family's set of relationships and that can assist families in garnering resources, strengthening kinship ties, negotiating the web of familial relationships, making difficult decisions and adapting problem-solving approaches.

The family's capacity to respond to the patient's needs is shaped by many unique features of every family system. Families are dynamic, interactional entities which are embedded in their social context and culture. They actively respond to events over time and are themselves constantly evolving. However, there are certain elements that characterize the family in our culture that significantly affect their capacity or will to manage the role of caregiver. These include the interrelationship or fit of illness-patient-family, family structure, family health beliefs and ethnicity, the stage in the family life cycle, family history of illness, loss, and adversity, and the ethical issues surrounding patient rights (Chachkes & Christ, 1996).

Families both affect and are affected by a patient's disability. More important is what has been termed the "fit" or lack of "fit" between the triad of 1) the needs, demand, and challenges of the disability, 2) who in the family is affected, and 3) the family's characteristics and coping abilities (Gitterman & Germain, 1980; Rolland, 1994). In this context, the goal of social work practice is to improve the fit by increasing the family's capacity to respond to the patient's needs and reducing unnecessary or ineffective efforts.

Families respond differently to different types of disabilities or stages of a particular disability and course of recovery. For example, some families have a more fatalistic approach to life and a limited sense of their own internal control over events, including illness and disability, and may not have sufficient determination or optimism to manage today's complex treatment protocols or to wholeheartedly believe in the efficacy of current treatment. Conversely, some families have a strong sense of their ability to control events, have experienced many life successes, and believe in the effectiveness of modern medical practices. They may function quite well with demanding treatment protocols during crises as well as with the rigorous demands of chronic illness and disability. Understanding these different responses is essential in providing appropriate help. The social worker must account for the unique constellation of strengths and vulnerabilities of families confronted with these increased and newer responsibilities.

Furthermore, family structures have changed in a number of ways that affect their capacity to cope with the illness of an individual member. For example, today's working women may have less time and emotional and financial resources available to fulfill their traditional caregiving role. The result may be difficulty in balancing multiple roles, work role strains, and work disruptions (Kramer & Kipnis, 1995).

At the same time, the extended family has become fragmented because of economic shifts, job reallocations, patterns of divorce and remarriage, and other social reasons. In addition, certain family structures have become much more prevalent in American society. These structures include those of the stepfamily or "blended family," domestic partnership, the geriatric family, the single parent family, and in higher concentrations in some areas of the country, the immigrant family. Families with these special structures tend to have particular vulnerabilities that influence their ability to cope with illness, especially if it is chronic or prolonged. Their unique characteristics often require that professionals develop inventive ways of assisting them in network building and providing them with effective educational strategies to accommodate their special needs (McGoldrick, Pearce, & Giordano, 1982; McGoldrick, Anderson, & Walsh, 1989).

The family's beliefs about disability, their familiarity with modern medicine, existing relationships with health care systems, their education, and general characteristics of resilience all have an effect on their capacity to understand, integrate, and utilize education and support. The impact of these beliefs is most vividly demonstrated in families who have recently emigrated from other countries. Language differences also can be a major barrier to compliance with today's sophisticated and complex treatment regimens.

The needs of the patient and family also are shaped by the stage of development of the family in the family life cycle. Carter and McGoldrick have developed a framework for understanding the family life cycle based on family life cycle stages that define predictable developmental tasks and life challenges. For example, if the mother of young children is the patient confronting a chronic disability, being able to identify ways of fulfilling her parenting role may be critical to her ability to utilize timely and effective treatment. She may deny her illness and postpone treatment if she fears the cost of separation from her children will have destructive effects. A 17-year-old young adult with a recent spinal cord injury that has rendered him quadriplegic will be dealing with increased dependency managing bathing, dressing, bowel and bladder care when maturational tasks should be centered on separation from family and establishing greater independence. Choosing a college, dealing with sexual and social relationships, critical issues in young adulthood, are disrupted by this injury and must be redefined within the context of greater physical dependency and emotional crisis (Carter & McGoldrick, 1989).

The patient's and family's ability to understand information about the disability and to follow treatment plans can be significantly affected by prior experiences of illness and loss. If the experience was very negative there can be an unrealistic pessimism and hopelessness even in the face of more optimistic treatment results. Or conversely, a good prior experience may make realistic acceptance of the limitations of functioning more difficult.

Realities of family function and family structures raise interesting questions about the realistic ability of some families to participate in these added responsibilities for caregiving. First of all, familial relationships are complicated. Traditional moral obligations to assume the burden of care have weakened and can break down under the pressures of more extensive caregiving. This has become more problematic as societal resources are less available In addition, there are multiple family needs competing for attention. The needs of the disabled person must be weighed along with the needs of the family unit. How much should families be expected to bear, how much is too much, and how much is too little? The ethical issues surrounding these concerns are a current topic of debate (Nelson & Nelson, 1995). Should families be forced to make extraordinary sacrifices or do they have the right to appeal? Should the health care system be held accountable and responsible when families cannot and should not shoulder these burdens?

Although the course of treatment and the crisis points of an illness have a significant impact on the family's capacity to manage effectively, insufficient attention often has been given to defining the trajectory of a disability for families and for patients. Families need to know the dimension of time and prognosis, that is, the duration and course of the disability and predicted outcome and phases, including the coping tasks they present (Aadalen & Kahn-Stroebel, 1981; Christ & Siegel, 1990; Rolland, 1994). This information is often not sufficiently communicated to families.

There are certain times when patients and families have more difficulty coping and around which supportive interventions can be particularly helpful. In rehabilitation, some important phases of the process include: the first months post onset of the disability when survival issues may be paramount and shock, panic, and denial prevail; the immediate post acute phase as the patient and family begin to recognize and understand the extent and limitations of the disability; the defining moments when certain treatments are discontinued, with accompanying patient/family anxiety, for example weaning from respirators; and when the patient has plateaued and further progress is not anticipated (Aadalen & Kahn-Stroebel, 1981).

Another critical aspect of helping the family of the rehabilitation patient is the acknowledgment that life does not return to normal but normal becomes redefined as the family struggles to integrate changed roles and dramatic alterations in functioning. Family caregiving is then not sporadic. Families must juggle trying to coordinate the patient's care, maintaining jobs and other responsibilities, and organizing the tasks of daily living. Some families handle this with a minimum of stress, whereas for others the experience is overwhelming, confusing, and troublesome.

It is critical not to downplay the essential contribution of family care and the level of expertise and commitment required to perform many of its most complex and demanding tasks (Levine, 1996). The family's enhanced role in health care must be acknowledged and legitimized. The social worker should be proactive in family intervention and not rely solely on the family to identify problems, locate the professionals who could give information, determine the timing for consultation, and formulate relevant questions. A proactive approach recognizes the family's role and responsibility, includes education and support as early as possible, and provides for follow-up monitoring of the family as well as the patient's functioning (Christ & Siegal, 1990; Fawzy et al., 1995).

Effective family interventions must also consider cultural issues. A patient/family must be understood within the context of cultural background and ethnicity. Cultural factors play an important role in how a patient maintains healthy behaviors, complies with medical regimens, and copes with the course of the disability.

All cultures and ethnic groups have systems of health beliefs, ways of explaining how illness occurs, how it can be cured or treated, and who should be involved in doing this. Culturally-based notions about family roles, gender issues, communication patterns, religious beliefs, and a range of other factors also influence how information is understood and processed.

Whatever cultural differences exist among peoples, cross-cultural variations also exist within cultures. Discussions about culture are generalizations, while individual behaviors are influenced by a variety of issues that include personality, temperament, and individual experiences. Differences in social classes within one country, which may reflect profound financial, educational, religious, and cultural influences, may be even more significant. Other influencing factors include the degree of mainstream cultural assimilation and acquisition of language.

The ability to provide appropriate care to culturally diverse populations demands an understanding of how these differences impact on the ways in which people use health care, respond to the health care system, and are able to adapt and conform to the expectations and values of mainstream American medical care (Chachkes & Christ, 1996).

Understanding cultural values is an important part of the psychosocial assessment and social work has been trained to identify relevant issues. Social work values promote respectful, culturally sensitive, and effective approaches to patient care and the enhancement of strengths in different cultures rather than being critical of them or labeling them as pathological.

EDUCATIONAL INTERVENTIONS

A MAJOR ASPECT of social work practice is psychosocial education, helping the patient and family to understand, integrate, and use information about diagnosis, the course of treatment, the expected outcomes, and factors related to self-care. This is a multidisciplinary function that has been long recognized as a critical element in the patient's recovery and the family's ability to cope successfully. In today's health care environment, with shortened lengths of stay and health care delivery taking place increasingly in the outpatient setting, there is a greater emphasis on patient preparation for care at home. In addition, biomedical advances have brought new treatments and new technologies into the health care arena. Managing these newer and more complex treatments at home without professional assistance creates a challenge even for the most competent and resourceful patients. With shorter lengths of stay in the acute rehabilitation setting, it has become more imperative to orient patients to the treatment modalities and activities that will be offered to them as part of their plan of care. Orientation to the setting, using educational materials, orientation groups, and other educational programs facilitate a more independent role and develop a partnership between clinicians, patients, and their families in achieving treatment goals. This supports the rehabilitation model that encourages patient participation and places the patient at the center of treatment planning. Helping people to be directly and actively involved in dealing with the problems that face them and making decisions and choices is an empowering process. The empowerment of vulnerable populations is a historic social work value and is at the core of the principles guiding social work interventions. Social work focuses on helping people feel more in control, having the knowledge, skill, and resources to make decisions and to take actions. The social work approach is strength-oriented, identifying personal assets and acknowledging the expertise gained from life experience. Social workers act as facilitators in helping people to actively engage in and utilize their skills in problem-solving and in reducing the feelings of dependency that the imbalance of power between patient and the "experts" engenders (Boehm & Staples, 2002).

Most of us do better when we are prepared. Knowing what to expect helps us to formulate the coping strategies that will support us in the face of impending crises. Sometimes it is necessary to learn new ways of doing things, which often means unlearning old ways that have been entrenched in our daily approach to situations. How patients integrate knowledge and change behaviors is complicated at best, and it is the focus of much professional attention. While good communication skills are imperative, it often is not enough to communicate well. Patients and families need time and repeated education in order to truly understand and integrate the information. This is particularly so because patients and families are being asked to integrate information at a time of vulnerability, when they are in crisis and anxious or afraid. Motivation, language skills, intelligence, comfort in asking questions, dealing with authority, and readiness to listen to information that may be new or anxiety-provoking are all influenced by individual reactions to events taking place. To make patient education relevant to a patient's life, it is important to understand the range of psychosocial and emotional issues that must be dealt with, including cultural perspectives and norms. All educational efforts, to be truly patient-centered, must include the patient's family, care partners, or others who are significant in the patient's daily life. Principles of adult learning and the skills needed for effective pedagogic communication are critical if health care providers are to be effective. Social work can play a critical role in identifying psychosocial barriers and facilitating the integration of knowledge. In many cases, the social worker is the educator, particularly when the information deals with psychosocial issues. The social worker provides the family with information about psychosocial processes, the predictable human experience of the disability, typical emotional reactions to phases of treatment and recovery, and typical crises and emergencies and strategies for their management (Vanetzian & Corrigan, 1995).

CASE MANAGEMENT

IT IS OFTEN difficult to distinguish between the case management role and the traditional social work discharge planning role, as there is necessarily some overlap in professional activities. Both include psychosocial assessment, establishment of a care plan, coordination of activities related to the implementation of the plan, documentation, and referrals to community resources. However, case management, in many settings, is an attempt to provide some continuity of care, allowing one professional to follow a patient throughout the stay in the particular setting as well as post discharge. Currently a number of disciplines have been designated as case managers, but notably they are most often social work and nursing. Frequently the two disciplines share this function. Case management has also been used as utilization management in an effort to monitor and ensure the appropriate use of medical resources and inpatient days. Counseling of the patient and family has generally remained separate from the case management role with its emphasis on reimbursement issues, insurance contracts, and the intricacies of capitated benefits (Opper, 1996).

DISASTER PREPAREDNESS

THE EVENTS OF September 11th highlighted the need to develop a psychosocial response to the impact of terrorism, war, and other traumatic events on health care providers as well as patients and their families. Hospital disaster plans have not typically addressed the psychosocial impact on their professional and ancillary staff who may be unsure about the degree of their own physical danger and/or who may have lost housing, personal possessions, and even loved ones during the event. They must continue, despite these concerns, to provide care to vulnerable patients. What was learned after the attack on the World Trade Center was the importance of establishing a work atmosphere that offers psychosocial services to staff to help comfort and calm and, when appropriate, clinical interventions for more acute reactions so that staff can continue to assist victims, patients, and families. It also became evident that hospitals need a disaster preparedness program, which integrates psychosocial aspects into the response to the needs of both staff and patients. Social workers, as part of the mental health team, can provide counseling and practical assistance to help staff cope with the crisis in order to continue to care for patients as well as to deal with the fears and anxieties of their patients. Social workers are knowledgeable about crisis intervention, debriefing and defusing techniques, stress management interventions, and posttraumatic stress counseling.

Patients in a rehabilitation program, particularly those who will remain functionally disabled, are concerned about their ability to manage should a disaster occur and about being in the community without the protection of the rehabilitation setting. They are worried about their safety, the ability to be evacuated, and their ability to obtain needed supportive services. Disaster preparedness should now be part of the overall preparation for transition from the rehabilitation setting to the community setting. For outpatients, information as well as discussion about disaster preparedness should be offered on a regular basis.

It is essential that any efforts to prepare for disasters, or to counsel those who have experienced them, emphasize that most reactions are normal and reflect what people generally experience in abnormal situations, such as terrorism and war. Most people do not see themselves as needing mental health services. Disaster counseling, therefore, uses strategies related to immediate problem-solving, preparedness for potential future events, and information on how to cope. Disaster counseling also identifies reactions that are more severe and require mental health treatments, offering tips on what signs and symptoms to look for and where to go for help (Everly, 2000; Galea, Ahern, Resnick, Kilpatrick, Bucuvalas, et al., 2002). Social workers can take a leadership role in organizing the mental health and psychosocial disaster preparedness program, in collaboration with other mental health providers such as psychologists, psychiatrists, and pastoral care workers.

LEADERSHIP

IN REHABILITATION MEDICINE, collaboration among professionals is a primary focus to ensure that patient needs and preferences remain the centerpiece of care. Each profession is expected to contribute fully to ensure that the patient receives the highest standards of care, not only through the interdisciplinary process but also through their overall contribution to the organization of services. The social work contribution to this mission is vital. Recently there has been much discussion within the profession of how to encourage an expanding leadership role for social workers, both for the provision of services as well as the development of policy (Berkman, 1995). Social workers are being called upon to use their knowledge and experience in developing new service-oriented programs, connecting to the community through expanded outreach activities, and using their skills in mediation, negotiation, and establishing consensus to maintain and enhance collaborative processes. These activities, which extend beyond the traditional role of direct patient care, demand leadership skills. Although historically social workers have struggled with professional self-esteem and identity, particularly within centralized and hierarchical organizations, an emphasis on assuming leadership roles has encouraged more confidence in professional skill and more comfort with assertiveness, a willingness to risk and to affirm professional expertise. Social workers have assumed responsibility for educational activities, research, marketing efforts, ethics consultations, employee and staff support, and wellness programs and new clinical roles in pain management, stress reduction, and mind-body interventions, among others (Glajchen, Blum, & Calder, 1995). These roles and activities provide increased opportunities for social work contributions to organizational well-being and patient care and contribute to a greater awareness of the professional expertise of social workers.

SUMMARY

SOCIAL WORK INTERVENTIONS in rehabilitation focus on the person in his/her environment. As such, psychosocial counseling, education, discharge planning, and case management all involve assisting patients and families to identify and mobilize both personal and interpersonal strengths in order to more successfully cope with and manage the impact of illness and disability on their lives. In addition, the social worker helps to strengthen the environment of care by identifying and linking people to community resources and protective support systems.

REFERENCES

Aadalen, S., & Kahn-Stroebel, F. (1981). Coping with quadriplegia. *American Journal of Nursing, 81*(8), 1471–1477.

Bartlett, H. (1961). *Social work in the health field.* Washington, DC: National Association of Social Workers.

Berkman, B. (1995). The emerging health care world: Implications for social work practice and education. *Social Work, 41*(5), 541–549.

Boehm, A., & Staples, L. (2002). The functions of the social worker in empowering: The voices of consumers and professional. *Social Work, 47*(4), 449–460.

Bracht, N. (1978). *Social work in health care.* New York: Haworth Press.

Brashler, R. (1994). Changes in practice intensify need to engage families in discharge planning. *Discharge Planning Update, 14*(3), 7–11.

Byrne, D., & Sauselein, G. (1994). Utilization review and discharge planning: Integration maximizes benefits. *Discharge Planning Update, 14*(3), 12–15.

Cabot, R. (1915). *Social service and the art of healing.* New York: Moffat, Yard and Company.

Carlton, T. (1984). *Clinical social work in health care settings.* New York: Springer Publishing Company.

Carter, B., & McGoldrick, M. (1989). Overview. In B. Carter & M. McGoldrick (Eds.), *The changing family cycle: A framework for family therapy.* Needham Heights, MA: Allyn & Bacon.

Chachkes, E. (1994). *A study of job satisfaction and turnover among hospital social workers.* Doctor of Social Work dissertation, Wurzweiler School of Social Work, Yeshiva University.

Chachkes, E., & Christ, G. (1996). Cross-cultural issues in patient education. *Patient Education and Counseling, 27,* 13–21.

Christ, G., & Siegel, K. (1990). Monitoring the quality of life needs of cancer patients. *Cancer, 65,* 760–765.

Compton, B., & Galaway, B. (1989). *Social work processes.* Belmont, CA: Wadsworth Publishing.

Everly, G. S., Jr. (Winter, 2000). Crisis Management Briefings (CMB): Large group crisis intervention in response to terrorism, disasters and violence. *International Journal of Emergency Mental Health, 2*(1), 53–57.

Fawzy, F., Fawzy, N., Arndt, L., & Pasnau, R. (1995). Critical review of psychosocial interventions in cancer care. *Archives of General Psychiatry, 52,* 100–113.

Galea, S., Ahern, J., Resnick, H., Kilpatrick, D., Bucuvalas, M., et al. (2002). Psychological sequelae of the September 11 terrorist attacks in New York City. *New England Journal of Medicine, 346*(13), 982–987.

Gitterman, A., & Germain, C. (1980). *The life model of social work practice.* New York: Columbia University Press.

Glajchen, M., Blum, D., & Calder, K. J. (1995). Cancer pain management and the role of social work: Barriers and interventions. *Health and Social Work, 20,* 200–206.

Kadushin, G., & Kulys, R. (1993). Discharge planning revisited: What do social workers actually do in discharge planning? *Social Work, 38*(6), 713–726.

Kramer, J., & Kipnis, S. (1995). Eldercare and work-role conflict: Toward an understanding of gender differences in caregiver burden. *Gerontologist, 35,* 340–359.

Lasker, R., & Weiss, E. (2003). Broadening participation in community problem solving: A multidisciplinary model to support collaborative practice and research. *Journal of Urban Health, 80*(1), 14–60. Bulletin of the New York Academy of Medicine.

Lawrence, F. (1988). Discharge planning: Social work focus. In P. Volland (Ed.),

Discharge planning: An interdisciplinary approach to continuity of care (pp. 119–152). Owings Mills, MD: National Health Publishing.

Levine, C. (1996). *Family caregiving in an era of change.* Background paper. New York: Nathan Cummings Foundation.

Loewenberg, F., & Dolgoff, R. (1992). *Ethical decisions for social work practice.* Itasca, IL: F. E. Peacock Publishers.

Mackelprang, R., & Salsgiver, R. (1996). People with disabilities and social work: Historical and contemporary issues. *Social Work, 41*(1), 7–14.

McGoldrick, M., Anderson, C., & Walsh, F. (1989). *Women in families: A framework for family therapy.* New York: W. W. Norton.

McGoldrick, M., Pearce, J., & Giordano, J. (Eds.). (1982). *Ethnicity and family therapy.* New York: Guilford Press.

National Association of Social Workers. New York City Chapter. (1996). *Social work: A unique profession vital to life and safety.*

Nelson, H., & Nelson, J. (1995). *The patient in the family: An ethics of medicine and families.* New York: Routledge Kegan-Paul.

Opper, R. (1996). Case management in rehabilitation: A logical transition for social work? *Continuum, 16*(6), 3–5.

Rehr, H. (1985). Medical care organizations and the social service connection. *Health and Social Work, 10,* 245–257.

Reiss, D., Steinglass, P., & Howe, G. (1993). The family's organization around the illness. In R. R. Cole & D. Reiss (Eds.), *How do families cope with chronic illness?* Hillsdale, NJ: Lawrence Erlbaum Associates.

Rolland, J. (1994). *Families, illness, and disability.* New York: Basic Books.

Russell, M. (1988). Clinical social work. In J. Goodgold (Ed.), *Rehabilitation medicine* (pp. 942–950). St. Louis, MO: The C. V. Mosby Company.

Sites, M. (1955). *History of the American Association of Medical Social Workers.* Washington, DC: American Association of Medical Social Workers.

Steinglass, P. (1992). Family systems theory and medical illness. In R. J. Sawa (Ed.), *Family health care.* Newbury Park, CA: Sage.

Steinglass, P., & Horan, M. E. (1988). Families and chronic medical illness. In F. Walsh & C. Anderson (Eds.), *Chronic disorders and the family.* New York: Haworth Press.

Vanetzian, E., & Corrigan, B. (1995). A comparison of the educational wants of family caregivers of patients with stroke. *Rehabilitation Nursing, 20*(3), 149–154.

Volland, P. (1988). *Discharge planning: An interdisciplinary approach to continuity of care.* Owings Mills, MD: National Health Publishing.

Young, R. (1994). Evolution of discharge planning in rehabilitation: A perspective. *Discharge Planning Update, 14*(3), 3–5.

31

Telerehabilitation— Solutions to Distant and International Care

ANDREW J. HAIG, MD

IT SEEMS PRETTY basic to say that people with disabilities have trouble getting around. For many, this is because of physical impairments that interfere with mobility. For others, cognitive or communication barriers require assistance. Unfortunately, for a disproportionate number, the ability to move around in society is also impaired by economic hardship, social isolation, and architectural barriers. Whatever the reason, the fact is that in rehabilitation, our patient population is uniquely challenged to show up at the doctor's office, the hospital, or the therapy clinic.

These people also challenge us because of our dual mission: Their typically complex medical situations are often best managed by highly expert specialists concentrated in larger centers, but their functional success depends on a full understanding of the resources and barriers of their local community.

So how do we see people who can't travel? How do we bring regional expertise into the local situation without wasted resources? Of course! Telerehabilitation. Bring the doctor/therapist/counselor/engineer/nurse to the patient without having the practitioner leave their workplace. Telerehabilitation involves the use of electronic media to perform rehabilitation functions at a distance from the patient.

One can imagine the uses—complex multidisciplinary assessment and planning with a team of clinicians, including the distant medical expert and the local social worker. Following medical issues like blood pressure, skin sores, spasticity medication effectiveness from a distance, yet more frequently than ever via remote monitors. Counseling patients from a distance yet in their own environment for an added effect of "situation specific learning." Teaching and monitoring gait, activities of daily living, or speech problems with semi-automated programs that gather more information than is possible in the clinic setting, yet with less therapist time.

The word "telerehabilitation" conjures up visions of all kinds of fancy computers, websites, video, audio, physiologic monitors, etc. That is certainly a part of telerehabilitation. But as the reader will find, the technology, as incredible as it may be, is only a tool in the larger area of telemedicine. In fact, telerehabilitation almost always succeeds or fails based on pragmatic human interaction. Technology rarely solves these social issues.

Questions that have to be answered are tough: Why should a specialist, comfortably situated in a big city office, want to spend the time and energy to reach out to people in a distant community? Why would local providers want to work with big medical centers that suck up the area's patients? Is there really a need, and is the need large enough for local and regional practitioners to consistently work together? Do they trust each other? Are practitioners comfortable with the quality of care they can provide without touching the patient? Who's going to pay, and is it affordable? Is it legal? When do the two sides connect with each other and how does that fit in with busy schedules?

This list of questions should be familiar. These issues come up in any business relationship. The answers to some of these questions are individual and personal. Others are generalizable and open to scientific inquiry. Still others are political/social in nature. This chapter will review many of the stories of success and failure in telerehabilitation. By reviewing the scientific and the less scientific issues, this chapter hopes to help readers implement previously successful models, begin their own telerehabilitation programs, and build scientific research related to telerehabilitation.

PATIENT ASSESSMENT AND TRIAGE

ASSESSMENT OF PATIENTS from a distance may be of great value. Wasted travel or missed opportunities for sophisticated solutions can be diminished. The challenge is to have the players know what their roles are and work effectively as a team. Arguably a team that meets face to face every week, bumps into each other in the halls, and never changes membership can muddle through without protocol. Telemedicine teams must have their roles defined, yet to be effective they must maintain their creativity and "transdisciplinary" interaction.

At the University of Michigan Rehabilitation Engineering Research Center and through a private company, Rehabilitation Team Assessments, LLC, we have worked extensively to standardize the assessment of complex disabilities, promoting the concept of "Standardized Multidisciplinary Assessment Protocols." These protocols are reproducible patient assessments involving multiple rehabilitation professionals, with decision making independent of any particular treatment program. Protocols have been worked out for back pain—the Spine Team Assessment (A. J. Haig, Geisser, Michel, Theisen, Yamakawa, et al., 2003; A. J. Haig, Geisser, Michel, Theisen, Yamakawa, et al., 2003), arm pain—the UPPER Assessment (Tong, Haig, Theisen, Smith, & Miller, 2001), severe neurologic or orthopedic disability—the Quick Program (Haig, Nagy, LeBreck, & Stein, 1985), and for pediatric disability—the Pediatric Evaluation and Rehabilitation Team (A. J. Haig, 1985). A template for these assessments is illustrated in Figure 31.1, and the hallmarks of good team interaction are shown in Table 31.1.

The Spine Team Assessment (STA) protocol has undergone extensive research, including face-to-face testing of over 1,000 patients and beta testing at outside clinics. In addition to the typical job of establishing norms and performance ranges for individual parts of the test, the

Pre-visit questionnaire	Individual assessments	Team meeting	Team report
Medical history	Physiotherapy	Codified reporting	Recommendations
Social history	Occupational therapy	Semi-structured roles	Goals
Function	Nurse	Creative but structured problem solving	Time frames
Goals	Social Worker	Sequencing and prioritizing	Resources
Resources	Physician	Consensus with patient	Person responsible
	Psychologist		Sequencing (copies to all stakeholders)
	(Vocational rehabilitation)		One week follow-up
	(Orthotics/prosthetics)		
	Speech-Language pathologist		

FIGURE 31.1 The Quick Program (A. J. Haig, Nagy, LeBreck, & Stein, 1993) illustrates the format for effective, creative, yet structured multidisciplinary assessment.

TABLE 31.1 Hallmarks of Good Team Assessments

Standardized data collection, with room for creativity

Standardized therapist reporting, with room for insight

Standardized team meeting format, with variations to improve collaboration

Standardized final report—goals, time frames, resources, person responsible, sequencing

Widespread distribution of results to all stakeholders

Follow-up after the assessment

research has also looked at team decision-making to establish a core "case law" set of hundreds of decision points the team may want to consider. For example, when a patient declines treatment that the team feels is in his or her best interest, numerous explanations (e.g., religious beliefs, poor knowledge base, influence of an attorney) lead to a larger group of intervention choices (e.g., for religious barriers, evaluate psychiatric possibilities, involve the patient's religious advisor, or eliminate the treatment recommendation). Thus a telemedicine team can consistently hold assumptions about actions to take regarding a clinical situation, and can "immediately" gain sophistication that typically takes years of face-to-face interpersonal work under talented leadership (Haig JOR in submission).

Barriers to implementation of the STA are illustrative of the issues in telemedicine. Rehabilitation Team Assessments, LLC, after extensive market research, found that the time, energy, and expertise required to build a business plan, train staff, develop clinical paperwork, and implement an outcome-based quality program were substantial, but could be minimized by developing specific software (Haig AJ, Haig DD).

Inter-rater reliability and validity studies are sorely needed if standardized assessments are to be used via telemedicine. Among the few small studies, Dreyer and others showed no substantial differences in four telerehabilitation subjects on two occupational therapy scales (Dreyer, Dreyer, Shaw, & Wittman, 2001). A few studies showed that nursing evaluation of pressure sores can be done via telerehabilitation (Mathewson, Adkins, & Jones, 2000; Vesmarovich, Walker, Hauber, Temkin, & Burns, 1999). Currently, with home health nursing, this is not so useful in the U.S., but with a nursing shortage or in areas where transportation to the nearest nurse is truly a challenge, there may be potential. Gourlay and others report on using a virtual reality kitchen in cognitive testing and training (Gourlay, Lun, & Liya, 2000).

Physiologic monitoring—of heart rate, oxygen levels, temperature, spasticity, skin pressure, and other measures—is important in some aspects of rehabilitation. Telemedicine collection and transmission of this data is well established due to the needs of "telecardiologists" and others. So, for instance, an advanced program of home-monitored cardiac rehabilitation with EKG and other monitoring is quite feasible (Ades et al., 2000).

Other potential uses of telerehabilitation assessment include obtaining expert second opinions, for example, for insurance company impairment ratings. There is also potential for pre-approval of patient transfer to an inpatient rehabilitation unit. The receiving service could get an actual look at the patient in addition to the laboratory information and medical records, and social workers could conference on discharge planning and other issues. Neither of these uses has been studied.

Finally, the physician, especially the rehabilitation physician, is often the rarest and least accessible member of the assessment team. Telemedicine in other fields has shown great promise in medical management issues. Evidence has shown that the physician-clinic staff can follow up on distant patients without travel, and perhaps with more efficient use of the physician time. Simple medical monitoring such as the management of anticoagulation may be done efficiently via telecommunication (Niiranen & Lamminen). The physician can follow up on medications and interventions via email or website. Physiologic measures, as noted above, can be monitored by the physician. The physician can interact with local "on the ground" health care partners including visiting nurses, therapists, social workers, family caregivers, and of course the patient. Actual time of interaction may be greatly shortened in some cases, making the telemedicine visit more efficient than a traditional office visit.

REHABILITATION THERAPIES

THE ACTUAL REHABILITATION, rather than patient assessment, has been the focus of much of the telemedicine research. Innovations occur in both communication and in protocol when telerehabilitation is attempted. There are opportunities for computerized learning and counseling, home-based assistive devices/training devices, telephone- or internet-based counseling, biofeedback training, and more detailed charting of progress via internet and computer use. Because the use of computers for communications involves a machine that is really designed to perform logical functions, it is natural that telemedicine projects often incorporate computer software that could be useful even in a face-to-face situation. For example, a computer-driven hand rehabilitation device designed by Popescu and others (Popescu, Burdea, Bouzit, & Hentz, 2000; Popescu, Burdea, Bouzit, Girone, & Hentz, 1999) is probably most valuable for its software and hardware design, rather than for the fact that it can be used from home vs. the clinic. The barrier between telerehabilitation and computerized rehabilitation is blurred.

Numerous demonstration projects have shown feasibility of various rehabilitation techniques, but randomized trials are rare and cost-effectiveness analysis is almost non-existent. Pain rehabilitation has been the subject of some research. One study in chronic pain patients showed that self-regulatory skills can be effectively taught via telephone or closed-circuit television (Appel, Bleiberg, & Noiseux, 2002). On the other hand, Andersson and others performed a randomized controlled trial of headache sufferers, in which half had frequent contact initiated by the counselor, while the other half initiated contact on a schedule. Dropout rates were about 1/3 regardless of group, and the effectiveness of treatment was not improved upon by therapist-initiated contact (Andersson, Lundstrom, & Strom, 2003).

Using games, exercises, and information, Reinkensmeyer, Pang, Nessler, and Painter (2002) demonstrated the feasibility of a stroke rehabilitation program, including measurement of compliance and improvement. Burdea and others have designed an orthopedic telerehabilitation system that shows promise, but was only tested in one subject (Burdea, Popescu, Hentz, & Colbert, 2000). A pediatric telerehabilitation has been developed (Connor, 1999).

It is quite realistic for persons with severe disability or reduced consciousness to be maintained at home, at great cost savings to society, but with substantial stresses on the family (Doble, Haig, Anderson, & Katz, 2003). A few randomized trials support the use of telemedicine to maintain patients at home. In 111 persons with spinal cord injuries, no difference was noted among those who received 9 weeks of telerehabilitation advice (either by video or telephone contact) compared to others in terms of quality of life, but there was a trend towards shorter subsequent hospitalizations in the telerehabilitation group (Phillips, Vesmarovich, Hauber, Wiggers, & Egner, 2001). A small survey of persons with traumatic brain injury suggested that there was good acceptability for telerehabilitation services, notably for assistance in cognitive areas and activities of daily living (Ricker et al., 2002). For a small group of five persons with Rancho level 1–3 traumatic brain injuries, video conferencing from home during the first 2 months after discharge from the hospital resulted in fewer ongoing family needs and more patients remaining at home at 6–9 month follow-up, compared to a control group (Hauber & Jones, 2002).

CLINICIAN EDUCATION

TELECOMMUNICATIONS OFFER SUBSTANTIAL opportunities for education of clinicians from a distance. These providers often seek knowledge in certain areas that is above the knowledge-base of their local peers, yet travel time, costs, and timeliness interfere with their access to traditional sources of learning, such as books or courses. Health care providers are also typically more literate in computer areas and more willing to access computers to seek information. A Canadian group targeted allied health professionals with their web-based modules on transfers, range of motion, and other rehabilitation skills, noting the relatively low expense of designing and posting this educational material (Lemaire & Greene, 2002).

Our group partnered with Ford Motor Company to bring University of Michigan educational resources to Ford physicians and health care providers throughout the world. The needs of the group were highly diverse, ranging from basic knowledge of diseases such as back pain to detailed calculations of occupational exposure rates. Their practice styles, cultural issues, and local plant needs required substantial diversity of content. We successfully launched a series of six Web-based modules covering back pain, arm pain, shoulder pain, noise exposure, workplace stress, and toxic exposures. Continuing medical education certificates were approved for American physicians, and although Ford chose not to include test performance in their physician performance approvals, this capability was available.

Maury Ellenberg, residency program director at Wayne State University, solved the problem of being in charge of residents all over Detroit by having daily educational conferences and group discussions via television (unpublished data). In interviewing the residents, the author was quite impressed that some who had not physically seen Dr. Ellenberg for a long time felt he was very involved in their training in a personal way.

We are currently working with a consortium of American residency training programs to build a sustainable, modular, web-based residency training program for universities and hospitals in developing regions of the world. The program steps include: seeking out and supporting a lead physician in the targeted country, seeking out and supporting an American counterpart, having them travel to each other's institutions and "bond" with each other. Choosing selected "modules" from the American residency training programs' collection of PowerPoint or other presentations. Developing distant mentorship of residents, especially in areas where the local lead is not a physiatrist (e.g., a developmental pediatrician or orthopedic surgeon). Providing evaluation tools such as multiple choice tests. Asking the local mentor to develop other modules to sustain the program. Networking between local mentors, and seeking sustainability.

BARRIERS TO ADOPTION

RASHID BASHUR, PHD, is considered by many to be one of the fathers of telemedicine. His work decades ago demonstrated feasibility of technical systems and ironed out many of the social/cultural aspects of use. Despite some exciting uses and demonstrations, the field did not take off until the advent of the Internet. The need for dedicated video lines or slow-transmission telephone lines was a substantial barrier, in part because of the cost and awkwardness, but perhaps even more because almost no clinician users had technical expertise. A technician was almost always required for setup and transmission.

The Internet changed all of that (Grimes et al., 2000). These days almost all younger clinicians and many older clinicians have great familiarity with the Internet. Their familiarity does not come from use of the Internet for clinical purposes, but from their use and experimentation in their daily lives.

Legal and payment barriers are really the main reason for slow adoption of telemedicine. Laws and interpretation are inconsistent and changing. In most places the patient care is judged to have taken place where the patient exists. So it is not clear in many cases whether a physician practicing in one state or country has a license to help a patient in another state or country. Insurers pay for services rendered in person. For example, Medicare criteria for payment includes "face-to-face" time with the patient. Some government insurance (Medicare, Medicaid) in the U.S. is now allowing telemedicine consultation at a discounted fee. Most private insurers do not. The unintended effect of laws on confidentiality is an increased perception of legal risk for those sending telemedicine information on the Internet.

Because of these confusions, telemedicine has been strongest in areas where confusing laws do not apply. Reflecting both the sparsely settled population and the presence of a national health system that is responsible for both care and costs, the Canadian and Australian systems have some advanced models of telerehabilitation in place (Liu & Miyazaki, 2000; Lemaire, Boudrias, & Greene, 2001; Logan & Radcliffe, 2000). The United States Armed Forces have very sophisticated telemedicine capabilities, though these are less developed for rehabilitation. One can appreciate the potential for abuse, but also the great cost savings if legal and financial incentives are in place.

In some cases telerehabilitation is best considered in the context of social services changes. For example, in Japan it has been proposed that the integration of occupational therapy telerehabilitation into community life centers for older patients will help the system to efficiently stretch occupational therapy resources (Tsuchisawa, Ono, Kanda, & Kelly, 2000).

Patients generally respond favorably to telerehabilitation interventions, but it is not known if this is an artifact of the novelty of the intervention or the added attention, rather than actual improvement in quality of care. Caregivers on the receiving end of expert advice also are generally delighted with the help received.

Specialists on the other end of the line seem less enthusiastic (Lemaire, Boudrias, & Greene, 2001). This may be an artifact of technophobia or related to the lack of some cues that the physicians find useful. Smell, touch, and some physical aspects of the interpersonal interactions are not transmitted via cable. Whether these are critical components of the examination or simply irrelevant but hard habits to break is an important consideration. Logan discussed the challenges of videoconferencing between rehabilitation team members who are distant. Physical contact, transfer of physical objects between members, and cultural aspects of care are challenging (Logan & Radcliffe, 2000).

Clearly, these days technological issues are far less important than social ones for successful telerehabilitation. Certainly some applications require high Internet bandwidth and are affected by delays in transmission, as may occur on the Internet. But most rehabilitation interventions are not so time-critical. Phillips and others did not find a difference between telephone and video conferencing (Phillips et al., 2001). Lemaire and others found low bandwidth video acceptable in transmitting rehabilitation information (Lemaire et al., 2001).

Typing skills remain a barrier to some persons who require help, especially the elderly, who typically have little typing or computer training. A Japanese group found good success in using a pen-type imaging sensor with home computers to provide social support to elderly clients served by a "home helper" office (Ogawa et al., 2003). This office transferred messages to helpers' mobile phones for timely responses.

TELEREHABILITATION RESEARCH POTENTIAL

THE NEED TO prove the effectiveness of telerehabilitation is critical (Palsbo & Bauer, 2000). Future work ranges from development of technology to validation of assessment measures, demonstrating new uses, randomized controlled clinical trials with long-term functional and costbased outcomes.

In addition to Canadian, Australian, and other international groups, American research has been supported primarily by the U.S. military, the U.S. Office of Telemedicine, and most prominently by the Rehabilitation Engineering Research Center for Telemedicine (Lathan, Kinsella, Rosen, Winters, & Trepagnier, 1999; Winters, 2002), funded by the National Institute for Disability and Rehabilitation Research.

THE POTENTIAL FOR INTERNATIONAL CARE

PERHAPS THE HIGHEST impact of telerehabilitation will be felt in developing and isolated countries. One could look, for example, at Nepal. According to UNICEF, 1.6% of the population of Nepal is severely disabled. Only 15% of people with disabilities in Nepal have ever been treated for their actual disability. More than 50% of disabilities onset before age 5 years. Sixty-eight percent have received no education, 82% were aware of rights but unable to access them, and 80% were unemployed. Minority populations, poor, and women were more effected than others. Superstition, magical causations, and discrimination are commonplace. Only 1% of people with disability perceive the utility of vocational training, and less than 1% have a flush toilet. There is only one listed member of the International Society for Physical and Rehabilitation Medicine in Nepal, and there is no residency training program for the specialty.

Yet there are numerous physicians and others who care about Nepal. For example the American Nepal Medical Foundation supports many projects and one of the medical schools. There are numerous examples of success with "community-based rehabilitation" consisting of families in conjunction with local briefly trained technicians. One could envision an "in-country" rehabilitation triage system in which the local technicians transmitted data to regional experts. One could imagine a residency training program primarily supported by Americans via web-based education and Internet mentoring. One could even see individual American physicians and therapists "adopting" a clinic, providing expertise, finding resources, and perhaps occasionally visiting. A case report of telemedicine management of intracerebral bleed from Nepal shows the potential for success (Nepal, Graham, Flynn, Cooke, & Patterson, 2001).

Numerous developing and isolated regions around the world have developed various aspects of telemedicine. Often in these countries the medical establishment focuses on disease rather than impairment and disability. Disabilities that ensue from AIDS, polio, leprosy, war trauma, and other devastating illnesses. As in all aspects of telemedicine, the problem is more one of awareness and responsibility than technological barriers.

Telerehabilitation is more than technology; it is communication. In the world of Internet and computing this kind of communication has great potential to improve care and cut costs. But success requires removal of barriers and requires research to prove the effectiveness of telerehabilitation.

REFERENCES

Ades, P. A., Pashkow, F. J., Fletcher, G., Pina, I. L., Zohman, L. R., & Nestor, J. R. (2000). A controlled trial of cardiac rehabilitation in the home setting using electrocardiographic and voice transtelephonic monitoring. *American Heart Journal, 139*(3), 543–548.

Andersson, G., Lundstrom, P., & Strom, L. (2003). Internet-based treatment of headache: Does telephone contact add anything? *Headache, 43*(4), 353–361.

Anonymous. (1999). "Telerehabilitation" may be in future of rehab care. *Hospital Case Management, 7*(12), 213–214.

Appel, P. R., Bleiberg, J., & Noiseux, J. (2002). Self-regulation training for chronic pain: Can it be done effectively by telemedicine? *Telemedicine Journal & E-Health, 8*(4), 361–368.

Burdea, G., Popescu, V., Hentz, V., & Colbert, K. (2000). Virtual reality-based orthopedic telerehabilitation. *IEEE Transactions on Rehabilitation Engineering, 8*(3), 430–432.

Conner, K. (1999). Technology through television. Pediatric telemedicine furthers rehab's continuum of care. *Rehab Management, 12*(2), 72–75.

Doble, J. E., Haig, A. J., Anderson, C., & Katz, R. (2003). Impairment, activity, participation, and life satisfaction and survival in persons with locked-in syndrome for over a decade. Follow-up on a previously reported cohort. *Journal of Head Trauma Rehabilitation, 18,* 435–444.

Dreyer, N. C., Dreyer, K. A., Shaw, D. K., & Wittman, P. P. (2001). Efficacy of telemedicine in occupational therapy: A pilot study. *Journal of Allied Health, 30*(1), 39–42.

Gourlay, D., Lun, K. C., & Liya, G. (2000). Telemedicinal virtual reality for cognitive rehabilitation. *Studies in Health Technology & Informatics, 77,* 1181–1186.

Graham, L. E., Flynn, P., Cooke, S., & Patterson, V. (2001). The interdisciplinary management of cerebral haemorrhage using telemedicine—A case report from Nepal. *Journal of Telemedicine & Telecare, 7*(5), 304–306.

Grimes, G. J., Dubois, H., Grimes, S. J., Greenleaf, W. J., Rothenburg, S., & Cunningham, D. (2000). Telerehabilitation services using web-based telecommunication. *Studies in Health Technology & Informatics, 70,* 113–118.

Haig, A. J. (1985). Unpublished trial, Pediatric Evaluation and Rehabilitation Team.

Haig, A. J. (2004). *Ford Motor Company-University of Michigan global physician education program.* Retrieved on April 23, 2004, from http://www.med.umich.edu/ford

Haig, A. J., & Haig, D. D. (2003). *Software to remove barriers to multidisciplinary rehabilitation assessment.* Prague: International Society for Physical and Rehabilitation Medicine (ISPRM).

Haig, A. J., Nagy, A., LeBreck, D. B., & Stein, J. (1995). Outpatient planning for persons with physical disabilities: A randomized prospective trial of physiatrist alone versus a multi-disciplinary team. *Archives of Physical Medicine Rehabilitation, 76,* 341–348.

Haig, A. J., Geisser, M. E., Theisen, M., Michel, B., & Yamakawa, K. (2000). The spine team assessment: Physical and psychosocial performance of 429 adults with chronic low back pain disability. American Academy of Physical Medicine and Rehabilitation Annual Assembly, San Francisco, California.

Haig, A. J., Theisen, M., Geisser, M. E., Michel, B., & Yamakawa, K. (2000). Team decision making for spine team assessment: Standardizing the multi-disciplinary assessment for chronic back pain. American Academy of Physical Medicine and Rehabilitation Annual Assembly, San Francisco.

Hauber, R. P., & Jones, M. L. (2002). Telerehabilitation support for families at home caring for individuals in prolonged states of reduced consciousness. *Journal of Head Trauma Rehabilitation, 17*(6), 535–541.

Kinsella, A. (1999). Disabled populations & telerehabilitation—new approaches. *Caring, 18*(8), 20–22, 24, 26—27.

Lathan, C. E., Kinsella, A., Rosen, M. J., & Winters, J. (1999). Trepagnier C. Aspects of human factors engineering in home telemedicine and telerehabilitation systems. *Telemedicine Journal, 5*(2), 169–175.

Liu, L., & Miyazaki, M. (2000). Telerehabilitation at the University of Alberta. *Journal of Telemedicine & Telecare, 6*(Suppl. 2), S47–S49.

Lemaire, E. D., & Greene, G. (2002). Continuing education in physical rehabilitation using Internet-based modules. *Journal of Telemedicine & Telecare, 8*(1), 19–24.

Lemaire, E. D., Boudrias, Y., & Greene, G. (2001). Low-bandwidth, Internet-based videoconferencing for physical rehabilitation consultations. *Journal of Telemedicine & Telecare, 7*(2), 82–89.

Logan, G. D., & Radcliffe, D. F. (2000). Supporting communication in rehabilitation engineering teams. *Telemedicine Journal, 6*(2), 225–236.

Mathewson, C., Adkins, V. K., & Jones, M. L. (2000). Initial experiences with telerehabilitation and contingency management programs for the prevention and management of pressure ulceration in patients with spinal cord injuries. *Journal of Wound, Ostomy, & Continence Nursing, 27*(5), 269–271.

Niiranen, S., & Lamminen, H. (2002). Feasibility of personal prothrombin time measurement in anticoagulant treatment follow-up. *Journal of Telemedicine & Telecare, 8*(6), 359–360.

Ogawa, H., Yonezawa, Y., Maki, H., Sato, H., Hahn, A. W., & Caldwell, W. M. (2003). A web-based home welfare and care services support system using a pen type image sensor. *Biomedical Sciences Instrumentation, 39,* 199–203.

Palsbo, S. E., & Bauer, D. (2000). Telerehabilitation: Managed care's new opportunity. *Managed Care Quarterly, 8*(4), 56–64.

Phillips, V. L., Vesmarovich, S., Hauber, R., Wiggers, E., & Egner, A. (2001). Telehealth: Reaching out to newly injured spinal cord patients. *Public Health Reports, 116*(Suppl. 1), 94–102.

Popescu, V., Burdea, G., Bouzit, M., Girone, M., & Hentz, V. (1999). PC-based telerehabilitation system with force feedback. *Studies in Health Technology & Informatics, 62,* 261–267.

Popescu, V. G., Burdea, G. C., Bouzit, M., & Hentz, V. R. (2000). A virtual-reality-based telerehabilitation system with force feedback. *IEEE Transactions on Information Technology in Biomedicine, 4*(1), 45–51.

Reinkensmeyer, D. J., Pang, C. T., Nessler, J. A., & Painter, C. C. (2002). Web-based telerehabilitation for the upper extremity after stroke. *IEEE Transactions on Neural Systems & Rehabilitation Engineering, 10*(2), 102–108.

Ricker, J. H., Rosenthal, M., Garay, E., DeLuca, J., Germain, A., Abraham-Fuchs, K., et al. (2002). Telerehabilitation needs: A survey of persons with acquired brain injury. *Journal of Head Trauma Rehabilitation, 17*(3), 242–250.

Tong, H. C., Haig, A. J., Theisen, M. E., Smith, C., & Miller, Q. (2001). Multidisciplinary team evaluation of upper extremity injuries in a single visit: The UPPER Program. *Occupational Medicine, 51*(4), 278–286.

Tsuchisawa, K., Ono, K., Kanda, T., & Kelly, G. (2000). Japanese occupational therapy in community mental health and telehealth. *Journal of Telemedicine & Telecare, 6*(Suppl. 2), S79–S80.

Vesmarovich, S., Walker, T., Hauber, R. P., Temkin, A., & Burns, R. (1999). Use of telerehabilitation to manage pressure ulcers in persons with spinal cord injuries. *Advances in Wound Care, 12,* 264–269.

UNICEF–Nepal. (2001). *A situational analysis of disability in Nepal.* Kathmandu, Nepal: UNICEF.

Winters, J. M. (2002). Telerehabilitation research: Emerging opportunities. *Annual Review of Biomedical Engineering, 4,* 287–320.

INTERNET RESOURCES

www.americantelemed.org

http://www.atnrc.org/rerc.html National Rehabilitation Hospital's Rehabilitation Engineering Research Center on telerehabilitation

http://www.brain-rehab.com/telerehab.htm Institute for Cognitive Prosthetics

www.engin.umich.edu/rerc Michigan Rehabilitation Engineering Research Center for Ergonomic Solutions to Employment

http://www.shepherd.org/shepherdhomepage.nsf Shepherd Center's Virginia C. Crawford Research Institute Telerehabilitation Program

http://www.smpp.northwestern.edu/MARS/telerehab.htm MARS (Machine Assisting Recovery from Stroke) at Northwestern University http://www.telerehab.net/ Missouri telerehabilitation Field Initiative Research Grant

http://www.wirelessrerc.gatech.edu/index.html Rehabilitation Engineering Research Center on Wireless Technology, University of Georgia

32

The Computer Revolution and Assistive Technology

LEONARD HOLMES, PHD

THE TERM "ASSISTIVE technology" was first coined in 1988
(Mendelsohn & Fox, 2002), but various forms of assistive technologies existed long before this term was used. Many conven-
iences that we now take for granted did not exist when that term was
first used. The computer revolution has accelerated the pace of change
in many fields. The field of assistive technology in rehabilitation has
benefited greatly from this revolution. Elsewhere in this volume Andrew
J. Haig discusses the field of telehealth and the rapid changes that we
have seen in this field. This chapter will focus on assistive technologies
and the remarkable changes that have occurred since the advent of personal computers. We will also get a glimpse of what the future holds.

Resources that are available online will be highlighted whenever possible to enhance the availability of this material. Online locations are
subject to change, however. If you cannot locate the material at the location specified try using only the root domain (such as http://www.able-
data.com without any additional directory information) or try searching
from one of the major search engines.

The Americans with Disabilities Act (ADA) (Americans with
Disabilities Act, 1990) requires employers to make reasonable accommodation for employees with disabilities. The act states in part:

No covered entity shall discriminate against a qualified individual with a disability because of the disability of such individual in regard to job application procedures, the hiring, advancement, or discharge of employees, employee compensation, job training, and other terms, conditions, and privileges of employment. (ADA, SEC. 102. DISCRIMINATION. 42 USC 12112. (a) General Rule, 1990)

This legislation has had an important influence on the development of assistive technology. Employers now have a strong incentive to hire persons with disabilities and to ensure their continued employment.

ASSISTIVE DEVICES FOR PHYSICAL DISABILITIES

ASSISTIVE TECHNOLOGY IS not a new field. The technology of the time has been used for centuries to assist persons who are disabled to live more normal lives. Prosthetics and assistive devices have existed since the beginning of recorded history. Canes, crutches, and peg legs are a part of our history. Antique manual wheelchairs still work, and they still provide improved mobility for persons with disabilities. The future promises wheelchairs that warn the user before hitting an object, and even models that shut down power to prevent the user from driving into objects (Kolar, 1996).

The 1990 U.S. census reported that more than 13.1 million people in the United States (over 5% of the population) used assistive technologies (Scherer & Galvin, 1996). This is more than double the 1969 figure of 6.2 million. The authors attribute this increase to three factors: longer lives resulting from greater rates of survival from trauma or disease, advances in microelectronics and computers, and the passing of legislation (such as the ADA) mandating assistive technology for persons with disabilities. (Figures from 2000 are unavailable because the questions asked in the census were changed.)

The relationship between the ADA and assistive technologies is actually even more complex. The rapid developments in assistive technology have allowed persons with severe disabilities to enter the workforce and participate more actively in society. Their participation was initially hindered by curbs, stairways, and employer attitudes. The ADA was needed as a response to these obstacles.

The pace of most technology has accelerated in recent years, and assistive technologies are no exception. Physical medicine and rehabilitation professionals now have a broad range of devices to choose from when working with a patient. This broad availability raises some interesting issues.

Surveys have found that around one third of assistive devices are abandoned and not used after a period of time (Phillips & Zhao, 1993). This finding has led to an increased emphasis on carefully matching the person with the proper assistive device. Marcia Scherer (2002) has edited an excellent volume reviewing all of the issues involved in this matching.

COMPUTERS AND DISABILITY

ONE DEVICE WHICH has revolutionized the lives of people with disabilities is the personal computer. Computers allow people to be gainfully employed without requiring them to be physically fit. Many assistive devices have been developed specifically to allow even persons with severe disabilities to use computers.

A computer was once a closet-sized machine kept in a climate-controlled room in a research facility. Since the 1970s computers have continued to shrink in size, and they have become more accessible to the population. Whole industries and career fields have been revolutionized by this rapidly changing technology. In addition to their integration into assistive devices, computers themselves have opened doors to persons with disabilities. Computers can assist an individual with a disability to perform a job which formerly required an able-bodied person. Computer skills have also become necessary in many jobs. This has resulted in a new generation of assistive devices which allow persons with disabilities to use computers.

Computers perform extremely rapid numeric calculations based on ones and zeros (on and off). All of a computer's other abilities are based on this simple core ability. Humans have to get data into and out of a computer in some manner. The devices which allow such interactions are known as input devices and output devices. Keyboards and mice are examples of input devices, and monitors and printers are examples of output devices. Persons with disabilities are often able to use computers using only these common input and output devices, but some disabilities necessitate other methods of input and output.

Most personal computers use keyboards as input devices. Modern computers often use a mouse, trackball, or other point-and-click device in addition to a keyboard. This creates obvious problems for persons with many different disabilities.

Persons who are visually impaired are able to use large monitors which project text and graphics onto a much larger screen. Many computer manufacturers now include monitors 19_ and larger as options when purchasing a new personal computer. Apple Computer has included a screen magnification program with its operating systems since 1989. Microsoft Windows and IBM OS/2 include similar programs. Braille output devices are also available, although they are generally limited to text output. Some newer devices allow for some graphics to be "displayed" by producing raised tactile images of line drawings on a special touch tablet. Text-to-speech software is also useful for this population.

Until recently the most common specialized input device for this population was the Braille keyboard. Voice recognition software is rapidly taking over this task, however. Such software is now sophisticated enough to convert fluent speech into text without requiring regular pauses.

Persons with physical disabilities are able to take advantage of a wide range of input and output devices. Individuals unable to use a standard keyboard have a variety of options available to them. Keyboard emulating devices take input from an alternative device and make it look like it came from a keyboard. In this manner persons with disabilities can operate "keyboards" by pointing their head in a certain direction, moving their eyes in a certain direction, using a mouth stick, sipping and puffing on a straw, or speaking commands. There are also special keyboards that include all keys in an arrangement for use by one hand. There are versions of these devices that also include the emulation of mouse movements and clicks. Many physically disabled persons also use voice recognition software.

Computers are also integrated into mechanical devices and environmental control systems. Cheatham and Magee (1997) review the devices that allow persons with disabilities to adjust room lighting, temperature control, and entertainment equipment. In a similar manner computers are becoming integrated into devices that aid in driving a car. These advances will someday allow the safe operation of a motor vehicle by people who cannot use the traditional hand and foot controls. Hearing aids are benefiting from digital signal processing based on computer technology. Research with monkeys has demonstrated that a robotic arm can be controlled directly by the brain (without intervening nerves and muscles) (Zimmer, 2004). This groundbreaking research being conducted at Duke and MIT may revolutionize assistive technologies in our lifetime. We have reached the point where it is difficult to identify where the computer ends and the assistive device begins.

It is easy to become overwhelmed by these assistive devices as they become more and more complex. The multidisciplinary team approach is essential in addressing this complexity. Each member of the team will be able to address different needs of the patient in order to assure that the technology is actually used. The Alliance for Technology Access (2000) has published an excellent guide to this field. This volume is written primarily for the consumer, with a forward by physicist Stephen Hawking—someone who has personally benefited from computerized assistive devices.

ASSISTING MOBILITY—
WHEELCHAIRS AND SCOOTERS

WHEN MANY OF us think of assistive devices we think of wheelchairs. Perry (1991) traces the history of wheelchairs to two-wheeled carts that were known in Sumeria and Assyria in 3500 bc. He reports that actual wheelchairs were not invented until the 5th century ad in China. By the 12th century they had been imported to Europe, where they gained acceptance. Perry reports that the first motorized wheelchair was developed in 1912, and that commercial production of motorized chairs began in 1916. Manual wheelchairs are still useful for many persons with disabilities, but high-tech wheelchairs and scooters, many of which incorporate computer technology, are increasingly extending the mobility of patients.

Cutter and Blake (1997) review the factors to consider in making a decision concerning the prescription of a wheelchair. Manual wheelchairs need to be both lightweight and durable. Nonfolding wheelchairs are generally stronger, but they are less easily transported. A wheelchair athlete may need an entirely different type of manual wheelchair than a more severely disabled person. Newer wheelchair models allow flexible placement of leg rests, arms, seats, wheels, and other parts. This allows the chair to change with the patient as rehabilitation progresses. Variables such as the distance between the axles, height, width, and wheel type affect the balance and stability of the chair. Many wheelchairs now allow the adjustment of rear wheel camber (which allows the tops of the wheels to be closer together than the bottoms of the wheels). Trudel, Kirby, Ackroyd-Stolarz, and Kirkland (1997) report that adjustable camber chair users report significantly higher incidents of instability than other users. Even the type of seat cushion used can be critical for the comfort and health of the user (Rosenthal et al., 1996).

Reclining wheelchairs are needed by some persons who have poor trunk stability or little ability to shift their weight. These chairs are heavier and bulkier than others. Computerized switches and controls have resulted in less bulk. The weight and bulk of any transportation device is important when community mobility is considered. A bulky scooter or reclining wheelchair is only useful in a shopping mall if you can transport it to the mall. Because of the ADA most communities in the United States provide public transportation for persons with disabilities. There are also funds available for some people who need to modify a van or automobile in order to transport a wheelchair or scooter. Persons who depend on manual wheelchairs for mobility often develop carpal tunnel syndrome and shoulder problems more frequently than the rest of the population. Recent improvements in wheelchair ergonomics are designed to address these problems.

Electrically powered wheelchairs and scooters sometimes incorporate some of the same assistive technology used in personal computer input devices. These chairs have traditionally been less portable than manual chairs, but they can be used by a much wider variety of persons. Joysticks are often used as the steering and acceleration mechanism on electric wheelchairs and scooters. If the person does not have the manual dexterity needed for such a control, a tongue control or a sip-and-puff system controls pneumatic switches that serve the same purpose. Voice actuated controls also exist, but they have not been widely used. Recent advances in speech recognition promise increasingly usable voice-actuated controls. Scooters are useful for persons with limited endurance, but they are seldom adequate if there is significant neuromuscular dysfunction. Letts (1991) wrote an excellent review of the state of power wheelchairs in 1991. Since that time power-assisted manual wheelchairs have emerged as a lightweight maneuverable alternative that is appropriate for some.

ASSISTING MOBILITY— ORTHOTICS AND PROSTHETICS

"ORTHOTICS" IS A term for applying something (an orthesis) to the outside of the body in order to straighten it or improve its function. These devices are usually considered independently of assistive devices, although the distinction is often blurred. Static ortheses are designed to immobilize a body part or to support it in a static position. Splints and casts that facilitate healing are examples. Dynamic ortheses are designed to assist joint mobility and paralyzed or weak muscles. Traditionally levers, pulleys, springs, elastics, and mobile power sources have been used. Computerization has resulted in the miniaturization of some of these components. J. F. Lehmann (1992) edited an excellent volume of articles that summarize the state of orthotics research and practice at that time.

Prosthetic devices are devices designed to aid persons who have lost a major limb. Prosthetics use has been recorded as far back in history as India's Rig-Veda period (from 3500–1800 bc) (Saunders, 1986). Although the exact number of amputations performed in the United States is unknown, the Amputee Coalition of America reported that there were 1,285,000 amputees in the US in 1996, representing 0.4% of the US population (Amputee Coalition of America, 2004). Over half of all lower-limb amputations occur in individuals with diabetes. Sixty percent of all amputations are due to vascular disease of one form or another.

Artificial limbs have become much more sophisticated and micro-electronic advances in computer technology allow some advanced prosthetics to be controlled by muscles which remain above the amputation. This allows improved mobility with the prosthesis. Such "myoelectric prostheses" are becoming much more popular. A set of electrodes in the prosthetic socket detects electrical signals from a voluntarily contracting muscle in the stump or residual limb. These signals are amplified and used to control an electric motor in the prosthesis. The "Utah Elbow" is an example of such a prosthesis. It utilizes two sets of electrodes along with microprocessor technology to provide elbow function and "terminal device operation" (Leonard & Meier, 1993). The terminal device on this prosthesis can be either a myoelectric artificial hand or a voluntarily opening metal hook. As previously mentioned, research is progressing on allowing direct nervous system control of prostheses. The C-leg system (Otto Bock & Co., 2004) is described by the company as

> the world's first completely microprocessor-controlled prosthetic knee/shin system with hydraulic swing and stance phase control. This product is so revolutionary that amputees who have been fitted with the device often state that its most obvious benefit is that "I don't have to think about walking any more." That's because the advanced microprocessor control does the thinking for them.

This is another rapidly moving area of technology; and one that will certainly have progressed even further by the time you read this. As with other assistive devices, the physician and patient have difficult decisions to make concerning which type of prosthesis to use. Sears (1991) provides some guidance on this question.

Computers are increasingly used in the design and manufacture of prosthetic devices (Lim, 1997). These methods reduce the problems of human error and accuracy loss in order to obtain a more perfect fit.

After an injury or amputation a patient is usually fitted with a temporary or preparatory prosthesis. This allows the patient to become accustomed to such a device at the same time as a custom permanent prosthesis is being prepared. The residual limb also needs time to stabilize before a final "definitive prosthesis" can be fitted. As with other assistive devices, prostheses are sometimes abandoned by their users. Advanced myoelectric prostheses are often quite heavy and can become uncomfortable after a period of time. Lighter devices are more comfortable but more limited in function. Matching the patient with the proper prosthesis is critical.

ASSISTIVE DEVICES FOR COGNITIVE IMPAIRMENTS

THE AMERICANS WITH Disabilities Act affects more than employers. Colleges and universities have also been required to make accommodations for students under the ADA. Learning disabilities and Attention Deficit Disorder are examples of cognitive disabilities which often require accommodation. More severe cognitive impairments such as mental retardation can also benefit from assistive devices. Computers with spell-checkers were some of the first assistive devices to be used with these populations. Other general software such as memory aids, reference software, and "word prediction" software is also useful for some members of these populations.

In addition to the use of these "general population" software packages, software has also been written especially for disabled populations. Brain-injured patients often need extensive cognitive retraining. This process can be repetitive and tedious, and computers are being used increasingly to assist. An example of these uses is a software program called Brain Train (Falconer, 2004) that is used by institutions as well as by patients and families. It consists of a set of 55 subprograms designed to assist in rehabilitation of cognitive and behavioral functions in brain-injured persons. It is claimed that the software can also assist with persons who are developmentally disabled or have learning disabilities. A second Brain Train volume focuses on vocational readiness, while a third volume adds over 20 newer subprograms. More information is available at http://www.brain-train.com.

Vanderheiden (1996) describes a hypothetical device called the Companion, which would incorporate many different functions into a true assistive device. He envisions this device as a combination of a calendar reminder system, cueing system, artificial intelligence system, global positioning system, mapping system, infrared link to communicate with computers and ATMs, smart card/debit card, and communications link to a central resource service. He described the use of this hypothetical device with the following scenario:

> Tim is awakened in the morning by his Companion, which reminds him what day it is and what he needs to do first. It also reminds him that he has a meeting tonight with his counselor and that he is supposed to appear at the alternate worksite this morning. Tim has worked out a routine with his Companion in which he sort of mumbles what he is doing as he is going through his morning routine, and the Companion notes whether any important activity seems to be missing or out of order and asks him simple questions as reminders. Tim walks out to the bus stop. As the buses pull up, he aims the Companion at the name on the bus

windshield display and pushes the trigger; the Companion reads the name of the bus to Tim and also tells him whether the buses seem to be ahead of or behind schedule. Tim's Companion also knows exactly which bus stop they are standing at (from the satellite GPS), whether Tim is where he should be, what time it is, and when to expect the bus.

When the correct bus arrives, Tim gets on board, authorizes his smart card by voice to transfer the proper fare to the bus, and takes his seat.

On his way home from the meeting with his counselor, Tim is very tired, falls asleep on the bus, and rides past his normal transfer stop. The Companion detects this and tries to wake him; it is tucked between Tim and the side of the bus, however, so it is muffled and Tim does not hear the signal over the noise of street construction. When Tim wakes up, he finds himself in an unfamiliar neighborhood. He panics and gets off the bus, which drives away. He further panics and presses the Help button on his Companion. The Companion runs through a standard set of questions and comments to calm Tim and help him apply his own problem-solving skills. Tim aims the Companion at a number of street signs, pushing the button to have them read to him. The Companion realizes where they are, but does not have any information about the safety or potential resources for Tim in this neighborhood. It advises Tim to call in, so Tim pushes the button to contact the central resource point. A specially trained resource person appears on the Companion's screen; by using the Companion's camera, the resource person can also see Tim. All of Tim's information is displayed directly on the screen in front of the resource person, along with whatever information the Companion can provide on the situation, including Tim's exact location. The resource person directs Tim to a local building that will be safe and calls a cab, since there are no buses that will easily get Tim back home from that location at this time of night. (Vanderheiden, 1996)

While the Companion is a hypothetical device, it illustrates the potential of computer technology to revolutionize assistive devices for cognitive impairments. Many aspects of its functionality are available in the VoiceNote GPS and the BrailleNote GPS (Pulse Data 2004). These devices allow persons with visual impairments and cognitive impairments to find their way in unfamiliar places and communicate more effectively with others.

THE INTERNET AND CONNECTIVITY

ANOTHER CHAPTER IN this book covers advances in telehealth and telemedicine. Most telehealth projects use high-speed networks that allow full-motion video and high quality audio to connect underserved healthcare populations with urban medical centers. A slower network, the Internet, connects people all over the world. This network allows people with disabilities to connect with each other and to obtain information that would otherwise require traveling to a library. In that sense the Internet is an assistive device.

Persons with disabilities are now able to communicate easily with each other across long distances. They are also able to access information that was once available only in libraries. Because the Internet is simply a large network of computers, its document locations are subject to change. A few of the more stable Internet resources related to disabilities will be listed in this chapter, but there is no guarantee that they will still be at these locations when you read this.

* http://www.usdoj.gov/crt/ada/ Americans with Disabilities Act information on the web. This site, sponsored by the U.S. Department of Justice, provides links to the text of the ADA along with various explanatory documents and technical manuals.
* http://www.abledata.com/ The web address for the Abledata database of assistive technologies. This database exists in various forms, but the online version is usually one of the most current. It is developed by The National Institute on Disability and Rehabilitation Research of the U.S. Department of Education.
* http://www.ataccess.org/ The Alliance for Technology Access is an organization devoted to cutting-edge assistive technology.
* http://codi.buffalo.edu/ Cornucopia of Disability Information is a site at the State University of New York at Buffalo which provides disability resources for consumers and professionals.
* http://www.naric.com/ The National Rehabilitation Information Center (NARIC) is a federally funded library and information center on disability and rehabilitation. NARIC collects and disseminates the results of federally funded research projects.
* http://www.healthfinder.gov/ Healthfinder is the U.S. government's consumer gateway site for health information on the World Wide Web.

THE FUTURE?

THERE IS A scene in one of the Star Trek movies where Mr. Scott attempts to talk to a 20th century computer. Nothing happens, of course. He then picks up the mouse and talks to the mouse. Again nothing happens. When he realizes that he must use his fingers to input information he grumbles about the antiquated technology.

In the near future we will all talk to our computers. Speech recognition has progressed to the point that it is truly useful. It will undoubt-edly play an even greater role in the assistive devices of the future. The Internet and similar networks will also revolutionize access to infor-mation. Wireless phones and Wi-Fi networks already allow remote con-nection to the Internet. This capability will likely be built into future assistive devices. The wheelchair of the future may come with built-in email. Database capability and global positioning systems (GPS) will also be integrated into future devices. Enhanced speech synthesis will allow much more lifelike speech for those who can't speak on their own. Artificial limbs will likely become even more capable than natural limbs, realizing the dream of the "Six Million Dollar Man" and the "Bionic Woman" of television fame.

Vanderheiden's (1996) previously cited description of the "Companion" is a brave prediction of the future of assistive devices for cognitive impairments. Devices like the Companion will integrate old and new technology in a comprehensive way, and allow a severely disabled per-son to lead a much more normal life. Since 1996 several aspects of his imaginary device, such as GPS technology, have become more com-monly used by all. Vanderheiden's vision of a comprehensive device is still unrealized.

As computer technology gets smaller, lighter, and faster, the most sophisticated assistive devices will get smaller, lighter, and more capa-ble. Space age polymers have already replaced metal in many devices, and this has helped them lose weight. Wearable computers are begin-ning to become practical. Power-assisted manual wheelchairs mean that we are no longer required to trade the portability of a manual wheel-chair for the improved mobility of a motorized wheelchair.

The best that we can really do is to predict the direction of things to come. If change continues at its current pace this chapter will be obso-lete before this book is revised. You, the reader, live in the future. You can see the future much more clearly than I.

REFERENCES

Alliance for Technology Access. (2000). *Computer and web resources for people with disabilities*. Alameda, CA: Hunter House Publishers.

Americans with Disabilities Act. (1990). Retrieved February 7, 2004, from http://www.usdoj.gov/crt/ada/statute.html

Amputee Coalition of America. (2004). *Limb loss FAQs*. Retrieved February 7, 2004, from http://www.amputee-coalition.org/nllic_faq.html

Cheatham, J., & Magee, K. (1997). Rehabilitation robotics and environmental control systems. *Physical Medicine and Rehabilitation State of the Art Reviews*, *11*(1), 133–150.

Cutter, N., & Blake, D. (1997). Wheelchair and seating systems: Clinical applications. *Physical Medicine and Rehabilitation State of the Art Reviews, 11*(1), 107–132.

Falconer, J. (2004). *Computers and brain injury: Some guidelines for rehabilitation.* Retrieved February 7, 2004, from http://www.brain-train.com/articles/computer.htm

Kolar, K. (1996). Seating and wheeled mobility aids. In J. C. Galvin & M. J. Scherer (Eds.), *Evaluating, selecting, and using appropriate assistive technology.* Gaithersburg, MD: Aspen Publishers.

Lehmann, J. F. (Ed.). (1992). Orthotics. *Physical Medicine and Rehabilitation Clinics of North America, 3,* 1.

Leonard, J., & Meier, R. (1993). Upper and lower extremity prosthetics. In J. DeLisa (Ed.), *Rehabilitative medicine principles and practice* (2nd ed., pp. 507–525). New York: J. B. Lippincott.

Letts. R. (1991). Power wheelchairs and other mobility aids. In R.M. Letts (Ed.), *Principles of seating the disabled* (pp. 263–286). Boca Raton, FL: CRC Press.

Lim. P. (1997). Advances in prosthetics: A clinical perspective. *Physical Medicine and Rehabilitation: State of the Art Reviews, 11*(1), 13–38.

Mendelsohn, S., & Fox, H. (2002). Evolving legislation and public policy related to disability and assistive technology. In M. Scherer (Ed.), *Assistive technology: Matching device and consumer for successful rehabilitation* (pp. 17–28). Washington, DC: American Psychological Association.

Otto Bock and Company. (2004). *C-Leg: New generation leg system revolutionizes lower limb prostheses.* Retrieved February 17, 2004, from http://www.ottobockus.com/products/lower_limb_prosthetics/c-leg_article.asp

Phillips, B., & Zhao, H. (1993). Predictors of assistive technology abandonment. *Assistive Technologies, 5,* 36–45.

Perry, A. (1991). The history of wheelchairs. In R. M. Letts (Ed.), *Principles of seating the disabled* (pp. 331–337). Boca Raton, FL: CRC Press.

Pulse Data. (2004). Retrieved February 17, 2004, from http://www.pulsedata.com/Products/Notetakers/BrailleNoteGPS.asp

Rosenthal, M., Felton, R., Hilean, D., Lee, M., Friedman M., & Navach, J. A. (1996). Wheelchair cushion designed to redistribute sites of sitting pressure. *Archives of Physical Medicine and Rehabilitation, 77*(3), 278–282.

Saunders, G. T. (1986). *Lower limb amputations: A guide to rehabilitation.* Philadelphia: F. A. Davis.

Scherer, M. (Ed.). (2002). *Assistive technology: Matching device and consumer for successful rehabilitation.* Washington, DC: American Psychological Association.

Scherer, M., & Galvin, J. (1996). An outcomes perspective of quality pathways to the most appropriate technology. In J. C. Galvin & M. J. Scherer (Eds.), *Evaluating, selecting, and using appropriate assistive technology.* Gaithersburg, MD: Aspen Publishers.

Sears, H. (1991). Approaches to prescription of body-powered and myoelectric prostheses. *Physical Medicine and Rehabilitation Clinics of North America, 2*(2), 361–371.

Trudel, M., Kirby, R., Ackroyd-Stolarz, S., & Kirkland, S. (1997). Effects of rear-wheel camber on wheelchair stability. *Archives of Physical Medicine and Rehabilitation, 78,* 78–81.

Vanderheiden, G. (1996). Computer access and use by people with disabilities. In J. C. Galvin & M. J.Scherer (Eds.), *Evaluating, selecting, and using appropriate assistive technology.* Gaithersburg, MD: Aspen Publishers.

Zimmer, C. (2004, February). Mind over machine. *Popular Science.* Retrieved February 8, 2004, from http://www.popsci.com/popsci/medicine/article/0,12543,576464,00.html

33

Trends in Medical Rehabilitation Delivery and Payment Systems

KRISTOFER J. HAGGLUND, PHD,
DONALD G. KEWMAN, PHD, NANCY E. WIRTH, MD,
AND STEVEN C. RIGGERT, PHD

OVER THE PAST 20 years, the U.S. health care system has been buffeted by explosive growth in utilization and costs of health care services. Both private and public payers have implemented a variety of controls on service and payment systems to slow the growth of spending. The changes in reimbursement systems have not always succeeded in reducing spending, but they have contributed to changes in the delivery of health care. Medical rehabilitation was initially protected from cost-containment forces, but it is now undergoing significant transformation. This chapter focuses on the current status and trends in the payment and delivery of medical rehabilitation services in the United States.

Rehabilitation care is evolving within the larger and complex health care system that continues to be shaped by changing demographics and economic forces. A principal characteristic of the changing health care landscape is the rapid rise in costs. The average annual per capita cost of health care in 1965 was $202, and total health costs consumed 5.7% of the U.S. gross domestic product (GDP). In 2002, the cost was $5440 and total health costs consumed 14.9% of the GDP or nearly 15 cents of every dollar spent in the U.S. (Levit, Smith, Cowan, Sensenig, & Catlin, 2003). This growth in the proportion of the GDP consumed by health care has alarmed citizens and other payers of health care benefits such as employers and government policy makers.

Growth in overall health care expenditures has been reflected in the growth of the rehabilitation field. For example, the number of free-standing rehabilitation hospitals increased from 68 in 1965 (Frederickson & Cannon, 1995) to 216 in 2002 (U.S. Department of Health and Human Services, 2003). There were also 936 rehabilitation units within health care facilities in 2003 (U.S. Department of Health and Human Services 2003). The number of skilled nursing facilities (SNFs) increased from 8,200 in 1989 (Frederickson & Cannon) to 14,755 in 2001 (U.S. Department of Health and Human Services).

Various factors have contributed to the tremendous growth in rehabilitation services. Advances in medical care have allowed more people to survive disabling conditions, thus increasing demand for services over longer periods of time. Buchanan, Rumpel, and Hoenig (1996) described an additional dynamic. They found that among Medicare recipients, growth in outpatient services from 1987 to 1990 was related to the availability of reimbursable services. Their analysis suggested that this growth was more highly attributable to good reimbursement to providers for their services and to provider decision-making, than to changes in demographics. Findings such as these were largely responsible for prompting the federal government (through Medicare) and private insurers to implement the substantial changes in service and payment systems described in this chapter.

CONTINUUM OF REHABILITATION CARE

INPATIENT CARE

REHABILITATION SERVICES ARE delivered in a variety of settings, including intensive or critical care units, acute hospital units, inpatient rehabilitation programs, outpatient clinics, and home care. A common entry point for patients into the rehabilitation settings is from acute inpatient medical settings. Ninety one percent of patients admitted to inpatient rehabilitation settings are from acute hospital care. Eighty-two percent of patients are discharged from inpatient rehabilitation to the community, 9% are discharged to nursing homes, 2% to a subacute facility, and 6% return to acute care settings (Deutsch, Fiedler, Granger, & Russell, 2002).

Patients sometimes receive rehabilitation services from part or all of the rehabilitation team when they are in an intensive care or acute medical unit. If they transfer to a comprehensive medical rehabilitation unit or facility, the services consume significant portions of the patients' days. In the case of Medicare and most other patients, this constitutes a minimum of 3 hours per day, due to insurer participation requirements. Typically, the interdisciplinary rehabilitation team will meet on a regular basis in "staffings" or patient care conferences to discuss each patient's progress, and to refine goals, treatment strategies, and discharge plans to ensure that services are delivered in a coordinated and efficient fashion.

Although the demand for inpatient rehabilitation services has remained strong, cost containment efforts have put pressure on providers to reduce the length of rehabilitation hospitalization. This has created an increased need for rehabilitation services following hospital discharge, and has been one reason for an increase in growth of subacute rehabilitation programs (Chan & Ciol, 2000), home-care services, and outpatient programs.

SUBACUTE REHABILITATION, SKILLED NURSING FACILITIES, AND RESIDENTIAL PROGRAMS

PATIENTS WHO CAN be safely discharged from the hospital but are not ready to return home may go to a subacute program, which is often a part of a skilled nursing facility (SNF) (Centers for Medicare and Medicaid Services, 2002). Alternatively, they may go to a regular nursing unit at a SNF or be admitted to a residential treatment program (sometimes licensed as an adult foster-care facility). Medicare recipients were more than twice as likely to be admitted to a SNF in 1999 than in 1994 (Centers for Medicare and Medicaid Services). Careful consideration of potential medical risks and patient safety in post-hospital placement decisions is an important part of discharge planning (Wright, Rao, Smith, & Harvey, 1996).

The least restrictive types of residential care are supervised living situations, where a person may live in an apartment alone or with a roommate. These persons live in the community, but require some assistance or supervision by a rehabilitation provider or other provider, who may have contact with them once or several times a day. A new and growing living option, especially for the elderly, is an assistive living facility (sometimes licensed as a home for the aged). Individuals usually live in apartment-like accommodations with assistance in homemaking chores and the availability of some supervision and personal assistance. These facilities are not regular venues for the delivery of rehabilitation services, but constitute a major growth market in housing options for elderly persons with disabilities who do not have significant nursing care needs. In 1999, 1.5% of Medicare beneficiaries were living in an assisted living setting (Centers for Medicare and Medicaid Services, 2002).

HOME CARE

THE FINAL STEP in the continuum of care is living at home with services provided either in an outpatient clinic or by home-care providers. These community-based services may include personal assistance services, skilled nursing, and/or other services, such as occupational or physical therapy. The likelihood of a Medicare recipient receiving contracted services from a home health agency increased 1.7 times between 1990 and 1998. In 2000, nearly 2.5 million Medicare recipients received home health agency services (Centers for Medicare and Medicaid Services, 2002). These home-based services may be combined with outpatient services from a rehabilitation clinic.

Personal assistance services are often a critical part of home care for persons with severe disabilities. These services usually include help with activities of daily living (ADLs), such as eating, bathing, grooming, and mobility. The availability of personal care assistance has been shown to have a positive relationship with physical and mental health for persons with stroke, spinal cord injury, or traumatic brain injury. These providers are typically not professionals, although a small percentage of them complete certification programs. Family members often provide services. When only family members provide personal assistance, the interpersonal relationships may become strained or "distorted." Combining the assistance of unrelated persons with that of family members seems to be associated with the best health outcomes (Nosek, 1993). The need to improve funding for such services in order to avoid unnecessary institutionalization has been a major goal of public policy activism by consumer groups of disabled persons.

OUTPATIENT CARE

OUTPATIENT REHABILITATION CLINICS may be hospital-based, or freestanding clinics that are privately owned by the providers working in the clinic (e.g., private practice clinic), or owned by a hospital, health system, or corporation that specializes in providing rehabilitative care. Some clinics may contain just one rehabilitation discipline, such as psychology or physical therapy. Other clinics may provide a range of rehabilitative services. The Medicare designation for the latter is a Comprehensive Outpatient Rehabilitation Facility (CORF). These settings are appropriate for patients who no longer require the same level of physician and/or skilled nursing support available in a hospital but need extensive therapy to improve functioning. Some outpatient facilities may contain programs where patients receive a specialized, highly interdisciplinary and integrated care, such as day treatment. These patients may include those with sports injuries, chronic musculoskeletal pain, traumatic brain injuries, work-related injuries, or those in need of vocational rehabilitation services. For those with work-related injuries or chronic musculoskeletal pain, the treatment venue may be the workplace, where individuals receive therapy guided by the rehabilitation staff in order to resume their previous job duties. In other cases, a periodic appointment with a single provider may meet the patient's needs.

TELEHEALTH

WITH MANY REHABILITATION centers and specialty programs residing in large metropolitan areas, and few programs in smaller cities and rural areas, accessibility to services remains a problem (see Haig, chapter 31). The transmission of voice, data, and images using telecommunications techniques has given rise to increased opportunities for rehabilitation providers to offer some specialized information and services to remote locations, such as the offices of less specialized rural providers or the homes of rehabilitation or disabled patients. Important services may include training and counseling, monitoring and assessment of rehabilitation progress, and therapeutic interventions. Various challenges remain to be overcome, such as reimbursement, licensing requirements in different states, privacy, and confidentiality, as well as improvement in the technology of the telecommunication devices. Telecommunication has the potential to augment care, as opposed to the view of it being a poor substitution for traditional care (Lathan, Kinsella, Rosen, Winters, & Trepagnier, 1999). Telehealth has begun to be used as a method for providing some rehabilitation services and education to persons with disabilities living in rural areas (Schopp, Johnstone, & Merveille, 2000).

INTERDISCIPLINARY REHABILITATION CARE

PATIENTS RECEIVE SERVICES from a variety of therapists to improve cognitive, behavioral, and physical functioning. The core rehabilitation team typically includes a physician (often a physiatrist, who is a physician practicing the specialty of physical medicine and rehabilitation), rehabilitation psychologist or neuropsychologist, social worker, nurse, physical therapist, occupational therapist, and speech/language pathologist. Various other professionals, such as case managers, orthotists, prosthetists, recreation therapists, dietitians, rehabilitation engineers, vocational rehabilitation counselors, and teachers may supplement the team.

In some inpatient programs, a team that specializes in a particular diagnosis, such as spinal cord injury or brain injury, may treat the patient. Specialized teams have been shown to reduce length of stay (e.g., Tator, Duncan, Edmonds, Lapczak, & Andrews, 1993) with equal or better outcomes, presumably through greater efficiencies in patient care. The goal of therapeutic intervention is maximal independence and discharge to the "least restrictive," and usually least costly, environment. Rehabilitation has been quite successful in this endeavor. Using spinal cord injury (SCI) as an example, a review of data collected from 1973–1996 reveals that 95.3% of individuals reside in private residences in the community following discharge and only 4.3% of persons with SCI are transferred to nursing homes. There is a recent rise in discharge of spinal cord injured patients to nursing homes, which may reflect both a change in case mix (older or ventilator-dependent people) and the trend for reducing the inpatient rehabilitation length of stay due to cost-containment considerations (DeVivo, 1999).

Technological aides that can assist persons with disability are a promising and increasingly important component of rehabilitative care (Symington, 1994). Rehabilitation engineers are sometimes involved in the evaluation and consideration of more elaborate, specialized equipment, such as environmental control units, computer systems, and power mobility devices that are customized to meet a particular patient's needs. Funding to purchase the more advanced assistive technology remains out of reach of many consumers. However, usage of more simple assistive technology, such as canes and walkers, results in fewer reported mobility difficulties in the disabled population (Agree, 1999).

Over the past 20 years, rehabilitation case managers have become a more significant part of the rehabilitation team. The role of case manager is often multifaceted, and may be carried out by individuals with specific roles on the team, such as a physician, nurse, psychologist, or social worker. In recent years, an individual who specializes in this activity and is not a direct treatment provider has often assumed this role. Most commonly, either the rehabilitation provider or the patient's insurance company employs this person. In some cases, there may be separate case managers associated with each of these interests.

Increasingly, these case managers play a pivotal role in recommending and arranging for the provision of needed care for the patient through the rehabilitation continuum. Also, this person may recommend against the approval or payment of services. This decision may be based on lack of insurance coverage for these benefits, lack of perceived need for the service, or the availability of a more cost-effective alternative. This role has led sometimes to friction between case managers and providers who see their professional judgment challenged, and with patients who resent being denied benefits to which they feel entitled.

Economic pressures have continued to mount for streamlining the rehabilitation team. This effort is taking several forms. For example, many rehabilitation hospitals no longer provide recreation therapy by a licensed recreation therapist. Also, some facilities rely more heavily on technicians or aides to provide a range of rehabilitation services. Sometimes referred to as "multi-skilling," this mode of providing services may cross traditional disciplinary lines, such as a technician or unlicensed assistant providing services usually provided by an occupational therapist. Multi-skilling has been criticized frequently because it was developed as a cost-containment method, and may lead to the provision of service by unqualified providers.

FUNDING SOURCES FOR MEDICAL REHABILITATION

PRIVATE PAYERS

EMPLOYERS PAY FOR or subsidize health care coverage for the majority of working Americans and their families. Over the last 2 decades, enrollment in managed care insurance plans has increased dramatically to approximately 95% of workers with health insurance (Henry J. Kaiser Family Foundation, 2004a). The most common types of managed care plans are health maintenance organizations (HMOs), preferred provider organizations (PPOs), and point-of-service plans (POSs). Although thorough descriptions of these types of managed care plans are beyond the scope of this chapter, the following summarizes the key differences between these plans.

HMOs are the oldest type of managed care plan, the most famous of which is Kaiser-Permanente. This HMO began its public operation in 1945 and now has 24% of all managed care enrollees (Henry J. Kaiser Family Foundation, 2004a). Traditional HMOs accept a capitation payment from the employer (or other payer) to deliver all the care necessary for its employees and their covered dependents. In a capitated contract, the HMO is paid a fixed sum of dollars for each member or enrollee of a plan, usually on a "per person per month" basis. The plan must meet the medical needs of all covered persons using the aggregate of this fixed dollar amount. Typically, each enrollee in a HMO selects a primary care provider, who coordinates all care and who authorizes all care that he/she doesn't provide, including specialty care, hospitalization, etc. The HMO may directly employ all, some, or none of the health care providers on their panel. If they are not employees of the HMO, the providers will usually have a contract with the HMO to provide care and share in the financial risks associated with the provision of care.

PPOs are plans where a managed care organization develops and contracts with groups of providers who agree to accept the plans' payment rates. The enrollee has a financial incentive to seek out the "preferred providers" because there may be no or lower co-payments. PPOs do not always have an assigned/selected primary care provider who authorizes services. Point-of-Service plans have both preferred (or "in-network") providers and "out-of-network" providers. Usually, enrollees select or are assigned a primary care provider who coordinates and authorizes care (often including out-of-network services). Again, the enrollee has a financial incentive to seek "in-network" services because the payment coverage is better.

Government Programs

Publicly financed health care programs accounted for nearly 46% of total national health care expenditures in 2002 ($713.4 billion; Levit et al., 2003). Medicare and Medicaid account for most of this spending, much of it directed to rehabilitation and other services for the elderly and people with disabilities. Patient populations at some rehabilitation facilities are composed primarily of Medicare and Medicaid recipients. Since their inception, both Medicare and Medicaid expenditures have consistently outpaced the rate of inflation and the rate of growth in expenditures of private funds. Federal and state legislative bodies have acted to slow this rapid growth rate through regulatory legislation and by encouraging experimentation in health care delivery models (Levit, Lazenby, & Braden, 1998). Health care delivery is being rapidly converted from fee-for-service (FFS) reimbursement to managed care, especially capitated contracts with commercial managed care organizations (MCOs).

Medicare

Title XVIII of the Social Security Act of 1965, otherwise known as Medicare, is the largest public payer of health care (Levit et al., 2003). Medicare is a social insurance program for persons over 65 years old, and for people with disabilities who have a sufficient work history to qualify for Social Security Disability Insurance (SSDI) for 24 consecutive months. In 2003, approximately 15% of Medicare beneficiaries (6 million) had a disability and were younger than 65 years old (Henry J. Kaiser Family Foundation, 2004b).

Part A of Medicare covers inpatient hospitalization, SNF care, home health care, and hospice care. Supplemental Medical Insurance (Part B) of Medicare is optional coverage that pays for physician and psychological services, and other services such as durable medical equipment, laboratory tests, medical supplies, and therapies (E. D. Hoffman, Klees, & Curtis, 2000). Contrary to popular belief, Medicare Part A expenditures are derived from mandatory payroll deductions from *current* wage earners. As health care costs rise and the population ages, Medicare Part A increasingly grows closer to financial insolvency. Depending on legislative action, Medicare Part A could exhaust its funds within the next few years. In order to slow down Medicare's cost inflation, federal legislation has encouraged experimental health care delivery programs and use of voluntary enrollment in managed care programs.

Medicaid

Medicaid (Title XIX of the Social Security Act) is a jointly sponsored program between the federal government and the states/territories. Within broad federal guidelines, each state establishes its own eligibility guidelines, determines the type and amount of services, sets provider payment rates, and administers its own program (E. D. Hoffman et al., 2000). States receive matching funds from the federal government to help offset the costs of care. The matching formula is based on the per capita income of each state/territory. Medicaid is the largest purchaser of health care services for the neediest and poorest people in the United States. In 2002, Medicaid covered approximately 47 million individuals, making it the most significant component of the "safety net." Medicaid's 2002 expenditures were $250.4 billion, representing approximately 35% of government expenditures for healthcare in the U.S. (Levit et al., 2003).

Approximately 8 million Medicaid recipients have a cognitive, psychiatric, or physical disability. A significant portion of Medicaid beneficiaries have multiple disabilities, further complicating health care service delivery. Furthermore, the elderly or disabled with low incomes who are eligible for Medicare are also eligible for supplemental Medicaid coverage. In 2002, there were approximately 7 million people who were dually enrolled in Medicaid and Medicare. In this era of cost containment and experimentation with health care delivery, it is important to remember that people under 65 years of age with disabilities comprise 16% of the enrollees in Medicaid, but spending for this group accounted for 43% of the costs in 2002 (Henry J. Kaiser Family Foundation, 2003c).

Limitations of the Medicare and Medicaid System for Persons with Disabilities

Overall, Medicare and Medicaid are critical and effective sources of health care for persons with disabilities. However, there are limitations of these programs that often exacerbate the health problems of persons with disabilities. Low reimbursement rates, limitations in coverage, and poor coordination of services place people with disabilities in a confusing and unfriendly health care maze. Furthermore, many people with disabilities have concomitant psychological and social problems, including affective and anxiety disorders, substance abuse/dependence, and social isolation (see, e.g., Heinemann, Keen, Donohue, & Schnoll, 1988). For many, behavioral difficulties, such as poor adherence to treatment regimens, result in costly complications and secondary disabilities. These problems are exacerbated by low income and difficulties meeting everyday basic living needs (Blendon et al., 1993). When psychological, social, and daily living needs go unmet, quality of life and medical status are worsened and health care costs are significantly increased (Friedman, Sobel, Myers, Caudill, & Benson, 1995). In addition, problems in obtaining health care worsen the health status and quality of life for persons with disabilities (Neri & Kroll, 2003).

As with Medicare, basic medical services are covered by Medicaid. The states, however, have wide discretion in providing "optional services," such as outpatient clinic services, diagnostic services, optometry, psychological care, rehabilitation, and physical therapy. Also, similar to Medicare, fee-for-service reimbursement is the traditional payment system in Medicaid. Medicaid costs have been rising dramatically over the last decade. State legislatures and governors, working with the federal government, have been rapidly converting their Medicaid systems from fee-for-service to managed care. Both reimbursement/payment methodologies have created problems for obtaining health care for people with disabilities. The health care needs of people with disabilities, combined with the low reimbursement to providers from Medicaid, contributes to many providers "not accepting Medicaid patients."

Furthermore, because of the recent dramatic reduction in revenues and increasing costs of Medicaid, every state has implemented changes to restrict Medicaid eligibility and benefits (Smith, Ramesh, Gifford, Ellis, & Wachino, 2003). The long-term effects of these changes are not yet known, but advocates are concerned that access to needed health care will be reduced for persons with disabilities.

CATASTROPHIC INSURANCE

LITTLE IS KNOWN about how health care changes will affect the delivery of rehabilitation services paid for by other forms of disability insurance, such as no-fault automobile catastrophic insurance, long-term disability insurance, and workers' compensation. Workers' compensation is different from most health programs because it provides for income replacement for injured workers as well as medical care. The significant costs associated with these benefits have led to tremendous efforts to rehabilitate workers and return them to the job. Workers' compensation carriers have used medical case management for many years in an attempt to control excessive costs secondary to overutilization of services. Prolonged disability is responsible for the greatest costs and involves medical, psychological, and socioecological issues that are best addressed from a multidisciplinary team. It is not clear, however, how often a rehabilitation model has been used effectively for temporarily or permanently disabled workers despite its proven efficacy with some groups of disabled persons.

Over the last 2 decades, workers' compensation costs rapidly rose to become a substantial business expense. Dembe and colleagues (Dembe, Himmelstein, Stevens, & Beachler, 1997) reported that workers' compensation costs rose 64% from 1984 to 1993, after adjusting for inflation, and made up 2.4% of the private sector payroll in 1991. Medical care costs overtook income replacement in total workers' compensation costs, something that had not happened in many years. Also, market competition among workers' compensation carriers, workers' demand for improved care, and employers' efforts to reduce costs and streamline administration have contributed to reform efforts. With these concerns in mind, more than 25 states began to enact legislation to reform workers' compensation, most of them authorizing or mandating managed care health delivery (Dembe et al.). Also, efforts have increased to link workers' compensation and general health care in order to reduce administrative costs, control cost shifting, and increase coordination of care, financing, and administration (Dembe et al.).

Only a few studies have examined either the short-term or long-term outcomes among people with disabilities using payer source, such as workers' compensation, as a variable. Tate and colleagues (1994), for example, examined the effects of payer type (Medicaid, catastrophic insurance, and private payer), extent of benefits, and independent living resources on functional, psychological, and social outcomes among 111 individuals with spinal cord injury. All participants were at least 2 years post-discharge from acute rehabilitation. Among the most significant findings was that people who had private insurance reported greater work and school activities compared to those with Medicaid or catastrophic no-fault insurance. Transportation benefits also were positively related to participation in work and school activities. Surprisingly, there was an inverse relationship between the extent of benefits and psychological and social outcome. The authors caution that the type of payment system and rules may foster dependency and poorer psychosocial outcome. Persons receiving catastrophic insurance benefits continually are forced to dramatize their needs to the insurance carrier or case manager in order to obtain benefits, sometimes creating a disincentive to increase independence. They suggested that a voucher system that allows personal choice of health care benefits might facilitate less dependency, improve psychological and social outcomes, and increase participation in functional activities, including work and school. The voucher system could be accompanied by an educational program to help individuals make choices of benefits that would maximize their independence and fit their unique situation.

FUNDING OF HEALTH CARE FOR CHILDREN WITH DISABILITIES

APPROXIMATELY 5% OF U.S. children and adolescents have a chronic health condition that interferes with one or more major life activities. Less than 1% of children have three or more chronic conditions, but developmental delays, learning disabilities, and emotional and behavioral problems are much more prevalent among this group of children with multiple chronic conditions (Newacheck & Stoddard, 1994). In general, children with chronic disabling conditions require coordinated specialized services, including occupational therapy, physical therapy, psychological and social services, speech and language therapy, and home care. As with adults, children with chronic disabling conditions are a relatively small percentage of all children, but they utilize a large percentage of health care services (Newacheck & Taylor, 1992). Medicaid covered approximately 2.1 million children with physical or mental disabilities and spent over $20 billion on health care for these children in 2000. This represented approximately 12% of the total Medicaid expenditures for 4% of the Medicaid population (Crowley & Elias, 2003). Also, children with special health care needs (CSHCN) such as those with chronic disabling conditions receive services funded by Title V programs (Social Security Act), through the Bureau of Maternal and Child Health, state health care programs, and school systems.

In addition to federal and state funded health care programs, approximately 60% of children with chronic disabling conditions receive services funded by private insurance. Often, these policies have restrictions on the type and scope of services, especially ancillary services and home care (Shonkoff et al., 1994). Also, many of these plans have annual or lifetime caps on benefits and/or cover only part of the costs of health care services. The children receiving health care through Medicaid and private insurance are rapidly being enrolled into managed care programs. The implications of these changes have yet to be fully realized, but many children's health care advocates have expressed concerns similar to those stated about the limitations of managed care for adults with disabilities.

Research has revealed mixed results on the effects of managed care on the outcomes of children with chronic disabling conditions. For example, Horwitz and Stein (1990) compared benefits for a sample of

HMOs with traditional indemnity insurers in Connecticut paying for services, to children on a fee-for-service basis. HMOs were found to offer more preventive care and increased access to care. However, both plans tended to have restrictions on services most commonly used by these children (mental health services and durable medical equipment). Case managers from both plans focused more on controlling costs than coordinating care. The study concluded that neither organization offered a comprehensive system of care to children with special health care needs.

Fox and Wicks (1993) conducted a cross-sectional survey of almost 700,000 children with disabilities due to chronic conditions. HMOs typically approved specialty care only when significant improvement could be documented within a short period of time. Other identified problems included difficulty accessing specialists, along with an insufficient number of specialists to provide consumer choice. Another survey (Fox, Wicks, & Newacheck, 1993) of state Medicaid offices documented that some HMOs were resistant to providing necessary mental health, speech, and occupational therapy services to children with special health care needs. For example, coordination of services for children at risk for serious emotional disturbance was hampered by the move toward managed care in one study (Hocutt, McKinney, & Montague, 2002). In general it was found that managed care plans for children with special health care needs who were Medicaid recipients referred the children to adult subspecialists more often than pediatric subspecialists. Also, long-standing provider relationships were disrupted in the transition to managed care. Furthermore, more parents of these children were dissatisfied with managed care than with fee-for-service Medicaid (Stroul, Pires, Armstrong, & Zaro, 2002).

STATE CHILDREN'S HEALTH INSURANCE PROGRAM

THE STATE CHILDREN'S Health Insurance Program (SCHIP), codified as Title XXI of the Social Security Act, was enacted as part of the Balanced Budget Act of 1997. The purpose of this law was to extend insurance/health care to approximately 40% of the uninsured children in the U.S. As a federal "grant-in-aid" program, this law encourages states to extend health care coverage either through Medicaid or through an alternative program to low-income, uninsured children. In return, the states may receive matching funds from the federal government. These programs increased the income threshold of eligibility for subsidized coverage to 214% of the federal policy level and insured 5.3 million children during FY 2002. In a sample of states, SCHIP enrolled a higher percentage of CSHCN, including children with a high level of unmet heath care needs, compared to the general child population (Szilagyi et al., 2003). These investigators suggest that SCHIP may need to consider a variety of financing mechanisms, including risk-adjustment funding strategies, high-risk pools, reinsurance mechanisms, and improved compensation for primary care practitioners, for case management of the severe CSHCN population within SCHIP.

Access to care under SCHIP is generally described as good for those enrolled in urban areas with managed care arrangements (Wooldridge et al., 2003). An important regulation of SCHIP for children with disabilities is that states may not deny enrollment or coverage because of preexisting conditions (Rosenbaum, Johnson, Sonosky, Markus, & DeGraw, 1998).

MANAGED CARE FOR PERSONS WITH DISABILITIES

THEORETICALLY, MANAGED CARE has the potential to improve care for medically complex, high-cost populations, such as people with disabilities (Reilly, Coburn, & Kilbreth, 1990) by employing organized delivery systems that emphasize timely, comprehensive, and community-based services. MCOs have traditionally avoided complex, high-cost populations and, therefore, have limited experience in implementing effective programs.

Evaluation studies of managed care performance in the general population have focused on utilization of services and costs. Rarely are these measures of performance paired with analyses of the health status of the population. The results of the performance of managed care on health outcomes have been mixed and there are virtually no data on functional health-related quality of life (Miller & Luft, 1994). This is particularly true of those with disabilities or chronic illness where there is a need for better outcome measures and evaluations that estimate the program effects (Ireys, Thornton, & McKay, 2002). Beatty and colleagues (2003) found few differences in access to care or outcomes across FFS or managed care payment systems for persons with arthritis, SCI, multiple sclerosis, or cerebral palsy.

The ability of a publicly funded managed care system in Tennessee to serve blind and disabled persons who receive Supplemental Security Income (SSI) was examined (Hill and Woolridge, 2003). They found that this disabled population had worse access to care (specialists, medication, & equipment) and less satisfaction with care compared to other managed care enrollees. Elderly Medicare managed care enrollees were also less satisfied with access to specialists, but more satisfied with costs compared to non-managed care enrollees (Iezzoni, Davis, Soukup, & O'Day, 2002).

In another study, Medicare beneficiaries in poorest health or most severely disabled perceived both access to care and cost difficulties irrespective of whether they were in managed care plans or had traditional FFS Medicare coverage (Beatty & Dhont, 2001). A qualitative study examining health care of people with cerebral palsy, multiple sclerosis, or spinal cord injury found that a lack of disability-specific knowledge, limited provider time, and poor communication among providers were obstacles to care coordination that were generally equally prevalent between persons in managed care and fee-for services health plans (Kroll & Neri, 2003). Porell and Miltiades (2001) found that Medicare managed care resulted in no adverse risk of decline in functional status in a large general population of Medicare recipients compared to FFS Medicare.

MANAGED CARE MODELS IN GOVERNMENT-FUNDED PROGRAMS

BOTH MEDICAID AND Medicare have been experimenting with health care delivery models that provide an alternative to the fee-for-services system. Medicaid's conversion to managed care has been much more rapid than that of Medicare. Additionally, the Medicare program is exclusively administered through the federal government, whereas Medicaid is essentially 56 separate programs. This creates numerous obstacles to developing and implementing model managed care programs for Medicare recipients with disabilities compared to Medicaid, where each state government has some latitude in experimenting with alternative delivery systems.

Although most states began converting fee-for-service Medicaid to managed care with the use of a primary-care case-management model, there has been rapid growth in risk-based managed care contracting since 1994. In this situation, a Medicaid agency contracts with an MCO to provide an agreed-upon set of services in exchange for a preset capitated payment for the entire health care needs of a patient. Payment is not contingent on the level of service provided, unless special services or programs (e.g., transplant services) are exempted from the contract and paid by Medicaid on a fee-for-service basis.

In many Medicaid programs, mental health services are also "carved out," creating a separate sub-capitation despite the fact that most policy analysts recommend complete integration of mental health services. For rehabilitation clients, this can result in a subcontract with a separate set of mental health providers, who may not be a part of the rehabilitation team and may lack specialized knowledge of the role of the person's disability. Savings incurred by this integration are also not available for use to fund non-mental health care. Until such services are integrated, the false distinction between mind and body will be perpetuated, and health care delivery will continue to be uncoordinated and ineffective. Also, Medicaid plans often do not include people who receive both Medicare and Medicaid. The regulations of the two programs are often incompatible, thereby complicating the coordination of health care services and financing. States can apply for waivers to combine the funding streams of these two programs in order to develop innovative health care delivery programs.

FOR-PROFIT VS. NOT-FOR-PROFIT SECTORS IN THE DELIVERY OF REHABILITATION CARE

MANY REHABILITATION CLINICS and hospital services are for-profit taxpaying businesses with accountability to owners/stockholders for profitability. This means that the less income that is paid out for patient care and administrative expenses, the more money there is to invest in the growth of the company or to pay owners/stockholders. A study of the impact of ownership arrangements and profitability in outpatient physical therapy clinics found that clinics jointly owned by physicians and physical therapists saw patients for 39%–45% more visits than in non-physician owned comprehensive rehabilitation facilities providing services, and concomitantly their revenue per patient was 30%–40% higher (Mitchell & Scott, 1992). Furthermore, it appeared that unlicensed personnel in the physician-owned practices delivered more care. Such findings have contributed to the regulations limiting the practice of physician referrals to rehabilitation facilities that they own. A study of home health agencies found that care was four times more expensive in for-profit proprietary agencies than in public agencies (Williams, 1994). When comparisons were made between for-profit and not-for-profit rehabilitation hospitals, for-profit hospitals showed higher net revenue and profits and employed fewer people than non-profit hospitals (McCue & Thompson, 1995). A large part of the growth in outpatient programs has been by for-profit corporations. Clearly, these companies have recognized the potential for profit and growth.

Non-profit entities do not pay corporate profits and do not answer to shareholders, but still face pressures to hold down costs and realize a positive financial margin to reinvest in the company's future. Some health care systems are owned and operated by local or state governments or the federal government. This includes city, county, or state health facilities and agencies as well as most public university medical centers. In addition, the military and veterans administration are one of the largest providers of rehabilitation services (Wilson & Kizer, 1997). The Veterans Administration Medical Centers (VAMC) rehabilitation departments are particularly well known for work with military service veterans with stroke, spinal cord injury, and those with amputations.

VAMCs offer comprehensive care including some options for care in nursing homes, residential placements, and home care. Coverage and benefits are dependent on several factors, including whether the health problem was incurred during or related to service in the military (i.e., service connected), and financial resources.

SPECIFIC COST-CONTAINMENT STRATEGIES

PROSPECTIVE PAYMENT AND CASE MIX GROUPS

AS MENTIONED EARLIER, much of the expansion in the continuum of rehabilitation care can be credited to a stable source of funding through Medicare and Medicaid. A decade ago, Medicare and Medicaid recipients comprised approximately half of patients seeking rehabilitation services (Aitchison, 1993). More recent statistics estimate that roughly 70% of all patients treated at inpatient rehabilitation facilities (IRFs) are Medicare beneficiaries (Centers for Medicare and Medicaid Services, 2004b). A second funding boon was the adoption of the Tax Equity and Fiscal Responsibility Act (TEFRA) in 1982, which allowed many rehabilitation hospitals and units to be reimbursed by Medicare based on the hospital's cost per discharge, rather than on what was considered a less lucrative prospective payment system (PPS) where facilities are reimbursed a predetermined fee for hospitalization based on the patient's diagnosis or diagnostic related groups (DRGs).

Exemption from prospective payment for rehabilitation facilities was done because DRGs did not account well for the high variability in hospital resource utilization for rehabilitation patients. An analysis by Schneider, Cromwell, and McGuire (1993) found that TEFRA limits were insufficient to account for increases in costs of providing care by rehabilitation facilities. However, the TEFRA payment system also provided a financial incentive for rehabilitation hospitals to discharge patients quickly (Chan et al., 1997). The hospital could collect incentive payments from Medicare for reducing its per-patient charge compared to a "base year." This could be accomplished by reducing length of patient stay, which did occur, but has caused the number of discharges from rehabilitation hospitals to skilled nursing facilities to increase 48% from 1992 to 1994 (Wynn). It also caused facilities to try to admit less complex and less severely disabled patients. In response to these issues, Congress passed a provision in the Balanced Budget Act of 1997 that mandated a revision for the entire post acute care (PAC) reimbursement system as a means of controlling costs (Cotterill & Gage, 2002). In the case of rehabilitation facilities, this mandated a change to a prospective payment system (PPS), which was originally scheduled for implementation on October 1, 2000. Subsequent modification of the Act by the Balanced Budget Refinement Act of 1999 and the Benefits Improvement Act of 2000 resulted in final adoption of an IRF PPS effective January 1, 2002.

When ultimately adopted, the PPS reflected a significant sea change from the previous retrospectively based TEFRA system. The new reimbursement system avoided per-diem charges, mandating instead a diagnostic-specific flat rate based on anticipated resources required for provision of patient rehabilitation services. Reimbursement rates were established for Case Mix Groups (CMGs) based on the patient's clinical characteristics as derived from the 21 defined Rehabilitation Impairment Categories (RICs), motor and cognitive level of function as defined by the Functional Independence Measure (FIM), and the patient's age. This classification scheme yielded 95 CMG categories with five additional categories for special situations. An additional important feature of the total reimbursement schedule is a three-tiered adjustment for comorbidities. Specific comorbidities have been defined by the Centers for Medicare and Medicaid Services (CMS) and can be classified as high cost (tier 1), medium cost (tier 2), or low cost (tier 3). The level of comorbidity provides a weighted adjustment to the overall prospective reimbursement rate. The only other adjustments to this rate are designed to address variations in cost due to geographic location, percentage of low-income patients, and rural location (Centers for Medicare and Medicaid Services, 2004b). Concern has also been expressed regarding the capacity of the new system to compensate appropriately for medically complex cases with higher acuity (Hoffman et al., 2003; Stineman, 2002). In general, IRF providers greeted the PPS with initial uneasiness. Most have faired well financially under the system (Schmelling, 2003), and the PPS is widely considered to be more equitable (Fowler, 2003).

An additional important goal for the PPS was to gather more and better information for purposes of improved future decision-making relative to rates and desired treatment locations. As part of the new PPS, patients are classified using a standard data collection instrument titled the Inpatient Rehabilitation Facility—Patient Assessment Instrument or IRF-PAI. Based on the Functional Independence Measure (FIM), the IRF-PAI provides a uniform set of patient data regarding admission and discharge levels of functional independence (Carter, Relles, Ridgeway, & Rimes, 2003). The IRF-PAI classification provides a reasonably uniform measure of time and resources required for inpatient rehabilitation. It has been described as one of the best CMS-designed prospective payment systems (Morrison, 2002). Beyond its utility as a classification measure, it provides a growing and comprehensive information base of standardized data for use in future decision-making.

The 75% Rule

THE CHANGE TO a PPS has indeed been a fundamental sea change in the character of reimbursement for IRFs. Yet, the enforcement of the long-standing "75% rule" represents perhaps a significantly greater threat to the capacity to provide patients with rehabilitation services as well as to the financial viability and ultimate survival of many inpatient facilities. As noted above, IRFs were exempted from participation in the earlier acute care prospective payment system (DRGs) due to the high variability in the resources needed for inpatient rehabilitation. A higher intensity of IRF services also resulted in generally higher reimbursement rates. However, as a condition for classification as an IRF, the provider was required to demonstrate that 75% of patients treated at the facility came from 10 diagnostic groups: stroke, spinal cord injury, congenital deformity, amputation, major multiple trauma, fracture of the femur (hip fracture), brain injury, polyarthritis (including rheumatoid arthritis), specified neurological disorders, and burns (Centers for Medicare and Medicaid Services, 2004b).

For a variety of reasons, the 75% rule was never consistently enforced. In particular, there has been considerable confusion regarding clear diagnostic classification, particularly for patients who undergo prosthetic joint replacement for severe arthritis (most frequently hips and knees). At question is whether individuals who have undergone such surgery still can be classified as experiencing arthritis in that joint. Also at question has been the adequacy of documentation of polyarthritis. Interestingly, it has been the improved quality of standardized data available from the IRF-PAI that has helped illuminate the inconsistencies in enforcement of this rule. According to CMS (2004b) estimates, only 13.35% of facilities were meeting the 75% rule. Nationally, only 50% of patients being served in the IRF setting fell into one of the 10 categories (Murer, 2002).

If enforced in the current environment, the financial consequences for patients and IRF providers has been described as severe (American Medical Rehabilitation Providers Association, 2004). Failure to meet the 75% rule would result in reclassification of the facility as an acute care facility with reimbursement at the substantially lower Inpatient Prospective Payment System rate (Centers for Medicare and Medicaid Services, 2004a). Given the significantly higher costs for the more intensive patient rehabilitation services (IPPS) and the significantly lower reimbursement rates in the IPPS, the consequences of such reclassification would be financially disastrous for an IRF. Enforcement of the 75% rule is slated for initiation on July 1, 2004. There were minor revisions to diagnostic categories that could be included under the 75% rule, and the rule was to be progressively phased in over 3 years with full implementation on July 1, 2007 (Centers for Medicare and Medicaid Services).

Implementation of this rule has raised widespread concern for IRF providers. The American Medical Rehabilitation Providers Association (American Medical Rehabilitation Providers Association, 2004) estimated that the impact could be catastrophic. The American Hospital Association cited statistics estimating that 94% of facilities would need to turn patients away, and that 90% of communities lack the capacity to serve patients in alternate settings (American Hospital Association, 2003). They estimated that 52% of patients would be harmed due to lack of access to inpatient rehabilitation facilities. In 2003, the American Hospital Association referenced estimates that only 157 of the current 1,210 IRFs would be eligible for licensing under the 75% rule. At this writing, vigorous efforts were underway to either reverse or substantially modify the enforcement provision of the 75% rule (American Medical Rehabilitation Providers Association).

DECREASED HOSPITALIZATION

WITH THE INCREASED penetration of managed care and the specter of additional cost-containment methodologies, traditional, institutionally based rehabilitation is undergoing significant changes in service delivery. Already, lengths of stay have been severely shortened. From 1986 to 1992, rehabilitation inpatient days declined by 3 to 4 days, or about 15% of the total rehabilitation stay (Wolk & Blair, 1994). This has resulted in a shorter time to reach rehabilitation goals. At the same time, occupancy rates have shown only slight changes, reflecting the increased number of patients admitted to most inpatient rehabilitation facilities even in the face of an increase in the number of inpatient programs. Decreased length of hospitalization has resulted in improved efficiency in the average patient's gains in functional status per week, with little negative effect on the total level of functional gains achieved during the rehabilitation stay during the 3-year period from 1990–1992 (Granger & Hamilton, 1994).

It can be anticipated that health care intensity and services will be tied to the reimbursement system that supports it. Cotterill and Gage (2002) noted that location for service provision (acute vs. acute rehab vs. SNF, etc.) tends to shift in response to reimbursement policies. As such, it is reasonable to assume that providers in all post-acute settings will seek to provide services in the most efficient and financially viable manner. If the Centers for Medicare and Medicaid Services' reform goals are to reduce costs and tie medical care to the realities of cost, it is reasonable to expect that services will adhere to the laws of the marketplace (Banja & DeJong, 2000). Ultimately, the challenge will be one of balancing the financial decisions with the needs for socially responsible medical care.

TREATMENT GUIDELINES

INCREASINGLY, CARE IS being provided based on guidelines or critical paths of care. This is an effort to provide cost-effective quality care by reducing variability in clinical practice by providers. In some settings, providers must justify deviations from such guidelines. This use of clinical guidelines increasingly involves the types of cases seen in rehabilitation, such as back pain (Low Back Pain Guideline Team, 1997), spinal cord injury (Consortium for Spinal Cord Medicine, 1997), or home care (Gingerich & Ondeck, 1995).

CONSUMER PROTECTION/RIGHTS

IN THE PAST, consumers have generally viewed their health provider as an advocate for their obtaining the best care possible. It has been understood by consumers that most providers were paid under a fee-for-service arrangement, where the more service that they delivered, the more money they were paid, and that they profited from caring for the patient. There was little reason to doubt that the provider would order everything that was medically necessary for the patient's care. Furthermore, because the provider made the decisions regarding care, they were legally liable for mistakes in decision-making or service delivery. At times, this led to the provision of excessive care and unnecessary health care costs for payers.

Now, the concern is the opposite. In a prepaid or capitated system, the provider of services may receive a fixed amount based on diagnosis, or have decisions regarding the kind or amount of treatment reviewed by payers or based on guidelines determined by others. In these managed health plans, the provider may be subject to strong financial incentives to limit care or provide less expensive care. In this case, the health care consumer can be less certain regarding the degree to which a treatment decision is motivated more by cost savings than by optimal care. In a poll commissioned by the American Psychological Association, 81% of adults sampled were very concerned about changes in the health care system. Thirty-six percent indicated that their main concern was quality of care, 25% indicated access or availability of care, and 21% were most concerned about cost (Newman, 1997). Non-elderly sick persons with managed health plans are significantly more likely than those with traditional fee-for-service insurance to complain of problems obtaining treatment, diagnostic tests, and uncaring physicians (Donelan, Blendon, Benson, Leitman, & Taylor, 1996).

These concerns have led to state and federal legislative and regulatory initiatives to safeguard consumer rights in key aspects of health care. In his 1998 State of the Union Address to Congress, President Clinton stated that physicians and not health plan "accountants" should make medical decisions. He called on Congress to pass a patients' Bill of Rights that includes many patient protections. As the century turned, there was considerable interest in a Patients' Bill of Rights. In fact, separate, though rather similar "Patient Protection Acts" were passed in both the House and Senate. Provisions included guidelines for access to services, choice of providers, continuity of care, appeal processes, and external review, among others. The largest differences between the bills involved definitions of liability for decision-making by insurance plans (Olsen, 2001). However, in the tragedy and aftermath of the World Trade Center attack on September 11, 2001, the Acts languished, as did almost all other legislation of the session. Although patient rights and responsibilities are defined to some extent by accrediting bodies such as the Joint Commission on Accreditation of Healthcare Organizations (JCAHO) and the Commission on Accreditation of Rehabilitation Facilities (CARF), further federal legislation has not been forthcoming.

Coalitions representing business and insurance interests assert that such regulation is not needed since the consumer is able to change health plans or providers if they are not satisfied with the care that they receive. In a perfect market system, this may be true, but this assertion ignores several important points. First, consumers may not always be able to judge when they are receiving inferior care, or be in a position to change health plans or providers when they experience poor care. Second, consumers who receive their health benefits through an employer may be at the mercy of limited options that the employer offers. Third, many persons receiving rehabilitative care require services that are very costly to managed health plans. Such plans may not have a financial incentive to keep such patients as part of their plan, and actually benefit if such a patient chooses another health plan.

There has been longstanding concern about the lack of consumer ability to influence factors that would allow marketplace forces to operate in an efficient manner in health care (Bingaman, Frank, & Billy, 1993). Kuttner (1997) indicates that consumers lack the "symmetrical" market power with providers of health care that would allow self-correcting for exploitative practices. Various solutions to rectifying this inequity have been proposed. These include publication of "report cards" on health plans and hospitals. Another suggestion is to establish consumer councils elected by consumers who work with the managers of health care plans to improve service (Rodwin, 1997).

In addition, there has been significant legislation affecting the privacy of medical information. In 1996, President Clinton signed into law the Health Insurance Portability and Accountability Act (HIPAA) as a measure to protect health insurance coverage for workers and their families when they lose or change jobs. To accomplish this, HIPAA also required the establishment of standards for electronic data transfer and management, as well as the security and privacy of health information (Centers for Medicare and Medicaid Services, 2002). The regulations were in many ways complex and far-reaching (Parver, 2001). Confusion was common following their implementation, though HIPAA was described by some commentators as manageable with knowledge, planning, and common sense (Murer, 2004).

THE FUTURE: A CONSUMER-DRIVEN SYSTEM OF HEALTH CARE

P EOPLE WITH DISABILITIES require health delivery systems designed specifically for their complex health care needs. As DeJong (1997) points out, people with disabilities have a "thinner margin of health" and need unique programs to engage in preventive and health maintenance practices. Also, they are more likely to acquire secondary conditions and have greater needs for access to specialists and ancillary services, such as durable medical equipment and assistive technologies (DeJong). The field of rehabilitation is uniquely suited to the needs of people with disabilities because of its focus on long-term outcomes.

However, traditional rehabilitation needs to be restructured. Rehabilitation providers and institutions are beginning to consider delivering comprehensive services under capitated, full-risk payment systems. The implications of these changes for people with disabilities and for the provision of rehabilitation services are profound and not yet fully understood. Initial evidence suggests that managed health care models designed specifically to meet the highly variable and complex health care needs of people with disabilities can successfully enhance long-term outcome and be cost-effective. This requires understanding the long-term needs and costs of people with disabilities, and delivering rehabilitation services in a cost-efficient but high-quality manner.

Community-based programs emphasizing preventive and health-promotion intervention will be integral to high-quality care that maximizes long-term outcomes and cost control. Additionally, the independent living movement has become more sophisticated and is making headway in convincing policy makers that a consumer-driven health care system is not only appropriate to promote independent living, but is likely to be cost-effective. For example, consumer-driven personal assistance programs are gaining popularity. A voucher system in which consumers exert greater control over where health care dollars are spent may be the next shift in reimbursement systems. This would force providers and managed care organizations to compete for limited dollars by improving services and emphasizing outcomes. Information and marketing will be a major component of health delivery systems, but it will need to be supported by research on the long-term success of interventions and organized delivery systems.

REFERENCES

Agree, E. (1999). The influence of personal care and assistive devices on the measurement of disability. *Social Science & Medicine, 48*(4), 427–443.

Aitchison, K. W. (1993). Rehabilitation at the crossroads: Financial and other considerations. *American Journal of Physical Medicine and Rehabilitation, 72*(6), 405–407.

American Hospital Association. (2003). The true cost of the proposed 75% rehab rule. *AHA News, 1*, 6.

American Medical Rehabilitation Providers Association (AMRPA). (2004, April 30). Statement of AMRPA. *Real-time outcomes reports* (news release).

Banja, J. D., & DeJong, G. (2000). The rehabilitation marketplace: Economics, values, and proposals for reform. *Archives of Physical Medicine and Rehabilitation, 81*(2), 233–240.

Beatty, P. W., & Dhont, K. R. (2001). Medicare health maintenance organizations and traditional coverage: Perspectives of health care among beneficiaries with disabilities. *Archives of Physical Medicine and Rehabilitation, 82*(8), 1009–1017.

Beatty, P. W., Hagglund, K. J., Neri, M. T., Dhont, K. R., Clark, M. J., & Hilton, S. A. (2003). Access to health care services among people with chronic or disabling conditions: Patterns and predictors. *Archives of Physical Medicine and Rehabilitation, 84*(10), 1417–1425.

Bingaman, J., Frank, R. G., & Billy, C. L. (1993). Combining a global health budget with a market-driven delivery system. Can it be done? *American Psychologist, 48*(3), 270–276.

Blendon, R. J., Donelan, K., Hill, C., Scheck, A., Carter, W., Beatrice, D., et al. (1993). Medicaid beneficiaries and health reform. *Health Affairs, 12*(1), 132–143.

Buchanan, J. L., Rumpel, J. D., & Hoenig, H. (1996). Changes for outpatient rehabilitation: Growth and differences in provider types. *Archives of Physical Medicine and Rehabilitation, 77*(4), 320–328.

Carter, G. M., Relles, D. A., Ridgeway, G. K., & Rimes, C. M. (2003). Measuring function for Medicare inpatient rehabilitation payment. *Health Care Financing Review, 24*(3), 25–44.

Centers for Medicare and Medicaid Services. (2002). *Overview of the Medicare program*. Retrieved from http://www.cms.hhs.gov

Centers for Medicare and Medicaid Services. (2004a). CMS announces changes in criteria for classifying inpatient rehabilitation facilities. CMS News (Press Release). Retrieved April 30, 2004, from http://www.cms.hhs.gov/media/press/release.asp

Centers for Medicare and Medicaid Services. (2004b). Changes to the criteria for being classified as an inpatient rehabilitation facility: Final rule. Washington, DC: Author.

Chan, L., & Ciol, M. (2000). Medicare's payment system: Its effect on discharges to skilled nursing facilities from rehabilitation hospitals. *Archives of Physical Medicine and Rehabilitation, 81*(6), 715–719.

Chan, L., Koepsell, T. D., Deyo, R. A., Esselman, P. C., Haselkorn, J. K., et al. (1997). The effects of Medicare's payment system for rehabilitation hospitals on length of stay, charges, and total payments. *New England Journal of Medicine, 337*(14), 978–985.

Consortium for Spinal Cord Medicine. (1997). *Acute management of autonomic dysreflexia: Adults with spinal cord injury presenting to health-care facilities*. Washington, DC: Paralyzed Veterans of America.

Cotterill, P. G., & Gage, B. J. (2002). Overview: Medicare post-acute care since the Balanced Budget Act of 1007. *Health Care Financing Review, 24*(2), 25–44.

Crowley, J. S., & Elias, R. (2003). Medicaid's role for people with disabilities. A report of the Kaiser Commission on Medicaid and the Uninsured. Retrieved from http://www.kff.org/medicaid

DeJong, G. (1997). Primary care for persons with disabilities. *American Journal of Physical Medicine and Rehabilitation, 76*(3 suppl.), S2–S8.

Dembe, A. E., Himmelstein, J. S., Stevens, B. A., & Beachler, M. P. (1997). Improving workers' compensation health care. *Health Affairs, 16*(4), 253–257.

Deutsch, A., Fiedler, R. C., Granger, C. V., & Russell, C. F. (2002). The Uniform Data System for Medical Rehabilitation Report of patients discharged from Comprehensive Medical Rehabilitation Programs in 1999. *American Journal of Physical Medicine and Rehabilitation, 81*(2), 133–142.

DeVivo, M. J. (1999). Discharge disposition from model spinal cord injury care system rehabilitation programs. *Archives of Physical Medicine and Rehabilitation, 80*(7), 785–790.

Donelan, K., Blendon, R. J., Benson, J., Leitman, R., & Taylor, H. (1996). All payer, single payer, managed care, no payer: Patients' perspectives in three nations. *Health Affairs, 15*(2), 254–265.

Fowler, F. J. (2003, August/September). Straight talk. *Rehab Management.*

Fox, H. B., & Wicks, L. B. (1993). Health maintenance organizations and children with special health needs: A suitable match? *American Journal of Diseases of Children, 147*, 546–552.

Fox, H. B., Wicks, L. B., & Newacheck, P. W. (1993). State Medicaid health maintenance organization policies and special needs children. *Health Care Financing Review, 15*(1), 25–37.

Frederickson, M., & Cannon, N. L. (1995). The role of the rehabilitation physician in the postacute continuum. *Archives of Physical Medicine and Rehabilitation, 66*(12 Suppl.), S5–S9.

Friedman, R., Sobel, D., Myers, P., Caudill, M., & Benson, H. (1995). Behavioral medicine, clinical health psychology, and cost offset. *Health Psychology, 14,* 509–518.

Gingerich, B. S., & Ondeck, D. A. (1995). *Clinical pathways for the multidisciplinary home care team.* Gaithersburg, MD: Aspen Publishers.

Granger, C. V., & Hamilton, B. B. (1994). The Uniform Data system for medical rehabilitation report of first admissions for 1992. *American Journal of Physical Medicine and Rehabilitation, 73*(1), 51–55.

Heinemann, A., Keen, M., Donohue, R., & Schnoll, S. (1988). Alcohol use in persons with recent spinal cord injuries. *Archives of Physical Medicine and Rehabilitation, 69*(8), 619–624.

Henry J. Kaiser Family Foundation. (2004a). Trends and indicators in the changing health care marketplace, 2004 Update. Retrieved June 10, 2004, from http://www.kff.org/insurance/7031/ti2004-2-3.cfm

Henry J. Kaiser Family Foundation. (2004b). Fact sheet: Medicare at a glance. Retrieved June 10, 2004, from http://www.kff.org/medicare/loader.cfm?url=/commonspot/security/getfile.cfm&PageID=33319

Henry J. Kaiser Family Foundation. (2004c). Fact Sheet: Medicaid Program at a glance. Retrieved June 10, 2004, from http://www.kff.org/medicaid/loader.cfm?url=/commonspot/security/getfile.cfm&PageID=30463

Hill, S. C., & Wooldridge, J. (2003). SSI enrollees' health care in TennCare. *Journal of Health Care for the Poor and Underserved, 14*(2), 229–243.

Hocutt, A. M., McKinney, J. D., & Montague, M. (2002). The impact of managed care on efforts to prevent development of serious emotional disturbance in young children. *Journal of Disability Policy Studies, 13*(1), 51–60.

Hoffman, E. D., Klees, B. S., & Curtis, C.A. (2000). Overview of the Medicare and Medicaid program. *Health Care Financing Review,* Medicare and Medicaid Supplement, 1–19.

Hoffman, J. M., Doctor, J. N., Chan, L., Whyte, J., Jha, A., & Dikmen, S. (2003). Potential impact of the new Medicare Prospective Payment System on reimbursement for traumatic brain injury inpatient rehabilitation. *Archives of Physical Medicine and Rehabilitation, 84,* 1165–1172.

Horwitz, S. M., & Stein, R. E. (1990). Health maintenance organizations versus indemnity insurance for children with chronic illness: Trading gaps in coverage. *American Journal of Diseases of Children, 144,* 581–586.

Iezzoni, L. I., Davis, R. B., Soukup, J., & O'Day, B. (2003). Satisfaction with quality and access to health care among people with disabling conditions. *International Journal for Quality in Health Care, 14*(5), 369–381.

Ireys, H. T., Thornton, C., & McKay, H. (2002). Medicaid managed care and working-age beneficiaries with disabilities and chronic illnesses. *Health Care Financing Review, 24*(1), 27–42.

Kroll, T., & Neri, M. T. (2003). Experiences with care co-ordination among people with cerebral palsy, multiple sclerosis, or spinal cord injury. *Disability & Rehabilitation, 25*(19), 1106–1114.

Kuttner, R. (1997). *Everything for sale: The virtue and limits of markets.* New York: Alfred A. Knopf.

Lathan, C., Kinsella, M. A., Rosen, M. J., Winters, J., & Trepagnier, C. (1999). Aspects of human factors engineering in home telemedicine and telerehabilitation systems. *Telemedicine Journal, 5*(2), 169–175.

Levit, K. R., Lazenby, H. C., & Braden, B. R. (1998). National health spending trends in 1996. *Health Affairs, 17*(1), 35–51.

Levit, K., Smith, C., Cowan, C., Sensenig, A., Catlin, A., & the Health Accounts Team. (2003). Health spending rebound continues in 2002. *Health Affairs, 23*(1), 147–159.

Low Back Pain Guideline Team. (1997). *Guidelines for clinical care: Acute low back pain.* Retrieved from http://www.med.umich.edu/i/oca/practiceguides/index.htm

McCue, M. J., & Thompson, J. M. (1995). The ownership difference in relative performance of rehabilitation specialty hospitals. *Archives of Physical Medicine and Rehabilitation, 76*(5), 413–418.

Miller, R., & Luft, H. (1994). Managed care plan performance since 1980: A literature analysis. *Journal of the American Medical Association, 271,* 1512–1519.

Mitchell, J. M., & Scott, E. (1992). Physician ownership of physical therapy services. Effects on charges, utilization, profits, and service characteristics. *Journal of the American Medical Association, 268*(15), 2055–2059.

Morrision, M. H. (2002, April). The positive spin. *Rehab Management, 24,* 26.

Murer, C. G. (2004, March). Trends and issues. *Rehab Management,* 46–48.

Neri, M. T., & Kroll, T. (2003). Understanding the consequences of access barriers to health care: Experiences of adults with disabilities. *Disability and Rehabilitation, 25*(2), 85–96.

Newacheck, P. W., & Stoddard, J. J. (1994). Prevalence and impact of multiple childhood chronic illnesses. *Journal of Pediatrics 124*(1), 40–48.

Newacheck, P. W., & Taylor, W. R. (1992). Childhood chronic illness: Prevalence, severity, and impact. *American Journal of Public Health, 82*(3), 364–371.

Newman, R. (1997, March). Keynote Address. Paper presented at the meeting of the American Psychological Association State Leadership Conference, Washington, DC.

Nosek, M. A. (1993). Personal assistance: Its effect on the long-term health of a rehabilitation hospital population. *Archives of Physical Medicine and Rehabilitation, 74*(2), 127–132.

Olsen, G. G. (2001, November). Legislative watch. *Rehab Management,* 43–44.

Parver, C. (2001, November). Protecting your patients and practice. *Rehab Management,* 74–75, 82.

Porell, F. W., & Miltiades, H. B. (2001). Disability outcomes of older Medicare HMO enrollees and fee-for-service Medicare beneficiaries. *Journal of the American Geriatrics Society, 49*(5), 615–631.

Reilly, P., Coburn, A. F., & Kilbreth, E. H. (1990). *Medicaid managed care: The state of the art.* Portland, ME: National Academy for State Health Policy.

Rodwin, M. A. (1997). The neglected remedy: Strengthening consumer voice in managed care. *The American Prospect, 34*, 45–50.

Rosenbaum, S., Johnson, K., Sonosky, C., Markus, A., & DeGraw, C. (1998). The children's hour: The State Children's Health Insurance Program. *Health Affairs, 17*(1), 75–89.

Schmelling, S. (2003, August/September). Trends and issues: Interview with Cherilyn G. Murer, JD, CRA. *Rehab Management.*

Schneider, J. E., Cromwell, J., & McGuire, T. P. (1993). Excluded facility financial status and options for payment system modification. *Health Care Financing Review, 15*(2), 7–30.

Schopp, L. H., Johnstone, B. R., & Merveille, O. C. (2000). Multidimensional tele-care strategies for rural residents with brain injury. *Journal of Telemedicine and Telecare, 6*(Suppl. 1), S146–S149.

Shonkoff, J., Sweeney, M., McManus, M., Corro, D., Skubel, E., & McPherson, M. (1994). *Meeting the needs of chronically disabled children in a changing health care system* (Issue Brief No. 651). Washington, DC: National Health Policy Forum, George Washington University.

Smith, V., Ramesh, P., Gifford, K., Ellis, E., & Wachino, V. (2003). States respond to fiscal pressure: State Medicaid spending growth and cost containment in fiscal years 2003 and 2004. Washington, DC: Kaiser Commission on Medicaid and the Uninsured. Henry J. Kaiser Family Foundation.

Stineman, M. G. (2002). Prospective payment, prospective challenge. *Archives of Physical Medicine and Rehabilitation, 83*(12), 1802–1805.

Stroul, B. A., Pires, S. A., Armstrong, M. I., & Zaro, S. (2002). The impact of managed care on systems of care that serve children with serious emotional disturbances and their families. *Children's Services: Social Policy, Research, & Practice, 5*(1), 21–36.

Symington, D. C. (1994). Megatrends in rehabilitation: A Canadian perspective. *International Journal of Rehabilitation Research, 17*(1), 1–14.

Szilagyi, P. G., Shenkman, E., Brach, C., LaClair, B. J., Swigonski, N., Dick, A., et al. (2003). Children with special health care needs enrolled in the State Children's Health Insurance Program (SCHIP): Patient characteristics and health care needs. *Pediatrics, 112*(6), e508–e520.

Tate, D. G., Stiers, W., Daugherty, J., Forchheimer, M., Cohen, E., & Hansen, N. (1994). The effects of insurance benefits coverage on functional and psychosocial outcomes after spinal cord injury. *Archives of Physical Medicine and Rehabilitation, 75*(4), 407–414.

Tator, C. H., Duncan, E. G., Edmonds, V. E., Lapczak, L. I., & Andrews, D. F. (1993). Neurological recovery, mortality and length of stay after acute spinal cord injury associated with changes in management. *Paraplegia, 33*(5), 254–262.

U.S. Department of Health and Human Services. (2003). *2003 CMS statistics.* CMS Publication no. 03445. Washington, DC: Author.

Williams, B. (1994). Comparison of services among different types of home health agencies. *Medical Care, 32*(11), 1134–1152.

Wilson, N. J., & Kizer, K. W. (1997). The VA health care system: An unrecognized national safety net. *Health Affairs, 16*(4), 200–204.

Wolk, S., & Blair, T. (1994). *Trends in medical rehabilitation.* Reston, VA: American Rehabilitation Association.

Wooldridge, J., Hill, I., Harrington, M., Kenney, G., Hawkes, C., & Haley, J. (2003). Interim evaluation report: Congressionally mandated evaluation of the State Children's Health Insurance Program. Report submitted to the U.S. Department of Health and Human Services. Retrieved from http://aspe.hhs.gov/health/schip/interimrpt/index.htm

Wright, R. E., Rao, N., Smith, R. M., & Harvey, R. F. (1996). Risk factors for death and emergency transfer in acute and subacute inpatient rehabilitation. *Archives of Physical Medicine and Rehabilitation, 77*(10), 1049–1055.

34

Legislation and Rehabilitation Professionals

Susanne M. Bruyère, PhD, and
Sara A. Van Looy

OVER THE COURSE of the past 3 decades, the field of rehabilitation has seen sweeping changes, as laws have been enacted to support the rights of individuals with disabilities, and subsequently the efforts of the professionals who provide services to these people have also changed. These legislative mandates have granted rights to persons with disabilities in accessibility of goods and services, transportation, telecommunications, housing, and employment (U.S. Department of Justice, 2002).[1] Although each of these areas is vital for accessing a full life as an American citizen, it is the area of employment that we focus on in this chapter. Not only rehabilitation legislation and legislation specifically targeted to persons with disabilities but other pieces of employment legislation also provide protections for persons with disabilities, and as such affect the functioning of rehabilitation professionals. For the purposes of this discussion, the laws that will be focused on are as follows: Titles I and V of the Rehabilitation Act of 1973 as amended, the employment provisions of the Americans with Disabilities Act (ADA) of 1990, the Ticket to Work and Work Incentives Improvement Act (TWWIIA), the Workforce Investment Act (WIA) of 1998, the Family Medical Leave Act (FMLA), the Occupational Safety and

Health Act (OSHA), the National Labor Relations Act (NLRA), and state workers' compensation laws.

Because rehabilitation professionals often come from varied backgrounds—psychologists, counselors or case managers, social workers, or others—their exposure to legislation impacting the rights of persons with disabilities will consequently be varied. Those who come from a psychology background may have had exposure to health or confidentiality requirements; those who have had rehabilitation counseling training should have had exposure to the Rehabilitation Act, the Individuals with Disabilities Education Act (IDEA), the ADA, TWWIIA, WIA, and other laws targeting the rights of persons with disabilities, such as the Fair Housing Act, the Architectural Barriers Act, and the Air Carrier Access Act. Those who come from an industrial, organizational, human resource, labor relations, or employment services background may have had exposure to employment and labor law regulations. This chapter will provide a common frame of reference across several of these pieces of legislation, particularly as it relates to the employment or return-to-work process, for rehabilitation professionals who serve persons with disabilities.

This chapter provides a brief overview of each law with an explanation of issues, concerns, or critical areas in service delivery that may arise from it. These are issues that have caused much consternation to employers attempting to fulfill their responsibilities under several—at times seemingly conflicting—pieces of disability and employment legislation (Gault & Kinnane, 1996). They are therefore of concern to the individual with a disability who is trying to either gain or maintain employment, as well as to rehabilitation professionals who serve people with disabilities The intent of this chapter is to contribute to the ability of rehabilitation professionals to assist employers and individuals with disabilities in navigating this maze. The authors offer a summary of some key strategies for operating effectively within this regulatory environment, which rehabilitation professionals can use either in coaching individuals about their rights or in providing consultation to employers about their responsibilities to persons with disabilities to lessen or eliminate discrimination in the employment process.

EMPLOYMENT LEGISLATION AFFECTING REHABILITATION SERVICE DELIVERY

THE REHABILITATION ACT OF 1973 AS AMENDED

TWO TITLES OF the Rehabilitation Act will be discussed here: Title I, which deals with employment and related support services available to

persons with disabilities as provided by the state-federal vocational rehabilitation system, and Title V, which prohibits discrimination on the
basis of disability in programs conducted by federal agencies, in programs receiving federal financial assistance, in federal employment, and
in the employment practices of federal contractors.

Title I of the Vocational Rehabilitation Act of 1973, as modified by
the Rehabilitation Act amendments of 1992 and 1998, has as its purpose:

> To assist States in operating statewide comprehensive, coordinated, effec-
> tive, efficient, and accountable programs of vocational rehabilitation,
> each of which is (A) an integral part of a statewide workforce investment
> system; and (B) designed to assess, plan, develop, and provide vocational
> rehabilitation services for individuals with disabilities, consistent with
> their strengths, resources, priorities, concerns, abilities, capabilities,
> interests, and informed choice, so that such individuals may prepare for
> and engage in gainful employment. (Sec. 100(a)(2)[2]

Some of the earliest legislative seeds for the vocational rehabilitation
service delivery system as we know it today were sown over 80 years
ago with the 1920 Civilian Rehabilitation (Smith-Fess) Act, Public Law
66-236 (Wright, 1980). The Rehabilitation Act has provided funds to states
on a formula basis since that time. In the years following the passage
of this legislation, vocational rehabilitation services have evolved and
greatly expanded to provide an extensive array of both public- and
private-sector services to address the employment and independent living needs of persons with disabilities.

Federal funding for the vocational rehabilitation service delivery system during fiscal year 2002 was over $2.4 billion. The state vocational
rehabilitation (VR) system is made up of 80 agencies in 56 states and ter-
ritories. Twenty-four states have two agencies; one designed for specific services to the blind and visually impaired, and the other providing
VR services to all other individuals with disabilities. The remaining 32
agencies offer combined services.[3] In fiscal year 2002, approximately
27,000 personnel staffed the 80 agencies. Examples of the services that
can be provided to persons with disabilities, as authorized under the
legislation, are as follows: vocational assessment, career counseling,
vocational training, job development and job placement, assistive technology, supported employment, and follow-along services. The legislative mandate requires that the order of selection for the provision of
vocational rehabilitation services shall be determined on the basis of
first serving those individuals with the most significant disabilities.
Individuals with disabilities, including individuals with the most significant disabilities, are generally presumed to be capable of engaging
in gainful employment, and the provision of individualized rehabilita-

tion services is designed to improve their ability to become gainfully employed. A successful outcome is considered to be placement in an integrated employment setting at a prevailing wage for a minimum of 90 days, although other vocational outcomes, such as homemaker and unpaid family worker, are accepted as legitimate closures for certain individuals who are deemed unable to seek competitive employment. During fiscal year 2002, 1.04 million individuals received services from state VR agencies, of whom 221,000 achieved employment outcomes.[4]

The following are the provisions of Title V of the Rehabilitation Act, which prohibits discrimination against persons with disabilities. Section 501 requires affirmative action and nondiscrimination in employment by federal agencies of the executive branch.[5] Section 503 requires affirmative action and prohibits employment discrimination by federal government contractors and subcontractors with contracts of more than $10,000.[6] Section 504 states that "no qualified individual with a disability in the United States shall, solely by reason of her or his disability, be excluded from, denied the benefits of, or be subjected to discrimination under" any program or activity that either receives federal financial assistance or is conducted by any executive agency or the U.S. Postal Service. Requirements include reasonable accommodation for employees with disabilities, program accessibility, effective communication with people who have hearing or vision disabilities, and accessible new construction and alterations.[7] Although the ADA does not apply to workplaces with fewer than 15 employees, a recent Tenth Circuit ruling confirmed that that limit does not apply to claims brought under the Rehabilitation Act against entities that receive federal funds (Hellwege, 2002). On June 25, 2001, accessibility requirements for federal electronic and information technology (EIT) took effect under Section 508 of the Rehabilitation Act. This law requires that such technology be accessible according to standards developed by the Architectural and Transportation Barriers Compliance Board (Access Board), which are now part of the federal government's procurement regulations.[8] Section 508 of the Rehabilitation Act applies to all federal agencies when they develop, procure, maintain, or use electronic and information technology. Section 508 was added to the Rehabilitation Act in 1986, but lacked teeth until 1998, when Congress pushed the Executive branch to develop accessibility standards. Those standards were completed in 2000, and gave the law the same kind of impact as ADA had in 1990, pushing forward the development of ways to access technology. Federal Web designers also have to make their sites accessible to users with disabilities, and anyone in government who develops or maintains technology products has to make sure that those technologies are accessible (Friel, 2002).

The standards for determining employment discrimination under the Rehabilitation Act are the same as those used in Title I of the ADA, and therefore the issues for rehabilitation professionals in dealing with how these rights play out in the workplace are similar. The implications for rehabilitation professionals are discussed in greater detail under the presentation of issues around implementation of Title I of the ADA, which follows.

THE AMERICANS WITH DISABILITIES ACT OF 1990

THE ADA IS a landmark piece of civil rights legislation that extends the prohibitions against discrimination on the basis of race, sex, religion, and national origin to persons with disabilities.[9] Individuals may have both rights and responsibilities under the law, depending on the roles they assume: as employers or consultants to employers, as practitioners providing health services to the public, or as individuals who today or in the future may be protected by the Act (O'Keeffe, 1994). Title I, the employment provisions of the ADA, applies to private employers with at least 15 employees and to state and local government employers. The ADA protects qualified individuals with disabilities from discrimination. A qualified individual with a disability is a person who meets the necessary prerequisites for a job and can perform the essential functions with or without reasonable accommodation. A reasonable accommodation is any modification or adjustment to a job, an employment practice, or the work environment that makes it possible for a qualified individual with a disability to participate in the job application process, perform the essential functions of a job, and/or enjoy benefits and privileges of employment equal to those enjoyed by employees without disabilities (U.S. Equal Employment Opportunity Commission, 2000).[10]

The ADA employment provisions make it unlawful to discriminate on the basis of disability in a wide range of employment-related actions, including recruitment, job application, hiring, advancement, compensation, benefits, training, and discharge. Title I prohibits both intentional discrimination and employment practices with discriminatory effect. Additionally, Title I limits the use of both pre-employment and post-employment medical examinations and inquiries. An individual with a disability may be subjected to a pre-employment medical examination and inquiry only after a conditional offer of employment has been made and only if all entering employees in the job category, regardless of disability, are subjected to such an examination. Post-employment medical examinations and inquiries must be job-related and consistent with business necessity. Employee medical information is to be maintained separately from other personnel information, treated in a confidential manner, and shared only with supervisors and managers who need to know about necessary restrictions on the work duties of the employee and necessary accommodations. First aid and safety personnel also can be given selected information if the disability might require emergency medical treatment, as can government officials investigating compliance with the ADA.

The reasonable accommodation requirement is central to the mandate of nondiscrimination against people with disabilities. Reasonable accommodation is not an entirely new concept. Reasonable accommodation is required under the Rehabilitation Act regarding the employment and participation of individuals with disabilities under federal contracts and programs, and under Title VII of the Civil Rights Act with respect to religious observances of employees. The ADA provides the following examples of reasonable accommodations: job restructuring; part-time or modified work hours; reassignment to a vacant position; acquisition or modification of equipment or services; appropriate adjustment or modifications of examinations, training materials, or policies; and provision of qualified readers or interpreters.

Employers are not, under the ADA, required to hire employees who may pose a "direct threat" to the workplace safety or health environment (U.S. Equal Employment Opportunity Commission [EEOC], 1992). The statutory definition of the term *direct threat* is "a significant risk to the health or safety of others that cannot be eliminated by reasonable accommodation" (U.S. EEOC). Employers may use the direct-threat defense only in cases where risk is significantly increased, and standards for determining how severe a risk is must be applied to all employees—both with and without disabilities (U.S. EEOC).

Despite these landmark civil rights employment protections for people with disabilities, enforcement of the law as originally intended has been problematic. The U.S. Equal Employment Opportunity Commission (EEOC) holds responsibility for receiving and investigating reports of disability-related employment discrimination. An ongoing concern is that the EEOC has had significant difficulty handling complaints that it receives in a timely fashion (Percy, 2001). In addition, in the last few years the Supreme Court has issued a number of decisions that have dramatically changed the way the ADA is interpreted (National Council on Disability, 2002). Decisions on the definition of disability, who can be considered "disabled," and the applicability of the statute to state governments have limited the application of the ADA in many cases (National Council on Disability, 2003). In addition, other questions of interpretation and application remain.

Over the past 10 years, questions and concerns about accommodations for persons with psychiatric disabilities have been voiced by employers and their legal representatives (Pechman, 1995), and employer surveys have found that the majority still hold patronizing or potentially discriminating attitudes (Scheid, 1998). In response to these concerns, the EEOC issued enforcement guidance on the ADA as it applies to persons with psychiatric disabilities (U.S. EEOC, 1997). This publication provides useful information to persons with disabilities as well as to rehabilitation practitioners who provide services to them, about the rights of persons with disabilities to accommodation and disclosure of disability under the ADA. However, this area continues to warrant further attention, as a study by Ullman, Johnson, Moss, and Burris (2001) of disability discrimination claims to the EEOC found that psychiatric illnesses were significantly less likely to be classified as Category A claims and fully investigated than were other disabilities.

When the ADA employment provisions first became effective, some industries were predominantly concerned about their hiring practices and restraints against being able to ask questions about prior injuries (Setzer, 1992); other employers responded with concerns about additional facets of employment that would be affected, such as the implications for insurance benefits and compensation (Huss, 1993; Nobile, 1996; & Zolkos, 1994). Now, with over 10 years of experience since the employment provisions became effective, employers also have become aware of the importance of examining how they treat job incumbents with disabilities. According to statistics kept by the U.S. Equal Employment Opportunity Commission, the federal agency that oversees compliance with the ADA employment provisions, of the 90,803 charges filed from July 26, 1992, through September 30, 1997, over half (52%) related to alleged unlawful discharge. In 2002, 60% of disability merit suits filed were based on unlawful discharge (U.S. EEOC, 2003). Thus, it appears that employers need assistance in navigating requirements for nondiscrimination across all phases of the employment process. Informed rehabilitation professionals can be of great assistance in this process both to these employers, and to job applicants and job incumbents with disabilities.

TICKET TO WORK AND WORK INCENTIVES IMPROVEMENT ACT OF 1999

THE TICKET TO Work and Work Incentives Improvement Act (TWWIIA), signed into law on December 17, 1999, was intended to provide beneficiaries and recipients of either Supplemental Security Income (SSI), Social Security Disability Insurance (SSDI), or both, the incentives and supports needed to either prepare for, attach to, or advance in work.[11] The goals of TWWIIA are to reduce and remove certain barriers to employment for individuals who receive SSI and SSDI and to encourage beneficiaries and recipients to access the services and supports needed to assist them in their pursuit of employment. At the heart of the Act was a desire by Congress to increase options available to beneficiaries of the Social Security Administrations (SSA) disability programs, by expanding upon the existing network of service providers available and creating a more comprehensive set of supports for people with disabilities considering work.[12] Whether these TWWIIA initiatives are successful or not will be measured by the impact they have on the benefit and return to work rates of beneficiaries and recipients (Roessler, 2002).

The Ticket to Work and Work Incentives Improvement Act includes three important titles: Ticket to Work and Self-Sufficiency, Expansion of Health Care, and Demonstration Projects/Studies. Title I expands vocational services options for persons with disabilities. The Ticket to Work and Self-Sufficiency Program is an important provision of Title I. This program replaces SSA's existing vocational rehabilitation program with an outcomes-based and market-driven program.

All SSI recipients and SSDI beneficiaries who have been determined to be disabled under SSA's adult definition of disability, are over 18 years of age, receive benefits, and, if expected to medically recover, have received a continuing disability review and are still considered disabled will receive a Ticket to Work. The Social Security Administration administers the provisions of Title I.[13]

The Ticket Program permits the individual beneficiary or recipient to choose from an array of service providers (called Employment Networks), placing control over provider selection in the hands of the consumer. The Ticket Program is purely voluntary and beneficiaries and recipients can choose to use their Ticket or not, decide who to deposit their Ticket with, and decide at any point to retract their Ticket from a provider if they feel the services they are receiving are inadequate.

The employment network (EN), an approved service provider under the Ticket Program, can be a private organization or public agency that agrees to work with SSA to provide vocational rehabilitation, employment, and/or other support services to assist a SSA beneficiary/recipient to prepare for, obtain, and remain at work. Under the Ticket Program, a service provider can elect to become an EN, become a service provider under another EN, or both. A state VR agency can be a part of multiple employment networks across a given state, but each EN must have an agreement with VR before initiating a referral to the designated state VR agency. An employment network that agrees to provide services can decide to receive either outcome payments for months in which a beneficiary does not receive benefits due to work activity (up to 60 months), or reduced outcome payments in addition to payments for assisting the beneficiary to achieve milestones connected with employment. In addition, state VR agencies can also elect to receive payment as they have in the past under the cost reimbursement option. This special status is in recognition of the fact that under the Rehabilitation Act of 1973 as amended, state VR agencies cannot deny services and supports to a consumer who is eligible. State VR agencies differ from other ENs in that the other ENs can make a decision to not accept someone's Ticket.

Title II of TWWIIA governs the provision of health care services to workers with disabilities. This section of the law attempts to reduce the disincentives to employment for people with disabilities posed by the threat of loss of health care benefits. Under this part of the Act, states are encouraged to improve access to health care coverage available under Medicare and Medicaid. Under this provision, new optional eligibility groups are established, creating two new eligibility categories, and also extending the period of premium-free Medicare Part A eligibility and requiring protection for certain individuals with Medigap. The Department of Health and Human Services, through the Centers for Medicare and Medicaid Services (CMS) (formerly Health Care Financing Administration [HCFA]), administers the health care provisions.[14]

WORKFORCE INVESTMENT ACT OF 1998 (WIA)

THE PURPOSE OF the Workforce Investment Act of 1998 (WIA)[15] is to consolidate workforce preparation and employment services into a unified system of support that is responsive to the needs of job seekers, employers, and communities (Public Law 105-220). Under Title I of the Act, a framework is provided for the delivery of workforce investment activities at the state and local level that provide services in an effective and meaningful way to all customers, including persons with disabilities. The new law is positioned not only to empower customers, but also to provide opportunities for business and human resource professionals to focus public programs on marketplace needs. If the restructuring called for under WIA succeeds, it will create the architecture needed to address the long-term challenges around retraining and upgrading the skills of the U.S. workforce (Pantazis, 1999).

WIA created a workforce development system that encourages and facilitates One-Stop service delivery (Workforce Investment Act of 1998, August 7, 1998). This employment and training system was intended to serve every job seeker through a central location that provides access to numerous workforce development programs. Core services—including assessment, basic job readiness, and help with job searches—are open to a universal population. For those who require further assistance finding employment, intensive services and job training are also available.

Title IV of the Workforce Investment Act reauthorizes the Vocational Rehabilitation (VR) program. The law specifically states that "linkages between the VR program and other components of the statewide workforce investment system are critical to ensure effective and meaningful participation by individuals with disabilities in workforce investment activities." Collaboration between the state units administering the VR program and generic workforce development services (Departments of Labor) is intended to produce better information, more comprehensive services, easier access to services, and improved long-term employment outcomes (Workforce Investment Act of 1998, Title IV, Section 403: 2).

To ensure such participation, WIA and the Department of Labor's Employment and Training Administration (ETA) stress the need for access and partnership when addressing the needs of people with disabilities. Universal access to one-stop services is a central component of WIA.[16] In a notice published in April 2000, the ETA stated: "the Department of Labor is committed to ensuring that the programs, services, and facilities of each One-Stop delivery system are accessible to all of America's workers, including individuals with disabilities" (U.S. Department of Labor, 2000). Every job seeker should have access to the core services available at their local One-Stop Center. Federal law mandates that all WIA activities, from core to intensive services, must be accessible to individuals with disabilities. While physical access to the One-Stop Center is important, access to all tools and services offered by the center—including virtual and computer-based resources—is critical if job seekers with disabilities are to benefit fully from the One-Stop system.

WIA mandates a series of partnerships in the One-Stop system, including Vocational Rehabilitation. VR has a seat on state and local Workforce Investment Boards and, ideally, is involved in the design of the workforce development system. States and local areas also can bring other disability organizations into the system as partners. The U.S. Department of Labor (DOL) encourages state and local policy makers to develop partnerships with disability-specific organizations to create an effective and universal workforce investment system.

FAMILY MEDICAL LEAVE ACT

THE FMLA (PUBLIC Law 103-3) went into effect on August 5, 1993.[17] It established, for employers with 50 or more employees, a minimum labor standard with regard to leaves of absence for family or medical reasons. The law's enactment was driven by concern to protect the needs of American workforces, while attending to the productivity concerns of employers.

Under the FMLA, an eligible employee may take up to 12 work-weeks of leave during any 12-month period for one or more of the following reasons: the birth of a child and to care for the newborn child; the placement of a child with the employee through adoption or foster care and to care for the child; to care for the employee's spouse, son, daughter, or parent with a serious health condition; and a serious health condition of the employee that makes the employee unable to perform one or more of the essential functions of his or her job.[18] An FMLA serious health condition is an illness, injury, impairment, or physical or mental condition that involves inpatient care or continuing treatment by a health care provider. During the FMLA leave, the employer must maintain the employee's existing level of coverage under a group health plan. At the end of FMLA leave, an employer must take an employee back into the same or an equivalent job. The FMLA does not require an employer to let an employee who is medically unable to do his job return to work, nor does it require modification of the job or reassignment to a new position.

Some of the questions that arise in use of the FMLA that relate to the functioning of rehabilitation professionals are in the interplay of FMLA leave with accommodation and return-to-work efforts (Scott, 1996; Shalowitz, 1993). In some cases, the FMLA leave itself can be an accommodation (FMLA Leave can be ADA Accommodation, 2002). In other situations, the FMLA may create difficulties for an employer attempting to get injured workers back to work and off benefits. Many employers have used "light duty" to bring an injured worker back to work within his/her medical restrictions. Light-duty jobs typically are very different from the job an employee was doing at the time of injury. Because the FMLA requires that a worker be restored to the same or an equivalent position on return from leave, an employer may not compel an injured worker to accept light-duty work in lieu of exercising his or her FMLA entitlement. Likewise, the Department of Labor has taken the position that an employer may not require an FMLA-eligible employee to accept reasonable accommodation instead of FMLA leave.

An employer may offer accommodation or light duty but may not compel it. On the other hand, if an employee rejects an offer of employment that is within his or her medical restrictions, an employer may contest the employee's entitlement to workers' compensation indemnity benefits. In addition, if an employee voluntarily accepts light duty, an employer may not designate time on light duty as FMLA leave, as the employee is working. However, time spent on light duty does not lessen an employee's right to be restored to the same or an equivalent position held at the time leave commenced.

Some employers raise questions about a perceived conflict between the FMLA provision allowing employers to ask for certification of a serious health condition and the ADA restrictions on disability-related inquiries by employees. The EEOC issued a fact sheet to address some of these most-often-asked questions about the ADA and FMLA interaction (EEOC answers, 1997).[19] This publication clarifies the point that when an employee requests leave under the FMLA for a serious health condition, employers will not violate the ADA by asking for the information specified in the FMLA certification form. The ADA allows medical inquiries that are "job-related" and consistent with business necessity.

The FMLA form requests only information relating to the particular serious health condition for which the person is seeking leave. An employer is entitled to know why an employee, who otherwise should be at work, is requesting time off under the FMLA. Medical inquiries that are strictly limited in this fashion are therefore not ADA violations (U.S. EEOC, 2000).

OCCUPATIONAL SAFETY AND HEALTH ACT

THE OCCUPATIONAL SAFETY and Health Act (OSHA) of 1970 represents the culmination of nearly a century of Congress's growing concern for workplace safety (Rothstein, 1990). The earliest laws concerning the health and safety of employees were enacted at the state level and were in place in some form in 46 states by 1921. These laws were not substantially preventive, and unfortunately their existence did little to curb the actual occurrence of incidents. However, workers' compensation schemes, also at the state level, made it possible for employees to recover damages from their employers for injuries incurred on the job, as well as allow the families of victims of industrial accidents some relief for their predicaments. Throughout the 20th century, laws were passed in response to specific workplace health issues: the Esch Act of 1912 curtailed phosphorus use in match factories; the Coal Mine Safety Act of 1952 was passed after 119 miners were killed in West Frankfort, Illinois a year earlier; the Construction Safety Act of 1969 addressed safety issues on construction sites of public works. Still, no piece of legislation covered all safety and health issues in every workplace for every employee until the passage of OSHA in 1970. Unlike some other employment regulation, OSHA is applied universally to all employers, regardless of the volume of business they conduct or the number of people in their employ (Rothstein).

At OSHA's core is the recognition that every worker has a right to a workplace that is free from recognized hazards. Therefore, when a potential hazard is identified, the OSH Administration, through the Labor Department, develops a standard against which workplace practices or conditions should be measured. Standards are issued by three procedures—one for interim standards, one for permanent standards, and one for emergency temporary standards. Investigation and evaluation of a standard-warranting situation begins when the OSH Administration becomes aware of pertinent information about that situation. With the exception of emergency hazards that require immediate precautionary treatment, a committee of no more than 15 members will be assigned to determine an appropriate standard within a 260-day period from the committee's assignment. The committee's recommendations are submitted and reviewed by all affected parties, comments are taken from interested persons, and a public hearing is held. The OSH Administration then decides to accept their recommended standard or to deny it based on stated reasons (Bureau of National Affairs, 1997).

After the implementation of a standard, the Labor Department can determine which workplaces will be inspected—either by the request of an employee in the particular workplace or at the OSH Administration's discretion. Inspections are conducted with the permission of the employer and according to OSHA guidelines. Violations of a standard are punishable by government-ordered abatement and monetary fines, set according to the size of the business, the seriousness of the violation, the good faith of the employer, and the record of prior violations. Violations that result in the death of an employee can be punished by criminal law (Bureau of National Affairs, 1997).

A major way in which this law may affect the functioning of rehabilitation professionals is its interplay with ADA requirements regarding employment screening prohibitions, medical confidentiality of records, and required accommodations. The ADA's limitations on employee testing can be in conflict with OSHA's need for testing in furtherance of workplace safety goals.

The ADA places significant restrictions on an employer's right to require pre-employment physicals, to make medical inquiries of employees and applicants, and to require that employees submit to physical examinations, and it restricts access to such information in an effort to prevent potential discrimination. The Occupational Safety and Health Act, in contrast, affirmatively requires employers to conduct testing in a variety of situations to assure safety. For example, employees exposed to high noise levels are required to be included within an audiometric testing program, which includes among other things annual hearing tests (Taylor, 1995). The ADA requires strict confidentiality of medical records. OSHA, on the other hand, requires employers to provide employees, their representatives with signed authorizations, and OSHA personnel access to such records in the interest of exposing potential hazards and their causes. By having the employee sign an information release, the employer can better assure that the information being released stays in the appropriate hands and that the ADA confidentiality requirements are not violated.

Although OSHA requirements can often take precedence over the ADA requirements to assure adherence to health and safety requirements, the reasonable accommodation element of the ADA can still be applied to OSHA-mandated policies and modifications. For example, an eyewash station, which may be required by OSHA for certain positions, must be installed in such a way that a wheelchair user would have access it.

The lines are not always so clear, however, particularly in terms of the direct-threat defense to ADA claims. Take, for example, the case of an employee with epilepsy working on an assembly line. The way an employer handles the situation is largely contingent on which legislation he or she believes is more likely to be invoked. Removal of the employee, satisfying the general duty clause of OSHA, may violate the ADA. The direct-threat defense is so difficult to prove that employers are likely to avoid the ADA claim at all costs, often leaving themselves in violation of OSHA standards. The complications arise when OSHA doesn't explicitly call for an action such as removal of an employee who has seizures. As a general rule, OSHA standards "trump" the ADA's duty to accommodate, but employers cannot rely on using OSHA as a defense to ADA claims unless the employment action in question was specifically called for by OSHA (Skoning & McGlothlen, 1994).

NATIONAL LABOR RELATIONS ACT

THE NATIONAL LABOR Relations Act (NLRA), also called the Wagner Act, was passed in 1935. It stands as the established framework for labor relations in the United States, covering union-management relations in almost every private firm in operation. The law protects workers from the effects of unfair labor practices by employers, and requires employers to recognize and bargain collectively with a union that the workers elect to represent them (Gold, 1998).

Among the main principles of the NLRA are the idea of exclusivity of representation, a policy against direct dealing, and the duty to provide information. Seniority rights gained through collective bargaining are also among the most valued benefits of having a unionized workplace (Gold, 1998). All of these areas may yield conflict for individuals seeking to invoke protection from laws such as the ADA, FMLA, or the Rehabilitation Act. These laws rely on making exceptions to or changes in terms and conditions of employment on an individual basis. Compliance with these laws may include dealing with the employer to discuss and secure those agreements that may fall outside the scope of the union's normal interactions, the unilateral implementation of an accommodation for an employee, and often the security of medical information, which the union may feel it has the right to access under the NLRA (Evans, 1992).

Reasonable accommodations for individuals with disabilities may present an especially problematic situation for employers and unions alike. Both parties are required by law to operate in a nondiscriminatory manner: the employer must accommodate a worker so that his or her essential job functions may be performed regardless of disability and must provide terms and conditions of employment that are free of discriminatory intent. The union must represent its constituency equally and consistently, as well as allow accommodations for people with disabilities to be implemented without unreasonable opposition (President's Committee, 1994).

Whenever a modification in the terms or conditions of employment is required, a review of the collective bargaining agreement would be advisable, as well as some kind of communication between the employer and the union concerning the accommodation and the potential effects it may have on the lives of other workers (President's Committee, 1994). An effective way to approach this is the use of joint labor-management teams (Bruyère, Gomez, & Handelmann, 1996).

In a unionized workplace, the rehabilitation professional can contribute to an injured worker's effective return to the workplace, taking into the account the interests of the employee, the employer, and the union to effect a successful reintegration. Organized labor has been an important part of the history of fighting for worker rights and against job discrimination, and these social issues are very important to workers with disabilities. Yet many employment professionals have little experience with unions and little knowledge of their purpose and structure (Bruyère, 1996). Adopting a position that favors both the person with a disability *and* the union will go a long way in the service delivery process to minimize conflict and maximize union support in the accommodation process.

Case law continues to develop in this area. A 2002 Supreme Court decision (*US Airways, Inc. v. Barnett*) ruled that employees with disabilities are not always entitled to reassignment to a job intended for workers with more seniority. The Supreme Court held that, in situations involving a conflict between a requested accommodation and an employer-created seniority system, the "seniority system will prevail in the run of cases." However, the court left open the possibility of an employee showing that reassignment would be a reasonable accommodation in a particular case despite the existence of a seniority system (Ford & Harrison, 2002).

WORKERS' COMPENSATION

WORKERS' COMPENSATION PROGRAMS are government-sponsored, employer-financed systems for compensating employees who incur an injury or illness in connection with their employment. They are designed to ensure that employees who are injured on the job receive timely compensation for their losses without proof of fault. Workers' compensation laws allow employees or their survivors to file claims for economic losses resulting from work-related injuries or occupational diseases. Benefits provided under workers' compensation laws include medical care, disability payments, rehabilitation services, survivor benefits, and funeral expenses. Employers who participate in workers' compensation programs usually are protected against tort actions that employees might otherwise pursue to redress their losses.

State workers' compensation statutes generally provide benefits to employees for job-related injuries, whether or not the injury is permanently disabling. In addition to medical care and treatment for job-related injuries, these statutes typically also provide benefits for temporary incapacity, scarring, and permanent impairment of specific parts of the body. Workers' compensation laws are maintained by all 50 states, the District of Columbia, American Samoa, Guam, the Virgin Islands, and Puerto Rico. In addition, the federal government administers workers' compensation programs authorized by the Federal Coal Mine Health and Safety Act, the Longshore and Harborworkers' Compensation Act, and the Federal Employers' Liability Act. Rehabilitation professionals working in private-sector rehabilitation and in the return-to-work process for persons with disabilities must interact with this system and its regulations regularly.

Although much attention was paid immediately after the passage of the ADA to disability nondiscrimination and the hiring process, some employers were already focusing on its impact on job incumbents with disabilities (Walworth, Damon, & Wilder, 1993). Now, even more attention is being paid to the ADA's impact on job retention aspects of the employment process. Of the ADA charges filed with the EEOC between 1992 and 1999, 16% were cited as being related to a back impairment (U.S. EEOC, 1999), which is a disability or injury often seen in the workers' compensation system. It is inevitable that the rehabilitation practitioner will deal with some persons for whom there will be an interplay of these two pieces of legislation.

Some authors have pointed out that disability nondiscrimination legislation such as the ADA appears to rest on very different principles than the workers' compensation system (Bell, 1994). The ADA is predicated on the premise that disability does not necessarily mean inability to work, and focuses on how accommodation can assist in removing barriers to employment caused by the interaction between functional limitations and the workplace. Workers' compensation legislation, however, focuses on the apparently contrasting premise that impairments are the cause of work limitations, and employees must prove loss of earning capacity because of injury.

Rehabilitation professionals in this area will need to concern themselves with clarifying for individuals with disabilities and for employers the significant aspects of workers' compensation legislation as it relates to protections provided by the ADA. These include such issues as the injured worker as a protected person under the ADA, queries by an employer about a worker's prior workers' compensation claims, hiring persons with a prior history of an occupational injury and application of the direct threat standard, reasonable accommodation for persons with disability-related occupational injuries, light-duty issue, and exclusive remedy provisions in workers' compensation laws. In response to a need for clarification of these issues, the EEOC issued enforcement guidance concerning the interaction between Title I of the ADA and state workers' compensation laws that can greatly assist rehabilitation professionals in responding to many of these employer questions (U.S. EEOC, 1996; Welch, 1996).

IMPLICATIONS FOR REHABILITATION SERVICE DELIVERY

To PREPARE PERSONS with disabilities appropriately for initial entry or reentry into the workplace, and to provide effective consultation to employers on disability nondiscrimination and equal access in the workplace, rehabilitation professionals must be apprised of state and federal legislation that affects both safety and equity practices in the workplace. The issues presented here in the implementation of specific pieces of legislation, and more specifically as they interrelate with disability nondiscrimination legislation, such as the ADA, and workforce preparation and benefits support, such as the Ticket legislation and WIA, point to areas where rehabilitation professionals need more knowledge and expertise and also where they can provide effective service. A listing of specific skill and knowledge areas needed by rehabilitation professionals in implementing the ADA as consultants were identified by Pape and Tarvydas (1994) as cutting across the following three distinct areas: core rehabilitation principles, knowledge, and functions; disability concepts, functions, and knowledge; and ADA knowledge and functions. The implications of disability nondiscrimination legislation specifically for the role of psychologists were addressed by Crewe (1994), who encourages specialized pre- or postdoctoral preparation in disability and rehabilitation for psychologists who are planning to apply their clinical or counseling psychology training to services for people with disabilities. The implications of disability nondiscrimination legislation such as the ADA for preparation of rehabilitation undergraduate and graduate professionals are discussed by Stude (1994), who encourages rehabilitation educators to include this information in existing coursework rather than isolating it into a specialized course. The importance of examining the gap between existing employment and disability policy and desired employment outcomes for persons with disabilities was the focus of a recent conference and resulting publication sponsored by the American Psychological Association and the National Institute of Disability and Rehabilitation Research (Bruyère et al., 2003).

The ADA has afforded rehabilitation professionals who contribute to employment opportunities for persons with disabilities a tool to more effectively combat discrimination in the recruitment, hiring, retention, and termination processes. Under the ADA, a significant service that vocational rehabilitation counselors might provide is assisting employers with job analyses, writing job descriptions, and helping develop or design the reasonable accommodations that will make initial hiring or return to work feasible for workers with disabilities (Walker & Heffner, 1992). Employers need assistance in the development of policies and procedures that do not discriminate against people with disabilities in the recruitment, hiring, health and other employment benefits, promotion and training, and termination processes.

The workers' compensation system is one that is cited as being difficult for both employees and employers, seemingly fanning the fires for a contentious and litigious relationship. One of the most important things rehabilitation professionals can do is to facilitate communication between the employer and the employee (Commerce Clearing House, 1997). Rehabilitation professionals can either themselves be that bridge with employers or serve as consultants to encourage supervisors and others in the workplace to address the employees' questions and provide supportive follow-up during disability leave. Rehabilitation professionals also can play a role in bringing human resource, safety, and health professionals within a given organization together to develop a unified approach to the ADA and workers' compensation (Walker & Hefner, 1992).

In all facets of this legislation, working both with individuals with disabilities and with employers and teaching them how to communicate their respective needs effectively is imperative. Often, when coached appropriately, both employees with disabilities and their supervisors or the human resources staff in a given organization can effectively address accommodation requests and resolve any conflicts that arise in negotiating final decisions on accommodations. Problems arise when there has been a prior history of poor performance, of poor relationship between supervisor and employee, or of general discord or conflict in a unit or workplace environment, creating a culture of mistrust in responding to employee needs.

SUMMARY

THE PURPOSE OF this chapter has been to provide rehabilitation professionals with a basic overview of some of the pieces of disability and employment legislation which may affect their functioning in the rehabilitation and return-to-work process. Several of these laws, such as the NLRA and the OSHA, are designed to protect workers' rights before injury occurs, and to emphasize employer responsibilities in the safety and equitable treatment of workers in all terms and conditions of employment. Regulatory requirements such as the FMLA, short-term disability leave requirements as dictated by state regulations, and workers' compensation legislation are designed to deal with the rights of employees once an injury or illness has occurred. These laws protect the right to a medical leave that gives the worker the time needed for the rehabilitation process and they assure the security of benefits to cover part of the medical costs and salary lost to time off work due to illness or injury, as well as a job upon their return. Legislation such as the Rehabilitation Act of 1973 as amended and the ADA focuses more specifically on the rights of workers with disabilities. These laws require equal access in the seeking and securing of employment, as well as retention and equitable access to other terms and conditions of employment. Regulatory requirements such as confidentiality of medical information also serve a role here, in terms of providing requirements for employers to keep confidential any medical diagnostic information on employees that they may gain access to. More recently, legislation such as the Social Security Administration's Ticket to Work and Work Incentives Improvement Act and the U.S. Department of Labor's Workforce Investment Act provide needed supports and services to remove barriers to employment and provide needed supports in the employment-seeking process.

Assisting the individual through the rehabilitation process to return to productive functioning in the community and in the workplace is the core of the rehabilitation professional's job. When employment outcomes are part of the rehabilitation goal, knowledge of the regulatory requirements that surround the workplace and have an impact on employer and employee behavior is vital for the rehabilitation professional to function effectively. This chapter has pointed out some of the possible areas of conflict or concern that may influence both worker and employer behaviors, and has provided a basic introduction for practitioners to pursue further information, given the nature of their services and interventions for persons with disabilities.

ACKNOWLEDGMENTS

The authors' efforts in writing this material were supported by a grant from the U.S. Department of Education National Institute on Disability and Rehabilitation Research for a Rehabilitation Research and Training Center for Economic Research on Employment Policies for Persons with Disabilities (Grant #H113B980038). The authors would like to acknowledge the work of Rebecca DeMarinis, a co-author on a prior version of this chapter published in 1999.

NOTES

1. A brief publication discussing these pieces of legislation, entitled *A Guide to Disability Rights Laws,* is available from the U.S. Department of Justice Civil Rights Division, Disability Rights Section, P. O. 66738, Washington, DC 20035-6738; (800) 514-0301 (voice), (800) 514-0383 (TTY). Or go to http://www.usdoj.gov/crt/ada/cguide.pdf to download the full publication.

2. See http://www.rcep6.org/rehabilitation_act.htm for complete text of the Rehabilitation Act.

3. For further information, visit the Council for State Administrators in Vocational Rehabilitation (CSAVR) at http://www.rehabnetwork.org, or contact the Executive Office: 4733 Bethesda Avenue, Suite 330, Bethesda, MD 20814; phone (301) 654-8414; fax (301) 654-5542.

4. Personal communication with Patricia Nash, Basic State Grants Branch, Rehabilitation Services Administration, U.S. Department of Education, February 5, 2004.

5. To obtain more information or to file a complaint, employees should contact their agency's Equal Employment Opportunity Office; call 1-800-669-4000 (voice), 1-800-669-6820 (TTY), or visit http://www.eeoc.gov.

6. For more information on section 503, contact Office of Federal Contract Compliance Programs, U.S. Department of Labor, 200 Constitution Ave., NW, Washington, DC 20210; (202) 693-0101. Visit http://www.dol.gov/esa/ofccp/ for a list of regional offices, section 503 information, and instructions for filing complaints.

7. For information on how to file complaints under section 504 with the appropriate agency, contact U.S. Department of Justice, 950 Pennsylvania Avenue, NW, Civil Rights Division, Disability Rights Section—NYAV, Washington, DC 20530; (800) 514-0301 (voice), (800) 514-0383 (TTY), or see http://www.ada.gov.

8. Information about these standards can be found at the Access Board web site at http://www.access-board.gov/news/508.htm.

9. Cornell University has developed an online guide to the ADA and reasonable accommodations for people with specific disabilities. See http://www.hrtips.org for more information.

10. A modification or adjustment is "reasonable" if it seems reasonable on its face, i.e., ordinarily or in the run of cases; this means it is "reasonable" if it appears to be "feasible" or "plausible." A deeper discussion of what is "reasonable" accommodation can be found in U.S. Equal Employment Opportunity Commission (2002).

11. For more information on the Work Incentives Improvement Act, see the

Social Security Administration (SSA) web site at http://www.ssa.gov/work/ Ticket/ticket_info.html

12. Cornell University has developed a series of Policy and Practice Briefs on Social Security issues, including one on the Ticket program. They can be found at http://www.ilr.cornell.edu/ped/dep/pp.html

13. Further information about the Ticket Program is available through the SSA on their toll-free number at 1-800-772-1213, or on the Social Security Administration web site at http://www.ssa.gov/work

14. Further information about the Medicaid Buy-In program can be found at the Centers for Medicare and Medicaid Services (CMS) web site at http://www.cms.hhs.gov/twwiia/factsh01.asp

15. For further information about the Workforce Investment Act, see http://www.doleta.gov/usworkforce/asp/wialaw.txt

16. The U.S. Department of Labor has developed an online toolkit (http://www.onestoptoolkit.org/) for One-Stops to help grantees ensure access for people with disabilities.

17. See http://www.dol.gov/esa/regs/statutes/whd/fmla.htm for the complete text of this law.

18. For additional information about the FMLA, or to file an FMLA complaint, individuals should contact the nearest office of the Wage and Hour division, Employment Standards Administration, U.S. Department of Labor. The Wage and Hour division is listed in most directories under U.S. Government, Department of Labor, or you can visit their Web site at http://www. dol.gov/esa/whd/. For further information, contact the Office of Legal Counsel's Attorney of the Day at (202) 663-4691.

19. The EEOC fact sheet, the *Family and Medical Leave Act, the Americans with Disabilities Act, and Title VII of the Civil Rights Act* can be ordered by writing or calling the EEOC's Office of Communications and Legislative Affairs at 1801 L St., NW, Washington, DC 20507; telephone (202) 663-4900, TTY (202) 663-4494, or at http://www.eeoc.gov/policy/docs/fmlaada.html on the EEOC Web site.

REFERENCES

Bell, C. (1994). The Americans with Disabilities Act and injured workers: Implications for rehabilitation professionals and the workers' compensation system. In S. Bruyère & J. O'Keeffe (Eds.), *Implications of the Americans with Disabilities Act for psychology* (pp. 137–149). New York: Springer Publishing & Washington, DC: American Psychological Association.

Bruyère, S. (Ed.). (1996). *A job developer's guide to working with unions: Obtaining the support of organized labor for the hiring of employees with disabilities.* St. Augustine, FL: Training Resource Network.

Bruyère, S., Erickson, W., VanLooy, S., Sitaras, E., Cook, J., Burke, J., et al. (2003). Employment and disability policy: Recommendations for a social sciences research agenda. In F. E. Menz & D. F. Thomas (Eds.), *Bridging gaps: Refining the disability research agenda for rehabilitation and the social sciences—Conference proceedings*. Menomonie: University of Wisconsin-Stout, Stout Vocational Rehabilitation Institute, Research and Training Centers.

Bruyère, S., Gomez, S., & Handelmann, G. (1996). The reasonable accommodation process in unionized environments. *Labor Law Journal, 48*, 629–647.

Bureau of National Affairs, Inc. (1997). Job safety and health (No. 228). In *The Laws in Brief: OSHA*. Washington, DC: Author.

Commerce Clearing House. (1997). Communication and concern help workers return to work. In *Workers' Compensation Business Management Guide* (pp. 299–301). Chicago: Author.

Crewe, N. (1994). Implications of the Americans with Disabilities Act for the training of psychologists. *Rehabilitation Education, 8*(1), 9–16.

EEOC answers biggest FMLA/ADA questions. (1997). *Disability Leave and Absence Reporter, 104*, 4.

Evans, B. (1992). Will employers and unions cooperate? *HR Magazine, 37*(11), 59–63.

FMLA Leave can be ADA Accommodation. (2002, September). *HR Focus, 79*(2), 2.

Ford & Harrison, LLP (2002, July 19). *Potential violation of collective bargaining agreement does not make requested accommodation unreasonable*. News release. Retrieved February 9, 2004, from http://www.fordharrison.com/fh/news/articles/07192002collective.asp

Friel, B. (2002). Access Granted. *Government Executive, 34*(7), 45–50.

Gault, R., & Kinnane, A. (1996). Navigating the maze of employment law. *Management Review, 85*(2), 9–11.

Gold, M. (1998). *An introduction to labor law*. Ithaca, NY: Cornell University, ILR Press.

Hellwege, J. (2002). Tenth Circuit blocks attempt to narrow Rehabilitation Act in disability cases. *Trial, 38*(12), 88–90.

Huss, A. (1993). ADA, insurance, and employee benefits. *Journal of the American Society of CLU & ChFC, 47*(5), 82–89.

National Council on Disability. (2002). *Supreme Court decisions interpreting the Americans with Disabilities Act*. Retrieved February 12, 2004, from http://www.ncd.gov/newsroom/publications/supremecourt_ada.html

National Council on Disability. (2003). The impact of the Supreme Court's ADA decisions on the rights of persons with disabilities. *The Americans with Disabilities Act Policy Brief Series: Righting the ADA*. Retrieved February 12, 2004, from http://www.ncd.gov/newsroom/publications/decisionimpact.html

Nobile, R. (1996). How discrimination laws affect compensation. *Compensation & Benefits Review, 28*(4), 38–42.

O'Keeffe, J. (1994). Disability, discrimination, and the Americans with Disabilities Act. In S. Bruyère & J. O'Keeffe (Eds.), *Implications of the Americans with Disabilities Act for psychology* (pp. 1–14). New York: Springer Publishing & Washington, DC: American Psychological Association.

Pantazis, C. (1999). The new Workforce Investment Act. *Training and Development, 53*(8), 48–50.

Pape, D., & Tarvydas, V. (1994). Responsible and responsive rehabilitation consultation on the ADA: The importance of training for psychologists. In S. Bruyère & J. O'Keeffe (Eds.), *Implications of the Americans with Disabilities Act for psychology* (pp. 169–186). New York: Springer Publishing & Washington, DC: American Psychological Association.

Pechman, L. (1995). Coping with mental disabilities in the workplace. *New York State Bar Journal, 67*(5), 22, 24–26, 49.

Percy, S. (2001). Challenges and dilemmas in implementing the Americans with Disabilities Act: Lessons from the first decade. *Policy Studies Journal, 29*(4), 633–640.

President's Committee on Employment of People with Disabilities. (1994). *Seniority and collective bargaining issues and the Americans with Disabilities Act—A strategy for implementation.* Final Report of the Seniority/Collective Bargaining Agreement Work Group. Washington, DC: Author.

Roessler, R. (2002). TWWIIAA initiatives and work incentives: Return-to-work implications. *Journal of Rehabilitation, 68*(3), 11–15.

Rothstein, M. A. (1990). *Occupational safety and health law* (3rd ed., pp. 1–25). St. Paul, MN: West Publishing Co.

Scheid, T. (1998). The Americans with Disabilities Act, mental disability, and employment practices. *Journal of Behavioral Health Sciences and Research, 25*(3), 312–324.

Scott, M. (1996). Compliance with ADA, FMLA, workers' compensation, and other laws requires road map. *Employee Benefit Plan Review, 50*(9), 20–30.

Setzer, S. (1992, February 24). Hiring restraints loom in disability law. *ENR News*, pp. 8–9.

Shalowitz, D. (1993, December 6). Return to work obstacle. *Business Insurance*, pp. 2, 53.

Skoning, G., & McGlothlen, C. (1994). Other laws shape ADA policies. *Personnel Journal, 73*(4), 116.

Stude, E. (1994). Implications of the ADA for master's and bachelor's level rehabilitation counseling and rehabilitation services professionals. *Rehabilitation Education, 8*(1), 17–25.

Taylor, R. W. (1995). Medical examinations under the ADA and OSH Act: A dilemma for employers. *Employment in the Mainstream, 20*(6), 23–25.

Ullman, M., Johnson, M., Moss, K., & Burris, S. (2001). The EEOC charge priority policy and claimants with psychiatric disabilities. *Psychiatric Services, 52*, 642–649.

U.S. Department of Justice. (2002). *A guide to disability rights laws.* Washington, DC: Author. Retrieved February 5, 2004, from http://www.usdoj.gov/crt/ada/cguide.pdf

U.S. Department of Labor. (2000, April 12). Training and Employment Information

Notice No. 16-99. Retrieved February 17, 2004, from http://wdsc.doleta. gov/disability/htmldocs/tein_16_99.cfm

U.S. Equal Employment Opportunity Commission. (1992). *A technical assistance manual on the employment provisions (Title I) of the Americans with Disabilities Act.* Washington, DC: Author.

U.S. Equal Employment Opportunity Commission. (1996). *EEOC enforcement guidance: Workers' compensation and the ADA.* Washington, DC: Author.

U.S. Equal Employment Opportunity Commission. (1997, March 25). *EEOC enforcement guidance on the Americans with Disabilities Act and psychiatric disabilities* (No. 915.002). Washington, DC: Author.

U.S. Equal Employment Opportunity Commission. (1999). *Cumulative ADA Charges, July 26, 1992—September 30, 1999.* Retrieved May, 2001, from http://www.eeoc.gov

U.S. Equal Employment Opportunity Commission. (2000). *The Family and Medical Leave Act, the Americans with Disabilities Act, and Title VII of the Civil Rights Act of 1964.* Retrieved February 4, 2004, from http://www.eeoc.gov/policy/docs/fmlaada.html

U.S. Equal Employment Opportunity Commission. (2003). *Annual Report, Fiscal Year 2002.* Retrieved February 5, 2004, from http://www.eeoc.gov/litigation/02annrpt.html

Walker, J., & Heffner, F. (1992). The Americans with Disabilities Act and workers compensation. *CPCU Journal, 45*(3), 151–152.

Walworth, C., Damon, L., &, Wilder, C. (1993). Walking a fine line: Managing the conflicting obligations of the Americans with Disabilities Act and workers' compensation laws. *Employee Relations, 19*(2), 221–232.

Welch, E. (1996). The EEOC, the ADA, and WC. *Ed Welch on Workers' Compensation, 6*(9), 178–179.

Wright, G. (1980). *Total rehabilitation.* Boston: Little, Brown.

Zolkos, R. (1994, July 18). Avoiding charges of bias. *Business Insurance,* p. 85.

35

Accreditation— A Quality Framework in the Consumer- Centric Era

BRIAN J. BOON, PhD

ARGUABLY, HEALTH CARE stands out as the most complex of service industries. As a sector within this industry, medical rehabilitation struggles with its many unique challenges. Downstream from acute care services, medical rehabilitation is now confronted with the task of demonstrating its value in a reimbursement environment that is directed toward more services for less money. Payment systems have not kept up to changes in service demand driven by patient's need and the rising requirement for specialized rehabilitation services.

In response to the many challenges in the rehabilitation industry, leadership is intensely focused on efforts to improve quality to demonstrate value to their many constituents. Although the use of formalized quality frameworks have been the norm in general industry, it is only in the last 20 years that the rehabilitation industry has employed with vigor the many quality frameworks available. Because practitioners in rehabilitation are key participants in quality improvement efforts conducted by organizations, it is a professional obligation that they critically understand features of the quality framework to be used, and where possible, influence decisions regarding which framework should be embraced. Often an administrator or business leader in an organization will lean toward a quality framework employed in other industries, such as manufacturing, and extended to health care because of their familiarity to quality programs or awards in terms of consumer products or services. For the rehabilitation industry, it is argued that a rehabilitation focused accreditation quality model is the best fit as a quality framework for advancing the performance of organizations who provide medical rehabilitation services.

To be comparable to other quality management alternatives, an accreditation model must include quality standards that reflect sound business practices, and address the systematization of continuous improvement efforts. However, to become a best-fit quality model in medical rehabilitation, quality standards must also include a prominent place for the person served and by extension, specific quality standards directed to advancing service to unique rehabilitation populations, such as persons with brain injury, spinal cord injury, chronic pain, and so on. It is these population-specific standards that differentiate accreditation as a quality framework from other frameworks as the best fit.

To understand and appreciate the value of accreditation for medical rehabilitation as a quality framework, it is important that accreditation be considered within its evolutionary context in relation to the dynamics of the broader health care industry. Accreditation as a quality framework was constructed by the rehabilitation industry in response to environmental pressures to demonstrate a commitment to quality. Since its inception in 1966, as the only rehabilitation specific accreditor, the Commission on Accreditation of Rehabilitation Facilities (CARF) has been the quality standards setting body for the broad rehabilitation industry, including medical rehabilitation. As the primary rehabilitation accreditor, CARF's quality standards have changed to meet the demands of the broader health care environment. Since 1966, many new quality management approaches have been trialed by the industry. It is argued that a rehabilitation-specific quality framework will continue to serve both the rehabilitation industry and its patients in that industry well into the future of consumer directed care. Further, the CARF quality model of accreditation will be compared and then differentiated through its unique focus on persons served, which is an orientation different from other "product" or "service to the consumer" quality management models. The other quality management frameworks include; the Malcolm Baldrige National Quality Program (Baldrige), the International Organization for Standardization (ISO), and the European Foundation for Quality Management (EFQM).

EVOLUTIONARY PHASES IN ACCREDITATION

THE EVOLUTIONARY PHASES of accreditation as a rehabilitation industry–specific quality management framework can be illustrated against the dynamic characteristics of the broader health care environment (Figure 35.1). One characteristic is the degree to which the environment is closed or exclusive. In contrast, an inclusive environment would optimize the involvement of many parties. Another characteristic is the degree to which an environment is transparent and therefore provides for an enhanced public accountability. A transparent environment often evolves in response to demands for greater accountability. As these environmental factors change, so do characteristics of the quality management framework. The continuum of these factors (exclusiveness to inclusiveness and low to high degrees of transparency) acts as reference points to the evolution of accreditation. Accreditation, as described through various eras, is influenced by environmental dynamics concurrent to the period of time or era. The described eras are not

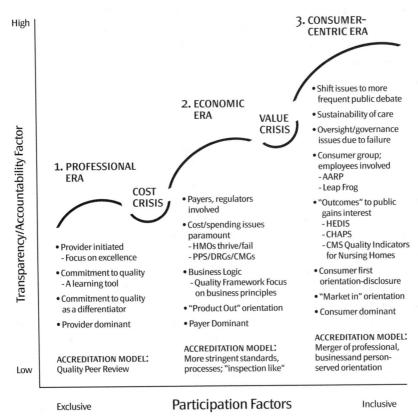

Figure 35.1 Evolutionary phases of accreditation

mutually exclusive and the features of one, in fact, can carry over to future eras. Over time, accreditation evolves to satisfy the demands of quality. As a unique quality framework and business orientation, accreditation is greatly positioned to optimize its impact on enhancing services to the lives of persons served (Stavert & Boon, 2003). Each of the following eras illustrates accreditation's evolutionary paths with reference specific to rehabilitation.

THE PROFESSIONS ERA (1960–1980)

IN ITS EARLY evolutionary steps, accreditation began as the result of the exclusive activity of the rehabilitation professions seeking to provide for a quality template and to pursue excellence in the delivery of service and care. Although certification, licensure, and various forms of regulation existed regarding the practice of care, these administrative requirements were not seen by rehabilitation professionals or regulators as guides to improving services or programs. As there existed no external benchmark for excellence, accreditation was sponsored as that guide to excellence. Many of the professional rehabilitation and health care associations supported and promoted accreditation as an industry-based quality initiative. CARF's current Board of Trustees is comprised of sponsoring members who represent many of the major professional organizations in the rehabilitation industry. Their sponsorship can be traced back to these early days.

During this era, quality standards were developed collegially, via expert consensus-based panels, and then endorsed by the community of providers. Accreditation processes took the form of on-site review visits or surveys of organizations to determine the degree of compliance/conformance to required standards. The act of preparing for and successfully completing accreditation demonstrated that an organization was committed to quality. This distinction was used to differentiate organizations from one another, sometimes allowing for those organizations that were accredited to claim specialty status. Being accredited by a neutral third party gave organizations the opportunity to proclaim that their organization met the standard of a quality-based organization. Accreditation was promoted as a voluntary initiative in rehabilitation, although it was also used as a supplement to regulation or rule requirements to receive certain payments. Peer-based accreditation maintained and advanced the privilege of the professions "regulating" themselves through this commitment to quality via accreditation.

The process of quality accreditation review by peers maintained provider autonomy and "control" over quality for a significant period of time. To some extent, during this period of provider dominance, consumers were, as a group, less organized or active and, to a degree, individually "passive" recipients of service or treatment. However, this apparent era of professional autonomy was soon challenged by the era of economics as costs began to challenge the collective system. Advances in the use of medical technology and pharmaceuticals, and a growing demand for more health care and specialized rehabilitation services resulted in rising costs. The challenges associated with these trends shifted the dynamics of the system from one predominated by professional direction and influence to one in which economics became a predominant factor in a changing and dynamic environment.

THE ECONOMIC ERA (1980–PRESENT)

COST-CONTAINMENT TACTICS

AS HEALTH CARE costs dramatically increased, discussions and concerns regarding the long-term affordability of health care and its impact on the delivery of quality service became a paramount industry and public-policy concern. While the rehabilitation industry continued to support accreditation, emerging environmental factors provided the opportunity for new management philosophies to be considered in the industry as it responded to the crisis in the "business" of health care. It was during this period that regulators and payers became more involved as the system and its faults became more transparent to the public. Health maintenance organizations evolved to control costs during this period while trying to maintain access to appropriate care. In response to economic crisis, health care leadership shifted to employing and adopting business logic to its health industry problems. Payers looked to alternative payment schemes and contract-management approaches to control costs. Providers experienced lower reimbursement rates or deep discount contracts, which resulted in fewer dollars per case and was part of the "rehabilitation carve-out" cost-management effort. The mantra of "doing more with less" was and remains a predominant theme in health care, much like the oft-heard phrase "funding dictates form."

With an increasing sensitivity to costs, accreditation was used as a vendor prequalification step in procurement of services by some payers. Some insurers used accreditation as a contract-management risk tool to ensure that quality rehabilitation service was embedded in their extended specialty-service provider networks (e.g., brain injury services). Insurers would only reimburse providers if they received third-party accreditation for their claimed specialty in rehabilitation. Insurers used accreditation to confirm those claiming to provide specialty rehabilitation services were qualified and ran programs to known quality standards. Similar logic was also employed by regulators and policy makers who may have passed rules, declarations, mandates, or directives regarding the requirements of accreditation for reimbursement and "quality" oversight purposes.

EMPLOYEES ENTER AS NEW PARTICIPANTS

IN RESPONSE TO THE cost crisis and the new business logic being employed, accreditation quality standards adjusted accordingly. Standards became longer, more stringent, and at times definitive or prescriptive. New programs/standards were added as outpatient rehabilitation or specialty services grew. By way of example, in response to the cost crisis in the workers compensation industry, CARF created "work hardening" standards to focus the provider, payor, and injured worker on the importance of return to work as an outcome of rehabilitation. The typical goals in rehabilitation, such as "improve strength" of the worker included the demands of its job to ensure return to work and ultimately contain costs. Quality rehabilitation standards relating to performance were also added, referencing measures of effectiveness, efficiency, or satisfaction. In an era of rising costs, results for dollars spent on quality standards relating to safety also became more of a priority with the increasing transparency of reported safety errors in the general health care system (Institute of Medicine, 1999). Errors in care are attributed to a fragmented system in an environment where there exist diminished trust and satisfaction of the consumer and the health professional. In partial response to the public-safety crisis, the accreditation process became a more rigorous or "inspective-like" quality-assurance exercise for organizations.

It was also during this era that the employer community became a more vocal and influential participant in the industry, even a proxy representative of their employees' health care quality concerns. Examples of this include the National Business Group on Health (NBGH), formerly known as the Washington Business Group on Health, and most recently The Leapfrog Group. The NBGH is a large employer group dedicated to finding innovative and forward-thinking solutions to health care issues (NBGH, 2004). It has recently initiated a council to look at employee health and quality metrics related to improved outcomes, enhanced quality, and managed costs. The Leapfrog Group (2004) is a coalition of 150 public and private organizations, Fortune 500 sourced, whose publicized priority tasks include improving safety of patient care or "saving lives," mobilizing employer purchasing power, recognizing and rewarding excellence in care through market-based incentives, and giving consumers information to make good choices about which hospital to use.

The stated motivations of both of these groups are to advance safer health care practice, manage costs, and extend the value of service to the benefit of the employer and its employees. For some employers, health care benefit expenses are cause for concern as they increase infrastructure costs. Higher health benefits result in a higher cost of goods or services delivered, placing in jeopardy an employer's competitive position in a cost-conscious global environment.

It is also during this era that cost concerns and the impact of cost-containment strategies on quality led to public discussions and debates. The cost crisis therefore creates greater transparency in various forms, such as commissions, agencies, institutes, and "think tanks" to consider potential remedies and changes to improve the system. As one example, the President's Advisory Commission on Consumer Protection and Quality in the Health Care Industry (1998) established by President Clinton studied health care quality and recommended improvement strategies to enhance health systems' responsiveness and effectiveness. Patient's rights legislation was one considered option from the report, the other being the established agency known as the National Forum for Quality Management and Reporting—an agency directed to establish common set performance indicators for the health system. In reference to the cost-management activity at the public level, even the Centers for Medicare and Medicaid Services (CMS) are trying to leverage its purchasing power to control costs (example: prospective payment system/"75-75%" rule) and demand involvement in public reporting of quality in systems of care (example: Nursing Home Compare). Significant public domain efforts signal collective unrest and potential changes in the environment, ultimately leading to a new era of health care delivery.

As the dynamics of the environment became more inclusive and open, and issues related to cost effectiveness, customer satisfaction, and safety became more prominent, the health care industry concurrently borrowed other industries' lessons and logic concerning quality. Health care/rehabilitation organizations began to employ quality frameworks (Counte & Meurer, 2001) such as ISO 9000, Baldrige, Total Quality Management (TQM), Continuous Quality Improvement (CQI), Quality Control Circles, Statistical Process Control (SPC), Balanced Scorecards/Reports, Process Reengineering, Management by Results, Outcome Management, etc. The Disney Institute even ventured into providing programs to health care organizations that wished to advance their customer-service approach. A good organization will always challenge itself to discover cost-effective methods of delivering quality rehabilitation service. All of the above-noted techniques quality, if implemented effectively, to help organizations "to do more with less."

Cost containment is a predominant theme within the economic era, and the resulting service reality for the rehabilitation field was to "do more with less." An employed business logic that embraced quality frameworks from other industries created a gap between leadership and those who provided direct services to persons served. Essentially, a gap of cultures was created between management and practitioners in relation to the methods of delivering high-quality care in a reducing reimbursement environment.

A prevailing countertrend to the economically driven cost-containment era was a more vigilant, autonomous, and empowered collective of consumer groups. Consumers fought the apparent restrictions to access and care practices imposed by managed care techniques. Employers, too, continued to be concerned by rising health-benefit costs with no end in sight. Over time, as more costs shift to employers and their employees, and overall there is less access to services for the masses, the public debate will begin regarding the value for dollars spent in the emerging, "to be dominant" consumer-centric marketplace. The "crisis of value" will challenge the industry to once again reorient and adjust to a new circumstance of environment dynamics. Payers, regulators, and providers will need to embrace the shifting influence that persons served will have in reshaping the future delivery of health care and rehabilitation.

CONSUMER-CENTRIC ERA (2000 AND BEYOND)

THE HEALTH AND human services industry is beginning to experience the early signs of fundamental change to their environment. Consumers or persons served are beginning to exercise choice, control, and with greater frequency, bear the financial cost for services received. This period, referenced as the consumer-centric era, is that time when the economic and service challenges in the health care system are so great, that the apparent sustainability of the health service system is at stake. The current federal and state fiscal crises, an aging population with growing health demands, and other industry factors will likely conspire to create a service crisis. Costs will remain a critical variable for ongoing management. The crisis of service, cost, and sustainability will shift debate from the private boardrooms of companies to the broader and transparent public arena, where concerns regarding accountability for quality are at the forefront of that debate.

It is during this period that the Internet-knowledgeable consumer will demonstrate unprecedented influence and create new demands in the health care system. Consumers will transition from relatively uninformed passive recipients of service to engaged and informed participants in their care and service plans. Consumers will be vigilant about timely access to affordable high-quality service with expected outcomes commensurate with experienced risk. Informed consumers will begin to advocate for improvements in the dimensions of rehabilitation, such as timely and friendly access to care, practice patterns consistent with established guidelines, and outstanding clinical and functional outcomes (Goonan, 1994). This social shift in influence already can be observed in the growing number of consumer-directed health plans, spending accounts, and service options that have become instituted with greater frequency in the marketplace. Pharmaceutical companies have also recognized the power of consumer authority as they begin marketing directly to consumers, often via television commercials, supplementing the traditional physician-only sales channels: "the 'blue pill' will allow you to golf pain-free like Tiger Woods!"

In an era of greater transparency, consumers will want access to information with respect to quality indicators of rehabilitation service. They also will demand more information over time in the form of "public report cards." Signs of increasing transparency already exist and, by extension, public accountability, which are illustrated in a set of first-generation public reports. Examples of these public reports include, to name a few, the Health Plan Employers Data and Information Set (HEDIS) is the tool used by the National Committee on Quality Assurance (NCQA, 2004), which is a group of measures designed to evaluate health plans' key processes; the Consumer Assessment of Health Plans (CAHPS) developed and managed by a consortium of organizations (Aging for Health Care Research and Quality, American Institutes for Research, Harvard Medicine School, RAND, and Westat); the CMS Nursing Home Compare; and general satisfaction questionnaires such as Health Grades, Inc., conducted by J. D. Power and Associates, (2004). Clearly, insurers/payers, regulators, and health organizations are focused on indices of quality as they relate to the consumer. Outcomes for services rendered will drive consumers and payers to select and reinforce the high-performance provider. Further, with the growing influence of consumers and greater health care costs being paid directly by consumers (Organization for Economic Cooperation and Development [OECD], 2003), the dominant social forces impacting human service systems will be consumer collectives. Consumer enclaves, in the traditional sense (e.g., American Association of Retired Persons) or via internet swarms (virtual collectives with common values and purpose), will create powerful social forces of significant magnitude to impact public policy, influence purchase trends, review quality, and ultimately assess the value of care via cost, service, and outcomes.

It is during this period of response to crises that key participants will reaffirm their primary focus on the task at hand—to organize systems, organizations, and services around persons served. If the explicit value of the system is to serve an engaged consumer, then services should be organized around the person served. A quality framework specific to rehabilitation should both support and advance this orientation. To be of value, quality frameworks must be inclusive and transparent to key participants in the system—provider, payor, and person served. With inclusive participation from key participants in the development of standards, rehabilitation accreditors can enhance their quality framework by importing the valuable knowledge the rehabilitation field, and persons served.

Industries outside of human services incorporate the customer requirement in their production or manufacturing process, to meet the customers' specifications. Quality is built into the design of the product. In an inclusive environment, a rehabilitation accreditor must also incorporate multiple-party input into the process of designing and promoting quality standards. Providers, payers, regulators, and persons served should be "at the table" when accreditors develop quality standards and establish the process to assess quality. They all participate in the rehabilitation system. This approach is inclusive, transparent, and leads to advancing accountability in the system. In turn, quality rehabilitation standards should also prominently recognize the unique role that the person served plays in the design, delivery, and outputs of care. The emerging consumer-centric environment will require that organizational practices are consistent with the values in rehabilitation to fully and meaningfully engage persons served. Further, this quality framework should reestablish the link between process and outcome, which recognizes the important role that both clinicians and persons served play in contributing to a quality result. Accreditation will provide the architecture for organizational service design and quality assessment and create an integrated, transparent, and value-based organization. In the consumer-driven era, a rehabilitation-specific accreditation quality framework will position organizations to shift their orientation by transitioning from pure business quality templates to accreditation quality templates in order to better serve individuals.

TRANSITION FROM A BUSINESS QUALITY MODEL TO AN ACCREDITATION QUALITY MODEL

HEALTH CARE AS an industry is a "big and complex business" in most developing countries. Internationally, health care spending continues to outpace economic growth in most industrialized countries (OECD, 2003), and in response, each country struggles with its own unique way to fund services through public, private, or variant hybrid payment systems. The magnitude of dollars spent on health care is poignantly reflected as a percentage of a country's gross domestic product (GDP). Utilizing data from OECD (2003), the proportion of GDP spent on health care in the United States reached 13.9%. In other countries, the numbers are almost as high: 10.9% for Switzerland, 10.7% for Germany, and Canada and France following with 9.7% and 9.5%, respectively. In the United States, costs continue to escalate. In the United States, health care spending reached $1.6 trillion in 2002 at a growth rate of 9.3% (CMS, 2003), representing 14.9% of GDP.

As previously noted, the overall environment of health care has recently and predominantly focused on cost relative to service. In an attempt to deal with the cost-to-quality issue, regulators, payers, and health care leaders in charge of health care plans or systems of care, including hospitals and rehabilitation settings, have tried to address the business complexity of health care by employing the logic necessary to survive in such a demanding environment. As a consequence, health care has employed and adapted a multitude of business-based quality tools, techniques, and principles. There exists some evidence that utilizing quality tools or techniques is perceived by management or organizational leadership as contributing to an organization's strategic or business goals (Yasin, Zimmerer, Miller, & Zimmerer, 2002). It is also interesting to note that the business-based quality frameworks are predated by accreditation-based quality framework methods (e.g., CARF accreditation—1966, ISO 9000—1987, Baldrige—1988). Why in some instances did the previously referenced quality management approaches emerge as a supplement or replacement to accreditation? It is plausible that accreditation business standards had not kept up with the business needs of organizations via its standards and therefore were no longer felt to be relevant or of value. An equally plausible reason is that the accreditation process was seen as a professional validation effort by clinicians to affirm that their processes were of high quality, resulting in clinical/functional gains. However, during an "economic squeeze" cycle, pure functional gains appear to be less relevant to cost-focused administrators and payers. Perhaps accreditation was really never perceived by administrators as a "true quality framework," but rather a requirement for payment or a clinically focused exercise. Further, in larger human service systems the accreditation of a rehabilitation program was rarely elevated to the attention of the President/CEO or Executive Director. In fact, if successful accreditation was realized repeatedly, it may have lost significance over time. Lastly, as the business challenges in health care grew, executives employed to lead health plans and hospitals had other management, industry, and educational experiences, and were more familiar with other quality models to advance the performance of their organization.

Since industry-based quality programs were known to help the competitiveness of industry globally, it was reasoned that these quality programs could help the health care industry to address its concerns. Industry quality frameworks were innovative, prestigious, and something new to many organizations. As a by-product of adopting the business quality techniques, it was hoped that these programs would create organizational spirit, trust, and renewal with staff. Undoubtedly, the opportunity for the clinician to become empowered in an organization to identify, discuss, and provide solutions to work problems can create a better service and work environment. However, while these quality programs were being introduced and business logic employed, the greatest long-term result of these organizational efforts, even if it was not appropriately implemented, was to create organizations comprised of leadership and practitioners that were "two minded and culturally disintegrated" (Goldsmith, 1998). In essence, the leadership and staff became disengaged from one another. This gap relates to an "orientation gap" in which the business-based quality framework fails to bridge the business with the rehabilitation care provided to persons with disability.

In the human services industry and especially in rehabilitation there are unique issues that are foreign to the typical manufacturing or service environments in which quality frameworks operate. As an illustration (Figure 35.2), in the manufacturing industry quality is a function of many causal factors, including worker, material, method, measurement, and machine (Ishikawa, 1985). These collectives of causal factors constitute a process that can be controlled via standardization to create

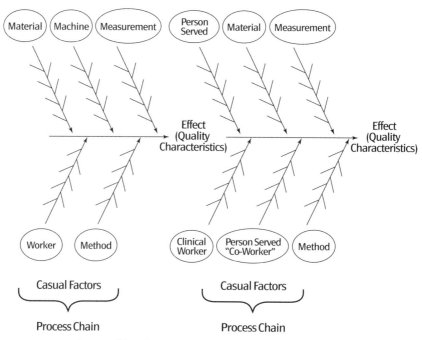

Figure 35.2   Cause-effect diagram.

a quality effect. In manufacturing, the effect is targeted quality—a certain level of designed quality. Quality of conformance is an indication of how far the actual product conforms to its quality target or design. Let us translate this quality formula to the human services industry and, specifically, to rehabilitation. The worker providing the services is the clinician. The method employed is his or her clinical intervention and/or process. The material is the person served, and the machine could be a pharmaceutical or technology that helps with functional restoration (e.g., a weight machine for strengthening exercise). However, the formula is even more complex in rehabilitation since an engaged consumer, or person served, is both the material *and* part worker or producer of an outcome. This is a unique factor that differentiates an accreditation quality framework from those employed by business where customer needs or requirements are defined and a product is produced or service generated to meet those desired needs and features. In the case of rehabilitation, the person served is both the coproducer of service and the recipient of service with an associated outcome. The rehabilitation process makes accommodations for this complex variable in the equation, and therefore a quality framework must emphasize this distinct point if it is to be relevant and of value. It is this distinction that those who provide direct services in the health and rehabilitation environment recognize and the reason why most employed business-based quality programs in health care are perceived as "foreign" or force-fitted into the health and rehabilitation industry.

An interesting note, in spite of the business philosophy employed during the economic era, is that health care and its delivery continued to remain fragmented, fragile, and an escalating cost factor for many employees and employers. The same observation can be made for accreditation, which also existed with its varied approaches during this period.

THE IMPORTANCE OF PROCESS
MEASURES AND PERSONS SERVED

THERE EXISTS THE desire by leaders in health and rehabilitation to ensure that human service systems meet the highest standards with respect to both business and clinical service excellence. Much study specific to assessing quality in health care has already been conducted. One well-known approach is to assess quality via its structure, processes, and outcomes (Donabedian, 1978, 1996). Structural assumptions of quality identify the necessary and enabling conditions that must be present in the provision of care or service, such as infrastructure and staff. Structural elements are necessary conditions but alone do not ensure quality. Process measures focus on the activities delivered according to accepted and predetermined standards; i.e., those standards related to care and the delivery of care within a program or organizational unit of analysis. Outcomes refer to the attainment of desired goals for the individual (e.g., return to work), at the level of the organization (e.g., reduced medical errors, patient satisfaction), or at a systems level (e.g., measures of community health, social participation). For organizational leadership, structure and outcomes factors are of more relevance and interest because they are more tangible for deliberation and debate. Process measures typically fall under the primary domain of interest for providers of health services. When outcomes can be linked to process, certainly providers are engaged as other parties in an evidenced-based or a promising practices approach. Persons served are also concerned with outcomes and the processes that they must participate in as well as those risks and consequences.

The advantages and disadvantages of process measures relative to outcome measures have been well articulated in other articles (Mant, 2001; Rubin, Provonost, & Diette, 2001). Outcomes measures are of relevance to persons served. However, quality frameworks again fail to recognize the role of persons served in producing an outcome, and therefore process measures are also relevant to persons served. Process measures have immediate appeal to clinicians in the health and rehabilitation environment. These measures identify exactly which processes are followed that are believed to result in an effective output or outcome. Measures that relate to process, the "science and art of doing," provide information that is observable and therefore function as a frame of reference for what needs to be changed to improve outcomes. Process measures utilized as standards of quality also reflect the care of service delivered, and therefore clinicians feel accountable for them because they have face validity—"it is what we do." Although outcomes are the desired goals of any rehabilitation process, it is recognized that many factors affect health care outcomes beyond the provider control, such as patient involvement and commitment to treatment regimens as well as many other external factors. There exists clinical comfort in using process measures. The challenge to a processes-only approach is confirming evidence that supports the relationship between a clinical process and outcome, which then puts the clinician and, by extension, persons served at risk in an environment where economics alone begin to influence the method, timing, and appropriateness of services. Where these links have been determined, all parties will focus on good process for expected outcomes. However, it is difficult to link of process to outcomes. This linkage is difficult to determine because of the necessity to provide for risk-adjusted outcomes to incorporate unique features of complex rehabilitation patient populations. Much research is needed to advance promising practices or the practice of evidence-based care and to advance the role of the person served as a critical resource in that process-outcome linkage analysis.

In order for an accreditation model to provide for a robust quality framework, it must appeal to the various key participants in the delivery system. Governance and executive leadership want a framework that is a template for the system of business (structure/process) and service performance (outcomes) of the organization that the excellence award programs typically provide. Clinical staff members desire a template to judge their care processes (process) and results (outcomes) achieved to some standard or benchmark. Persons served want input, participation (process), and assurances of quality (outcomes) results. The drive of the collective then is to ensure that organizations are assessed against the framework of structure, process, and outcomes. In relation to these dimensions, accreditation will be assessed in reference to three other respected business-quality frameworks (Baldridge, ISO, and EFQM) and then will be differentiated against these frameworks to demonstrate the best fit within the rehabilitation industry and in the consumer-centric era.

QUALITY IMPROVEMENT FRAMEWORKS AND THE ACCREDITATION MODEL OF QUALITY

CLEARLY THE SUCCESS of any business enterprise is dependent upon how an organization manages its resources to create effective and efficient delivery systems of service. In an effort to meet this challenge, health care organizations have implemented a variety of respected quality frameworks previously referenced. Further, many organizations simultaneously pursue accreditation for purposes of "deemed status," mandates, or the extended philosophy of continuous improvement in the rehabilitation setting. The CARF accreditation model of quality will be compared to three predominant and respected business-quality frameworks: the Malcolm Baldrige National Quality Program—Health Care Criteria for Performance Excellence (2004), the International Organization for Standardization—ISO 9000: 2000 Quality Management Principles (2000), and the European Foundation for Quality Management (EFQM)—Excellence Model (1999). The accreditation model used is the Commission on Accreditation of Rehabilitation Facilities (CARF)—Medical Rehabilitation Standards (2004). The comparison approach has been adapted from an international review of business excellence and award programs (Calingo, 2002). The author would also like to underscore that all these models are excellent for organizations that wish to advance their business and service practices. Further, all of these frameworks are complementary and can be employed as a holistic step-wise model to enhance business and service improvement.

All of the selected quality frameworks have a directional purpose, which is to advance the success of the organization employing the respective framework (see Table 35.1). The Baldrige and EFQM models evolved in response to industry concerns regarding quality in an increasingly competitive national and global economy. The Baldrige approach was extended to health care in 1999, and the EFQM has been employed as a guide in the health industry via the EFQM International Health Sector Group. The CARF model, the oldest of the quality models, has since its inception been directed to "enhancing the lives of persons served" as a quality framework in the human services. ISO, like other quality frameworks, has been equally utilized in health along with many other industry sectors (see Table 35.2). The orientations of these programs also differ. Both Baldrige and EFQM focus on advancing an organization's practices, capabilities, and results. The award process, which includes self-assessment and external scoring, could include a site visit if the potential

TABLE 35.1   Purpose of Quality Framework

Framework	Inception–revisions	Orientation	Percentage of applicant sites visited	Outcome
Baldrige	1988, Health in 1999 (annual revisions)	Recognition of organizational excellence and best practice promotion	20	Award
ISO 9000	1987, 1994, 2000 (originated in 1947)	Requirements for quality management systems and guidance for performance improvement	100	Certification, follow-up surveillance audits on corrective actions, option for scheduled audits
EFQM	1991	Recognition of organizational excellence and best practice promotion	20	Award
CARF	1966-many	Recognition that an organization demonstrates quality, value, and optimal outcomes of services through continuous improvement focused on enhancing lives of persons served	100	Accreditation, follow-up quality improvement plan and ongoing annual conformance to quality reports

TABLE 35.2 Adaptation to Sectors

Framework	Adaptation	Number of sectors
Baldrige	Unique but equal criteria for sectors: business, education, and health care	3
ISO 9000	Multiple industries and increased depth (example: ISO 9001 criteria is applied)	Multiple Industry
EFQM	Unique but equal criteria for sectors: large commercial, subsidiary operating units, small to medium enterprise, public sector	4
CARF	Equal business criteria, multiple sector specific criteria—aging services, employment and community, behavioral health, medical rehabilitation and increased depth by program within sector	Medical rehabilitation subsectors programs: * Comprehensive integrated inpatient * Spinal cord system of care * Interdisciplinary pain * Brain injury * Outpatient medical * Home and community * Case management * Health enhancement * Pediatric family centered * Occupational rehabilitation

of finalist status exists. An ISO outcome is the status of certification that demonstrates compliance with quality-management system principles via specific 9001 requirements, and thus requires that all organizations be assessed via site visit. In CARF accreditation, organizations must demonstrate their conformance to business and service/care standards, confirmed by site visit in order to receive an accreditation outcome. CARF requires ongoing conformance—the sustainability of quality. By far, ISO is the largest of the quality framework models comprising 148 national standards bodies and 2,981 technical bodies, reflecting the scope of this organization. As of December 2002, 562,000 conformity certificates were issued by 750 certification bodies in 159 countries (ISO, 2004).

Each of the quality frameworks also recognizes that there exist many

TABLE 35.3   Levels of Quality Recognition

Framework	Number of Levels	Description
Baldrige	1	Points > 700 usually trigger award
ISO 9000	1	Certification of compliance
EFQM	3	Commitment to Excellence, Recognition of Excellence (350 points), European Quality Award (> 750 points)
CARF	3	Time based—3 year, 1 year, or non-accreditation

pathways to performance improvement and operational excellence. The excellence benchmarks in Baldrige and EFQM are found both in their scoring structure and evaluative dimensions. A points system is employed in Baldrige and EFQM. Those exceeding a cumulative 700 points in Baldrige or a 750 cumulative point threshold in EFQM are typically eligible as finalists to receive a quality award (Table 35.3). The EFQM Excellence Model also provides gradients in the evolution of excellence via its stepwise approach: commitment to excellence, recognition of excellence status, and award status. The European Quality Award (EQA) signifies the best of excellent performing organizations. ISO 9000 compliance is audited on-site via a checklist guide reflecting the audit 9001 criteria. Compliance is either met or not met—the resulting outcome leading to a certificate of compliance that extends to 3 years. CARF accreditation has two determined outcomes, accreditation or nonaccreditation. The accreditation outcome is based on the degree of conformance (Table 35.4) to standards as determined by surveyor via checklist. However, there are levels of accreditation that are time-based.

TABLE 35.4   Evaluation Dimensions

Framework	Dimension Structure
Baldrige	Process: Approach, deployment, learning, and integration Results: Current level, rate and breadth, performance comparison, and linkage of results to process and action plan requirements ISO 9000
EFQM	For enablers and results criteria the following apply: Results, approach, deployment, assessment, and review
CARF	Conformance rating: Non, partial, substantial, exemplary

A 1-year level of accreditation outcome signifies that there is organizational conformance to many standards, however, deficiencies are noted requiring correction, and therefore a return site visit in 1 year. A 3-year outcome is awarded if the organization exemplifies substantial conformance to standards—both in policy and practice. Both Baldrige and EFQM review their respective criteria of quality along the evaluative dimensions of whether an organization plans and deploys improvement strategies in the organizations, links the results to action, and learns and integrates information to further improve organizational performance. The notion of this "approach, deployment, results, learning, and integration" sequence is embedded within the structure of CARF's standards, which are scoreable because of their unidimensional and measurable design. In all four quality frameworks, the "review" is conducted by a third party or neutral agent to the organization seeking an award, certification, or accreditation (Table 35.5). In the case of Baldrige, EFQM, and CARF, awards or accreditation is provided by the quality organization that conducts and manages the reviews/accreditation process. In contrast, ISO utilizes its 148 national standard body organizations to accredit registration bodies that employ auditors to determine ISO compliance and certification. ISO does not directly certify ISO compliance.

Lastly, each quality framework also employs set criteria or standards. While the scope of the chapter is not to review the details of each framework's criteria, there exist both notable high-level similarities and differences (see Table 35.6). All frameworks recognize the importance of leadership, focus on customer, involvement of staff/human resources, continuous improvement utilizing information, and performance. The Baldrige and EFQM frameworks have well-formulated Leadership/ Strategic Planning standards that reinforce the need to set short/long term direction, and the deployment of plans with follow-up, compari-

TABLE 35.5   Reviewer Categories

Framework	Title of Reviewers	Number of Reviewers	Training Time
Baldrige	Examiner	> 400	3 days, inclusive of 30–40 hour case study
ISO 9000	Registrars—Auditor	—	—
EFQM	Assessor	≈ 169	2.5 days
CARF	Surveyor	1,400	5 days and intern program

TABLE 35.6   Criteria of Quality Frameworks

Baldrige: 2004	ISO 9000: 2000	EFQM— Excellence Model	CARF
Leadership	Customer focus	Leadership	Input from persons served
Strategic planning	Leadership	People	Accessibility
Focus on patients, other customers, and markets	Involvement of people	Policy and strategy	Information management and performance improvement
Measurement, analysis, knowledge, and management	Process approach	Partnership and resources	Rights of persons served
Staff focus	Systems approach management	Processes	Health and safety
Process management	Continued improvement	People results	Human resources
Organizational performance results	Factual approach to decision making	Customer results	Leadership
	Mutually beneficial supplier relationship	Society results	Legal requirements
		Key performance results	Financial planning and management
			Rehabilitation process for persons served

son, and revision. Key organizational performance results are also well-emphasized in Baldrige/EFQM, including results for patients, financial results, staff and operating results. Baldrige, EFQM, and ISO focus on higher-order system measures (example: financial results, market share measures, etc.). EFQM also includes results for society, extending the notion of social responsibility to an outcome for the organization. The other quality frameworks also address results in similar ways.

CARF also has a well-defined organizational performance section that requires an organization to focus on organizational metrics of efficiency, effectiveness, service access, and satisfaction from the perspective of persons served and other stakeholders. CARF's accreditation focus looks at the business components of an organization and drills down to the organizational unit (program) delivering rehabilitation to persons served. CARF requires that effectiveness (example: work status at 1-month postdischage) to persons served also be measured at a point in time following service to measure true long-term effectiveness or the specific organizational outcomes related to persons served. CARF's other accreditation criteria, such as input from persons served, accessibility, and rights of persons served, also differentiate CARF from the other quality frameworks.

Other quality frameworks typically lack standards that detail the quality standards to protect the rights of persons served, such as requirements to demonstrate a commitment to recognize diversity (culture), to exceed policies to ensure confidentiality and privacy, to provide access to information and ensure informed choice, and so on. The key stakeholders who have contributed to CARF's medical rehabilitation standards development have placed the persons served at the center of an organization's quality assessment. It has been this way since its inception almost 38 years ago. This approach affirms that in rehabilitation, quality is influenced by the inclusiveness of persons served as key participants in the output or outcome of the process. Hence, service or treatment planning includes shared responsibility and commitment between provider and persons served. As an example of a measured substandard, treatment goals are to be written in the words of persons served in order that the person is engaged and understands the purpose and goals of service. Further, the rehabilitation practitioner is aware of the reasons why the person is seeking services, what goals he or she wants to achieve, and the activities in which they wish to participate.

The person-centric theme or approach has been similarly referenced in a publication written by the Institute of Medicine (2001), which identified that one of the aims for health care improvement is to include a patient-centered approach that is customized to patient needs/values, where the patient is the source of control and in a system that is transparent in its efforts. In the behavioral health sector of rehabilitation, a similar theme has also emerged in the final report of the President's New Freedom Commission on Mental Health (2003), which also affirmed that mental health services and treatment should be consumer and family centered in order to promote and ensure that individualized care plans are directed to enhancing full community participation. Social responsibility and value of rehabilitation also come to the forefront via CARF's focus on accessibility. Accessibility standards, which are directed to promoting access to services and removing barriers for persons with disability, such as attitudinal or environmental barriers in order to effect a positive outcome for persons served as active participants in society. This single feature differentiates CARF and its rehabilitation-industry values from the other reputable and noteworthy quality frameworks.

To further instill the person-served orientation, the organization and its leadership must also demonstrate that they promote and protect the rights of persons served as part of their business/service focus. The accreditation-based quality framework emphasizes that enhanced communication efforts to the consumer, the creation of programs and services appropriate to the diversity of the population served, and a demonstration of cultural competency will differentiate providers in the future. Accreditation standards focused on consumer input go beyond mere assessment of input forums of persons served, satisfaction surveys, or market analysis of customer requirements. These are all excellent exercises to better serve customers. Quality frameworks in rehabilitation should advance the orientation to persons served within the organizational business context to organizations that seek to provide high-quality service to people in an era where there will be no alternative to the benchmark of assessed value. Rehabilitation organizations of the future must embrace their responsibility to persons served to ensure value and quality in their privileged position of service. Those organizations, leadership and staff, that embrace this orientation will be well prepared for the consumer-centric era.

The last differentiator in the CARF quality framework is the standard related to the rehabilitation process—specific "process-based" standards often defined by the person served population (example: persons with brain injury). A quality framework in rehabilitation must outline process standards that are directed to effecting positive change in the functional ability of persons served. Based on the specific rehabilitation population served, the composition of the rehabilitation team, scope of services, program goals, assessment or diagnostic services rendered, establishing treatment plans and goals, and community reintegration planning all vary dramatically based on the person served. CARF's accreditation quality model outlines specific quality protocols for such processes that do not exist in other quality frameworks (see Table 35.2).

A quality framework that also provides rehabilitation relevant consensus standards creates an additional point of reference for organizations to design new rehabilitation programs or to offer more services in their community. Further, a quality framework can serve as a reference point to experiment and assess outcomes when deviating from the designed rehabilitation standard or targeted quality. Standards can act as blueprints for design, as process controls, and as benchmarks for internal or external comparison. These kinds of standards have "face validity" for clinicians and persons served and/or their families in the rehabilitation community not offered by other quality frameworks. It is the accreditation-based quality framework with its unique orientation to persons served and sector specificity that differentiates it from other quality frameworks.

THE EXTENDED VALUE OF ACCREDITATION

ALL OF THE previously referenced quality frameworks, techniques, and philosophies offer the discipline of thought and action necessary to improve the performance of an organization. Accreditation, with its unique history, depth of rehabilitation-specific standards, and persons-served orientation, offers an extended value beyond the accreditation site visit to the benefit of key participants in the system. The extended value of accreditation can be seen in the benefits to persons served, organizations, payers, regulators, and society (Table 35.7).

TABLE 35.7 Extended Value in Accreditation

Society

General
* Maintains the importance of quality in the "human services" in world of competing interests
* Quality and excellence in systems lead to greater access for people
* Systems focused on people, perform well, create participation opportunities for persons with disabilities; these outcomes contribute to thriving communities/nations
* A well-performing rehabilitation sector reduces stigma of disability, enhances participation for persons
* Congruence with laws (example: ADA, Olmstead decision, etc.)

Regulators General
* Allows experts and public to determine quality indicators in "specialty" areas; done by a third party accreditator
* Highest priority risks can be focused of quality oversight by regulator
* Accreditation template provides systems with quality benchmarks across a continuum of services
* Accreditation, with specificity built into programs, sets service standards expectation regardless of location, size, etc. All people deserve high-quality care regardless of location/site (standardize quality)
* Supports public's demand for enhanced quality

Payer
* Requirement that providers be accredited demonstrates commitment to quality on behalf of accounts/lives covered
* Accreditation standards can be used for service protocols/management practices/cost models/etc.
* Accreditation used as external confirmation of declared specialty, assuring best care/outcome/service expectation for all stakeholders
* Accreditation requirement of all providers to establish information and outcome management system could be leveraged to establish system improvement efforts; contribute to report cards
* Standards used to create quality continuum of service to better serve accounts/lives concerned

(Continued)

TABLE 35.7 *(Continued)*

Organization

Governance/Executive
* Another third-party review enhances accountability disclosure/quality assurance/risk management function
* Snapshot of human service/business competencies
* Maintains corporate vigilance to society/persons served
* Public demonstration of commitment to quality; can be used as promotional tool
* Bridges "the business with the care" to learn and improve
* May fulfill legal and regulatory requirements
* Balances long-term/short-term business and care priorities

Clinician
* Maintains prominence of persons served as co-creator of outcomes, helps to focus on person-based outcomes
* Program standards act as process templates (face validity), expedite program/service development
* Standards represent embedded knowledge of profession and service of those who participate, at different levels, in the service system
* Standards can be used to appropriately minimize or extinguish undesirable variations in service; enhance learning
* Standards can be translated to technology platform to enhance practice

Person Served
* Reasonable assurance of quality, focus on person orientation
* Expectation of individualized approach, participation; that rights and dignity will be maintained
* In rehabilitation, designation of specialty states if program accredited (example, spinal cord injury)

To persons served, accreditation offers a reasonable assurance that the services they are to receive meet "current industry standards" with respect to quality and that they will be engaged in care processes and decisions that affect them. Organizations benefit by knowing that they practice their trade against known standards, endorsed by experts and consumers alike. Accreditation creates and confirms the "business and service to person served" alignment. Organizations which maintain their commitment to quality via third-party accreditation, specifically designed and conducted for their rehabilitation-specific business, commit to an accountability framework—both internal and external. In an era of transparency, post-Enron, public trust can be further fortified by organizations that undergo additional third-party review. The accreditation process also bridges the business with the clinical care of components of rehabilitation service delivery. Payers can participate in quality systems by endorsing the requirement of quality service via accreditation as part of their extended service strategy, rebuilding public confidence to well-run and well-intended health service organizations. The opportunity also extends beyond a public relations exercise if accreditation is used to employ service protocols and aid in contract management practices inclusive of incentives for performance and the collection of data for system improvement opportunities.

Person served, providers, and payers must integrate their efforts in the long run if the system is to achieve a desired state of sustained performance and enhanced access. Regulators who utilize accreditation as a partial oversight function are also afforded the opportunity to focus on their highest priorities, relieving providers of administrative review processes that are duplicative to accreditation and outside their area of expertise. Most importantly, a hallmark differentiator of the value of accreditation specific to rehabilitation is confirmed in its social responsibility function, which links results for the individual served to the greater society. As one of many available quality frameworks, only accreditation maintains the importance of rehabilitation to broader society. With its intense focus on persons served, accreditation standards act as "reference grids" to create effective systems of service and set goals focused on enhancing community participation opportunities for persons with disabilities (e.g., work) to minimize the stigma and barriers associated with disabilities. This clarity of purpose afforded by accreditation is the extended thread of value from persons served to society as a whole.

CONCLUSIONS

ACCREDITATION HAS EVOLVED over many years in response to different trends in the health and rehabilitation industry. Many indicators suggest discontinuous change in the health care and rehabilitation field. The engaged and informed consumer will continue to challenge the entire service delivery system—its leadership and skilled health professionals. The internet will become of greater use to consumers as they make decisions about care and service options. Report cards will be accessed by the masses. Payers and employers are likely to facilitate the development of incentives to reward providers for quality and excellence. Excellence awards and accreditation models in principle will remain focused on their similar intent to improve and guide organizations to performance excellence. Quality frameworks utilized by organizations will be required to embrace the changing and unique features specific to the business of delivering health care and rehabilitation services. Valued quality frameworks will need to recognize the importance and role of persons served both as contributors to the health and rehabilitation process, and as recipients of the output or outcomes. This factor alone requires a unique quality framework that accreditation can provide. Further, the accreditor who builds a model of quality and standards through an inclusive process will create greater face validity and value within the broader community served—the community of citizenship.

To be of value and relevant, accreditation must also evolve to the needs of its customers. Accreditors are in a unique position of having many beneficiaries, such as accredited organizations, state agencies that mandate third-party accreditation, payers, and to some extent the general public. The general public will insist that accountability be created in our health system. One "check and balance" process that employs the necessary integrity is the accreditation process and the outcome or "seal of quality." As not-for-profit entities, accreditors must serve a higher purpose in view of the direct recipients of service, the persons served. That higher-order purpose is a moral obligation. In the collective sense, persons served are the community, the country, and the nation served. Since the wealth of any nation is no greater than its health, creating efficient and effective quality-based delivery systems is to the ultimate to the benefit of society. Efficiency, effectiveness, and satisfaction regardless of the quality framework employed creates capacity in the human services system for greater access to those who may not be privileged to receive the best of care. It also stands to reason that the health of any nation and the quality of its health care is no greater than its access to that care. A commitment to quality, therefore, is a commitment to all persons served.

REFERENCES

Baldrige National Quality Program. (2004). *Health care criteria for performance excellence*. Gaithersburg, MD: National Institute of Standards and Technology.

Calingo, L. M. R. (2002). National quality and business excellence awards: Mapping the field and prospects for Asia. In L. M. R. Calingo (Ed.), *The quest for global competitiveness through national quality and business excellence awards* (pp. 21–40). Tokyo: Asia Productivity Organization.

Center for Medicare and Medicaid Services. (2003). Retrieved from *http://cms.hhs.gov*

Commission on Accreditation of Rehabilitation Facilities. (2004). *Medical rehabilitation standards manual*. Tucson, AZ: Author.

Counte, M. A., & Meurer, S. (2001). Issues in the assessment of continuous quality improvement implementation in health care organizations. *International Journal for Quality Health Care, 13*, 197–207.

Donabedian, A. (1978). The quality of medical care. *Science, 200,* 856–864.

Donabedian, A. (1996). Evaluating quality of medical care. *Millbank Quarterly,* 44, 166–206.

European Foundation for Quality Management. (1999). *The EFQM excellence model 1999*. Tilburg, Netherlands: Pabo Prestige Press.

Goonan, K. J. (1994). Using quality assurance systems to change behaviour. In T. W. Granneman (Ed.), *Review, Regulate or Reform? What works to control workers' compensation medical costs* (pp. 247–267). Cambridge: Workers' Compensation Research Institute.

Institute of Medicine. (1999). *To err is human*. Washington, DC: National Academy Press.

Institute of Medicine. (2001). *Crossing the quality chasm. A new health system for the 21st century*. Washington, DC: National Academy Press.

International Organization for Standardization. (2000). *ISO 9000—2000 (E)*. Geneva, Switzerland: Author.

Ishikawa, K. (1985). *What is total quality control. The Japanese way*. Englewood Cliffs, NJ: Prentice-Hall.

J. D. Power and Associates. (2004). Retrieved from http://www.jdpower.com

Leapfrog Group. (2004). Retrieved from http://www.leapfroggroup.org

Mant, J. (2001). Process versus outcome indicators in the assessment of quality of health care. *International Journal of Quality Health Care, 13,* 475–480.

Moeller, J. (2001). The EFQM excellence model. German experiences with the EFQM approach in health care. *International Journal for Quality in Health Care, 13,* 45–49.

Mycek, S. (1997). Getting beyond industrial logic: Renewing our truth in the value of health. *Health Care Forum Journal, 16,* 18–20.

National Business Group on Health. (2004). Retrieved from http://www.wbgh.org

National Committee on Quality Assurance. (2004). Retrieved from http://www.ncqua.org

New Freedom Commission on Mental Health. (2003). *Achieving the promise: Transforming mental health care in America. Final Report*. Rockville, MD: Department of Health and Human Services.

Organization for Economic Cooperation and Development. (2003). *Health at a glance 2003—OECD countries struggle with rising demand for health spending*. Retrieved from http://www.oedc.org

President's Advisory Commission on Consumer Protection and Quality in the Health Care Industry. (1998). *Quality first: Better care for all Americans*. Washington, DC: U.S. Government Printing Office.

Rubin, H. R., Provonost, P., & Diette, G. B. (2001). The advantages and disadvantages of process-based measures of health care quality. *International Journal for Quality in Health Care, 13,* 469–474.

Stavert, D., & Boon, B. J. (2003). Listening to consumers . . . CARF Canada opens. *International Journal of Heath Care Quality Assurance Incorporating Leadership in Health Service, 16*(3), 1–9.

Yasin, M. M., Zimmerer, L. W., Miller, P., & Zimmerer, T. W. (2002). An empirical investigation of the effectiveness of contemporary management philosophies in a hospital operational setting. *International Journal of Health Care Quality Assurance, 15*, 268–276.

36

Outcomes Measurement and Quality Improvement in an Acute Inpatient Rehabilitation Setting

ORA EZRACHI, PHD

I N AN ERA of mediated access to health care and increasing requests for accountability in the delivery of health care services from both payers and consumers, it has become imperative that all health care providers submit evidence of the various impacts of their efforts. Approaching this task has necessitated the formalization of procedures for documentation and interpretation of outcomes of clinical service delivery, as well as for the implementation and ongoing monitoring of performance improvement activities. Information and outcomes management systems, as these procedural systems are labeled, have developed uniquely in particular facilities or settings, but encompass an underlying philosophy, usually following guidelines suggested by some accrediting body, of focusing on collecting outcome data and eliciting feedback from the consumer, or person served, and using that information to enhance the performance improvement process.

Outcomes management (utilizing the data-driven methodology of program evaluation) is a means of ensuring an objective assessment of the effectiveness and efficiency of the delivery of medical rehabilitation services. The Commission on the Accreditation of Rehabilitation Facilities (CARF) defines outcomes measurement and outcomes management as follows (*CARF Standards Manual*, 2002):

> A systematic procedure for determining the effectiveness and efficiency of results achieved by the persons served during service delivery or following service completion, as well as the individuals' satisfaction with those results. An outcomes management system measures outcomes by obtaining, aggregating, and analyzing data regarding how well the persons served are functioning after exit/discharge from a specific service. Outcomes measures should be related to the goals that recent services were designed to achieve. (p. 320)

CARF *Standards Manual*, (2002) also provides a principle for Information and Outcomes Management Systems:

> Information is gathered and analyzed to measure and manage outcomes. The information gathered is relevant to the core values and mission of the organization and to the needs of all stakeholders. Analyzed information is used to improve performance in a variety of areas. It is the responsibility of the organization to share relevant information with stakeholders at a frequency that meets their needs. The information shared with stakeholders accurately reflects the performance of the organization and considers the requests and inputs of stakeholders. (p. 50)

Outcomes measurement is an essential component for evaluating the efficacy and efficiency of treatment intervention in rehabilitation. (For an excellent introduction, see Dittmar and Gresham (1997) and the related web-based slide presentation on the Uniform Data System for Medical Rehabilitation (UDSMR) website, www.udsmr.org.) Outcomes measurement is useful, however, only to the degree that it allows for reliable and valid assessment of treatment effects and leads to initiatives aimed at quality and performance improvement. As a primary example in the field of rehabilitation, CARF, the Commission on the Accreditation of Rehabilitation Facilities, offers a consultative accreditation process that promotes the implementation and integration of information and outcomes management systems within rehabilitation facilities. Facilities that apply for CARF accreditation are required to conform to various standards for the delivery of services and documentation of performance.

CARF (Standards Manual, 2002) also provides facilities with objectives and guidelines for (a) the types of information to be gathered; (b) the level at which the information is gathered, i.e., the level of the person served and the programmatic level; (c) maintaining the integrity of the information collected; (d) focusing the analysis of the information, i.e., relevance and use in the decision-making process, comparison against expected levels of performance; (e) performance improvement activities, in terms of both information to be collected to determine the nature of the problem, and a monitored performance improvement plan; and (f) communication with stakeholders, e.g., consumers, payers, referral sources, the community.

It is essential that data on functional outcomes be routinely collected, preferably using reliable, valid, nationally recognized benchmark measures (such as the Functional Independence Measure, FIM™, see below) along with instruments developed and adapted to target results of a particular institution's specific programmatic efforts. Data need to be collected on an ongoing basis, from all persons served, at several points in the rehabilitation continuum, for example, admission to program, discharge from program, some time (e.g., 3 months) after discharge from program. Findings from consumer satisfaction measures must also be integrated into the system so that they can guide performance improvement efforts.

In most acute inpatient rehabilitation facilities, data are collected in accordance with the Uniform Data System for Medical Rehabilitation, which was established in 1983 to meet a long-standing need to document severity of patient disability and the outcomes of medical rehabilitation. The most widely used instrument for the assessment of the functional impact of treatment interventions, the Functional Independence Measure (FIM™), was developed to address this need and to provide a uniform approach to the functional assessment of persons receiving inpatient rehabilitation services. [See Hamilton, Granger, Sherwin, Zielezny, and Tashman (1987) and selected bibliography list at the end of this chapter.]

> The FIM includes a seven-level scale that designates major gradations in behavior from dependence to independence. This scale provides for classification of patients by their ability to carry out an activity independently, versus their need for assistance from another person or device. If help is needed, the scale quantifies that need. The need for assistance (burden of care) translates to the time/energy that another person must expend to serve the dependent needs of the disabled individual to achieve and maintain a certain quality of life. (*Guide for the Uniform Data Set for Medical Rehabilitation (Adult FIM), Version 5.0,* effective January 1, 1997, pp. III-1–III-47)

The FIM™ instrument was designed as a discipline-free measure, so data are usually derived from ratings and input from a variety of rehabilitation professionals, e.g., nurses, physical therapists, occupational therapists, social workers, speech-language pathologists, and physicians. The data set also includes items that document patient demographic characteristics, such as age, gender, living setting, as well as diagnoses, impairment groups, comorbidities, length of inpatient hospital stay, and discharge disposition.

It is also recognized that the FIM™, although primarily useful as a measure of changes in motoric function and activities of daily living, may not always capture the effects of other types of intervention, e.g., psychological, social work, therapeutic recreation, or the effects of intervention in those impairment groups where motoric functioning per se is not the primary deficit, e.g., patients undergoing post-cardiac surgery rehabilitation, where the major deficit may be endurance-related rather than level of motor functioning, or where the motoric deficits fall in a narrow area of activity, e.g., post-joint replacement patients where the primary deficit is in locomotion. In these instances, it is essential that other, more relevant measures be utilized to allow for appropriate and valid assessment of the effects of intervention.

The Rusk Institute of Rehabilitation Medicine has been CARF-accredited since the early 1980s. It has also developed an exemplary Outcomes Management System (OMS) that integrates several approaches to meet the objectives of an effective information and outcomes management system. The approach presented herein is derived from over 10 years of experience with the Rusk Institute OMS, and provides a schematic for the translation of the desired objectives into an operational approach.

TABLE 36.1 Burden of Care

Burden of care (rated on a 7-point scale where 1 = totally dependent and 7 = totally independent) is assessed on 18 activities in 6 areas as shown below.

Area	Activity
Self-Care	Eating, Grooming, Bathing, Dressing—Upper, Dressing—Lower, Toileting
Sphincter Control	Bladder Management, Bowel Management
Transfers	Bed/Chair/Wheelchair, Toilet, Tub/Shower
Locomotion	Walk/Wheelchair, Stairs
Communication	Comprehension, Expression
Social Cognition	Social Interaction, Problem Solving, Memory

Along with the FIM™, additional program effectiveness measures are used to capture the impact of services delivered either for specific populations or in therapeutic areas not sensitively captured by the FIM™. For example, cardiac rehabilitation patients may be additionally assessed using measures of oxygen consumption at admission and at discharge from program to evaluate degree of improvement and impact of programmatic efforts. For therapeutic recreation, the Leisure Competence Measure, modeled after the FIM™ but focusing on rating of participation in leisure activities, can be used to assess changes in this area (Klosik & Crilly, 1997). Development and use of special indicators in areas such as nursing, speech-language pathology, psychology, and social work services are also useful.

An exemplary outcomes management system rests on a well-designed, focused, and comprehensive approach to the collection, analysis, and interpretation of quantitative and qualitative data. Data collection is usually focused in four major areas:

Patient descriptors, which include demographic data, diagnostic categories, and discharge dispositions.

Functional status assessment, using the FIM™ and additional instruments to measure changes in functioning between admission and discharge.

Satisfaction with services and participation in planning program, using assessments during the inpatient stay and post-discharge. These include measures of satisfaction with treatment and length of treatment for each therapeutic modality, as well as with facilities and amenities, e.g., environment and food services. (See below for more detailed information and examples.)

Post-discharge follow-up using the FIM™, which tracks maintenance of functional outcomes achieved during the inpatient stay after return to the community, and community integration and participation measures, to allow for tracking individuals' return to community and activities.

In order to provide a context for the collection and interpretation of data, the system must initially develop program objectives. Program objectives are usually organized within three major areas: effectiveness, efficiency, and consumer satisfaction. Where feasible, there should also be follow-up objectives for community reintegration.

Effectiveness reflects the benefits derived from having received inpatient services. Program objectives, e.g., increased independence, are measured in terms of the degree of movement (or progress) toward achieving program goals as derived from ratings at inpatient admission and discharge. Measurement is usually reflected as change in a score that measures level of functioning, or burden of care, between admission and discharge. Data should be examined and analyzed on a timely and regular basis, e.g., quarterly, and compared to regional and national benchmarks where appropriate or available. Additionally, it is imperative to include feedback mechanisms to relevant responsible parties and to request and monitor corrective action and performance improvement activities.

Efficiency relates to utilization of resources, both institutional and by the persons served. These are measured using indicators such as length of stay, costs, and discharges to non-institutional settings. As with effectiveness data, these data also need to be examined and analyzed on a regular and timely basis, e.g., quarterly, compared to regional and national benchmarks, and corrective actions should be applied as necessary.

Consumer satisfaction focuses on feedback from the persons served. Program objectives provide indicators of how well the programs/services are received by the persons served. For example, objectives can include (a) maintaining/increasing consumer satisfaction with inpatient services, and (b) maintaining/increasing consumer participation in planning inpatient programs.

These objectives can be measured by examining responses to patient satisfaction surveys and questions focusing on (a) whether the persons served felt they had benefited from their treatment, (b) whether they would recommend the particular facility to others, (c) how satisfied they were with the overall care received, and (d) whether they were able to participate in planning their treatment program.

Patient satisfaction measures are often used as marketing tools to highlight a particular facility's strengths relative to other facilities with which it may be competing. Although a useful and perhaps essential approach, facilities must also use consumer feedback intelligently to drive their performance improvement efforts. Patient satisfaction surveys should provide a systematic method for the collection, analysis, and utilization of quantitative ratings and qualitative comments from consumers of inpatient rehabilitation services. Using both consumer and professional input, items should be selected and developed that both cover the range of services delivered and elicit responses to specific aspects and components of the treatment experience. This specificity allows the facility to focus performance improvement efforts on targeted areas of weakness. In addition to rating individual items on a scale ranging from *very satisfied* to *very dissatisfied*, respondents are also encouraged to provide comments regarding both positive and negative experiences.

Satisfaction surveys should be mailed to all inpatients 1–2 weeks post-discharge. It is assumed that contacts with all patients soon after discharge will yield an accurate representation of consumer satisfaction. The survey should be accompanied by a cover letter, co-signed by a hospital administrator and the medical director, and a pre-addressed postage paid reply envelope. A follow-up thank you/reminder postcard can be mailed 1 week later. (The use of the postcard generally increases the response rate.) The postcard thanks former patients if they have already returned the survey, reminds them if they haven't, and tells them whom to call to get another copy of the survey. At the Rusk Institute we have found response rates averaging around 35% with this procedure.

Reports are generated quarterly. For each quarter, both quantitative ratings and qualitative comments are tabulated. Quantitative ratings are summarized and reported by item within each service area. Qualitative comments are tabulated verbatim, annotated as to whether they are positive, negative, neutral, or mixed, and organized by service area.

At the Rusk Institute, a Consumer Input Steering Committee was established to review all patient satisfaction data (i.e., surveys, letters, etc.). This committee receives the report and distributes quantitative ratings and relevant qualitative ratings to individual departments for comment and corrective action plans. The quantitative summaries are also included in the quarterly Rusk Institute OMS Report.

The results of the survey are distributed at various levels within the facility, e.g., clinical staff, administration, board, at varying levels of detail. Providing survey results to consumers is also an essential component of the system and includes the use of a consumer-focused newsletter to report on program outcomes (e.g., case mix, average FIM™ changes) and patient satisfaction data, and regular use of the facility website.

Follow-up objectives for community reintegration indicate how well functional gains are maintained and transfered to the post-discharge setting. They are measured by comparing discharge status with status at follow-up, usually 3–6 months post-discharge. Again, data should be examined on a regular and timely basis, e.g., quarterly, compared to regional and national benchmarks, and corrective actions should be applied as necessary.

Sampling and Analysis. Data on effectiveness, efficiency, consumer satisfaction, and community integration should be collected on all persons served where possible. If this is not possible due to various constraints, e.g., volume, resources, then sampling should be stratified by case mix. That is, the sampling of persons served should reflect, proportionately, the distribution of impairment groups seen in the facility.

This is essential when the data are aggregated across impairment groups for analysis. It is also necessary to examine and analyze findings separately by impairment group, to be able to detect differential responses to treatment and/or levels of satisfaction. At times it is also useful to collect subsets of data on specific subgroups, e.g., functional communication measures on persons with stroke.

Feedback systems. An absolutely essential component for an outcomes management system is the feedback loop, the mechanism for allowing the information gathered to be summarized and re-directed back in a focused way to allow for the development of performance improvement activities. An outcomes management system should provide varied feedback to both the institution and consumers. There are several levels of institutional feedback (e.g., quarterly management reports, reports to peer review committees), and several approaches used to disseminate findings to consumers (e.g., consumer newsletter, consumer satisfaction data on website).

Management reports should be generated quarterly and summarized annually to report the findings of the previous survey period and include results and discussion of outcome analyses with summary and recommendations. In addition, recommendations should be made for issues requiring follow-up review and further action. This information reaches various levels of clinical and administrative staff through committee pathways. Consumers should be provided with information on functional outcomes and patient satisfaction through quarterly newsletters distributed to all inpatients, and via the facility website.

Results of OMS reviews should be distributed to all relevant clinical departments. Specific information is provided for cases where identified outcomes require review and follow-up. Departments are encouraged to formulate performance improvement efforts to address areas where program objectives are not being met or could be enhanced. Recommendations are also made for additional measures/indicators that can be incorporated into the OMS for survey, analyses, and follow-up.

The OMS serves as a resource for clinical and administrative data needs by providing analyses and specialized reports on request, e.g., short and long length of stay cases for the Inpatient Utilization Review Committee, patient satisfaction results for the Consumer Input Steering Committee and Marketing Committee. The OMS manager also works with administrative and clinical staff continuously to develop targeted indicators and performance improvement initiatives.

An annual review of the OMS serves as a formal mechanism for assessing the performance and adequacy of the system. It provides an opportunity for all staff affected by the system to offer feedback and suggestions regarding system efficiency, effectiveness, methods, and procedures, and to recommend revisions to the OMS to ensure meaningful and practical outcome results which can assist the institution in providing high-quality rehabilitation care in a cost-effective environment.

SUMMARY

THIS OVERVIEW WAS intended to provide the reader with a perspective on the importance of an outcomes management system for the monitoring of organizational performance in acute rehabilitation settings, as well as an approach to implementation and a schematic view of the process. This area is full of opportunity and lends itself to creativity in problem solving. Most importantly, it is difficult to overstate the need for the feedback loop in the process. The collection of data is necessary, but not sufficient. The circle is only complete when data are actually examined and used to further performance improvement activities.

REFERENCES AND SELECTED BIBLIOGRAPHY

Baldridge, R. B. (1993). Functional assessment of measurements. *Neurology, 17*(4), 3–10.

Carf Standards Manual,Medical Rehabilitation. (2002) Commission on Accreditation on Rehabilitation Facilities (CARF). Tucson, AZ.

Carey, R. (1990). Integrating case management, program evaluation, and marketing for inpatient and outpatient rehabilitation programs. *Advances in Clinical Rehabilitation, 3,* 219–249.

Chang, W. C., & Chan, C. (1995). Rasch analysis for outcomes measures—some methodological considerations. *Archives of Physical Medicine & Rehabilitation, 76*(10), 934–939.

Crewe, N. M., & Dijkers, M. (1995). Functional assessment. In L. A. Cushman & M. J. Scherer (Eds.), *Psychological assessment in medical rehabilitation. Measurement and instrumentation in psychology* (vol. XV, pp. 101–144). Washington, DC: American Psychological Association.

Dickson, H. G., Hodgkinson, A., & Kohler, F. (1994). Inpatient quality assurance by local analysis of uniform data set data. *Journal of Quality in Clinical Practice, 14*(3), 145–148.

Dittmar, S., & Gresham, G. E. (1997). *Functional assessment and outcome measurement for the rehabilitation health professional.* Gaithersburg, MD: Aspen.

Dodds, T. A., Martin, D. P., Stolov, W. C., & Deyo, R. A. (1993). A validation of the functional independence measure and its performance among rehabilitation patients. *Archives of Physical Medicine & Rehabilitation, 74*(5), 531–536.

Drew Cates, J. (1995). Functional assessment. In M. Stanley & P. G. Beare (Eds.), *Gerontological nursing* (pp. 91–97). Philadelphia: F. A. Davis.

Fiedler, R. C., & Granger, C. V. (1996). The Functional Independence Measure: A measurement of disability and medical rehabilitation. In N. Chine & J. L. Melvin (Eds.), *Functional evaluation of stroke patients* (pp. 75–92). Tokyo: Springer-Verlag.

FIMware(r) User Guide and Self-Guided Training Manual, Version 5.20 (1999). Buffalo: State University of New York at Buffalo.

Fisher, W. P., Harvey, R. F., Taylor, P., Kilgore, K. M., & Kelly, C. K. (1995). Rehabits: A common language of functional assessment. *Archives of Physical Medicine & Rehabilitation, 76*(2), 113–122.

Forer, S. (1992). How to make program evaluation work for you: Utilization for program service. *NeuroRehabilitation, 2,* 52–71.

Frattali, C. M. (1993). Perspectives on functional assessment and its use for policy making. *Disability and Rehabilitation, 15*(1), 1–9.

Fricke, J. (1993). Measuring outcomes in rehabilitation: A review. *British Journal of Occupational Therapy, 56*(5), 217–221.

Fuhrer, M. J. (1988). Rehabilitation research in the 1980s. *Advances in Clinical Rehabilitation, 2,* 232–256.

Glass, R. M. (1989). Program evaluation. In B. England, R. M. Glass, & C. H. Patterson (Eds.), *Quality rehabilitation: Results-oriented patient care* (pp. 19–37). Chicago: American Hospital Association.

Goldstein, T. S. (1995). Measuring function. In *Functional rehabilitation on orthopedics* (pp. 183–215). Gaithersburg, MD: Aspen Publishers.

Gonnella, C. (1992). Program evaluation. In G. F. Fletcher, J. D. Banja, B. B. Jann, & S. L. Wolf (Eds.), *Rehabilitation medicine: Contemporary clinical perspectives* (pp. 243–268). Philadelphia: Lea and Febiger.

Granger, C. V., & Brownscheidle, C. M. (1995). Outcome measurement in medical rehabilitation. *International Journal of Technology Assessment in Health Care, 11*(2), 262–268.

Granger, C. V., Cotter, A. C., Hamilton, B. B., & Fiedler, R. C. (1993). Functional assessment scales: A study of persons after stroke. *Archives of Physical Medicine & Rehabilitation, 74*(2), 133–138.

Granger, C. V., & Gresham, G. E. (1993). Functional assessment in rehabilitation medicine. *Physical Medicine and Rehabilitation Clinics of North America, 4*(3), 417–423.

Granger, C. V., Hamilton, B. B., Keith, R. A., Zielezny, M., & Sherwin, F. S. (1986). Advances in functional assessment for medical rehabilitation. *Topics in Geriatric Rehabilitation, 1*(3), 59–74.

Granger, C. V., Kelly-Hayes, M., Johnston, M., Deutsch, A., Braun, S., & Fiedler, R. C. (1996). Quality and outcome measures in medical rehabilitation. In R. L. Braddom (Ed.), *Physical medicine and rehabilitation* (pp. 239–253). Philadelphia: W. B. Saunders.

Guide for the Uniform Data Set for Medical Rehabilitation (including the FIM™ instrument), Version 5.0. (1997). Buffalo: State University of New York at Buffalo.

Hamilton, B. B., & Granger, C. V. (1994). Disability outcomes following inpatient rehabilitation for stroke. *Physical Therapy, 74*(5), 494–503.

Hamilton, B. B., Granger, C. V., Sherwin, F. S., Zielezny, M., & Tashman, J. S. (1987). Uniform national data system for medical rehabilitation. In M. J. Fuhrer (Ed.), *Rehabilitation outcomes: Analysis and measurement* (pp. 137–147). Baltimore: Paul H. Brookes Publishing Co.

Heinemann, A. W., Linacre, J. M., Wright, B. D., Hamilton, B. B., & Granger, C. V. (1994). Prediction of rehabilitation outcomes with disability measures. *Archives of Physical Medicine & Rehabilitation, 75*(2), 133–143.

Johnston, M. V., & Granger, C. V. (1994). Outcomes research in medical rehabilitation: A primer and introduction to a series. *American Journal of Physical Medicine & Rehabilitation, 73*(4), 296–303.

Johnston, M. V., & Keith, R. A. (1993). Measurement standards for medical rehabilitation and applications. *Physical Rehabilitation and Medicine Clinics of North America, 4*(3), 425–449.

Johnston, M. V., Keith, R. A., & Hinderer, S. (1992). Measurement standards for interdisciplinary medical rehabilitation. *Archives of Physical Medicine & Rehabilitation, 73*(suppl.), S3–S23.

Johnston, M. V., Wilkerson, D. L., & Maney, M. (1993). Evaluation of the quality and outcome of medical rehabilitation programs. In J. DeLisa, B. M. Gans, & D. M. Currie (Eds.), *Rehabilitation medicine: Principles and practice* (pp. 240–268). Philadelphia: J. B. Lippincott.

Keith, R. A., Granger, C. V., Hamilton, B. B., & Sherwin, F. S. (1987). The Functional Independence Measure: A new tool for rehabilitation. *Advances in Clinical Rehabilitation, 1,* 6–18.

Landrum, P. K., Schmidt, N. D., & McLean, A. (Eds.). (1995). *Outcome-oriented rehabilitation: Principles, strategies, and tools for effective program management.* Gaithersburg, MD: Aspen Publishers.

Merbitz, C., Morris, J., & Grip, J. C. (1989). Ordinal scales and foundations of misinference. *Archives of Physical Medicine & Rehabilitation, 70*(4), 308–312.

Stineman, M. G., & Granger, C. V. (1994). Outcome studies and analyses: Principles of rehabilitation that influence outcome analyses. In G. Felsenthal, S. J. Garrison, & F. U. Steinberg (Eds.), *Rehabilitation of the aging and elderly* (pp. 511–522). Baltimore: Williams and Wilkins.

Wade, D. T. (1992). *Measurement in neurological rehabilitation* (pp. 218–223). Oxford, England: Oxford University Press.

Wagner, K. A. (1987). Outcome analysis in comprehensive medical rehabilitation. In M. J. Fuhrer (Ed.), *Rehabilitation outcomes: Analysis and measurement* (pp. 19–28). Baltimore: Brookes.

Wilkerson, D. L., Batavia, A. I., & DeJong, G. (1992). Use of functional status measures for payment of medical rehabilitation services. *Archives of Physical Medicine & Rehabilitation, 73,* 111–120.

Wilkerson, D. L., & McDermott, M. (1994) Critical function and process pathways in medical rehabilitation—Outcome-to-process analysis. *Archives of*

Index

A

B

F

T

X

Xeroxstomia, 589
X-linked disorders, 401
X-rays, as diagnostic tool, 160, 206, 395, 549-550

Y

YAG (yttrium aluminum garnet)laser, 709
Yellow marrow, 47
Yoga, 727, 731

Z

Zero Acceptance of Pain (ZAP) Quality
    Improvement Project, 231
Zinc deficiencies, 464